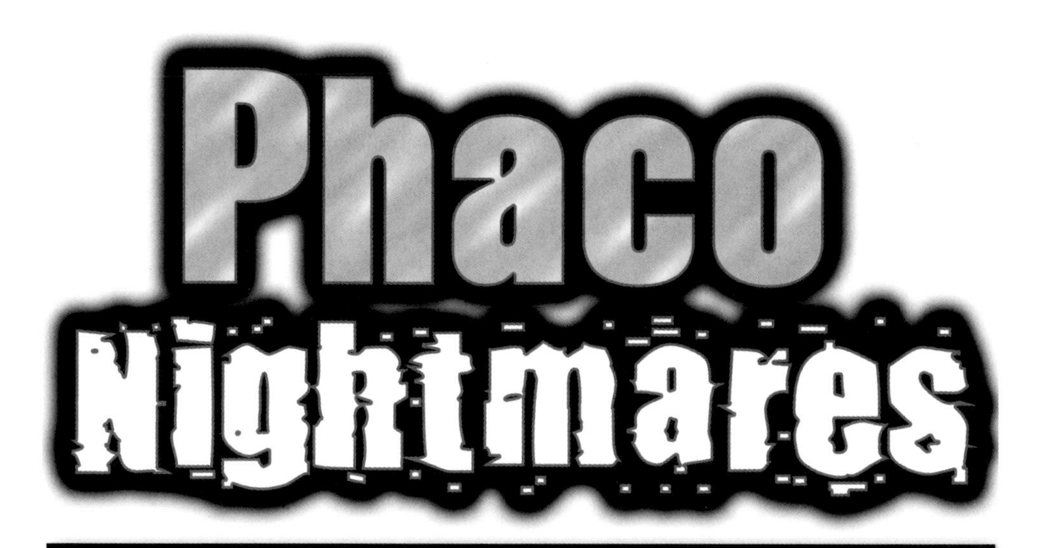

Conquering Cataract Catastrophes

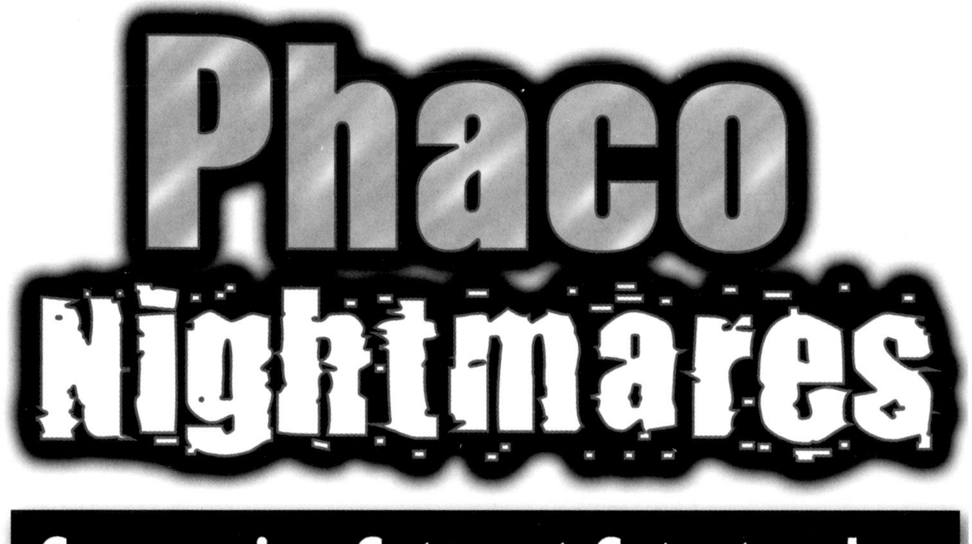

Edited by

Amar Agarwal, MS, FRCS, FRCOphth
Dr. Agarwal's Eye Hospital
Chennai, India

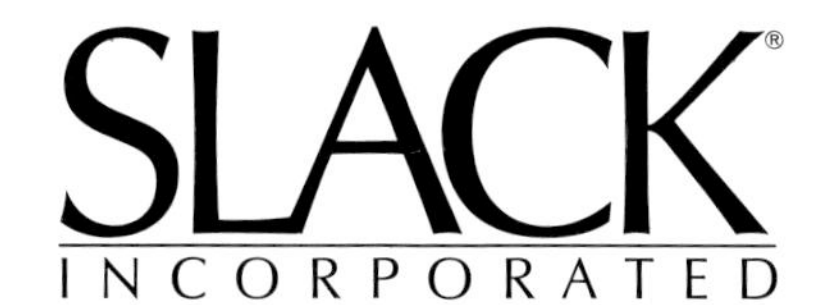

Delivering the best in health care information and education worldwide

PGL WW260 P441A
KHA

www.slackbooks.com

ISBN-10: 1-55642-772-7
ISBN-13: 978-1-55642-772-5

Copyright © 2006 by SLACK Incorporated

All rights reserved. No part of this book may be reproduced, stored in a retrieval system or transmitted in any form or by any means, electronic, mechanical, photocopying, recording or otherwise, without written permission from the publisher, except for brief quotations embodied in critical articles and reviews.

The procedures and practices described in this book should be implemented in a manner consistent with the professional standards set for the circumstances that apply in each specific situation. Every effort has been made to confirm the accuracy of the information presented and to correctly relate generally accepted practices. The authors, editor, and publisher cannot accept responsibility for errors or exclusions or for the outcome of the material presented herein. There is no expressed or implied warranty of this book or information imparted by it. Care has been taken to ensure that drug selection and dosages are in accordance with currently accepted/recommended practice. Due to continuing research, changes in government policy and regulations, and various effects of drug reactions and interactions, it is recommended that the reader carefully review all materials and literature provided for each drug, especially those that are new or not frequently used. Any review or mention of specific companies or products is not intended as an endorsement by the author or publisher.

SLACK Incorporated uses a review process to evaluate submitted material. Prior to publication, educators or clinicians provide important feedback on the content that we publish. We welcome feedback on this work.

Published by: SLACK Incorporated
6900 Grove Road
Thorofare, NJ 08086 USA
Telephone: 856-848-1000
Fax: 856-853-5991
www.slackbooks.com

Contact SLACK Incorporated for more information about other books in this field or about the availability of our books from distributors outside the United States.

Library of Congress Cataloging-in-Publication Data

Phaco nightmares : conquering cataract catastrophes / edited by Amar Agarwal.
p. ; cm.
Includes bibliographical references and index.
ISBN-13: 978-1-55642-772-5 (alk. paper)
ISBN-10: 1-55642-772-7 (alk. paper)
1. Cataract--Surgery--Complications. 2. Phacoemulsification--Complications. 3. Eye--Surgery--Complications.
[DNLM: 1. Phacoemulsification. 2. Cataract Extraction--methods. 3. Phacoemulsification--adverse effects. WW 260 P5309 2006] I. Agarwal, Amar.

RE451.P53 2006 617.7'42059--dc22

For permission to reprint material in another publication, contact SLACK Incorporated. Authorization to photocopy items for internal, personal, or academic use is granted by SLACK Incorporated provided that the appropriate fee is paid directly to Copyright Clearance Center. Prior to photocopying items, please contact the Copyright Clearance Center at 222 Rosewood Drive, Danvers, MA 01923 USA; phone: 978-750-8400; website: www.copyright.com; email: info@copyright.com

Printed in the United States of America.

Last digit is print number: 10 9 8 7 6 5 4 3 2 1

Dedication

This book is dedicated to Samuel Masket.

Contents

Section IV: Posterior Segment—Worst Case Scenarios

Section V: Bimanual Phacoemulsification

Acknowledgments

A book of this nature would not be possible without the help of the Almighty, who helps us tide over all nightmares.

About the Editor

Dr. Amar Agarwal is the pioneer of phakonit, which is **phako** with a **n**eedle **i**ncision **t**echnology. This technique became popularized as bimanual phaco, microincision cataract surgery (MICS), or microphaco. He is the first to remove cataracts through a 0.7 mm tip with the technique called microphakonit. He has also discovered no anesthesia cataract surgery and FAVIT, a new technique to remove dropped nuclei. The air pump, which was a simple idea of using an aquarium fish pump to increase the fluid into the eye in bimanual phaco and co-axial phaco, has helped prevent surge. This built the basis of various techniques of forced infusion for small incision cataract surgery. He was also the first to use trypan blue for staining epiretinal membranes and publishing the details in his four- volume *Textbook of Ophthalmology*. His latest discovery is a new refractive error called aberropia.

Dr. Agarwal has received many awards for his work in ophthalmology, most significantly the Barraquer Award and the Kelman Award. He has also written more than 33 books, which have been published in various languages—English, Spanish, and Polish. He also trains doctors from all over the world in his center on phaco, bimanual phaco, LASIK, and retina. The website for Dr. Agarwal's Eye Hospital is http://www.dragarwal.com.

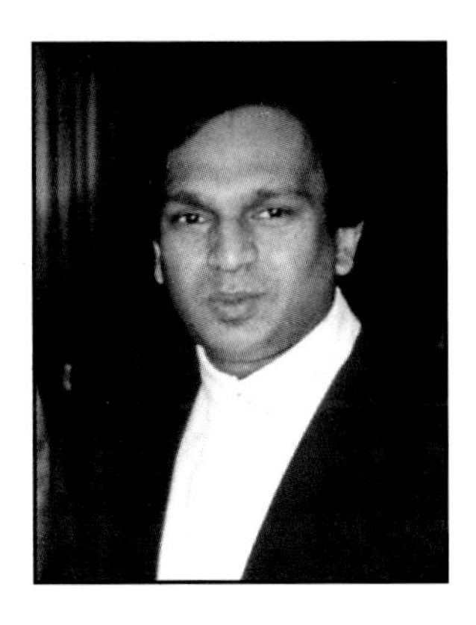

About the Contributors

Athiya Agarwal, MD, FRSH, DO
Dr. Agarwal's Group of Eye Hospitals and Eye Research Centre
Chennai, Bangalore, India

Sunita Agarwal, MS, FSVH, DO
Dr. Agarwal's Group of Eye Hospitals and Eye Research Centre
Chennai, Bangalore, India

Cristela F. Aleman, MD
Director, Cataract Department
Director, Clinica Boyd
Panama, R.P.

Jorge L. Alio, MD, PhD
Instituto Oftalmológico De Alicante
Refractive Surgery and Cornea Department
Miguel Hernández University Medical School
Alicante, Spain

David J. Apple, MD
John A. Moran Eye Center
University of Utah
Salt Lake City, Utah

Aritz Bidaguren, MD
Department of Ophthalmology
Hospital Donostia
Basque Health Service-Osakidetza
Donostia-San Sebastián
Spain

Benjamin F. Boyd, MD, FACS
Consultant Editor
Highlights of Ophthalmology
Panama, R.P.

Samuel Boyd, MD
Director, Laser Department
Associate Director, Clinica Boyd
Panama, R.P.

Scott E. Burk, MD, PhD
Cincinnati Eye Institute
Cincinnati, Ohio

Clement K. Chan, MD, FACS
Medical Director
Southern California Desert Retina Consultants, M.C.
and Inland Retina Consultants
Palm Springs, California
Associate Clinical Professor
Department of Ophthalmology
Loma Linda University
Loma Linda, California

David F. Chang, MD
Los Altos, California

William J. Fishkind, MD, FACS
Tucson, Arizona

Yolanda Gallego, MD
Department of Ophthalmology
Hospital Donostia
Basque Health Service-Osakidetza
Donostia-San Sebastián
Spain

Cristina Irigoyen, MD
Department of Ophthalmology
Hospital Donostia
Basque Health Service-Osakidetza
Donostia-San Sebastián
Spain

Soosan Jacob, MS, DNB, FRCS, MNAMS, FERC
Dr. Agarwal's Group of Eye Hospitals and Eye Research Centre
Chennai, Bangalore, India

Christopher Khng, MD
Cincinnati Eye Institute
Cincinnati, Ohio

Ashok Kumar, MD, DO, FERC
Dr. Agarwal's Group of Eye Hospitals and Eye Research Centre
Chennai, Bangalore, India

Steven G. Lin, MD
Southern California Desert Retina Consultants, M.C.
Inland Retina Consultants
Palm Springs, California

Luis W. Lu, MD, FACS
Eye Physician and Surgeon Director
Pennsylvania Eye Consultants
Saint Marys, Pennsylvania

Anthony J. Maloof, MBBS, MBiomedE, FRANZCO, FRACS
Intraocular implant Unit
Sydney Hospital and Sydney Eye Hospital
Sydney, Australia

John W. McAvoy, PhD
Save Sight Institute Research Laboratories
Save Sight Institute
The University of Sydney
Sydney, Australia

Javier Mendicute, MD
Chairman, Department of Ophthalmology
Hospital Donostia
Basque Health Service-Osakidetza
Begitek Clínica Oftalmológica
Donostia-San Sebastián
Spain

E. John Milverton, MBBS, DO, FRANZCO, FRCOphth
Intraocular Implant Unit
Sydney Hospital and Sydney Eye Hospital
Sydney, Australia

Herminio Negri, MD
Instituto Oftalmológico De Alicante
Refractive Surgery and Cornea Department
Miguel Hernández University Medical School
Alicante, Spain

Robert H. Osher, MD
Cincinnati Eye Institute
Cincinnati, Ohio

Suresh K. Pandey, MD
Assistant Professor
John A. Moran Eye Center
Department of Ophthalmology & Visual Sciences
University of Utah
Salt Lake City, Utah
Ophthalmic Surgeon, Intraocular Implant Unit
Sydney Hospital & Sydney Eye Hospital
Sydney, Australia
Scholar to the University of Sydney
Save Sight Institute and Discipline of Ophthalmology
Sydney, Australia

Pandelis A. Papadopoulos, MD, PhD, FEBO
Director, Ophthalmology Department
Athens Metropolitan Hospital
Director, Diagnostic & Therapeutic Eye Center
Ophthalmo-Check Ltd
General Secretary, Hellenic Society of Cataract and Refractive Surgery
Athens, Greece

Shetal M. Raj, MS
Iladevi Cataract & IOL Research Centre
Raghudeep Eye Clinic
Ahmedabad, India

Mahipal Singh Sachdev, MBBS(AIIMS), MD Ophthal(AIIMS)
Centre for Sight
New Delhi, India

Michael E. Snyder, MD
Cincinnati Eye Institute
Cincinnati, Ohio

R. Sujatha, DO, FERC
Dr. Agarwal's Group of Eye Hospitals and Eye Research Centre
Chennai, Bangalore, India

Brighu Swamy, MBBS (Hons), M Med (Clin Epi)
Sydney Eye Hospital & Save Sight Institute
University of Sydney
Sydney, Australia

Alejandro Tello, MD
Fundación Oftalmológica Vejarano
Popayán, Colombia
Department of Ophthalmology
Universidad del Cauca
Popayán, Colombia

Marta Ubeda, MD
Department of Ophthalmology
Hospital Donostia
Basque Health Service-Osakidetza
Donostia-San Sebastián
Spain

Abhay R. Vasavada, MS, FRCS
Iladevi Cataract & IOL Research Centre
Raghudeep Eye Clinic
Ahmedabad, India

L. Felipe Vejarano, MD
Fundación Oftalmológica Vejarano
Popayán, Colombia
Department of Ophthalmology
Universidad del Cauca
Popayán, Colombia

Liliana Werner, MD, PhD
John A. Moran Eye Center
University of Utah
Salt Lake City, Utah

M. Edward Wilson, MD
N. Edgar Miles Center for Pediatric Ophthalmology
Storm Eye Institute
Medical University of South Carolina
Charleston, South Carolina

Preface

Have you ever wondered why some surgeries go so smoothly, and other times you are just struggling and then something even worse happens, and your biggest nightmare becomes a reality? Think about that fine line between triumph and tragedy. Eastern philosophy always knew these answers, however, the Western scientific mind has just started to ponder the possibilities. With quantum physics, the more we understand, the little we really know. This has often been explained in science as the Uncertainty Principle and was known to the originators of Western science—Zeno and the early Greek philosophers in the 5th century.

We have understood over the years that the most primordial of energy forms in the physical world is magnetism. If there is chemical energy being used then electrical energy will be playing a role somewhere; if there is electrical energy being read then there will be magnetic energy in play too. Today we understand that the human body functions with all these energies. However, the magnetic energy is so low that it is often ignored. In Eastern philosophy, the subtle energies have been given a great role to play, that of cause and effect, or the law of karma. And all of us in the physical world are subject to this universal law.

Somewhere down the road, we are all using this subtle energy to perform any task. Whether it is capsulorrhexis, nuclear fragmentation, or IOL insertion, our energy through our eyes, hands, and all parameters are focused at all times on the patient's welfare. If for one small moment our attention is diverted, the result is a catastrophe. Now why did that moment of carelessness come? Was it our doing, was it that we were not able to throw enough energy or was there something repelling our energy—the patient's own energy field? With years and years of searching and researching the genesis of this problem, a clearer understanding came with the learning of quantum physics. When two waves of magnetic energy clash with each other, many other things happen: reflection, refraction, penetration, and interaction. When these happen in symbiosis, we have smooth sailing in that particular eye of that particular patient. When for any reason these waves clash and some former imprint has created a knot in the wave form, our attention might slip, the patient may move, or some other problem can cause a phaco nightmare. This in essence is the law of cause and effect: the cause created the knot in the energy wave form, the effect helped in creating the disaster.

Whatever the reasons, through multitudes of surgeries performed through perfect hands the world over, the contributors of this book have gathered together their worst case scenarios to help you better understand how to treat these situations. There are five sections in this book: the basic understanding of the dynamics involved, difficult situations, anterior and posterior segment disasters, and finally the newest trajectory in our world of cataracts —bimanual phaco.

Dear reader, please view these scientific endeavors only so that it may make your hands stronger and so the next time you face a disaster, you may still realize there are many more ways to have paradise regained.

Amar Agarwal, MS, FRCS, FRCOphth
Dr. Agarwal's Eye Hospital
Chennai, India
dragarwal@vsnl.com

Foreword

It takes a unique person to "show his dirty laundry" in front of peers and students just to illustrate teaching points in the name of education. But education has become the mantra of Amar Agarwal. He has spent the better portion of his life unselfishly teaching others in his writings and in live surgery. Several years ago, he authored five textbooks in ophthalmology in one year! Microincision bimanual surgery (Phakonit) performed with no anesthesia has become a technique known worldwide and was pioneered and taught by Dr. Agarwal.

In this book, Dr. Agarwal has assembled a world-class group of surgeons to discuss a wide variety of difficult and challenging cases in phacoemulsification. *Phaco Nightmares: Conquering Cataract Catastrophes* is a comprehensive text that will guide beginning and experienced phaco surgeons alike. Current issues such as Floppy Iris Syndrome and old nemesis problems like nanophthalmos and posterior polar cataracts are addressed. Complicated cases that few would feel comfortable taking on are discussed in detail and addressed in a way that gives you the confidence and clearer understanding of the issues at hand and what might lay ahead for you should you decide to tackle the case yourself.

Just as Dr. Agarwal has built a world-renowned Eye Hospital for ophthalmic care, research, and education in the shape of a human eye, he has produced a text herein that will help give this generation of ophthalmic surgeons the experience and knowledge to meet the challenges of difficult and challenging cataract surgery into the 21st century. I applaud his dedication to our profession.

Stephen S. Lane, MD
Adjunct Professor of Ophthalmology
University of Minnesota
Minneapolis, MN
USA

I

Phacoemulsification: Machine and Technique

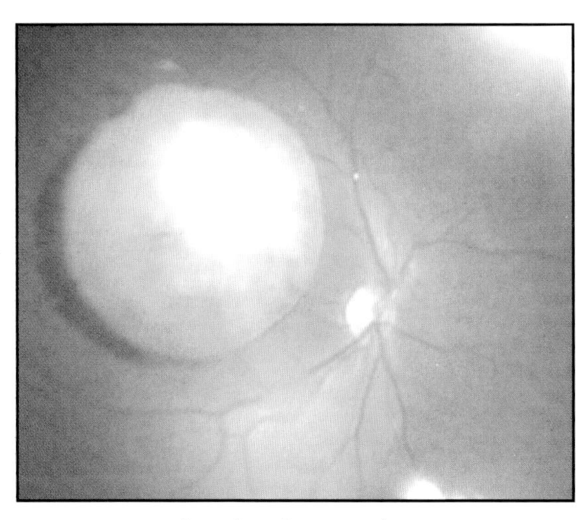

Dropped nucleus lying on the retina.

Chapter 1

Avoiding Problems With the Phacoemulsification Machine

William J. Fishkind, MD, FACS

Introduction

All phaco machines consist of a computer to generate ultrasonic impulses, and a transducer and piezo electric crystals to turn these electronic signals into mechanical energy. The energy thus created is then harnessed, within the eye, to overcome the inertia of the lens and emulsify it. Once turned into emulsate, the fluidic systems remove the emulsate, replacing it with balanced salt solution (BSS).The recent trend in phaco surgery is to minimize power utilizing new power modalities, and maximize the use of fluidics to remove the cataractous lens.

Power Generation

Power is created by the interaction of frequency and stroke length. Frequency is defined as the speed of the needle movement. It is determined by the manufacturer of the machine. Presently, most machines operate at a frequency of between 35,000 cycles per second (Hz.) to 45,000 cycles per second. This frequency range is the most efficient for nuclear emulsification. Lower frequencies are less efficient and higher frequencies create excess heat.

Frequency is kept constant by tuning circuitry that is designed into the machine computer. Tuning is vital because the phaco tip is required to operate in varied media. For example, the resistance of the aqueous is less than the resistance of the cortex, which in turn, is less than the resistance of the nucleus. As the resistance to the phaco tip varies, to maintain maximum efficiency, small alterations in frequency are created by the tuning circuitry in the computer. The surgeon will subjectively determine good tuning circuitry by a sense of smoothness and power.

Stroke length is defined as the length of the needle movement. This length is generally 2 to 6 mils (thousandths of an inch). Most machines operate in the 2 to 4 mil range. Longer stroke lengths are prone to generate excess heat. The longer the stroke length, the greater the physical impact on the nucleus, and the greater the generation of cavitation forces. Stroke length is determined by foot pedal excursion in position 3 during linear control of phaco.

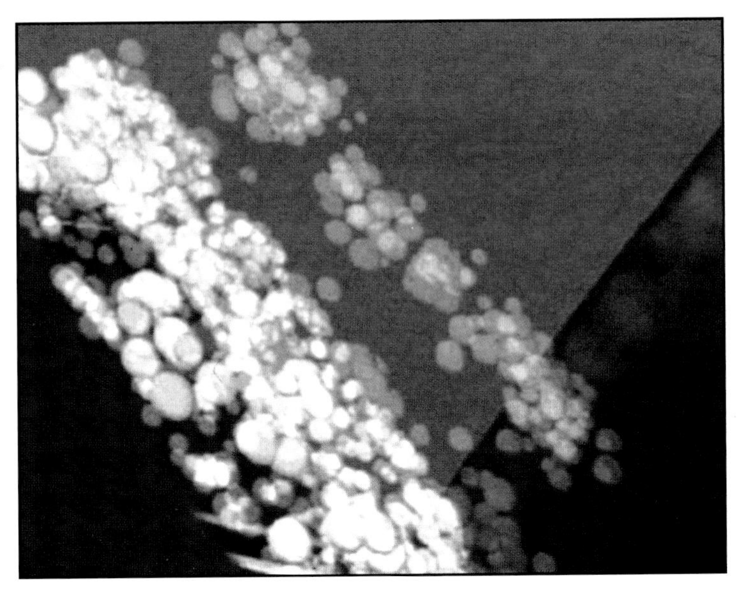

Figure 1-1. Micro bubbles generated at the phaco tip.

ENERGY AT THE PHACO TIP

The actual tangible forces that emulsify the nucleus are thought to be a blend of the "jackhammer" effect and cavitation.[1] The "jackhammer" effect is merely the physical striking of the needle against the nucleus. The cavitation effect is more convoluted. Recent studies indicate that there are two kinds of cavitational energy. One is transient cavitation and the other is sustained cavitation.

Transient Cavitation

The phaco needle, moving through the liquid medium of the aqueous at ultrasonic speeds, creates intense zones of high and low pressure. Low pressure, created with backward movement of the tip, literally pulls dissolved gases out of solution, thus giving rise to micro bubbles. Forward tip movement then creates an equally intense zone of high pressure. This produces compression of the micro bubbles until they implode. At the moment of implosion, the bubbles create a temperature of 13000 degrees and a shock wave of 75,000 PSI. Of the micro bubbles created, 75% implode, amassing to create a powerful shock wave, radiating from the phaco tip in the direction of the bevel with annular spread. However, 25% of the bubbles are too large to implode. These micro bubbles are swept up in the shock wave and radiate with it. Transient cavitation is a violent event. The energy created by transient cavitation exists for no more than 6 to 25 milliseconds. It is this form of cavitation that is thought to generate the energy responsible for emulsification of cataractous material (Figure 1-1).

The cavitation energy thus created can be directed in any desired direction as the angle of the bevel of the phaco needle governs the direction of the generation of the shock wave and micro bubbles.

The author has developed a method of visualization of these forces, called "enhanced cavitation". Using this process, it can be seen that with a 45° tip, the cavitation wave is generated at 45° from the tip and comes to a focus 1 mm from it. Similarly, a 30° tip generates cavitation at a 30° angle from the bevel, and a 15° tip 15° from the bevel (Figure 1-2). A 0° tip creates the cavitation wave directly in front of the tip and the focal point is 0.5 mm from the tip (Figure 1-3). The Kelman tip has a broad band of powerful cavitation that radi-

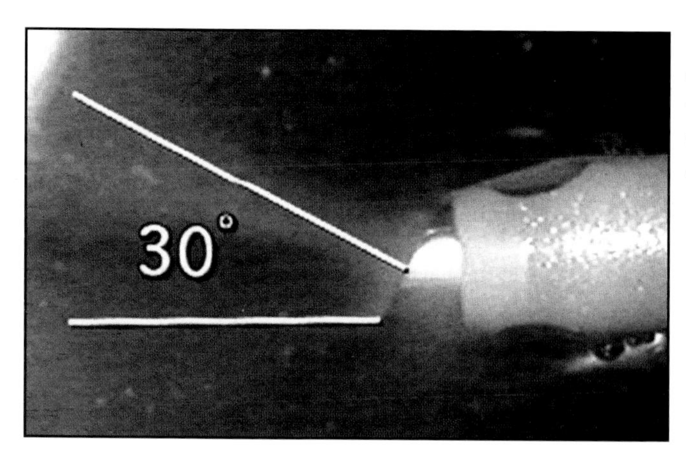

Figure 1-2. 30° tip. Enhanced cavitation shows ultrasonic wave focused 1 mm from the tip, spreading at an angle of 30°.

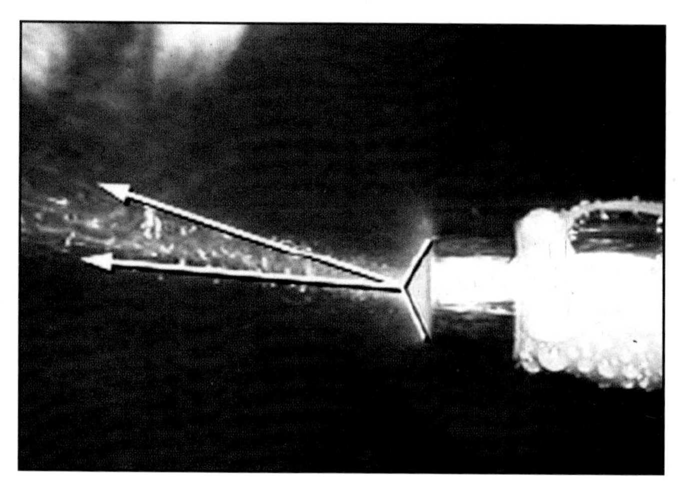

Figure 1-3. 0° tip. Enhanced cavitation shows ultrasonic wave focused .5 mm in front of the tip, spreading directly in front of it.

ates from the area of the angle in the shaft. A weak area of cavitation is developed from the bevel but is inconsequential (Figure 1-4).

Taking into consideration analysis of enhanced cavitation, it can be concluded that phacoemulsification is most efficient when both the jackhammer effect and cavitation energy are combined. To accomplish this, the bevel of the needle should be turned toward the nucleus, or nuclear fragment. This simple maneuver will cause the broad bevel of the needle to strike the nucleus. This will enhance the physical force of the needle striking the nucleus. In addition, the cavitation force is then concentrated into the nucleus rather than away from it. Finally, in this configuration, the vacuum force can be maximally exploited as occlusion is encouraged (Figure 1-5). This causes energy to emulsify the nucleus and be absorbed by it. A 0° tip automatically focuses both the jackhammer and cavitational energy directly in front of it (Figure 1-6). When the bevel is turned away from the nucleus, the cavitational energy is directed up and away from the nucleus toward the iris and endothelium (Figure 1-7).

Sustained Cavitation

If phaco energy is continued beyond 25 milliseconds, transient cavitation with generation of micro bubbles and shock waves ends. The bubbles then begin to vibrate, without implosion. No shock wave is generated. Therefore there is no emulsification energy produced. Sustained cavitation is ineffective for emulsification of the cataractous lens (Figure 1-8).

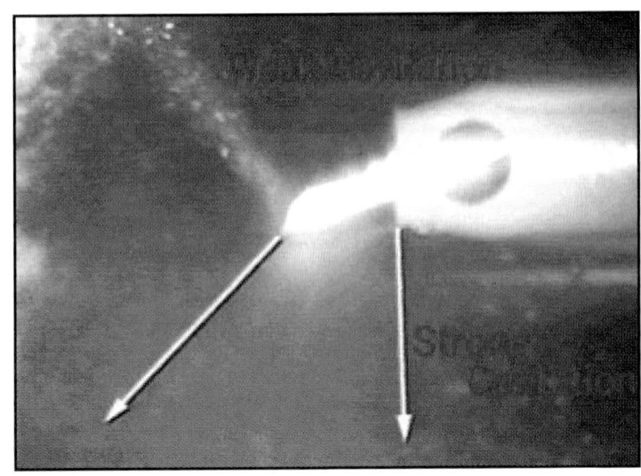

Figure 1-4. Kelman tip. Enhanced cavitation shows broad band of enhanced cavitation spreading inferiorly from the angle of the tip. A weak band of cavitation spreads from the tip.

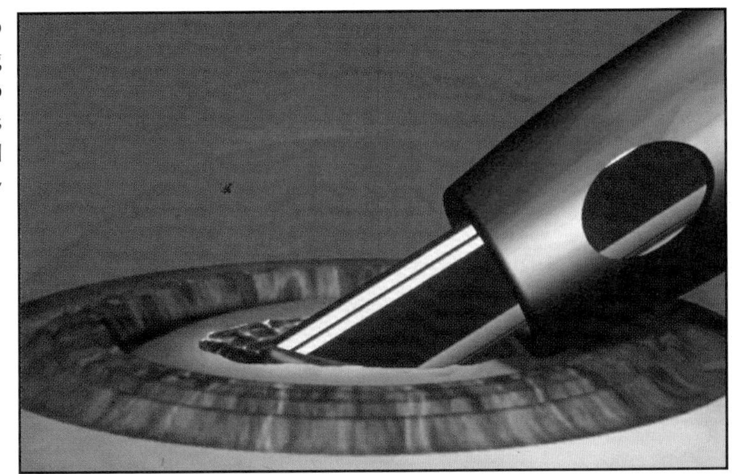

Figure 1-5. 30° tip bevel down. Turning the bevel of the phaco tip toward the nucleus focuses cavitation and jackhammer energy into the nucleus.

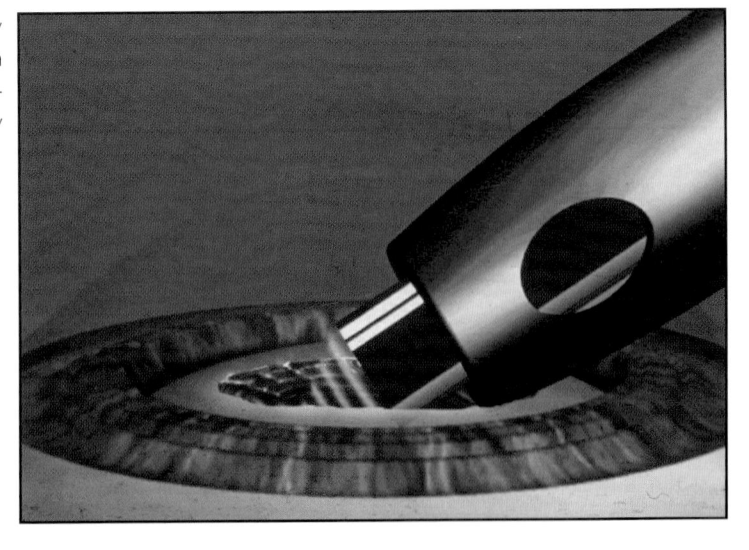

Figure 1-6. The 0° tip, by its design, focuses both jackhammer and cavitation forces directly ahead into the nucleus.

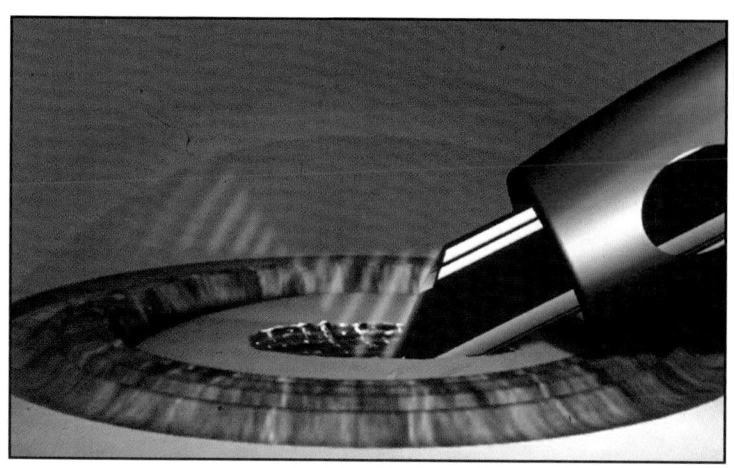

Figure 1-7. 30° tip bevel up. The bevel is turned away from the nucleus. Cavitation energy is wasted and may damage iris and endothelium.

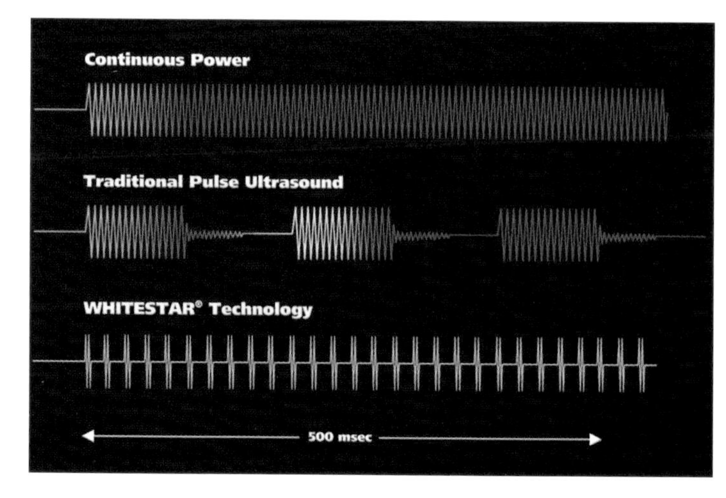

Figure 1-8. Transient cavitation energy is shown in red, stabilized cavitational energy shown in blue. Continuous power: Only the initial energy is transient. The remainder is stabilized energy. In a 50-millisecond pulse, only the initial 25 milliseconds is transient. In micro pulse phaco, the entire pulse is transient energy. (Photo courtesy of Mark E. Schafer, PhD, AMO.)

Water bath, hydrophonic studies indicate that transient cavitation is significantly more powerful than sustained cavitation. With this information in mind, it would appear that continuous phaco is best used to emulsify the intact nucleus, held in place by the capsular bag, as one does during the sculpting phase of divide and conquer or stop and chop. Transient cavitation is maximized during micro pulse phaco. This is best used during phaco of the nuclear fragments in the later phase of the above two procedures, or during phaco chop procedures.

Modification of Phaco Power Intensity

Application of the minimal amount of phaco power intensity necessary for emulsification of the nucleus is desirable. Unnecessary power intensity is a cause of heat with subsequent wound damage, endothelial cell damage, and iris damage with alteration of the blood-aqueous barrier. Phaco power intensity can be modified by: 1) alteration in stroke length, 2) alteration of duration, and 3) alteration of emission.

Alteration of Stroke Length

Stroke length is determined by foot pedal adjustment. When set for linear phaco, depression of the foot pedal will increase stroke length and therefore power. New foot pedals, such as those found in the Allergan Sovereign and the Alcon Infinity, permit surgeon adjustment of the throw length of the pedal in position three. This can refine power application. The Bausch & Lomb Millennium dual linear foot pedal permits the separation of the fluidic aspects of the foot pedal from the power elements.

Alteration of Duration

The duration of application of phaco power has a dramatic effect on overall power delivered. Usage of pulse or burst mode phaco will considerably decrease overall power delivery. New machines allow for a power pulse of duration alternating with a period of aspiration only. Burst mode (parameter is machine dependent) is characterized by 80 or 120 millisecond periods of power combined with fixed short periods of aspiration only. Pulse mode utilizes fixed pulses of power of 50 or 150 milliseconds with variable short periods of aspiration only.

Micro Pulse

Recently, through the development of highly responsive and low mass piezo crystals, combined with software modifications, the manufacturers of phaco machines have shortened the cycle of on and off time. This process, patented by AMO (Advanced Medical Optics), is called "micro pulse." This technology is now available in most phaco machines.

A duty cycle is defined as the length of time of power on combined with power off. The short bursts of phaco energy followed by a short period without phaco energy allows two events to occur. First, the period without phaco energy permits the nuclear material to be drawn toward the phaco tip with increased efficiency. Second, the absence of power allows for cooling of the phaco tip. This cool phaco tip has been termed "cold phaco." This is a misnomer as the phaco tip is not cold, but warm. However, studies indicate that it will not develop a temperature greater than 55 degrees Celsius, the temperature required to create a wound burn.

Phaco techniques such as phaco chop utilize minimal periods of power in pulse mode, or micro pulse mode, to reduce power delivery to the anterior chamber. In addition, the use of pulse mode, or micro pulse mode, to remove the epinucleus provides for an added margin of safety. When the epinucleus is emulsified, the posterior capsule is exposed to the phaco tip and may move toward it due to surge. Activation of pulse phaco, or micro pulse phaco, will create a deeper anterior chamber to work within. This occurs because, as noted previously, each period of phaco energy is followed by an interval of no energy. During the interval of absence of energy, the epinucleus is drawn toward the phaco tip, producing occlusion, and interrupting outflow. This allows inflow to deepen the anterior chamber immediately prior to onset of another pulse of phaco energy. The surgeon will recognize the outcome as operating in a deeper, more stable anterior chamber.

Alteration of Emission

The emission of phaco energy is modified by tip selection. Phaco tips can be modified to accentuate: 1) power, 2) flow, or 3) a combination of both.

1. Power intensity is modified by altering bevel tip angle. Noted previously, the bevel of the phaco tip will focus power in the direction of the bevel. The Kelman tip will produce broad powerful cavitation directed away from the angle in the shaft. This tip is excellent for the hardest of nuclei. New flare and cobra tips direct cavitation into the opening of the bevel

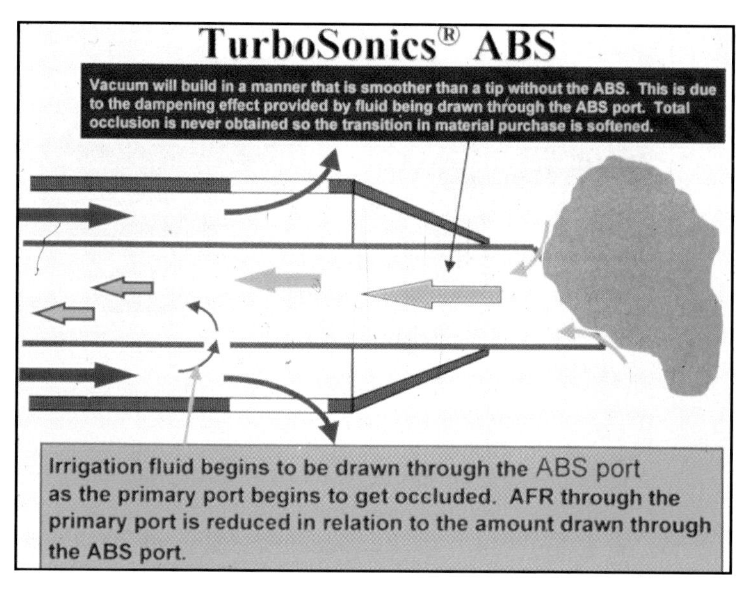

Figure 1-9. A 0.175 mm hole drilled in the shaft of the ABS tip provides an alternate path for fluid to flow into the needle when there is an occlusion at the phaco tip. (Photo courtesy of Alcon.)

of the tip. Thus random emission of phaco energy is minimized. Designer tips such as the "flathead" designed by Dr. Barry Seibel and power wedges designed by Mr. Douglas Mastel modify the direction and focus delivery of phaco energy intensity.

2. Power intensity and flow are modified by utilizing a 08 tip. This tip will focus power directly ahead of the tip and enhance occlusion due to the smaller surface area of its orifice. Small diameter tips, such as 21 gauge tips, change fluid flow rates. Although they do not actually change power intensity, they appear to have this effect, as the nucleus must be emulsified into smaller pieces for removal through the smaller diameter tip.

   The Alcon ABS (aspiration bypass system) tip modification is available with a 08 tip, a Kelman tip, or a flare tip. The flare is a modification of power intensity and the ABS a flow modification. In the ABS system, a 0.175 mm hole in the shaft permits a variable flow of fluid into the needle, even during occlusion. Therefore occlusion is never allowed to occur (Figure 1-9). This flow adjustment serves to minimize surge.
3. Finally, flow can be modified by utilizing one of the microseal tips. These tips have a flexible outer sleeve to seal the phaco incision. They also have a rigid inner sleeve or a ribbed shaft configuration to protect cooling irrigant inflow. Thus a tight seal allows low flow phaco without danger of wound burns. Phaco power intensity is the energy that emulsifies the lens nucleus. The phaco tip must operate in a cool environment and with adequate space to isolate its actions from delicate intraocular structures. This portion of the action of the machine is dependent upon its fluidics.

Fluidics

The fluidics of all machines are fundamentally a balance of fluid inflow and fluid outflow. Inflow is determined by bottle height above the eye of the patient, and irrigation tubing diameter. It is important to recognize that with recent acceptance of temporal surgical approaches, and modifications of the surgical table, the eye of the patient may be physically higher than in the past. This requires that the irrigation bottle be adequately elevated. A shallow, unstable anterior chamber will otherwise result.

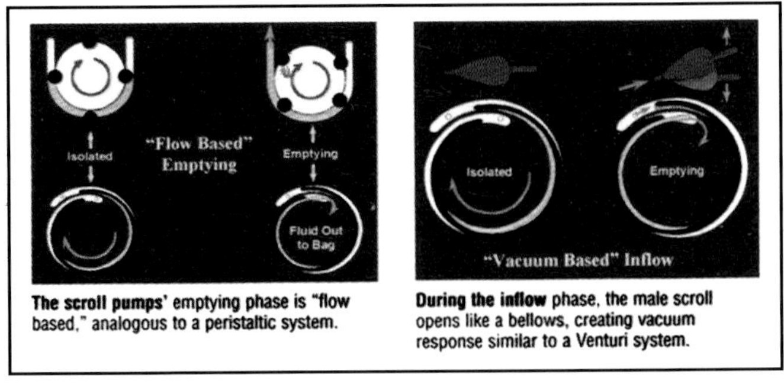

Figure 1-10. Concentrix pump showing flow based mechanics. (Photo courtesy of Bausch & Lomb.)

Outflow is determined by the sleeve-incision relationship, as well as the paracentesis size, aspiration rate, and vacuum level commanded. The incision length selected should create a snug fit with the phaco tip selected. This will result in minimal uncontrolled wound outflow with resultant increased anterior chamber stability.

Aspiration rate, or flow, is defined as the flow of fluid, measured in cc/min, through the tubing. With a peristaltic pump, it is determined by the speed of the pump. Flow determines how well particulate mater is attracted to the phaco tip. Aspiration level or vacuum is a level and measured in mmHg. It is defined as the magnitude of negative pressure created in the tubing. Vacuum is the determinant of how well, once occluded on the phaco tip, particulate material will be held to the tip.

Vacuum Sources

There are three categories of vacuum sources or pumps. These are flow pumps, vacuum pumps, and hybrid pumps.

1. The primary example of the flow pump type is the peristaltic pump. These pumps allow for independent control of both aspiration rate (flow) and aspiration level (vacuum).
2. The primary example of the vacuum pump is the venturi pump. This pump type allows direct control of only vacuum level. Flow is dependent upon vacuum level setting. Additional examples are the rotary vane and diaphragmatic pumps.
3. The primary example of the hybrid pump is the AMO Sovereign peristaltic pump or the Bausch & Lomb Concentrix pump (Figure 1-10). These pumps are interesting as they are able to act like either a vacuum or flow pump depending on programming. They are the most recent supplement to pump types. They are generally controlled by digital inputs creating incredible flexibility and responsiveness. They are rapidly becoming the standard type of pump for modern phaco.

The challenge to the surgeon is to balance the effect of phaco intensity, which tends to push nuclear fragments off the phaco tip, with the effect of flow, which attracts fragments toward the phaco tip, and vacuum, which holds the fragments on the phaco tip. Generally low flow slows down intraocular events, and high vacuum speeds them up. Low or zero vacuum is helpful during sculpting of hard or large nucleus, where the high power intensity of the tip may be applied near the iris or anterior capsule. Zero vacuum will prevent inadvertent aspiration of the iris or capsule, avoiding significant morbidity.

Surge

A principal limiting factor in the selection of high levels of vacuum or flow is the development of surge. When the phaco tip is occluded, flow is interrupted and vacuum builds

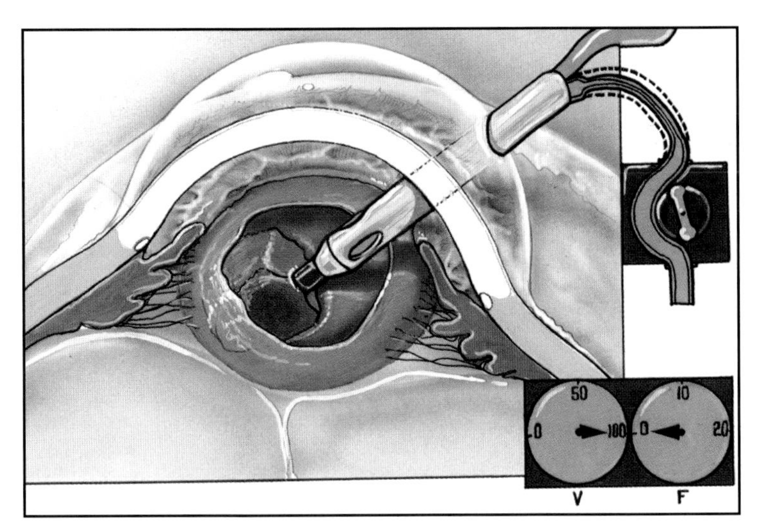

Figure 1-11. Occlusion: vacuum builds, flow falls toward zero, tubing collapses. (From Fishkind WF. *Complications in Phacoemulsification*. New York, NY: Thieme Publishers; 2002. Reprinted with permission.)

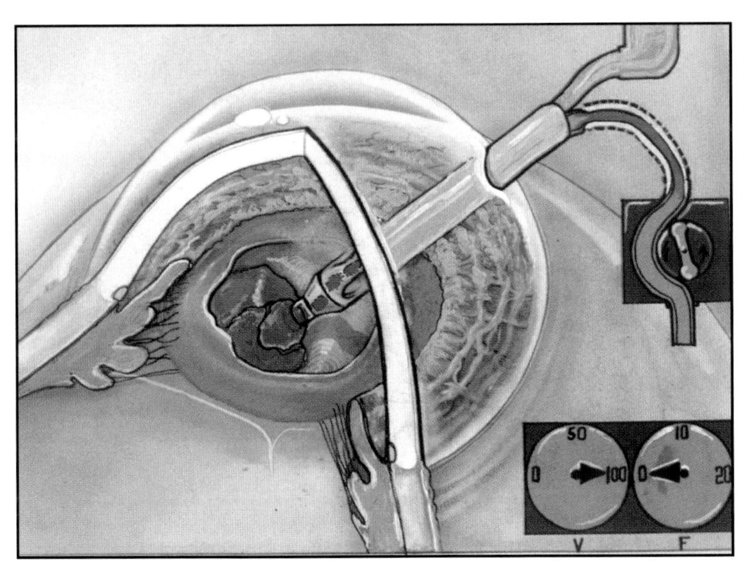

Figure 1-12. Occlusion break: vacuum drops to zero. Flow rapidly increases to preset. Tubing expands. Outflow exceeds inflow. Anterior chamber begins to shallow. (From Fishkind WF. *Complications in Phacoemulsification*. New York, NY: Thieme Publishers; 2002. Reprinted with permission.)

to its preset level (Figure 1-11). Emulsification of the occluding fragment then clears the occlusion. Flow immediately begins at the preset level in the presence of the high vacuum level. In addition, if the aspiration line tubing is not reinforced to prevent collapse (tubing compliance) the tubing will have constricted during the occlusion. It then expands on occlusion break. The expansion is an additional source of vacuum production. These factors cause a rush of fluid from the anterior segment into the phaco tip. The fluid in the anterior chamber may not be replaced rapidly enough by infusion to prevent shallowing of the anterior chamber. Therefore, there is subsequent rapid anterior movement of the posterior capsule. This abrupt forceful stretching of the bag around nuclear fragments may be a cause of capsular tears. In addition, the posterior capsule can be literally sucked into the phaco tip, tearing it. The magnitude of the surge is contingent on the presurge settings of flow and vacuum (Figure 1-12).

Surge is therefore modified by selecting lower levels of flow and vacuum. The phaco machine manufacturers help to decrease surge by providing noncompliant aspiration tubing. This will not constrict in the presence of high levels of vacuum. More important are noteworthy new technologies:

1. AMO Sovereign—Microprocessors sample vacuum and flow parameters 50 times a second creating a "virtual" anterior chamber model. At the moment of surge, the computer senses the increase in flow and instantaneously slows or reverses the pump to stop surge production. The Alcon Infinity works in a similar manner.
2. Bausch & Lomb Millennium—The dual linear foot pedal can be programmed to separate both the flow and vacuum from power. In this way, flow or vacuum can be lowered before beginning the emulsification of an occluding fragment. The emulsification therefore occurs in the presence of a lower vacuum or flow so that surge is minimized.
3. Alcon Infinity/Legacy—The Aspiration Bypass System (ABS) tips have mm holes drilled in the shaft of the needle. During occlusion, the hole provides for a continuous alternate fluid flow. This will cause dampening of the surge on occlusion break.

Preocclusion Phacoemulsification

Another way to avoid surge is to prevent occlusion entirely. By definition, a surge requires occlusion. In preocclusion phaco utilizing micro pulse, the nuclear fragment is emulsified before it can occlude the phaco tip. Therefore, vacuum never builds to maximum and surge is avoided. This appears to be an extremely efficient method of emulsification. It allows for fragment removal with minimal energy level and duration, in a deep and controlled anterior chamber.

Neosonics technology (Alcon) also creates preocclusion phaco. The oscillatory movement of the phaco tip mechanically knocks the fragments off the phaco tip. This will prevent occlusion.

Phacoemulsification Technique and Machine Technology

The patient will have the best visual result when total phaco energy delivered to the anterior segment is minimized. Additionally, phaco energy should be focused into the nucleus. This will prevent damage to iris blood vessels and endothelium. Finally, proficient emulsification will lead to shorter overall surgical time. Therefore a lesser amount of irrigation fluid will pass through the anterior segment. The general principles of power management are to focus phaco energy into the nucleus, vary fluid parameters for efficient sculpting and fragment removal, and minimize surge.

Divide and Conquer Phaco

Sculpting

To focus cavitation energy into the nucleus, a 0° tip or a 15° or 30° tip turned bevel down should be utilized. Zero or low vacuum (depending on the manufacturer's recommendation) is mandatory for bevel down phaco. This will prevent occlusion. Occlusion, at best, will cause excessive movement of the nucleus during sculpting. At worst, occlusion occurring near the equator is the cause of tears in the equatorial bag early in the phaco procedure, and occlusion at the bottom of a groove will cause phaco through the posterior capsule. Once the groove is judged to be adequately deep, the bevel of the tip should be rotated to the bevel up position to improve visibility and prevent the possibility of phaco through the posterior nucleus and posterior capsule. If micro pulse phaco is used, duty cycles with longer power on than off should be selected. This will allow phaco to proceed with clean emulsification and avoid pushing the nucleus away from the phaco tip, potentially damaging zonules.

Quadrant and Fragment Removal

The tip selected, as noted above, is retained. Vacuum and flow are increased to reasonable limits subject to the machine being used. The limiting factor to these levels is the development of surge. The bevel of the tip is turned toward the quadrant or fragment. Low pulsed or burst power is applied at a level high enough to emulsify the fragment without driving it from the phaco tip. "Chatter" is defined as a fragment bouncing from the phaco tip due to aggressive application of phaco energy.

Epinucleus and Cortex Removal

For removal of epinucleus and cortex, the vacuum is decreased while flow is maintained. This will allow for grasping of the epinucleus just deep to the anterior capsule. The low vacuum will help the tip hold the epinucleus on the phaco tip, without breaking off chunks due to high vacuum, so that it scrolls around the equator and can be pulled to the level of the iris. There, low power pulsed phaco is employed for emulsification. If cortical cleaving hydrodissection has been performed, the cortex will be removed concurrently.

Stop and Chop Phaco

Groove creation is performed as noted above under Divide and Conquer sculpting techniques. Once the groove is adequate vacuum and flow are increased to improve holding ability of the phaco tip. The tip is then burrowed into the mass of one hemi nucleus using pulsed linear phaco. The sleeve should be 1 mm from the base of the bevel of the phaco tip to create adequate exposed needle length for sufficient holding power. Excessive phaco energy application is to be avoided, as this will cause nucleus immediately adjacent to the tip to be emulsified. The space thus created in the vicinity of the tip is responsible for interfering with the seal around the tip and therefore the capability of vacuum to hold the nucleus. The nucleus will then pop off the phaco tip, making chopping more difficult. With a good seal, the hemi nucleus can be drawn toward the incision and the chopper can be inserted at the endonucleus–epinucleus junction. After the first chop, a second similar chop is performed. The pie-shaped piece of nucleus thus created is removed with low power pulsed phaco as discussed in the Divide and Conquer section. Epinucleus and cortex removal are also performed as noted above.

Phaco Chop

Phaco chop requires no sculpting. Therefore, the procedure is initiated with high vacuum and flow and linear pulsed phaco power. For a 0° tip, when emulsifying a hard nucleus, a small trough may be required to create adequate room for the phaco tip to burrow deep into the nucleus. For a 15° or a 30° tip, the tip should be rotated bevel down to engage the nucleus. The phaco tip should be buried into the endonucleus with the minimal amount of power necessary. If the phaco tip is inserted into the nucleus with excess power, the adjacent nucleus will be emulsified creating a poor seal between nucleus and tip. This will make it impossible to remove fragments as the tip will just "let go" of the nuclear material (Figure 1-13). Additionally, the bevel should be turned toward the fragment to create a seal between tip and fragment, allowing vacuum to build and create holding power (Figure 1-14).

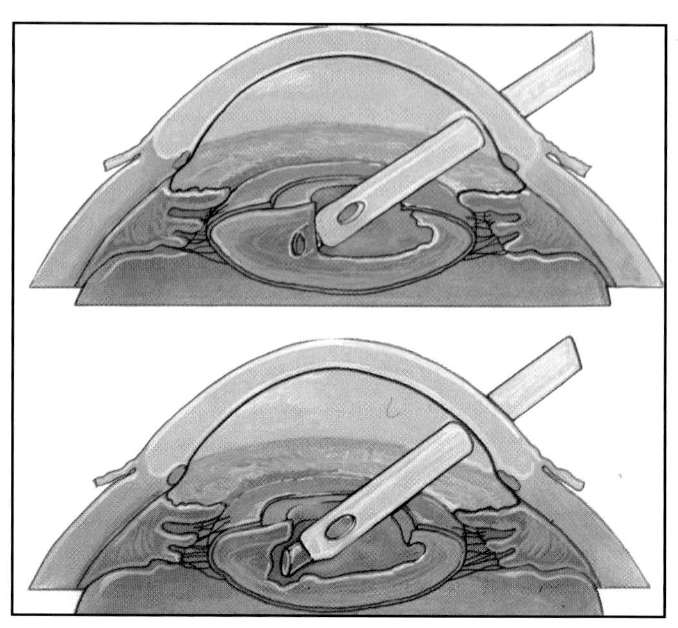

Figure 1-13. Top: Power adequate to enter nucleus but maintain seal between the tip and nucleus. This will allow the tip to maneuver the nucleus. Bottom: Excessive power causes the nucleus around the tip to be emulsified. There is no seal around the phaco tip. The nucleus cannot be maneuvered by the tip. (From Fishkind WF. *Complications in Phacoemulsification*. New York, NY: Thieme Publishers; 2002. Reprinted with permission.)

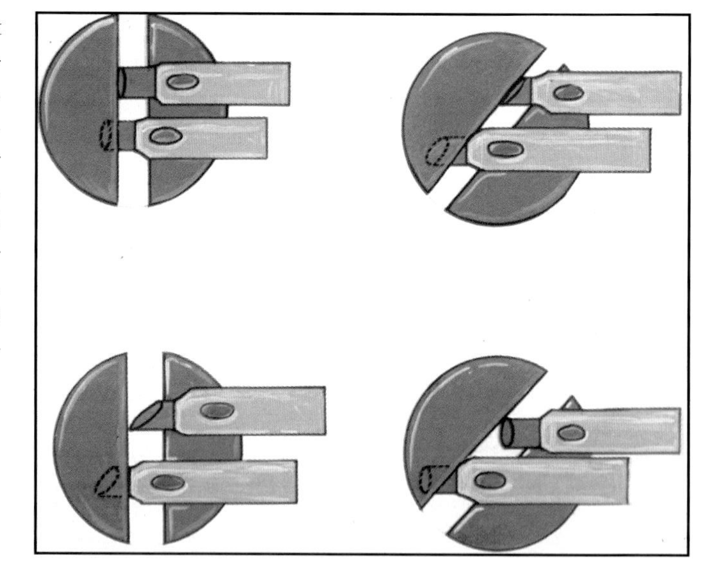

Figure 1-14. Top: Correct position of nucleus in relation to the phaco tip. Occlusion is effortless. Bottom: Incorrect orientation. Occlusion is difficult. (From Fishkind WF. *Complications in Phacoemulsification*. New York, NY: Thieme Publishers; 2002. Reprinted with permission.)

Horizontal Chop

A few bursts or pulses of phaco energy will allow the tip to be buried within the nucleus (Figure 1-15). It then can be drawn toward the incision to allow the chopper access to the epi-endo nuclear junction. If the nucleus comes off the phaco tip, excessive power has produced a space around the tip, impeding vacuum holding power as noted above. The first chop is then produced. Minimal rotation of the nucleus will allow for creation of the second chop. The first pie-shaped segment of nucleus is mobilized with high vacuum and elevated to the iris plane. There it is emulsified with low linear power, high vacuum, and moderate

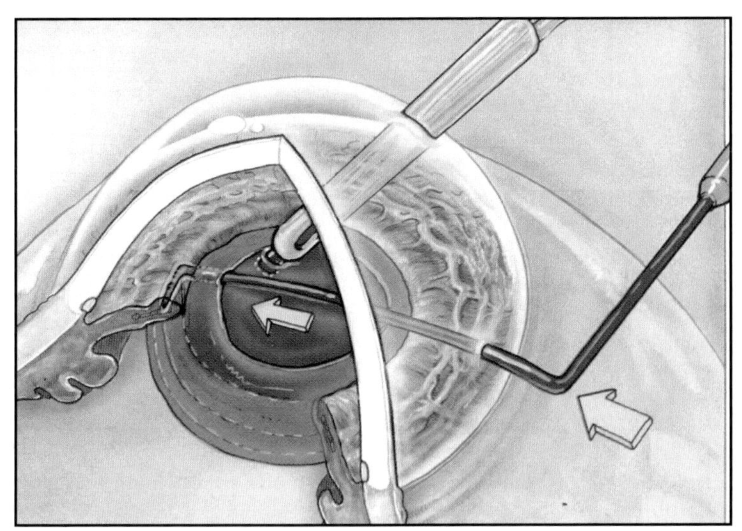

Figure 1-15. Horizontal chop. The phaco tip is drawn toward the wound and the chopper is placed into the epinucleus-endonucleus junctions, often under the anterior capsule. (From Fishkind WF. *Complications in Phacoemulsification*. New York, NY: Thieme Publishers; 2002. Reprinted with permission.)

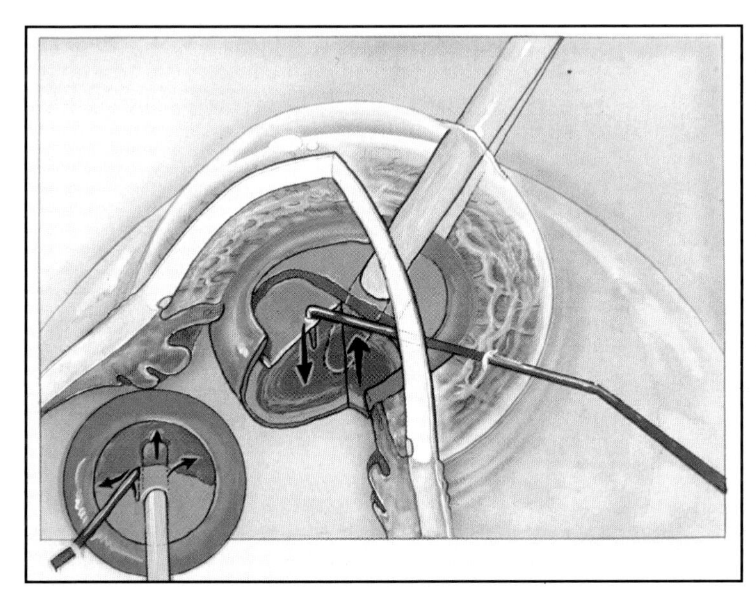

Figure 1-16. Vertical Chop. The sharp chopper is placed adjacent to the phaco tip and plunged into the substance of the endonucleus. (From Fishkind WF. *Complications in Phacoemulsification*. New York, NY: Thieme Publishers; 2002. Reprinted with permission.)

flow. The process of chopping and segment removal is continued until the endonucleus is removed.

Vertical Chop

Once the phaco tip is embedded within the nucleus, a sharp chopper (Nichamin made by Katena) is pushed down into the mass of the nucleus at the same time the phaco tip is elevated (Figure 1-16). The chopper is then advanced down and left and the phaco tip, up and right. This creates a cleavage in the nucleus. The process is repeated until the entire nucleus is chopped. The segments thus created are then elevated to the plane of the pupil and emulsified.

Bimanual Microincisional Phaco

The development of micro pulse ("cold phaco") has led to the performance of phaco with an unsleeved tip. This allows for two 20-gauge 1.4 mm incisions or 21-gauge 1.2 mm incisions. The instrumentation for this procedure is important and the relationship between the instrument and incision size is essential. If the wound is too tight, it is difficult to manipulate the instruments. If the wound is too large, excessive outflow permits chamber shallowing. Micro incision phaco is reportedly more efficient than standard as the flow from irrigating chopper in the direction of the phaco tip captures fragments and carries them toward the phaco tip. The small incisions cause less disruption of the blood aqueous barrier, and are more stable and secure. With insertion of an intraocular lens (IOL) through the 1.4 mm incision, there is less disruption of ocular integrity with immediate return to full activities and less risk of postoperative wound complications.

Irrigation and Aspiration

Similar to phaco, anterior chamber stability during irrigation and aspiration (I/A) is due to a balance of inflow and outflow. Wound outflow can be minimized by employing a soft sleeve around the I/A tip. Combined with a small incision (2.8 to 3 mm), a deep and stable anterior chamber will result. Generally, a 0.3 mm I/A tip is used. With this orifice, a vacuum of 500 mmHg. and flow of 20 cc/min is excellent to tease cortex from the fornices. Linear vacuum allows the cortex to be grasped under the anterior capsule and drawn into the center of the pupil at the iris plane. There, in the safety of a deep anterior chamber, vacuum can be increased and the cortex aspirated. Alcon has developed a steerable silicone I/A tip. This tip allows for maneuverability in the anterior chamber to remove hard to reach cortex, such as sub-incisional cortex. Additionally, the soft orifice will not tear the posterior capsule even if it is aspirated.

Vitrectomy

Most phaco machines are equipped with a vitreous cutter that is activated by compressed air or by electric motor. As noted previously, preservation of a deep anterior chamber depends upon a balance of inflow and outflow. For vitrectomy, a 23 gauge cannula, or chamber maintainer, inserted through a paracentesis, provides inflow. Bottle height should be adequate to prevent chamber collapse. The vitrector should be inserted through another paracentesis. If equipped with a Charles Sleeve, this should be removed and discarded. Utilizing a flow of 20 cc/min, vacuum of 250 mmHg, and a cutting rate of 250 to 350 cuts/min, the vitrector should be placed through the tear in the posterior capsule, orifice facing upward, pulling vitreous out of the anterior chamber. The vitreous should be removed to the level of the posterior capsule (Figure 1-17).

Alternatively, the vitrector can be inserted through a pars plana incision 3 mm posterior to the limbus. In an effort to better visualize the vitreous for thorough vitrectomy, unpreserved sterile prednisone acetate (Kenalog) can be injected into the vitreous. The prednisone particles adhere to the vitreous strands, making the invisible, visible.

Conclusion

It has been said that the phaco procedure is a blend of technology and technique. Awareness of the principles that influence phaco machine settings is a prerequisite for the performance of a proficient and safe operation. Additionally, often during the procedure, there is a demand for modification of the initial parameters. A thorough understanding of fundamental principles will enhance the capability of the surgeon for appropriate response

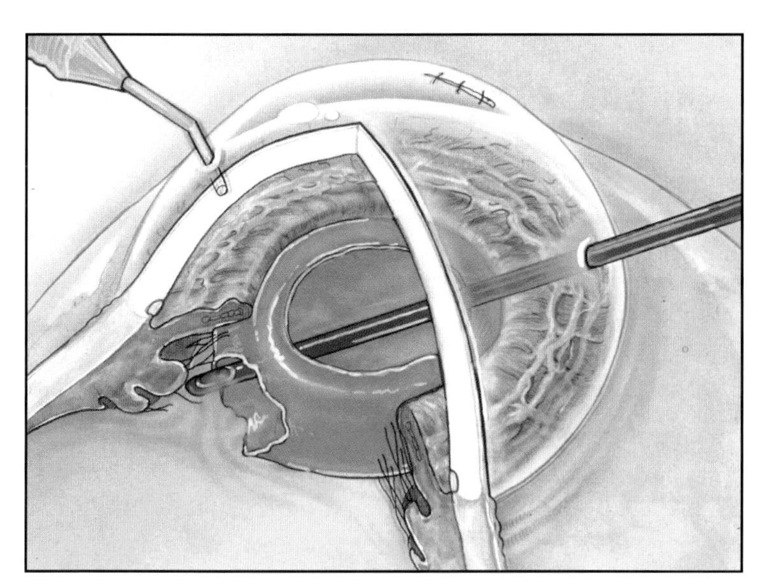

Figure 1-17. The vitrector is placed through a new paracentesis deep to the rent in the posterior capsule. Irrigation is via a cannula. (From Fishkind WF. *Complications in Phacoemulsification*. New York, NY: Thieme Publishers; 2002. Reprinted with permission.)

to this requirement. It is a fundamental principle that through relentless evaluation of the interaction of the machine, and the phaco technique, the skillful surgeon will find innovative methods to enhance technique.

Key Points

1. All phaco machines consist of a computer to generate ultrasonic impulses, and a transducer and piezo electric crystals to turn these electronic signals into mechanical energy. The energy thus created is then harnessed, within the eye, to overcome the inertia of the lens and emulsify it.
2. Power is created by the interaction of frequency and stroke length. Frequency is defined as the speed of the needle movement. It is determined by the manufacturer of the machine. Stroke length is defined as the length of the needle movement.
3. The actual tangible forces that emulsify the nucleus are thought to be a blend of the "jackhammer" effect and cavitation.
4. Recently, through the development of highly responsive and low mass piezo crystals, combined with software modifications, the manufacturers of phaco machines have shortened the cycle of on and off time. This process, patented by AMO (Advanced Medical Optics), is called "micro pulse." This technology is now available in most phaco machines.
5. A principal limiting factor in the selection of high levels of vacuum or flow is the development of surge.

References

1. Buratto L, Osher RH, Masket S, eds. *Cataract Surgery in Complicated Cases*. Thorofare, NJ: SLACK Incorporated; 2001.
2. Fishkind WJ, ed. *Complications in Phacoemulsification: Recognition, Avoidance, and Management*. New York: Thieme Publishers; 2001.
3. Fishkind WJ. Pop Goes the Microbubbles. ESCRS Film Festival Grand Prize Winner, 1998.
4. Fishkind WJ, Neuhann TF, Steinert RF. *The Phaco Machine in Cataract Surgery Technique: Complications & Management*. 2nd Ed. Philadelphia: W.B. Saunders and Co; 2004.
5. Seibel BS. *Phacodynamics: Mastering the Tools and Techniques of Phacoemulsification Surgery*. 3rd ed. Thorofare, NJ: SLACK Incorporated; 2000.

Chapter 2

Gas-Forced Infusion: The Solution for Surge

Sunita Agarwal, MS, FSVH, DO

History

The main problem we had in bimanual phaco/phakonit was the destabilization of the anterior chamber during surgery. We solved it to a certain extent by using an 18-gauge irrigating chopper. Then this author suggested the use of an antichamber collapser, which injects air into the infusion bottle. This pushes more fluid into the eye through the irrigating chopper and also prevents surge. Thus, we were able to use a 20 gauge or 21 gauge irrigating chopper as well as solve the problem of destabilization of the anterior chamber during surgery. Now with microphakonit because of gas forced infusion we are able to remove cataracts with a 0.7 mm irrigating chopper. Subsequently, we used this system in all our co-axial phaco cases to prevent complications like posterior capsular ruptures and corneal damage.

Introduction

Since the introduction of phacoemulsification by Kelman,[1] it has been undergoing revolutionary changes in an attempt to perfect the techniques of extracapsular cataract extraction surgery. Although advantageous in many aspects, this technique is not without its attending complications. A well-maintained anterior chamber without intraocular fluctuations is one of the prerequisites for safe phacoemulsification and phakonit.[2]

When an occluded fragment is held by high vacuum and then abruptly aspirated, fluid rushes into the phaco tip to equilibrate the built-up vacuum in the aspiration line, causing surge.[3] This leads to shallowing or collapse of the anterior chamber (Figure 2-1). Different machines employ a variety of methods to combat surge (Figure 2-2). These include usage of noncompliant tubing,[4] small bore aspiration line tubing,[4] microflow tips,[4] aspiration bypass systems,[4] dual linear foot pedal control,[4] and incorporation of sophisticated microprocessors[4] to sense the anterior chamber pressure fluctuations.

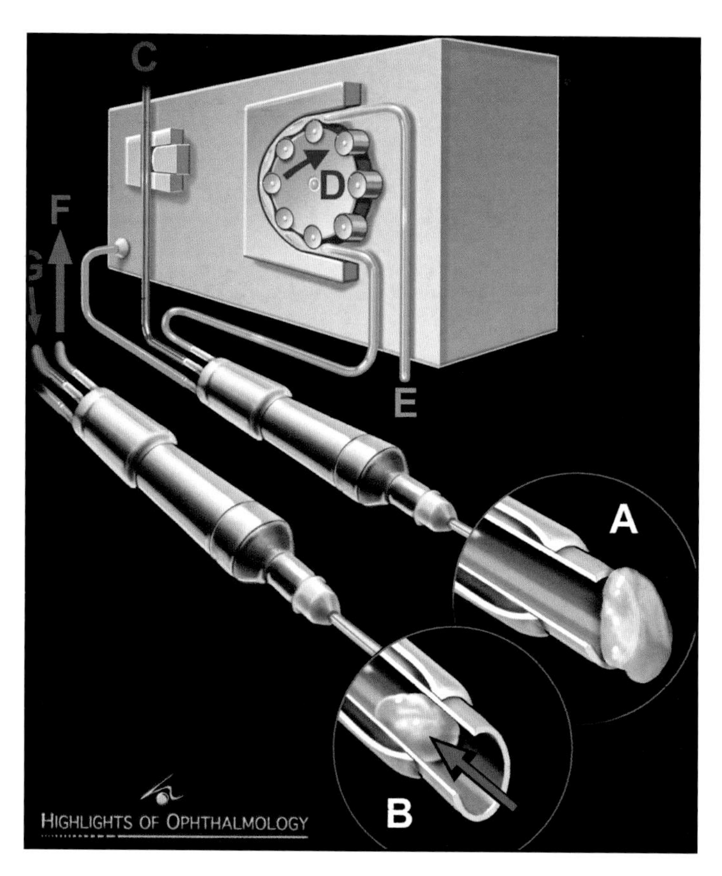

Figure 2-1. Mechanism of the undesirable surge phenomenon. One problem area of the closed phaco system occurs during abrupt dislodging of an occluding piece of lens material so that it no longer occludes the aspiration port of the phaco tip. A sudden drop in intraocular pressure (IOP) occurs as the fluid rate into the eye fails to immediately match the sudden fluid rate out of the eye. This is known as the "surge phenomenon". (A) Shows a piece of lens material occluding the aspiration port of the phaco tip and is held in place by vacuum pressure created by the operating pump (D). Note there is no drainage (E) from the blocked system. Infusion from the irrigating bottle (C) has ceased, but is still providing controlled IOP due to its elevated position above the eye. With sufficient vacuum pressure from the pump and/or emulsification from the ultrasonic energy, the nuclear piece will abruptly enter the aspiration port and the fluid system will once again open (B). Because the plastic infusion/aspiration lines and the eye walls are flexible in absorbing the sudden inflow/outflow pressure differential, there occurs a moment when the infusion fluid (G-small arrow) does not effectively enter the eye fast enough to replace the fluid suddenly moving out of the unblocked system (F-large arrow). Outflow rate from the force of the pump is momentarily greater than the replacing infusion rate. This out of balance system (out of balance in not providing constant IOP) in which the eye momentarily absorbs the inflow/outflow rate differential, may traumatically collapse the eye for a short period. (Courtesy of Benjamin F. Boyd, Ed. *The Art and the Science of Cataract Surgery*. Highlights of Ophthalmology, English Edition, 2001.)

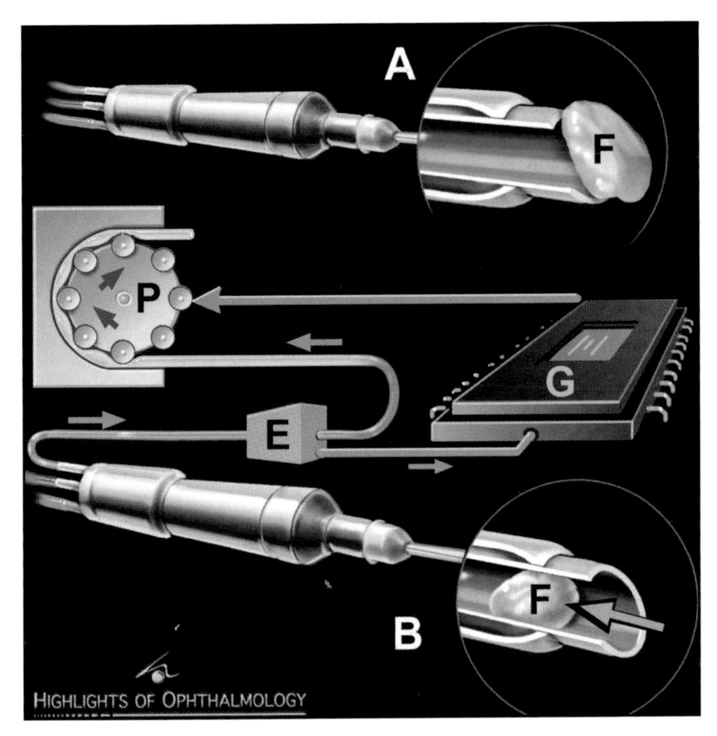

Figure 2-2. Technical solution to prevent the undesirable surge phenomenon. One technical solution for eliminating the surge phenomenon involves the use of a high-tech microprocessor (A). When a nuclear piece (F) occludes the aspiration port and then suddenly (B) is aspirated (F-arrow) by the vacuum pressure of the pump (P), a sensor (E) located on the aspiration line signals a microprocessor (G) in the unit that an abrupt surge in aspiration flow has begun to take place. Within milliseconds, the microprocessor directs the motor of the pump (P) to slow down. The reduction in aspiration rate resulting from the slowed pump occurs before the eye can collapse from any volume differential encountered between sudden inflow and outflow rates. The potentially dangerous surge phenomenon is avoided. This elimination of the surge phenomenon allows the surgeon to safely use higher vacuum rates (necessary in some situations) with a reduction in the need to use potentially damaging high ultrasonic power settings. Surgery becomes safer and faster. (Courtesy of Benjamin F. Boyd, Ed. *The Art and the Science of Cataract Surgery*. Highlights of Ophthalmology, English Edition, 2001.)

The surgeon-dependent variables to counteract surge include good wound construction with minimal leakage,[5] and selection of appropriate machine parameters depending on the stage of the surgery.[5] An anterior chamber maintainer has also been described in literature to prevent surge, but an extra side port makes it an inconvenient procedure.

We herein describe a simple and effective method to prevent anterior chamber collapse during phacoemulsification and phakonit by increasing the velocity of the fluid inflow into the anterior chamber. This is achieved by an automated air pump which pumps atmospheric air through an air filter into the infusion bottle thereby preventing surge. We stumbled upon this idea when we were operating cases with Phakonit[6] where we wanted more fluid entering the eye, but now also use it in all our phaco cases.

Air Pump

Various methods have been used to combat surge during phacoemulsification. We describe a simple device that can be used with any phacoemulsification machine to minimize surge during phacoemulsification. An automated air pump is used to push air into the infusion bottle, thus increasing the pressure with which the fluid flows into the eye. This increases the steady-state pressure of the eye, making the anterior chamber deep and well maintained during the entire procedure. It makes phakonit and phacoemulsification a relatively safe procedure by reducing surge even at high vacuum levels.

Technique

A locally manufactured automated device, used in aquariums to supply oxygen, is utilized to forcefully pump air into the irrigation bottle. This pump is easily available in aquarium shops. It has an electromagnetic motor that moves a lever attached to a collapsible rubber cap. There is an inlet with a valve that sucks in atmospheric air as the cap expands. On collapsing, the valve closes and the air is pushed into an intravenous (IV) line connected to the infusion bottle (Figure 2-3). The lever vibrates at a frequency of approximately 10 oscillations per second. The electromagnetic motor is weak enough to stop once the pressure in the closed system (ie, the anterior chamber) reaches about 50 mm of Hg. The rubber cap ceases to expand at this pressure level. A micropore air filter is used between the air pump and the infusion bottle so that the air pumped into the bottle is clean of particulate matter.

Method

1. First, the BSS bottle is placed in the IV stand.
2. Now an air pump (as described above) is plugged into the electrical connection.
3. An IV set now connects the air pump to the infusion bottle. The tubing passes from the air pump and the end of the tubing is passed into the infusion bottle.
4. When the air pump is switched on, it pumps air into the infusion bottle. This air goes to the top of the bottle and because of the pressure, it pumps the fluid down with greater force. The fluid now flows from the infusion bottle to reach the phaco handpiece or irrigating chopper. The amount of fluid now coming out of the handpiece is much more than what would normally come out and with more force (Figures 2-4 and 2-5).
5. An air filter is connected between the air pump and the infusion bottle so that the air being pumped into the bottle is sterile.
6. This extra amount of fluid coming out compensates for the surge that would otherwise occur.

Continuous Infusion

Before we enter the eye, we fill the eye with viscoelastic. Once the tip of the phaco handpiece in phaco or irrigating chopper in phakonit is inside the anterior chamber, we shift to continuous irrigation. This is very helpful, especially for surgeons who are starting phaco or phakonit. This way, the surgeon never comes to position zero and the anterior chamber never collapses. Even for excellent surgeons this helps a lot.

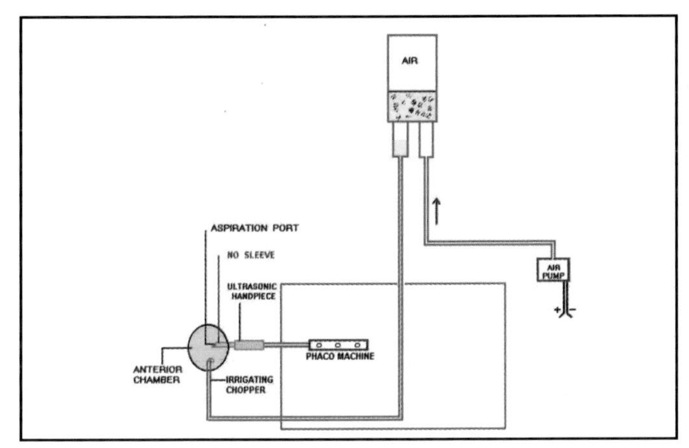

Figure 2-3. Diagrammatic representation of the connection of the air pump to the infusion bottle.

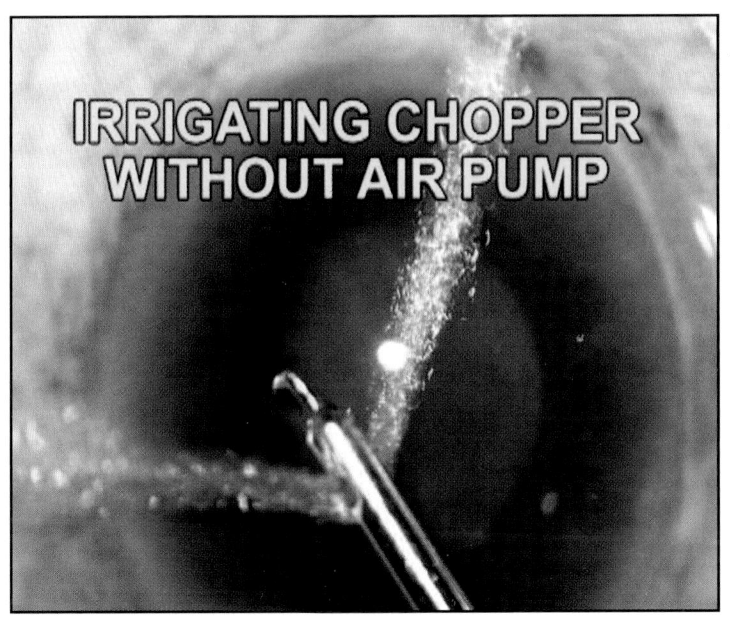

Figure 2-4. Flow of fluid through the irrigating chopper without an air pump.

ADVANTAGES

1. With the air pump, the posterior capsule is pushed back and there is a deep anterior chamber.
2. The phenomenon of surge is neutralized. This prevents the unnecessary posterior capsular rupture.
3. Striate keratitis postoperatively is reduced, as there is a deep anterior chamber.
4. One can operate hard cataracts (Figure 2-6) quite comfortably, as striate keratitis does not occur postoperatively.
5. The surgical time is shorter as one can emulsify the nuclear pieces much faster because surge does not occur.
6. One can easily operate with the Phakonit technique as quite a lot of fluid now passes into the eye. Thus, the cataract can be removed through a smaller opening.
7. It is quite comfortable to do cases under topical or no anesthesia.

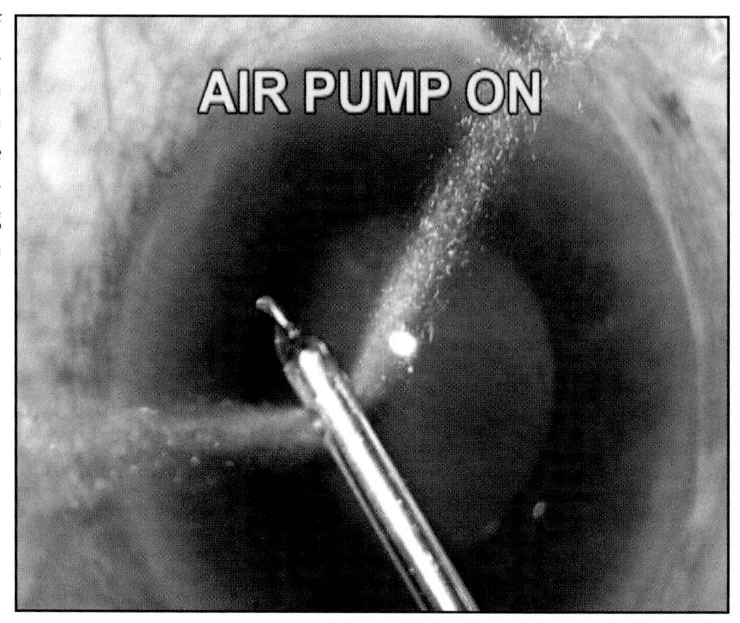

Figure 2-5. Flow of fluid through the irrigating chopper with an air pump. Note when the air pump is on, the amount of fluid coming out of the irrigating chopper is much greater.

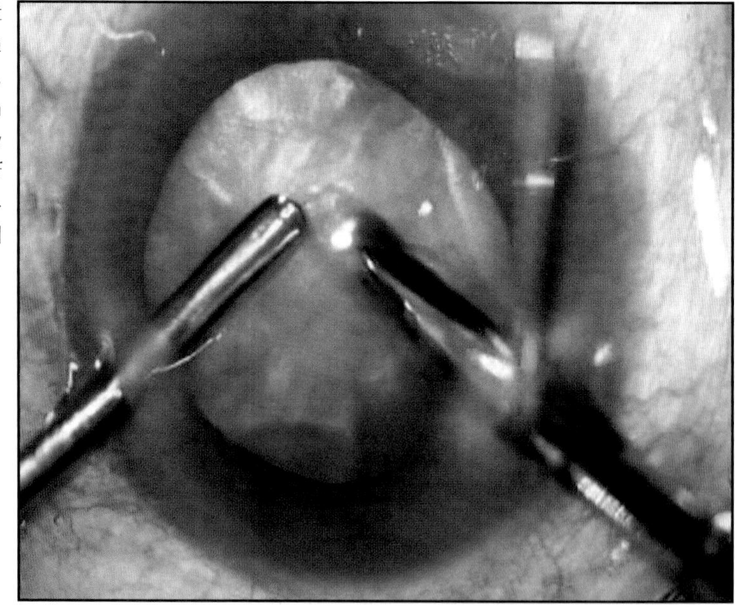

Figure 2-6. Phakonit being performed in a mature brown cataract. Such difficult cases can be operated upon by phakonit because of the air pump. It deepens the chamber and prevents any surge.

Topical or No Anesthesia Cataract Surgery

When one operates under topical or no anesthesia, the main problem is that the pressure is high, especially if the patient squeezes the eye. In such cases, the posterior capsule comes up anteriorly and one can produce a posterior capsular rupture. To solve this problem, surgeons tend to work more anteriorly, performing supracapsular phacoemulsification/phakonit. The disadvantage of this is that striate keratitis tends to occur.

With the air pump, this problem does not occur. When we use the air pump, the posterior capsule is quite far back, as if we are operating a patient under a block. In other words, there is a lot of space between the posterior capsule and the cornea, preventing striate keratitis and inadvertent posterior capsular rupture.

Internal Gas-Forced Infusion

This was started by Arturo Pérez-Arteaga from Mexico. The anterior vented gas-forced infusion system (AVGFI) of the Accurus surgical system is used.

This is a system incorporated in the Accurus machine that creates a positive infusion pressure inside the eye; it was designed by the Alcon engineers to control the IOP during anterior and posterior segment surgery. It consists of an air pump and a regulator inside the machine. The air is pushed inside the bottle of intraocular solution, and so the fluid is actively pushed inside the eye without raising or lowering the bottle. The control of the air pump is digitally integrated in the Accurus panel; it also can be controlled via the remote. The footswitch can be preset with the minimum and maximum of desired fluid inside the eye so that the surgeon can go directly to this value with the simple touch of the footswitch. Pérez-Arteaga recommends presetting the infusion pump at 100 to 110 mmHg to perform a phakonit. This parameter is preset in the panel and also as the minimum irrigation force in the footswitch; then he recommends presetting the maximum irrigation force at 130 to 140 mmHg in the foot pedal, so if a surge exists during the procedure, the surgeon can increase the irrigation force by touching the footswitch to the right. With the AVGFI, the surgeon has the capability to increase these values even more.

Discussion

Surge is defined as the volume of the fluid forced out of the eye into the aspiration line at the instant of occlusion break. When the phacoemulsification handpiece tip is occluded, flow is interrupted and vacuum builds up to its preset values. Additionally, the aspiration tubing may collapse in the presence of high vacuum levels. Emulsification of the occluding fragment clears the block and the fluid rushes into the aspiration line to neutralize the pressure difference created between the positive pressure in the anterior chamber and the negative pressure in the aspiration tubing. In addition, if the aspiration line tubing is not reinforced to prevent collapse (tubing compliance), the tubing, constricted during occlusion, then expands on occlusion break. These factors cause a rush of fluid from the anterior chamber into the phaco probe. The fluid in the anterior chamber is not replaced rapidly enough to prevent shallowing of the anterior chamber.

The maintenance of steady-state IOP[2] during the entire procedure depends on the equilibrium between the fluid inflow and outflow. The steady-state pressure level is the mean pressure equilibrium between inflow and outflow volumes. In most phacoemulsification machines, fluid inflow is provided by gravitational flow of the fluid from the balanced salt solution (BSS) bottle through the tubing to the anterior chamber. This is determined by the bottle height relative to the patient's eye, the diameter of the tubing, and most importantly by the outflow of fluid from the eye through the aspiration tube and leakage from the wounds.[2]

The inflow volume can be increased by either increasing the bottle height or by enlarging the diameter of the inflow tube. The IOP increases by 10 mmHg for every 15 cm increase in bottle height above the eye.[5]

High steady-state IOPs increase phaco safety by raising the mean IOP level up and away from zero, ie, by delaying surge-related anterior chamber collapse.[2]

Air pump increases the amount of fluid inflow thus making the steady-state IOP high. This deepens the anterior chamber, increasing the surgical space available for maneuvering and thus prevents complications like posterior capsular tears and corneal endothelial damage. The phenomenon of surge is neutralized by rapid inflow of fluid at the time of occlusion break. The recovery to steady-state IOP is so prompt that no surge occurs and this enables the surgeon to remain in foot position 3 through the occlusion break. High vacuum phacoemulsification/phakonit can be safely performed in hard brown cataracts using an air pump. Phacoemulsification or phakonit under topical or no anesthesia[6,7] can be safely done, neutralizing the positive vitreous pressure that occurs due to squeezing of the eyelids.

Summary

The air pump is a new device that helps to prevent surge. This prevents posterior capsular rupture, helps deepen the anterior chamber, and makes phacoemulsification and phakonit safe procedures even in hard cataracts.

Key Points

1. The air pump is a simple and effective method to prevent anterior chamber collapse during phacoemulsification and bimanual phaco/phakonit by increasing the velocity of the fluid inflow into the anterior chamber.
2. This is achieved by an automated air pump that pumps atmospheric air through an air filter into the infusion bottle, thereby preventing surge.
3. A micropore air filter is used between the air pump and the infusion bottle so that the air pumped into the bottle is clean of particulate matter.
4. Surge is defined as the volume of the fluid forced out of the eye into the aspiration line at the instant of occlusion break.
5. The air pump helps to prevent surge. This prevents posterior capsular rupture, helps deepen the anterior chamber, and makes phacoemulsification and phakonit safe procedures even in hard cataracts.
6. The main advantage of gas-forced internal infusion is that the surgeon can use the same machine and avoid the use of an external air pump. The main disadvantage is that not all phaco machines contain an air pump.

References

1. Kelman CD. Phacoemulsification and aspiration: a new technique of cataract removal. A preliminary report. *Am J Ophthalmol.* 1967;64:23–25.
2. Wilbrandt RH. Comparative analysis of the fluidics of the AMO Prestige, Alcon Legacy, and Storz Premiere phacoemulsification systems. *J Cataract Refract Surg.* 1997;23:766–780.
3. Seibel B. *Phacodynamics: Mastering the Tools and Techniques of Phacoemulsification Surgery.* 4th ed. Thorofare, NJ: SLACK Incorporated; 2004.
4. Fishkind WJ. The Phaco Machine: How and why it acts and reacts? In: *Agarwal's Textbook of Ophthalmology.* Jaypee Brothers: New Delhi; 2000.

5. Seibel B. The fluidics and physics of phaco. In: Agarwal S, Agarwal A, Sachdev M, et al, eds. *Phacoemulsification, Laser Cataract Surgery and Foldable IOLs*. 2nd ed. Jaypee Brothers: New Delhi; 2000: 45–54.
6. Agarwal A, Agarwal A, Agarwal S. Phakonit and laser phakonit. In: Agarwal S, Agarwal A, Sachdev M, et al, eds. *Phacoemulsification, Laser Cataract Surgery and Foldable IOLs*. 2nd ed. Jaypee Brothers: New Delhi; 2000; 204–216.
7. Agarwal A. No anaesthesia cataract surgery with karate chop. In: Agarwal S, Agarwal A, Sachdev M, et al, eds. *Phacoemulsification, Laser Cataract Surgery and Foldable IOLs*. 2nd ed. Jaypee Brothers: New Delhi; 2000: 217–226.

Chapter 3

Mastering the Transition to Phacoemulsification: Avoiding Nightmares

Samuel Boyd, MD; Benjamin F. Boyd, MD, FACS; Cristela F. Aleman, MD

Introduction

The transition from planned extracapsular extraction to phacoemulsification fundamentally refers to the gradual change that the ophthalmic surgeon who already masters the planned extracapsular must undertake in order to dominate the new technique of phaco, which is equipment-dependent. This transition should be progressive and atraumatic. This learning curve is achieved with effort, dedication, and proper training to perform each phase of the transition well.

Surgical Techniques in the Transition

Anesthesia

During the transition, it is advisable that the surgeon utilize the type of anesthesia with which he feels more safe and in better control. It is unnecessary to add a new source of stress or immediate change at this stage of the procedure. Nevertheless, when the surgeon is in charge of the situation and masters the phaco technique, it is ideal to use topical anesthesia because of its ability to provide immediate visual recovery.

Role of the Ancillary Incision

This is an important step. Although there are techniques to perform it with only one hand, phaco is fundamentally a two-handed procedure. The ancillary incision is made before the main incision is performed. This incision serves as an entry for a second instrument, which is necessary for maneuvers to remove the nucleus. At the end of surgery, the ancillary incision also serves to inject fluid into anterior chamber to test for leaks in the wound.

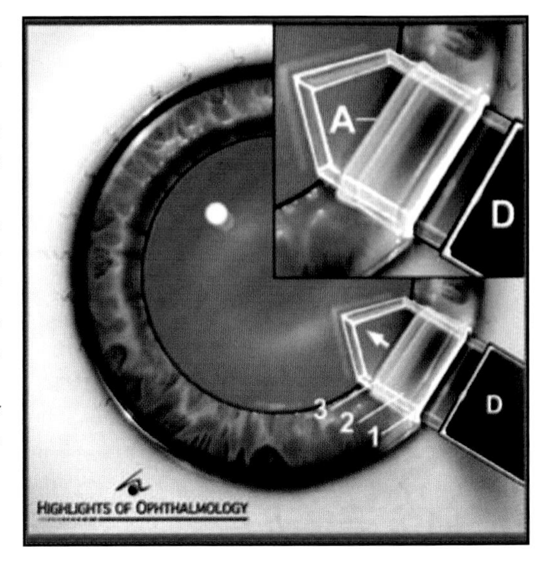

Figure 3-1. Final step of self-sealing, stepped, valvulated tunnel incision at the limbus performed with the diamond knife—surgeon's view. A diamond knife blade (D) enters the first incision (1), the second tunnel incision (2), and is then directed slightly oblique to the iris plane and advanced (arrow) into the anterior chamber. This forms the internal aspect of the incision into the chamber (A). This is the third step (3) in the three-step self-sealing incision. (Courtesy of Benjamin F. Boyd, Ed. *The Art and the Science of Cataract Surgery*. Highlights of Ophthalmology, English Edition, 2001.)

The Main Incision

During the early stages of the transition, the surgeon should plan to start the operation as a phaco but learn how to convert to the planned extracapsular he or she is accustomed to doing successfully if this becomes necessary. This will provide additional comfort and confidence. The surgeon may start with a small stepped limbal valvulated incision slightly larger than the phaco tip (Figure 3-1), even though he knows that he plans to convert to his usual planned extracapsular. It is not advisable to start the transition with a corneal incision because, upon enlarging it, the resulting astigmatism may be severe. The more anteriorly located the incision, the more astigmatism the patient may end up with. By starting the transition with a limbal incision, the surgeon will use the same area for the incision that he is accustomed to use in his planned extracapsular but will make the incision valvulated (stepped) and smaller than the usual extracapsular. The surgeon must master the technique of the small incision valve like incision at the limbus, so that it can be part of his armamentarium in the future. Once the surgeon is certain that he will not need to convert from phaco to planned extracapsular and therefore will not need to enlarge the incision, he may choose to make a corneal incision if he wishes, but not before. This is what we refer to as a safe transition from a large to a small incision, a transition that must be undertaken step by step as the surgeon progresses in his learning curve. Later, as he learns to master phacoemulsification, the surgeon is ready to make two significant changes in the technique: 1) operate from an oblique position and make the incision temporally, and 2) perform a corneal incision instead of a limbal incision.

Anterior Capsulorrhexis

This is a vital step in the transition. Changing from the can opener capsulotomy to the anterior continuous circular capsulorrhexis (CCC) is one of the fundamental steps in the transition (Figures 3-2, 3-3, and 3-4). The surgeon must learn first by practicing capsulorrhexis on the skin of a grape or by using a very thin sheet of plastic wrap such as the one that covers some chocolate candies. Once the surgeon understands the concept of the technique and can do it in the laboratory, he or she may begin to use it for the patient.

It is highly recommended to make the capsulorrhexis under sufficient viscoelastic. The latter should be injected into the anterior chamber before trying the capsulorrhexis. It

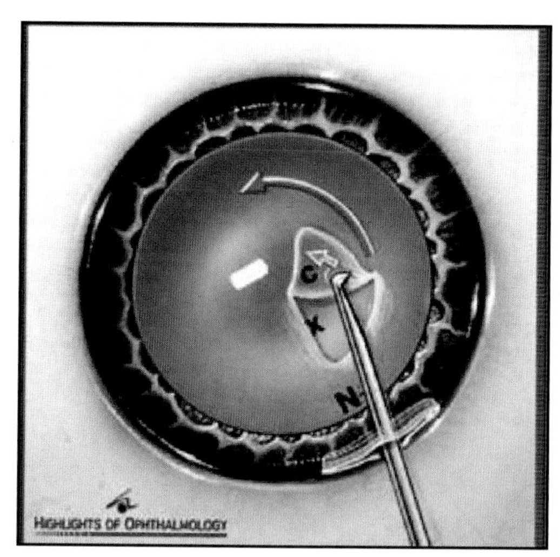

Figure 3-2. Continuous curvilinear anterior capsulorrhexis with cystitome—step 1. Anterior capsulorrhexis is one of the steps of phacoemulsification that is practically the same both for the surgeon beginning the transition or for the more advanced surgeon, with the exception that some advanced surgeons prefer to do a smaller capsulorrhexis. The technique shown here is the initial step performed with the cystitome needle. In the transition, it should be continued with forceps. With an irrigating cystitome, the center of the anterior capsule is punctured, creating a horizontal V-shaped tear. The tear is extended toward the periphery and continued circumferentially in the direction of the arrow. (Courtesy of Benjamin F. Boyd, Ed. *The Art and the Science of Cataract Surgery.* Highlights of Ophthalmology, English Edition, 2001.)

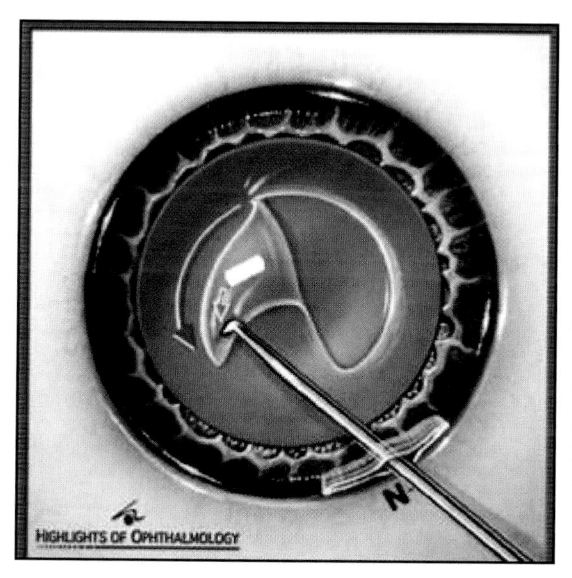

Figure 3-3. Continuous curvilinear anterior capsulorrhexis with forceps—step 2. After the initial tear of the anterior capsule is made with an irrigating cystitome in the center of the anterior capsule, the tear is extended toward the periphery in a circular direction, this time utilizing a forceps as shown in this figure. The tear is extended toward the periphery and continues circumferentially in a continuous manner for the remaining 180 degrees, as initially described by Gimbel. (Courtesy of Benjamin F. Boyd, Ed. *The Art and the Science of Cataract Surgery.* Highlights of Ophthalmology, English Edition, 2001.)

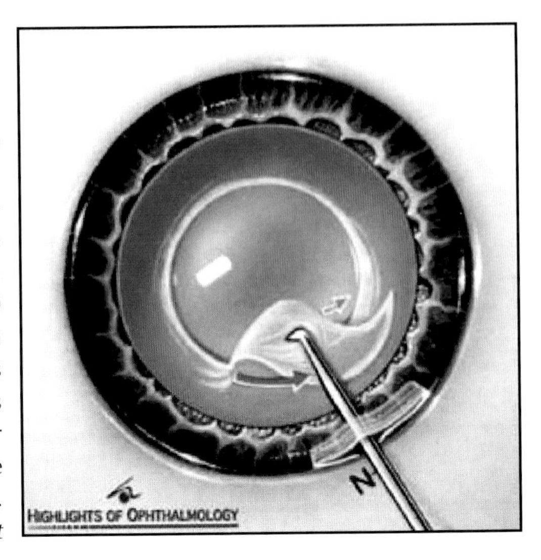

Figure 3-4. Continuous curvilinear anterior capsulorrhexis with forceps—step 3. The flap of the capsule is flipped over on itself. The forceps engage the underside of the capsule. The tear is continued toward its radial segment. In the transition, beginning surgeons are encouraged to use forceps in order to perform the CCC. Viscoelastic is essential in this maneuver. The correct size of the CCC is 5.5 mm to 6.0 mm. For the early steps of the transition, when the surgeon may have to convert to ECCE, it is important to perform two relaxing incisions radially at 10 and 2 o'clock in the anterior capsule in order to facilitate the removal of the complete nucleus in an ECCE if necessary. (Courtesy of Benjamin F. Boyd, Ed. *The Art and the Science of Cataract Surgery*. Highlights of Ophthalmology, English Edition, 2001.)

is also fundamental not to begin with dense, hard cataracts where it is difficult to see the edge of the capsulorrhexis. It is prudent to try performing this procedure over and over again in cataracts that are less dense until the surgeon is able to perform them in eyes with poor visualization of the edge of the capsule.[1] A better method is to use trypan blue in all cases, which helps the surgeon visualize the rhexis clearly.

Because the surgeon, in the initial stages that we are discussing here, will most probably need to convert to extracapsular extraction (ECCE), it is important that he perform two relaxing incisions radially in the anterior capsule at 10 and 12 o'clock following the CCC in order to facilitate the removal of the complete nucleus with a planned manual extracapsular extraction. If these relaxing incisions in the anterior capsule are not done, the surgeon may confront serious problems in removing the nucleus.

Staining of the Anterior Capsule

Over the red reflex observed through the microscope, the anterior capsule and the border of the progressively performed CCC can be very well visualized. This allows the completion of the circle under adequate visual control. On the other hand, when the surgeon is dealing with white, hypermature cataracts that have either been allowed to get into that advanced stage or have been produced by trauma, the details and border of the CCC cannot be well visualized because this white cataract interferes with fundus reflex. Consequently, the step by step progress in the performance of the CCC is not well visualized.

These important considerations have led to the development of a very effective technique to control the performance of the CCC in white cataracts. It involves staining the anterior capsule of the lens in order to adequately visualize the details during the performance of the CCC (Figure 3-5). Without the dye, it is nearly impossible to see the anterior capsule. These cataracts are risky. It is very difficult to distinguish the anterior capsule from the underlying cortex. This technique should be useful even when the surgeon is in the capsulorrhexis learning process, no matter the density of the cataract.

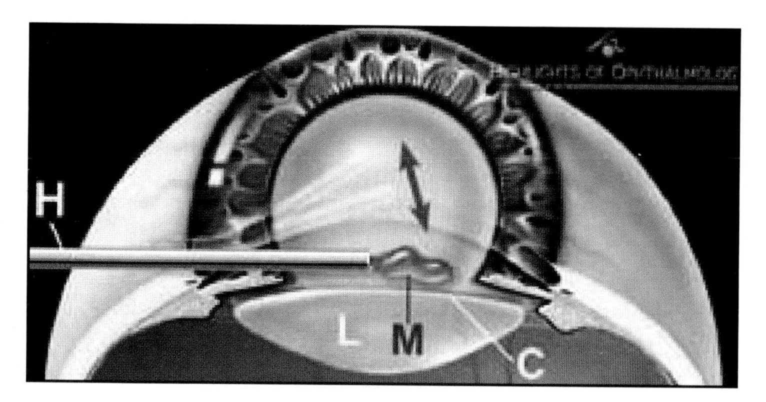

Figure 3-5. Staining the anterior capsule in dense cataracts to perform adequate CCC. White cataracts (L) present a problem because the red reflex is not present, making the capsulorrhexis quite difficult and risky. A viscoelastic is first injected into the anterior chamber, immediately followed by the injection of a bubble of air that partially displaces the viscoelastic from the anterior chamber. This leaves the corneal endothelium lubricated with the viscoelastic. A hydrodissection cannula (H) is introduced through the corneal incision over the anterior capsule (C) filled with a few drops of Trypan blue to be instilled over the anterior capsule. (Courtesy of Benjamin F. Boyd, Ed. *The Art and the Science of Cataract Surgery*. Highlights of Ophthalmology, English Edition, 2001.)

Hydrodissection

Once the surgeon is able to perform a CCC without problems, he is ready to go into the next step, which is hydrodissection (Figure 3-6). This step should not be undertaken before mastering the capsulorrhexis[2] because tears in the anterior capsule may extend towards the equator when performing the injection with fluid to do the hydrodissection. With this maneuver, by using waves of liquid, we try to separate the anterior and posterior capsules from the cortex and the nucleus from the epinucleus.[3] When this is achieved, the nucleus is liberated so that it will be free for the ensuing maneuvers of rotation, fracture, and emulsification. As long as the surgeon is not sure that the nucleus has been freed of its attachments through the hydrodissection and will rotate easily, he should not try to rotate it mechanically because this may lead to rupture of the zonules.[4] Also, if the nucleus is not separated from the cortex by hydrodissection (Figure 3-7), the surgeon should not proceed to apply the phaco ultrasound to the nucleus because he or she may well meet with complications by extending the effects of ultrasound not only to the nucleus but peripherally to the cortex. This can lead to the feared rupture of the posterior capsule. Instead, the surgeon should decide to convert to a ECCE.

The Mechanics of the Phaco Machine

Optimal Use of the Phaco Machine

Several surgeons and teachers describe the three main functions of the phaco machine: 1) irrigation, 2) aspiration, and 3) emulsification of the nucleus fragments (Figure 3-8). Irrigation is done with the irrigation bottle, aspiration with the aspiration pump, and emulsification with ultrasonic energy through the titanium needle present in the phaco tip of the

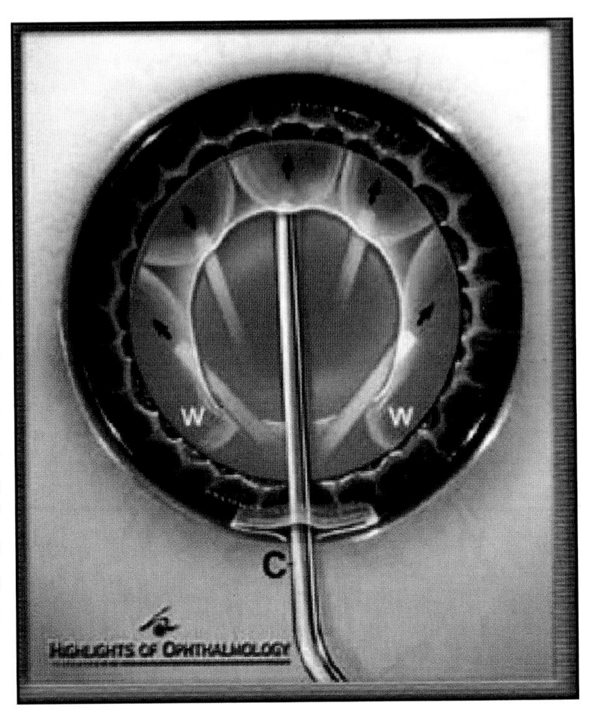

Figure 3-6. Hydrodissection of the lens capsule from the cortex during phacoemulsification—surgeon's view. Following circular curvilinear anterior capsulorrhexis, a cannula (C) is inserted into the anterior chamber. The cannula tip is placed between the anterior capsule and the lens cortex at the various locations shown in the ghost views. BSS is injected at these locations (arrows) to separate the capsule from the cortex. The resultant fluid waves (W) can be seen against the red reflex. These waves continue posteriorly to separate the posterior capsule from the cortex. (Courtesy of Benjamin F. Boyd, Ed. *The Art and the Science of Cataract Surgery*. Highlights of Ophthalmology, English Edition, 2001.)

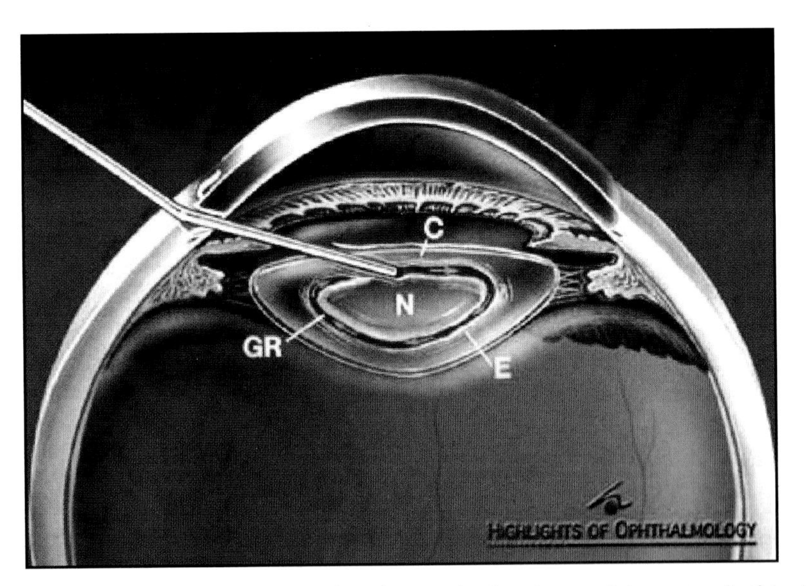

Figure 3-7. Hydrodissection—separation of nucleus and epinucleus and the cortex. In this stage, the cannula is advanced beneath the cortex (C) and the infusion with BSS is started in order to separate the nucleus (N) from the epinucleus (E). The pink arrows between these two structures, nucleus (N) and epinucleus (E), show the flow of fluid. The gold "ring" of fluid separating the nucleus from the epinucleus is identified as GR. (Courtesy of Benjamin F. Boyd, Ed. *The Art and the Science of Cataract Surgery*. Highlights of Ophthalmology, English Edition, 2001.)

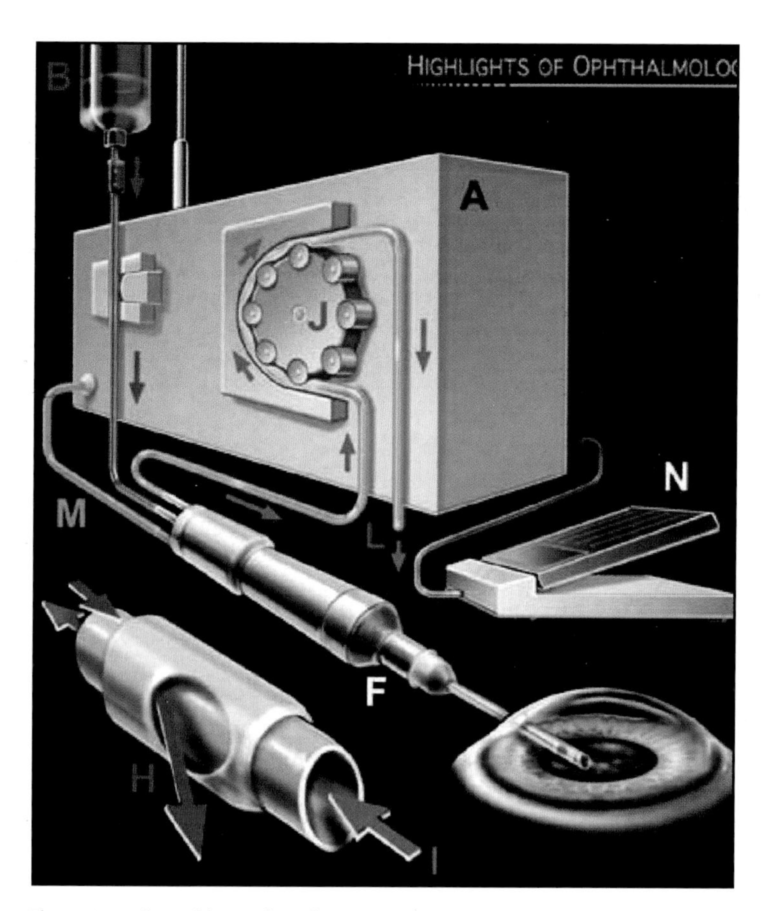

Figure 3-8. The principles of how the phaco machine works. This conceptual view shows the three main elements of most phaco systems. 1) The **irrigation** (red): IOP is maintained and irrigation is provided by the bottle of BSS (B) connected via tubing to the phaco handpiece (F). It is controlled by the surgeon. Irrigation enters the eye via an infusion port (H) located on the outer sleeve of the bi-tube phaco probe. Height of the bottle above the eye is used to control the inflow pressure. (2) **Aspiration** (blue): (I) enters through the tip of the phaco probe, passes within the inner tube of the probe, travels through the aspiration tubing and is controlled by the surgeon by way of a variable speed pump (J). The peristaltic type pump is basically a motorized wheel exerting rotating external pressure on a portion of the flexible aspiration line that physically forces fluid through the tubing. Varying the speed of the rotating pump controls rate of aspiration. Aspirated fluid passes to a drain (L). (3) **Ultrasonic energy** (green) is provided to the probe tip via a connection (M) to the unit. All three of these main phaco functions are under control of the surgeon by way of a multi-control foot pedal (N). (Courtesy of Benjamin F. Boyd, Ed. *The Art and the Science of Cataract Surgery*. Highlights of Ophthalmology, English Edition, 2001.)

handpiece. Many types of phaco tip shapes have been created to more efficiently handle nuclear extraction. A command pedal, which is controlled by the surgeon's foot, guides the machine into the following four positions: 0 (zero) is at rest; position 1 for irrigation, position 2 for irrigation–aspiration, and position 3 for irrigation, aspiration, and emulsification (Figure 3-9).

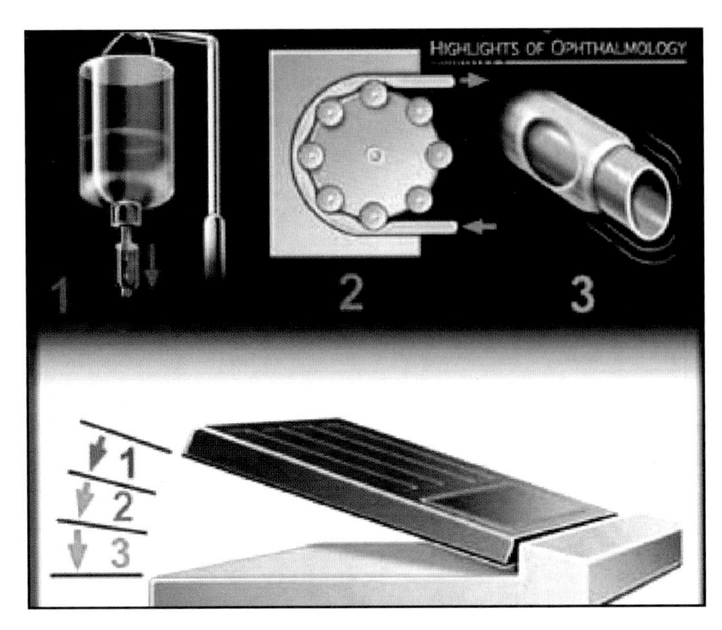

Figure 3-9. Basic phaco foot pedal functions. The foot pedal controls inflow, outflow, and ultrasonic rates. With the foot pedal in the undepressed position, the inflow valve is closed, the outflow pump is stationary, and there is no ultrasonic energy being delivered to the phaco tip. With initial depression of the pedal (1), the **irrigation** line from the raised infusion bottle is opened. Further depression of the pedal (2), starts and gradually increases the flow rate of the **aspiration** pump to a maximum amount preset by the surgeon. Further depression of the pedal (3) turns on increasing **ultrasonic power** to the phaco tip for lens fragmentation. (Courtesy of Benjamin F. Boyd, Ed. *The Art and the Science of Cataract Surgery*. Highlights of Ophthalmology, English Edition, 2001.)

The first function (irrigation), controlled by the foot pedal, is provided by a bottle with BSS. The liquid flows by gravity. The amount of liquid that reaches the anterior chamber depends on the height of the bottle, the diameter of the tubing, and the pressure already existing in the anterior chamber. The flow rate into the eye is determined by the balance of the pressure in the tubing—regulated by the height of the bottle, and the back pressure in the anterior chamber. When the two are equal, there is no flow. If there is leakage or aspiration of fluid from the anterior chamber, the pressure there drops, and fluid in the tubing flows in to restore the pressure in the anterior chamber, and indirectly, the volume. The tubing is purposely made wide enough so that it impedes the flow of the BSS only slightly under normal rates of flow. It does limit maximum flow, eg, during anterior chamber collapse.

The second function, aspiration, is provided by a pump, which creates a difference in pressure between the aspiration line and the anterior chamber. The pump may be a peristaltic pump, a Venturi pump, a diaphragm pump, a rotary vane pump, or a scroll pump. The peristaltic pump has become the most widely known and used. Many feel it is safer. Just like inflow, a base level of suction occurs whenever the pump is activated, depending on how hard the pump is working. When there is occlusion of the tip with the foot pedal in the aspiration position (position 2), the pump will continue to pump and create more and more suction until the material provoking the occlusion is aspirated, or until the suction in the tubing reaches the maximum that the surgeon has preset on the control

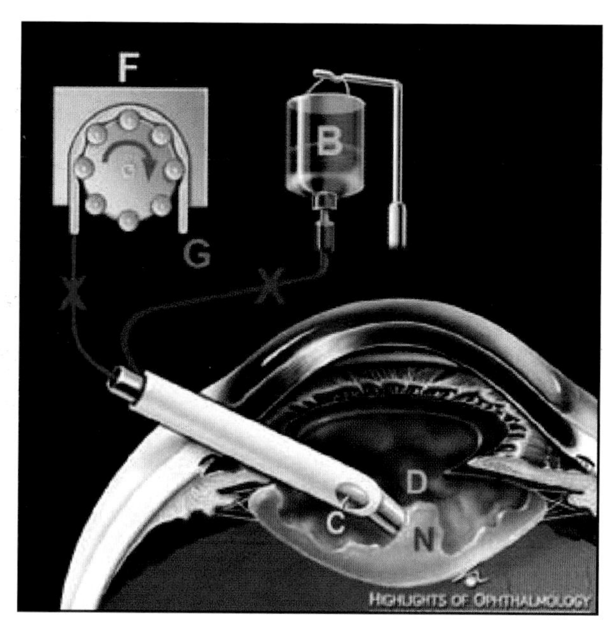

Figure 3-10. Fluid dynamics— balance of inflow and outflow during phacoemulsification—tip occluded with lens material—hydrostatic closed system. When the tip of the phacoemulsification probe is occluded with nuclear material, the vacuum pressure rises to a level to which the machine is set (table—arrow—1), and the inflow and outflow rates go down. With the aspiration port occluded, no fluid can enter or exit the eye. (Courtesy of Benjamin F. Boyd, Ed. *The Art and the Science of Cataract Surgery.* Highlights of Ophthalmology, English Edition, 2001.)

panel (Figure 3-10). This latency period before reaching maximum suction level provides a greater security margin, allowing the surgeon to take immediate action in case the tip grasps (and sucks in) the iris or the posterior capsule instead of grasping the lens mass. The reason for limiting the maximum suction pressure is to limit the rush of fluid out of the eye the moment the fragment that occluded the tip is aspirated. This provides the surgeon the opportunity to stop aspiration and avoid collapse of the anterior chamber.

The third function of the phaco machine—the production of ultrasonic vibrations leading to emulsification of the lens—is carried out by a crystal transducer located in the handpiece, which transforms high frequency electrical energy into high (ultrasonic) frequency mechanical energy. The crystal drives the titanium tip of the phaco unit to oscillate in its anterior-posterior axis. It is precisely the anteroposterior oscillation of the phaco tip which produces the emulsification (Figure 3-11).

Parameters of the Phaco Machine

These parameters need to be set and reset depending on the type of cataract—soft, medium-hard, hard; the stage of the operation; and also, importantly, the various situations that the surgeon must solve.[5] These parameters are:

1. The amount of ultrasonic energy applied to the nuclear material for its emulsification. It is expressed as a percentage of the phaco machine's available power and it determines the turbulence that is generated in the anterior chamber during surgery. It is ideal to use the least amount of power possible during the operation. This is achieved by combining other functions of the machine and maneuvers within the nucleus to facilitate fracture and emulsification of the lens. The use of excess phaco energy may result in damage to structures beyond the nucleus, such as the posterior capsule and the endothelium.
2. The aspiration flow rate. This measures the amount of liquid aspirated from the anterior chamber per unit of time. In practical terms, this determines the speed with which the lens material is sucked into the phaco tip. This is synonymous with

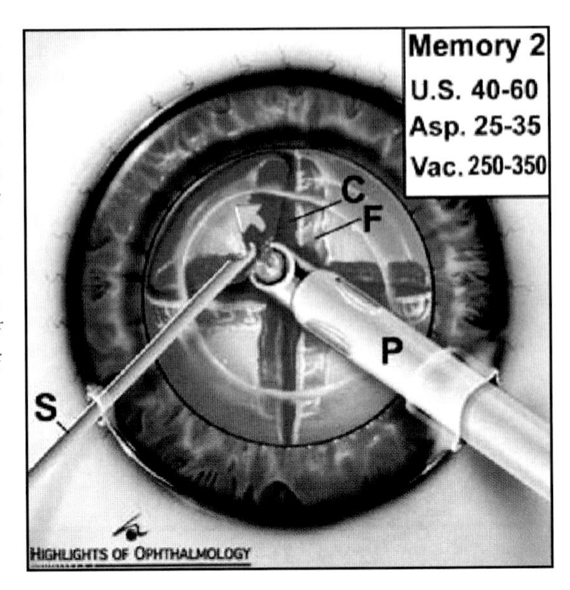

Figure 3-11. Emulsification of lens fragments. This surgeon's view shows the management of the lens quadrants. The apex of each of the four loose quadrants is lifted, the ultrasound phaco tip is embedded into the posterior edge of each, and by means of aspiration the surgeon centralizes each quadrant for emulsification. (Courtesy of Benjamin F. Boyd, Ed. *The Art and the Science of Cataract Surgery*. Highlights of Ophthalmology, English Edition, 2001.)

the power of "attraction" or suction of the lens fragments into the irrigation-aspiration handpiece. High maximum flow rates may result in collapse of the anterior chamber if the irrigation cannot keep up.

3. The third parameter measures the vacuum or negative pressure created in the aspiration line and actually determines the force with which the material is fixated onto the orifice in the phaco tip. This is known as fixation power or grasp and depends on the aspiration force. The higher the aspiration pressure, the more rapid the aspiration flow, and the less time it takes to obtain the maximum vacuum power. If the occlusion at the tip is broken or interrupted due to the negative pressure in the aspiration line, fluid is rapidly sucked out of the eye. This may lead to collapse of the anterior chamber with risk of damage to the corneal endothelium as well as the posterior capsule. This is known as the "surge phenomenon" (Figure 3-12).

Fluid Dynamics During Phaco

Michael Blumenthal, MD, has made profound studies on this most important subject.[6] Its understanding really makes a difference between success and failure in small incision cataract surgery, particularly in phacoemulsification. There are two factors specifically involved: 1) the amount of inflow and 2) the amount of outflow during any given period of the surgery. Fluid dynamics are responsible for the following intraocular conditions during surgery: a) fluctuation in the anterior chamber depth; b) turbulence; c) IOP.[7]

Fluctuation in the anterior chamber depth is the consequence of the following conditions: the amount of outflow exceeds the amount of inflow in a given period. As a result, the anterior chamber is reduced in depth or collapses. When the amount of outflow is reduced below the amount of inflow, the anterior chamber depth is recovered. This phenomenon, when repeating itself, increases fluctuation. When fluctuation occurs abruptly, as in the sudden release of blockage of the phaco tip in aspiration, this is called "surge". The new machines are equipped with special sensors that prevent the possibility of this unpleasant event.

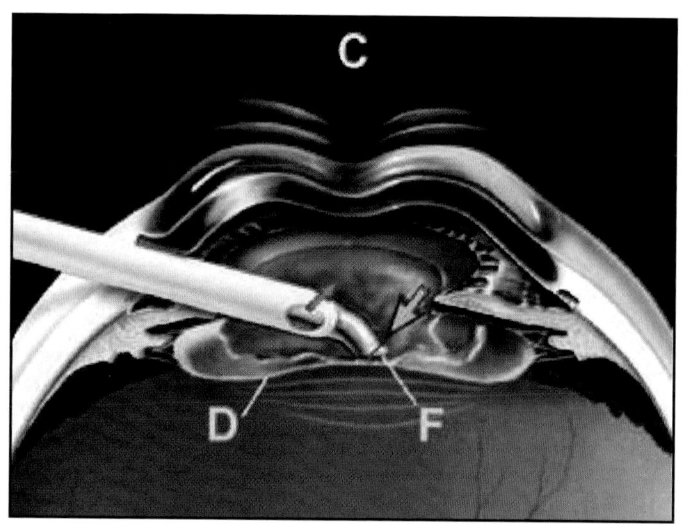

Figure 3-12. Physical problems caused by surge. During the surge phenomenon when a nuclear piece (F) is abruptly aspirated from the eye, the anterior chamber may collapse due to a sudden loss of intraocular fluid. The cornea (C) may cave in, resulting in possible endothelial cell damage if it comes near the phaco probe. The posterior capsule (D) may also be damaged from anterior displacement toward the instrument. The fluid outflow rate must be brought under control, and the inflow rate (small red arrow) and outflow rate (large blue arrow) are again equalized with the eye repressurized, to reestablish a balanced system with a constant and controlled IOP. (Courtesy of Benjamin F. Boyd, Ed. *The Art and the Science of Cataract Surgery*. Highlights of Ophthalmology, English Edition, 2001.)

Nucleus Removal and Application of Phaco

Fracture and Emulsification

This is really when the surgeon begins to utilize the ultrasound energy in the phaco machine and apply it within the patient's eye. During the transition period, this is a step that should be preceded by a good number of hours of practice in the experimental laboratory until the surgeon is confident in the application of the ultrasound energy. It implies that he or she has been able to successfully perform all the previous steps over and over again in different patients. This experience will serve the surgeon as the requisite basis for success in the emulsification and removal of the nucleus in the present patient.[8]

In removing the nucleus, the surgeon first attempts to divide the nucleus by fragmenting it into smaller portions that in due time will then be emulsified individually (Figure 3-13). If the fracture or division of the nucleus has been incomplete and has resulted in large pieces or incomplete fractures, the surgeon will not be able to perform the phacoemulsification successfully or he will need to use so much ultrasound energy that there may be endothelial damage. Present techniques of phacoemulsification are precisely geared to avoiding the use of large amounts of ultrasound energy.

There are different techniques for the fracture of the nucleus. In the end, the surgeon will decide which one he prefers or feels more secure with. Often, it depends on the type and maturity of the cataract. At this stage of the transition, when the surgeon is only beginning his experience with fracturing and dividing the lens to apply the ultrasound, the most rec-

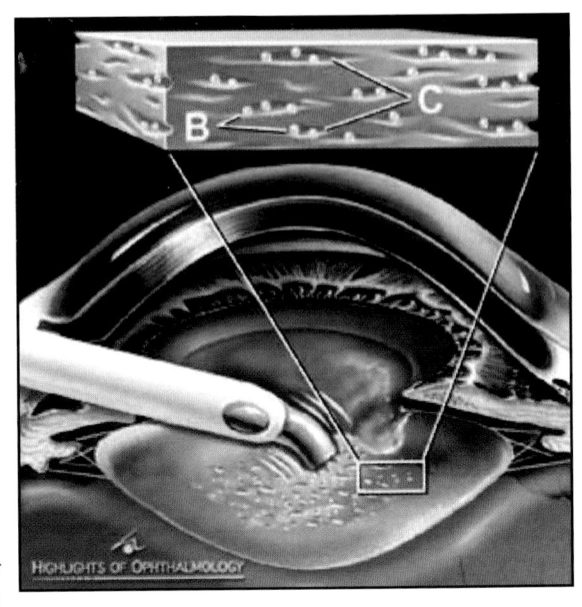

Figure 3-13. The role of cavitation in breaking the cataract inside the bag. There are two forces involved in emulsifying a cataract: 1) the mechanical force of the ultrasound, and 2) the mechanism of cavitation. The magnified section of cataract presented here shows that as the phaco tip makes its tiny ultrasonic movements, the energy releases bubbles (B) inside the nucleus, creating cavities (C). The build-up of bubbles inside the nucleus creates new hollow spaces (C) in the lens structure, the phenomenon of cavitation. This cavitation facilitates the break-up and destruction of the cataract. (Courtesy of Benjamin F. Boyd, Ed. *The Art and the Science of Cataract Surgery*. Highlights of Ophthalmology, English Edition, 2001.)

ommended procedure is to divide it into four quadrants, the well-known "Divide and Conquer" first presented by Gimbel. Later, the surgeon will be able to utilize other modern techniques that also use high vacuum and low phaco, but which may be too difficult in the transition.

At this stage of division or fracturing of the lens in the transition, it is recommended that the surgeon use a discretely high amount of ultrasound, low or no vacuum, low aspiration and the conventional height of the bottle (65 to 72 cm).

The Divide and Conquer Technique

In the Divide and Conquer technique, the phacoemulsification instrument is used to create a deep tunnel in the center or the upper part of the nucleus. The nucleus is split into halves, sometimes fourths, and even occasionally into eighths. Splitting the nucleus is safer for the endothelium and easier to learn, especially for the less experienced ophthalmologist converting from planned extracapsular surgery to phacoemulsification. It is easier to keep smaller particles away from the endothelium without having to push them against the posterior capsule than it is to emulsify a large, cumbersome nucleus.[9]

The nuclear fracturing techniques developed by Gimbel are in part possible because of the CCC technique that Gimbel and Neuhann originated. The mechanical fracturing of the lens causes extra physical stress within the capsule, and that cannot be done without risk of tears extending around posteriorly unless you have a proper CCC. There is almost an interdependence of these two methods. The fracturing techniques have not only provided more efficiency in phacoemulsification in routine cases, they have also made phacoemulsification in difficult cases safer and more feasible.

Gimbel clarifies that not only are there lamellar cleavage planes corresponding to the different zones of the lens, but also there are radial fault lines corresponding to the radial orientation of the fibers. Until the development of these nuclear fracturing techniques, we

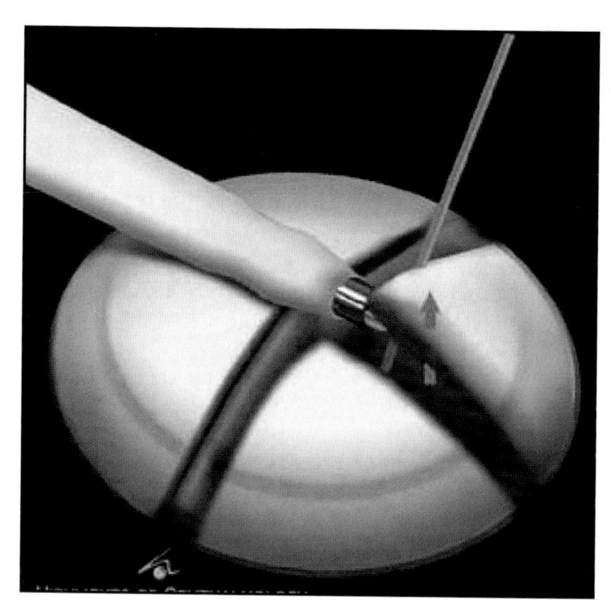

Figure 3-14. This cross section view shows the phacoemulsification probe removing the nucleus fragments within the capsular bag. Note the apex of one of the fragments created in the nucleus being lifted with the second instrument (arrow) and the ultrasound tip embedded into the posterior edge of each segment ready for emulsification. The epinucleus and cortex will then be removed during the phaco process. If we operate on a softer cataract, the freed fractured pieces are emulsified immediately. (Courtesy of Benjamin F. Boyd, Ed. *The Art and the Science of Cataract Surgery*. Highlights of Ophthalmology, English Edition, 2001.)

had not taken advantage of this construction. The lens fractures quite readily in radial or pie-shaped segments. To accomplish this radial fracturing, the surgeon must sculpt deeply into the center of the nucleus and push outwards. Sculpting is used to create a trench or trough in the nucleus. Then the surrounding part is divided into two hemisections. The separation must occur in the thickest area of the lens located at the center of the nucleus.

An additional consideration with these types of nuclear fractures is whether the segments should be left in place until all the fracturing is complete or whether they should be broken off and emulsified as soon as they are separated. With a lax capsule and particularly with a dense, or brunescent nucleus, Gimbel considers that it is safer to leave the segments in place to keep the posterior capsule protected.[10] The segments are easier to fracture if they are held loosely in place by the rest of the already fractured segments still in the bag (Figure 3-14).

Emulsification of the Nuclear Fragments

If the surgeon has been successful in the fragmentation of the nucleus, the next step is to emulsify the pieces of segments of the divided nucleus. He may do this with the linear continuous mode or with the pulse mode. The latter done during the transition provides more security for the surgeon and allows him to use less ultrasound, which is the definite tendency at present.

The surgeon may later slowly begin to utilize other more specialized techniques known as the different "chop" techniques, which we will discuss later. These techniques facilitate the emulsification of the segments or pieces of the fractured nucleus more than the Divide and Conquer, but they are a little more complex. During this step of emulsification of the nuclear fragments, the surgeon may deliver low ultrasound, high vacuum, and a larger flow of aspiration, with a conventional height of the bottle.

Aspiration of the Epinucleus

During this specific step, there is a higher incidence of rupture of the posterior capsule for the surgeon in the period of transition. This is due to his lack of familiarity with handling large fragments of epinucleus and cortex because in the planned ECCE he is accustomed to removing a large and complete nucleus that includes all the epinucleus and a significant amount of cortex. During the transition, the surgeon has to manage safely the irrigation-aspiration handpiece. Later, when he masters the technique, he may aspirate the epinucleus and cortex by maintaining the aspiration with the tip of the phaco handpiece. For this stage of the aspiration of the epinucleus, the surgeon will use very low or no ultrasound power, a moderate to high vacuum, and high flow of aspiration, with the bottle of fluid maintained at the conventional height.

Aspiration of the Cortex

This step is closely related to the previous one. There can also be a larger incidence of posterior capsule rupture during this stage because the surgeon does not have the epinucleus as a barrier, which up to a few seconds before was protecting the posterior capsule. The surgeon should use a larger quantity of viscoelastic whenever required with the purpose of protecting the posterior capsule. During the transition period, he may help his maneuvers by using the Simcoe cannula, with which the planned extracapsular surgeon usually feels safe. This cannula may be introduced through the ancillary incision. The Simcoe cannula has the disadvantage, though, that the aspiration hole or aperture is smaller than that of the irrigation-aspiration handpiece of the phaco machine. Consequently, the aspiration of the masses of cortex may become more difficult and slow. During this stage, the surgeon should use zero (0) phaco power, maximum vacuum, and the highest flow of aspiration as compared with all the previously mentioned methods. The fluid bottle is maintained at the conventional height. The aspiration of the cortex is also performed with the bimanual aspiration technique, which is very useful, especially in the subincisional cortex aspiration process.

Intraocular Lens Implantation

Implanting the Lens

The preferred intraocular lens (IOL) implantation is performed as shown in Figure 3-15.

Removal of Viscoelastic

Throughout the different stages of this procedure, the presence of viscoelastic in the anterior chamber is always a measure to keep in mind in order to prevent or minimize damage to the surrounding structures during surgical maneuvers, particularly the corneal endothelium. When removing viscoelastic from the anterior chamber, the phaco machine must be in zero phaco or ultrasound, high vacuum, very low aspiration and the bottle of fluid should be significantly lower. After all the surgical steps have been accomplished, it is important, as we all know, to remove the viscoelastic in order to avoid a high IOP postoperatively, with subsequent corneal edema, blurred vision, and pain during the first postoperative days.

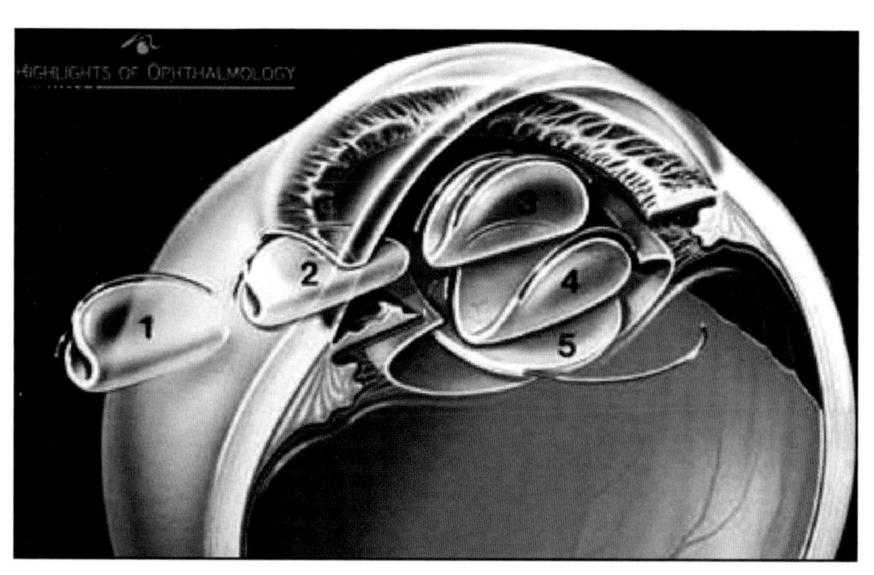

Figure 3-15. This cross section view shows the movement of the foldable IOL during insertion. Folding forceps removed for clarity. (1) Folded lens outside the eye. (2) Folded lens passing through small incision. (3) Folded lens placed posteriorly into the capsular bag through anterior capsule opening and then rotated 90 degrees. (4) Lens slowly unfolded in the bag. (5) Final unfolded position of lens within the capsular bag. (Courtesy of Benjamin F. Boyd, Ed. *The Art and the Science of Cataract Surgery*. Highlights of Ophthalmology, English Edition, 2001.)

Closure of the Wound

If a good incision has been made, valve-like, self-sealing and waterproof, no suture will be absolutely necessary even in those cases where the wound has been extended to an arc of 5.2 mm for IOL implantation. As long as these two requisites are met, that is, extending the incision to 5.2 mm with a special knife blade of that size and maintaining a valve-like, self-sealing incision, there is little danger of complications without sutures. Nevertheless, if the surgeon is not sure he has made a valvulated incision from the beginning, even a 3 mm incision with no sutures will leak. If so, to leave the patient without any sutures would be to take an unnecessary risk. It is more prudent to place one or two 10-0 nylon sutures in the wound and they may be removed early in the postoperative stage. This decision really depends on the ability of the surgeon to create a valve-like, self-sealing incision.

Key Points

1. During the transition, it is advisable that the surgeon utilize the type of anesthesia with which he or she feels more safe and in better control.
2. Once the surgeon is certain that he will not need to convert from phaco to planned extracapsular and therefore will not need to enlarge the incision, he may choose to make a corneal incision if he wishes, but not before.
3. The surgeon must learn first by practicing capsulorrhexis on the skin of a grape or by using a very thin sheet of plastic wrap.
4. Fluctuation in the anterior chamber depth is the consequence of the amount of outflow exceeding the amount of inflow in a given period. As a result, the anterior chamber is reduced in depth or collapses.

References

1. Carreño E. From can opener to capsulorrhexis: the crucial step in the phaco transition. Course on how to shift successfully from manual ECCE to machine-assisted small incision cataract. American Academy of Ophthalmology, Oct. 1999.
2. Barojas E. Importance of hydrodissection in phaco. In: Boyd B. *The Art and the Science of Cataract Surgery.* Panama: Highlights of Ophthalmology; 2001.
3. Carreño E. Hydrodissection and hydrodelineation. In: Boyd B. *The Art and the Science of Cataract Surgery.* Panama: Highlights of Ophthalmology; 2001.
4. Koch PS. *Simplifying Phacoemulsification.* 5th ed. SLACK Incorporated; 1997: 87–98.
5. Seibel BS. *Phacodynamics: Mastering the Tools and Techniques of Phacoemulsification Surgery.* 3rd ed; 1999.
6. Blumenthal M, Kansas P. Fluidics during cataract surgery. *Small Incision Manual Cataract Surgery—Mini-Nuc and Fluidics Phacosection and Viscoexpression.* 2004;2:7-27.
7. Seibel SB. The fluidics and physics of phaco. In: Agarwal A. et al. Phacoemulsification, laser cataract surgery and foldable IOL. Second edition. Jaypee Brothers: New Delhi; 2000;45–54.
8. Benchimol S, Carreño E. The transition from planned extracapsular surgery to phacoemulsification. *Highlights of Ophthalmol.* 1996;24:3.
9. Centurion V. The transition to phaco: a step by step guide. *Ocular Surgery News.* 1999.
10. Boyd BF. Preparing for the transition. In: Boyd BF, ed. *The Art And Science of Cataract Surgery.* Panama: Highlights of Ophthalmology; 2001:93.

Chapter 4

Preventing Complications Using No Anesthesia Cataract Surgery With the Karate Chop Technique

Amar Agarwal, MS, FRCS, FRCOphth

Introduction

On June 13th, 1998 at Ahmedabad, India the first no anesthesia cataract surgery was done by the author as a live surgery at the Phako & Refractive Surgery conference. This has opened up various new concepts in cataract surgery.[1-4] In this surgery, the karate chop technique was used.

Nucleus Removal Techniques

Since the introduction of phacoemulsification as an alternative to standard cataract extraction technique, surgeons throughout the world have been attempting to make this new procedure safer and easier to perform while ensuring good visual outcome and patient recovery. The fundamental goal of phaco is to remove the cataract with minimal disturbance to the eye using the least number of surgical manipulations. Each maneuver should be performed with minimal force and maximum efficiency should be obtained.

The latest generation of phaco procedures began with Dr. Howard Gimbel's divide and conquer nuclear fracture technique in which he simply split apart the nuclear rim. Since then we have evolved through the various techniques namely four quadrant cracking, chip and flip, spring surgery, stop and chop and phaco chop.

Karate Chop

Unlike the peripheral chopping of Nagahara or other stop and chop techniques, we have developed a safer technique called "central anterior chopping" or "karate chop". In this method, the phaco tip is embedded by a single burst of power in the central safe zone and after lifting the nucleus a little bit (to lessen the pressure on the posterior capsule) the chopper is used to chop the nucleus. In soft nuclei, it is very difficult to chop the nucleus. In most cases, one can take it out in toto. But if the patient is above 40 years of age, one might have to chop the nucleus. In such cases, we embed the phaco probe in the nucleus and then with the left hand cut the nucleus as if we are cutting a piece of cake. This movement should be done three times in the same place. This will chop the nucleus.

Soft Cataracts

In soft cataracts, the technique is a bit different. We embed the phaco tip and then cut the nucleus as if we are cutting a piece of cake. One should embed slightly as the nucleus is very soft. This should be done 2 to 3 times in the same area so that the cataract gets cut. It is very tough to chop a soft cataract, so this technique helps in splitting the cataract.

28 Gauge Agarwal Chopper

We have devised our own chopper. The other choppers, which cut from the periphery, are blunt choppers. Our chopper has a sharp cutting edge. It also has a sharp point. The advantage of such a chopper is that you can chop in the center and need not go to the periphery. This is a 28-gauge chopper, so it can easily pass through the side port without enlargement.

By going directly into the center of the nucleus without any sculpting, the ultrasound energy required is reduced. The chopper always remains within the rhexis margin and never goes underneath the anterior capsule. Hence, it is easy to work with even small pupils or glaucomatous eyes. Since we don't have to widen the pupil, there is little likelihood of tearing the sphincter and allowing prostaglandins to leak out and cause inflammation or cystoid macular edema. In this technique, we can easily go into even hard nuclei on the first attempt.

Karate Chop Technique

Incision

A temporal clear corneal section is made. If the astigmatism is plus at 90 degrees then the incision is made superiorly. Always make the incision at the plus axis because the incision would flatten, whereas a suture would steepen the case. First, a needle with viscoelastic is injected inside the eye in the area where the second site is made (Figure 4-1). This will distend the eye so that when a clear corneal incision is made, the eye will be tense and one can create a good valve. Now a straight rod is used to stabilize the eye with the left hand. With the right hand, the clear corneal incision is made (Figure 4-2).

When we started making the temporal incisions, we positioned ourselves temporally. The problem with this method is that every time the microscope is turned, it would affect the cables connected to the videocamera. Further, the operating room staff would get confused between the right eye and left eye. To solve this problem, we decided on a different strategy. We have operating trolleys on wheels. The patient is wheeled inside the operation room and for the right eye the trolley is placed slightly obliquely so that the surgeon does not change his or her position. The surgeon stays at the 12 o'clock position. For the left eye, the trolley with the patient is rotated horizontally so that the temporal portion of the left eye comes at 12 o'clock. This way the patient is moved and not the surgeon.

Rhexis

Capsulorrhexis is then performed through the same incision (Figure 4-3). While performing the rhexis, it is important to note that the rhexis is started from the center and the needle moved to the right and then downward. This is important because concepts of tem-

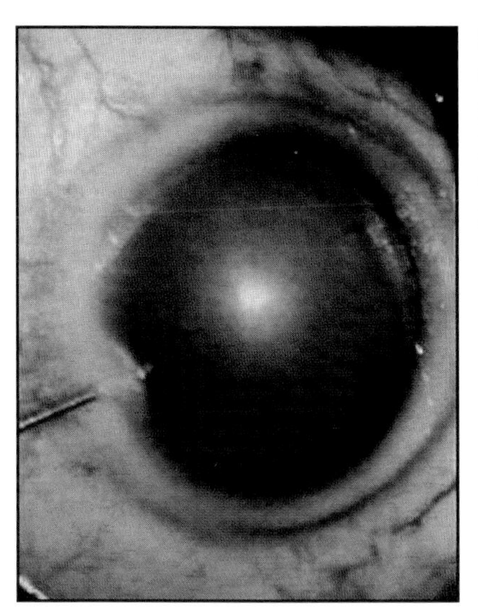

Figure 4-1. Eye with cataract. Needle with viscoelastic entering the eye to inject the viscoelastic. This is the most important step in no anesthesia cataract/clear lens surgery. This gives an entry into the eye through which a straight rod can be passed to stabilize the eye. Note no forceps holds the eye.

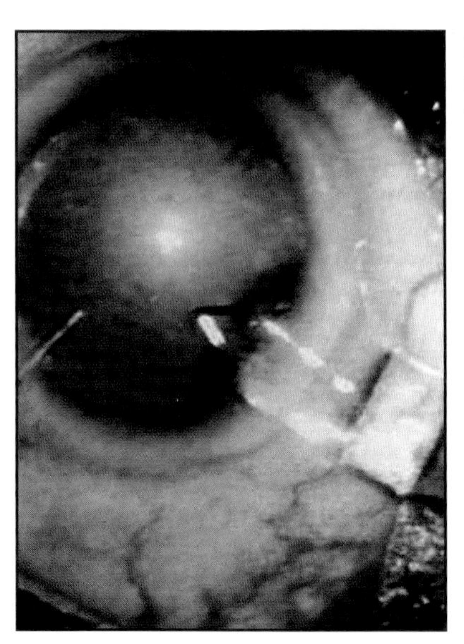

Figure 4-2. Clear corneal incision. Note the straight rod inside the eye in the left hand. The right hand is performing the clear corneal incision. This is a temporal incision and the surgeon is sitting temporally.

poral and nasal have changed. It is better to remember it as superior or inferior, right or left. The weakest point of the rhexis is generally where you finish it. In other words, the point where you tend to lose the rhexis is near its completion. If you have done the rhexis from the center and moved to the left, then you might have an incomplete rhexis on the left-hand side inferiorly. Now, the phaco probe is always moved down and to the left. So every stroke of your hand can extend the rhexis posteriorly creating a posterior capsular rupture. Now, if we perform the rhexis from the center and move to the right and then push the flap inferiorly—then if we have an incomplete rhexis near the end of the rhexis it will be superiorly and to the right. Any incomplete rhexis can extend and create a posterior capsular tear. But in this case, the chances of survival are better. This is because we are moving the phaco probe down and to the left, but the rhexis is incomplete superiorly and to the right.

Note: If you are left-handed, start the rhexis from the center and move to the left and then down.

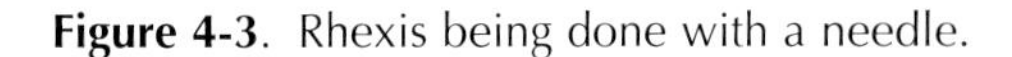

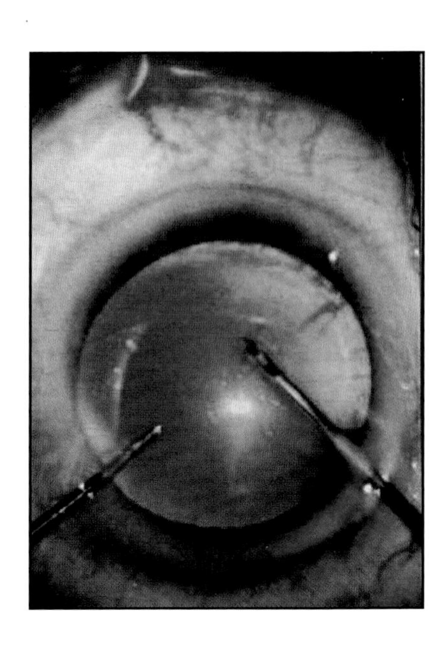

Figure 4-3. Rhexis being done with a needle.

HYDRODISSECTION

Hydrodissection is then performed. We watch for the fluid wave to see that hydrodissection is complete. We do not perform hydrodelineation unless operating on a posterior polar cataract. In such a case we do only hydrodelineation and not hydrodissection. Viscoelastic is then introduced before inserting the phaco probe. In mature cataracts, one cannot see the fluid wave, so in such cases just watch the nucleus moving anteriorly.

KARATE CHOP—TWO HALVES

We then insert the phaco probe through the incision slightly superiorly to the center of the nucleus (Figure 4-4). At that point, apply ultrasound and see that the phaco tip gets embedded in the nucleus. The direction of the phaco probe should be obliquely downward toward the vitreous and not horizontally towards the iris. Then only the nucleus will get embedded. The settings at this stage are 70% phaco power, 24 ml/minute flow rate, and 101 mm Hg suction. By the time the phaco tip gets embedded in the nucleus, the tip would have reached the middle of the nucleus. We prefer a 15° tip but any tip can be used.

Now phaco ultrasound is stopped and the surgeon brings his foot to position 2 so that only suction is being used. The nucleus is lifted. When we say lift, it means just a little so that when we apply pressure on the nucleus with the chopper, the direction of the pressure is downward. If the capsule is a bit thin, as in hypermature cataracts, the posterior capsule may rupture and create a nucleus drop. So when we lift the nucleus the pressure on the posterior capsule is lessened. Now, with the chopper the surgeon cuts the nucleus with a straight downward motion (Figure 4-5) and then moves the chopper to the left when the center of the nucleus is reached. In other words, the left hand moves the chopper like a laterally reversed L.

Remember, do not go to the periphery for chopping, but do it at the center.

Once a crack is created, the surgeon splits the nucleus till the center, then rotates the nucleus 180° and cracks again, so that there are two halves of the nucleus. In brown cataracts, the nucleus will crack but sometimes in the center the nucleus will still be attached. The nucleus must be split totally in two halves and the posterior capsule should be seen throughout.

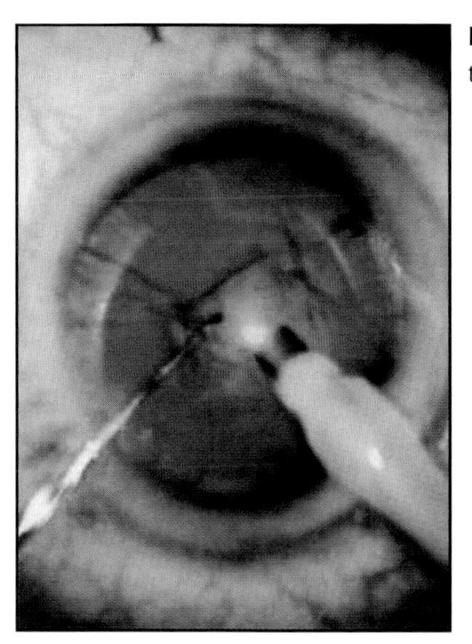

Figure 4-4. Phaco probe placed at the superior end of the rhexis.

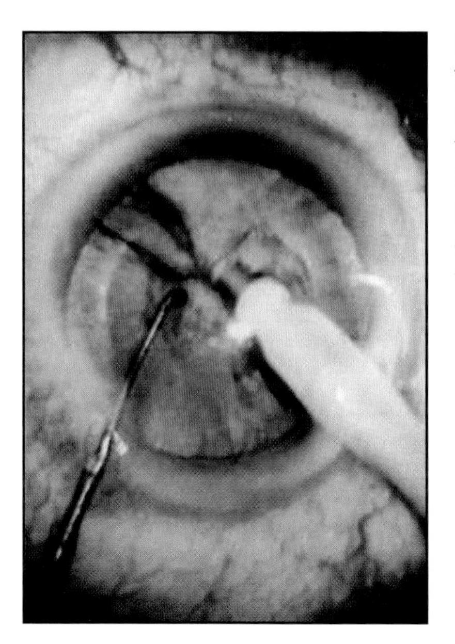

Figure 4-5. Phaco probe embedded in the nucleus. The phaco probe tip embedding started from the superior end of the rhexis and it embedded in the middle of the nucleus. If we had started in the middle, we would have embedded only inferiorly, ie, at the edge of the rhexis and chopping would be difficult. Left hand chops the nucleus and splits like a laterally reversed L, that is downwards and to the left.

Karate Chop–Further Chopping

Now that there are two halves, there is a shelf to embed the probe. The probe is placed with ultrasound into one half of the nucleus (Figure 4-6). The probe can be passed horizontally because of the shelf. The probe is embedded, then pulled a little bit. This step is important so that there is an extra bit of space for chopping. This will prevent the surgeon from chopping the rhexis margin. The force of the chopper is applied downwards. Then the chopper is moved to the left so that the nucleus gets split. Again, the posterior capsule should be seen throughout to assure that the nucleus is totally split. The probe is released, as the probe will still be embedded into the nucleus. In this manner, three quadrants are

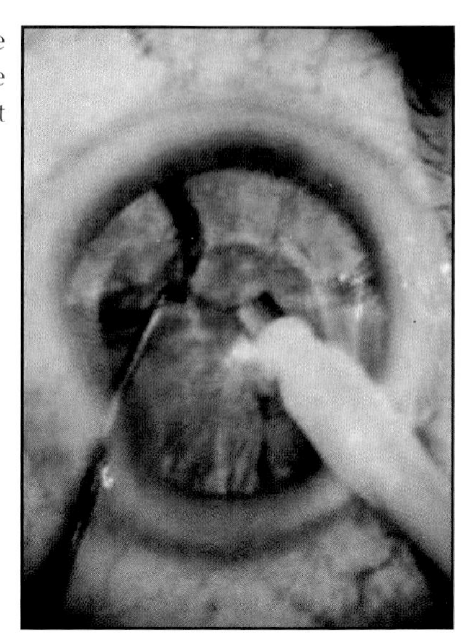

Figure 4-6. Phaco probe embedded in one half of the nucleus. Go horizontally and not vertically as you have now a shelf of nucleus to embed. Chop and then split the nucleus.

created in one half of the nucleus. Then another three halves are created with the second half of the nucleus. Thus, there are now six quadrants or pie-shaped fragments. The settings at this stage are 50% phaco power, 24 ml/minute flow rate, and 101 mm Hg suction.

Remember 5 words—embed, pull, chop, split, and release.

Pulse Phaco

Once all the pieces have been chopped, take each piece out one by one and in pulse phaco mode aspirate the pieces at the level of the iris. Do not work in the bag unless the cornea is preoperatively bad or the patient is very elderly. Always use the air pump at this stage as surge is prevented and the chamber becomes deep. The setting at this stage can be phaco power 50 to 30%, flow rate 24 ml, and suction 101 mm Hg.

Remember: it is better to have striate keratitis than posterior capsular rupture.

Cortical Washing and Foldable Intraocular Lens Implantation

The next step is to do cortical washing (Figure 4-7). Always try to remove the subincisional cortex first, as that is the most difficult. Note the left hand has the straight rod controlling the movements of the eye. If necessary use a bimanual irrigation aspiration technique. Then inject viscoelastic and implant the foldable IOL.

Stromal Hydration

At the end of the procedure, inject the BSS inside the lips of the clear corneal incision. This will create a stromal hydration at the wound. This will create a whiteness that will disappear after 4 to 5 hours. The advantage of this is that the wound gets sealed better.

No Pad or Subconjunctival Injections

No subconjunctival injections or pad are put in the eye. The patient walks out of the operating room and goes home. The patient is seen the next day and after a month glasses are prescribed.

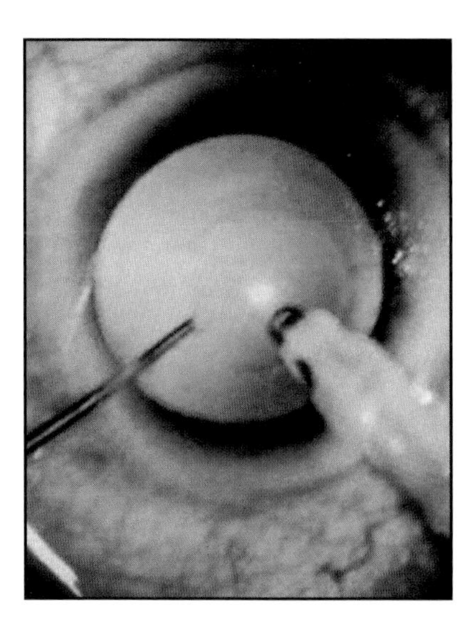

Figure 4-7. Cortical aspiration completed. Note the straight rod in the left hand that helps control the movements of the eye.

NO ANESTHESIA CATARACT SURGERY

We had been wondering whether any topical anesthesia is required, so we operated on patients without any anesthesia. In these patients, no xylocaine drops were instilled. The patients did not have any pain. It is paradoxical because we have been taught from the beginning that we should apply xylocaine. We never use any one-tooth forceps to stabilize the eye. Instead we use a straight rod, which is passed inside the eye to stabilize it when we are performing rhexis, etc. The first step is very important. We first enter the eye with a needle and inject viscoelastic inside the eye. This is done in the area of the side port. Now we have an opening in the eye through which a straight rod can be passed to stabilize it. Francisco Gutierrez-Carmona from Spain modified the technique using cold fluid and called it "cryoanalgesia".

AIR PUMP TO PREVENT SURGE

One of the main problems of phacoemulsification is surge.[1] The problem is that as the nuclear piece gets occluded in the phaco tip and we emulsify it, surge occurs. Many people have tried various methods to solve this problem. Some phaco machines have been devised to solve this problem. Others have tried to use an anterior chamber maintainer to get more fluid into the eye. The problem with the anterior chamber maintainer is that another port has to be made. In other words, we have three ports and if you are doing the case under topical or no anesthesia (as we do in our hospital), it becomes quite cumbersome. Another method to solve surge is to use more phacoaspiration and chop the nuclear pieces with the nondominant hand. The problem with this is the surgical time decreases and if the case is a hard brown cataract, phacoaspiration will not suffice.

Surge occurs when an occluded fragment is held by high vacuum and is then abruptly aspirated with a burst of ultrasound. What happens is that fluid from the anterior chamber rushes into the phaco tip and this leads to a collapse of the anterior chamber. Sunita Agarwal thought of a method to solve surge using an air pump (see Chapter 2). We got this idea when we were using phakonit. We wanted more fluid entering the eye. Now, we routinely use the air pump to solve the problem of surge.

Conclusion

As in any other field, progress is inevitable in ophthalmology, even more so in cataract surgery. We have started to look at cataract surgery as a craft and should constantly try to improve our craft and become better every day. By this, we will be able to provide good vision to more people than anyone dared dream a few decades ago. If a patient is not cooperative, do give a peribulbar block and do the case. Any anesthesia that suits the patient and the surgeon should be used.

Key Points

1. In "central anterior chopping" or "karate chop," the phaco tip is embedded by a single burst of power in the central safe zone and after lifting the nucleus a little bit (to lessen the pressure on the posterior capsule), the chopper is used to chop the nucleus.
2. In soft cataracts, the technique is a bit different. Embed the phaco tip and then cut the nucleus as if cutting a piece of cake. This should be done 2 to 3 times in the same area so that the cataract gets cut.
3. The Agarwal chopper has a sharp cutting edge and a sharp point. The advantage of such a chopper is that you can chop in the center and need not go to the periphery.
4. Never use one-tooth forceps to stabilize the eye. Instead use a straight rod, which is passed inside the eye to stabilize it when performing rhexis.
5. Routinely use the air pump to solve the problem of surge.

References

1. Agarwal A, Agarwal A, Sachdev MS, Mehta KR, Fine IH, Agarwal A. *Phacoemulsification, Laser Cataract Surgery, and Foldable IOLs*. 2nd ed. Delhi, India: Jaypee Brothers; 2000.
2. Agarwal A, Agarwal S, Agarwal A. No anesthesia cataract surgery with the karate chop technique. In: Agarwal A, ed. *Presbyopia: A Surgical Textbook*. Thorofare, NJ: SLACK Incorporated; 2002: 177–185.
3. Agarwal A, Agarwal S, Agarwal A. No anesthesia cataract and clear lens extraction with karate chop. In: Agarwal A, ed. *Phako, Phakonit and Laser Phako: A Quest for the Best*. Panama: Highlights of Ophthalmology; 2002: 113–120.
4. Agarwal A, Agarwal S, Agarwal A. No anesthesia cataract and clear lens extraction with karate chop. In: Boyd, Agarwal. *LASIK and Beyond LASIK*. Panama: Highlights of Ophthalmology; 2001: 451-462.

Chapter 5

Using Safe Horizontal Chopping to Prevent Ruptures

L. Felipe Vejarano, MD; Alejandro Tello, MD

Introduction

Since the initial description by Nagahara in 1993,[1] chopping techniques have been progressively displacing the previous techniques of central bowling or cracking (divide and conquer), because they have been shown to require less ultrasound energy, operative time, and intraocular manipulation, without an increase in intraoperative or postoperative complications.[2–4] However, phaco chop also showed some points of concern. Sometimes it was difficult to achieve the first fracture. Also, when the nucleus was already fragmented, the nuclear pieces sometimes fitted together, as in a jigsaw puzzle, making it difficult to get the first piece out of the bag. Surgeons began to modify Nagahara´s original technique, and Koch described the "stop and chop" technique.[5,6] This technique combines Gimbel's[7,8] and Shepherd's[9,10] nucleus preparation for divide and conquer nucleofractis technique and Nagahara's chop to break up the nucleus. Although some authors have found no significant differences between non-stop phaco-chop and stop and chop techniques,[11] in other studies Can and coauthors found that horizontal pure phaco chop techniques used less ultrasound and had less loss of endothelial cells, with faster visual recovery and return to preoperative pachymetry.[12] Although stop and chop involves chopping, non-stop phaco chop is a pure chopping technique, thus eliminating all sculpting and saving ultrasound energy. Moreover, we agree with Chang when he states that while making grooves, the force to hold the nucleus is provided by the zonules and capsule, causing stress of those structures, especially in hard cataracts. We think that stop and chop is a very good technique for surgeons making the transition from cracking to chopping, but we believe that non-stop chop is more efficient, and, as Chang states, not only for standard cases, but especially for complicated surgeries, such as those with small pupils, loose zonules, brunescent nuclei, or mature white lenses.[13]

The last annual surveys of the American Society of Cataract & Refractive Surgery show an increasing interest in the chopping technique, which was being used by 24% of respondents. However the preferred technique is still the nucleofractis, divide and conquer (54%).[14] We think that one reason for this is that phaco chop is more difficult to learn because the most difficult skills are performed with the nondominant hand. Therefore, the learning curve may be longer than people anticipate, and some may give up before mastering the technique. Another point of concern with phaco chop is the rupture of the edge of the continuous curvilinear capsulorrhexis (CCC). This is one of the possible complications of phaco chop, using Nagahara's horizontal technique, secondary to chopping anteriorly to the anterior capsule. It is especially probable in a surgeon with little experience in chopping. The technique we describe herein, Vejarano's safe chop, developed by one of the authors (L. Felipe Vejarano, MD), greatly reduces the possibility of tearing the edge of the CCC during phaco chop.

A crucial recent breakthrough in phacoemulsification has been to perform the surgery through a microincision (1.0 to 1.5 mm), yielding the further advantages of such a small wound. Independently, Agarwal in India and Tsuneoka in Japan began that technique in 1998 and 1999, respectively.[15,16] Agarwal coined the term "phakonit", which stands for phacoemulsification (Phako) performed with a needle opening (n) via an ultrasmall incision (i) with the sleeveless ultrasound tip (t).[17] Alió has called this technique "microincisional cataract surgery" (MICS).[18] We have reported very good results in Phakonit/MICS using Vejarano's safe chop technique.[19–20]

Preliminary Technique

For standard coaxial phaco, a 1.0 mm side-port incision is made with a Diamond lancet (Accutome, Malvern, Pennsylvania) approximately 80° to the left of the main incision (right-hand surgeons). Main incision (2.8 to 3.0 mm length for standard coaxial phaco, depending on the size of the tip used) location is chosen according to the preoperative astigmatism and surgeon's preference. In our group, its location is usually corneal and temporal. When the surgeon is used to a superior approach, frequently he or she will feel that with a temporal approach the hands are lacking the support provided by the patient's forehead and eyebrow, but when surgeons learn how to take advantage of the better maneuverability and angle of attack of the tip to the nucleus and fragments, they do not return to the superior approach. We have two different approaches for making the main incision: a biplanar or a triplanar incision. The surgeons that use the triplanar incision make initially a groove of around 250 to 350 microns before constructing the tunnel with a short dissection using a crescent blade. The advantages[21] are that it avoids irregular cut at the corners (dog-ears), which sometimes may be formed in a biplanar approach, and that when planning to widen the incision to insert a rigid PMMA IOL, this technique allows a better apposition of the wound edges. The drawback is that it is more time consuming.

The tunnel must be around 1.5 mm long. If the tunnel is too long (longer than 2.00 mm) passing the phaco tip through it and turning the tip downward to perform the procedure creates undue striae and makes visualization difficult. Moreover, you can get oarlocked as you try to manipulate the phaco needle, and the increased wound distortion will pose the risk of incisional burn. If the tunnel is too short (shorter than 1.4 mm), with a premature entry into the anterior chamber, the anterior chamber will tend to shallow, and it will lead to iris prolapse. To avoid this situation, when making the tunnel, direct the blade anteriorly.

In MICS/Phakonit, a trapezoidal 0.8/1.2 mm side-port incision is made using a Diamond lancet (Accutome) and 0.3 ml intracameral lidocaine 2% administered in cases of topical anesthesia; Viscoat and Provisc (Alcon, Fort Worth, Texas) are injected through the side-port incision using Arshinoff's soft shell technique.[22] The main incision, 0.8/1.2 mm length, is performed using the same trapezoidal Diamond knife.

A 5.5 mm CCC is created using the Micro Incision Capsulorhexis Forceps, 23g (Accutome or MicroSurgical Technology [MST], Redmond, Washington) in phakonit cases or with a regular Utrata forceps in standard phaco cases. In order to keep the anterior chamber pressurized so that the anterior face of the lens is flattened, avoid egress of fluid or viscoelastic through the wound due to an excessive instrument pressure on the posterior incision lip, or an oversized incision or a tight lid speculum. In cases of white hypermature cataracts, if there is liquefied cortex, the resulting intralenticular fluid pressure may also encourage peripheral extension of the capsular tear, and in this setting it is even more important to keep the anterior capsule flattened. Cohesive viscoelastics perform better in flattening the anterior capsule surface than dispersive viscoelastics, but dispersives are more retentive. Using both of them with the Arshinoff's soft shell technique is a good option.[22]

In white and brunescent cataracts, the capsule may be very thin and friable, and due to the presence of a poor red reflex or even absence of it, it is difficult to distinguish the capsule from the cortex and to follow the leading edge. Currently, the best way to maximize visualization and improve control is using an anterior capsule staining method. Trypan blue and ICG are effective in staining the capsule.[23–26]

Hydrodissection is performed. We prefer to allow some amount of viscoelastic out of the eye before injecting the BSS for hydrodissection in order to avoid sudden increase in IOP. This is especially important when performing phakonit. Hydrodelineation is optional, but helps to isolate the nucleus, allowing the surgeon to work with the tip in a safer area, and the golden ring may serve as a guide for the point where the chopper must be placed before making the division of the nucleus, leaving the epinucleus and cortex as a cushion protecting the equator of the capsular bag. Currently, we are using the Infiniti vision system (Alcon, Fort Worth, Texas). For standard cases, we use the Rosen phaco chopper (Katena Products, Denville, NJ), and in phakonit cases we use Vejarano's Irrigating Chopper (Accutome) designed by Dr. Vejarano.

Safe Chop in Coaxial Phaco

Using burst mode or hyperpulses, the phaco tip (Table 5-1) is buried into the nucleus core, close to the proximal edge of the rhexis, attacking the nucleus at an angle of approximately 45°. It is possible to use the tip bevel down, so that the ultrasound energy is directed far from the corneal endothelium. When the tip is buried, the foot pedal is switched to position two and the chopper is slid beneath the anterior capsule, 180° away from the side port, with the tip tilted, to occupy less space. This maneuver is much easier to perform than sliding it under the anterior capsule just in front of the phaco tip, since it requires just a forward movement and is along the axis of the shaft of the chopper (Figure 5-1). The chopper is displaced until the equator of the nucleus is reached, and then the chopper's tip is rotated to reach its vertical position, moved inside the bag and along the equator, to a peripheral point in front of the phaco tip. In this position, the chopping maneuvers will take place (Figure 5-2). In hard cataracts, we hold the nucleus between the two instruments for a moment, and apply a small amount of additional pulse or burst mode ultrasound energy, so that the tip penetrates deeper in the nuclear material. This allows us to gain improved control of the whole nucleus during the chopping process, since it doesn't become easily dislodged, as long as the high vacuum and the deep position of the tip maintain a tight occlusion seal around the tip. An optional variation of the technique, practiced by one of the authors (AT), is that initially, before burying the phaco tip into the nucleus, he slides the chopper below the rhexis edge and places it in position. This maneuver has been described by Drs. Fine[27–29] and Chang,[30,31] and Dr. Tello has found that combining it with Vejarano's safe chop, provides very good control for the first fracture of the nucleus, which is usually the most difficult to achieve. However, sometimes the nucleus does not divide. This is more common in cases of soft rubbery cataracts or rock hard nucleus, or when the surgeon places the chopper or the phaco tip too superficially. In this situation, a

Table 5-1.

Settings for Standard Phacoemulsification With the Infiniti (Alcon)

Cataract Type	*Step*	*Power Lineal (%)*	*Burst ms*	*Pulses*	*% On*	*Neosonix (Amplitude)*	*Neosonix (Threshold)*	*Vacuum Lineal (mm Hg)*	*Aspiration Flow Fixed (cc min)*
Soft	*Chop*	20–30	30*	20	20–30	30	0	450	30
	Quadrants	10–20		20	20–30	30	0	400	45
	Epinucleus	10–20		20	20–30	30	0	400	30–60
Medium	*Chop*	40	50*	30	40	50	0	450	30
	Quadrants	40		30	40	50	0	400	45
	Epinucleus	20–30		20	40	30	0	400	30–60
Hard	*Chop*	80	100*	30–40	50	100	0	450	30
	Quadrants	80		40	50	100	0	400	45
	Epinucleus	30–40		20–30	40	30–40	0	400	30–60

* According to surgeon's preferences, burst or hyperpulses may be used.

**In soft cataracts and for the epinucleus, NeoSonix usage is optional.

***According to the anterior chamber stability, the surgeon may choose to use the higher levels and fixed flow, or the lower ones and linear flow.

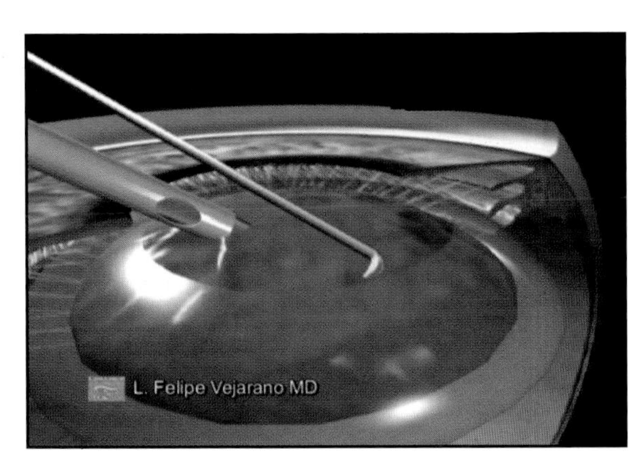

Figure 5-1. The chopper is slid in a longitudinal movement from the side port and enters beneath the capsulorrhexis 180° from the paracentesis, approximately 100° from the main incision.

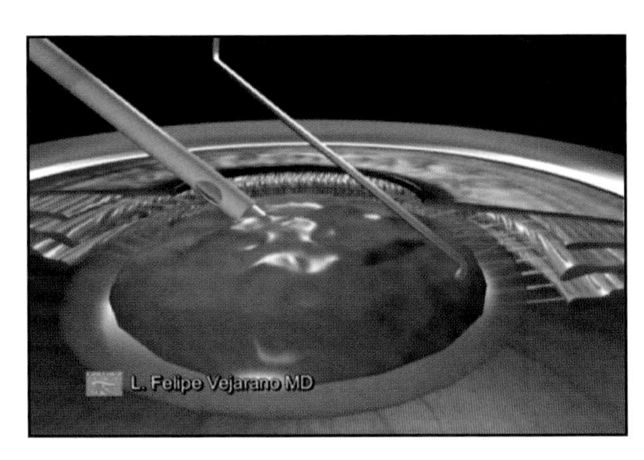

Figure 5-2. The chopper is moved inside the capsular bag, along the lens' equator, and placed in front of the phaco tip. At that moment, additional pulsed ultrasound is applied, so that the tip buries deeper in the nucleus, before performing the chopping.

crater, or even a small groove, is created in the place where the tip was buried. The best option is to rotate 90° and penetrate the tip inside this crater, facing the wall of nuclear material, and after impaling the nucleus make a new attempt to chop it. This maneuver almost always will be successful.

After dividing the nucleus in halves, we rotate it 45° to get the first piece of heminucleus. The phaco tip is rotated so that the bevel faces the vertical wall of nuclear material of the distal heminucleus, making occlusion easier, pushing the tip gently toward the heminucleus. High vacuum and hyperpulses, 30 to 50% "on" ultrasound energy, and "dynamic rise time" on 4 are used. For surgeons just beginning chopping, the rise time may be set in 0 to 2. When the tip is holding the heminucleus, the foot pedal is switched to position 2, and in this moment the phaco chopper is slid through the space between the two nuclear halves, moved beneath the anterior capsule up to the nucleus equator, and then again displaced inside the bag to the position in front of the phaco tip (Figure 5-3). In this maneuver, the chopper will find almost no resistance, since the fracture gives room for a very smooth displacement of the instrument. It is very important to reach the lens' equator, so that the movement of the chopper may be done without affecting the nucleus held by the phaco tip. It is usually not necessary to pull the heminucleus toward the surgeon, after holding it with the phaco tip, in order to place the phaco chopper in position. The subsequent fragments are managed in the same way, sliding the phaco chopper along the fracture lines into the capsular bag, toward the lens' equator. When several nuclear fragments have been emulsified, the amount of nuclear material is less, and we have more room in the center, so it is not usually necessary to go beneath the anterior CCC in order to chop them.

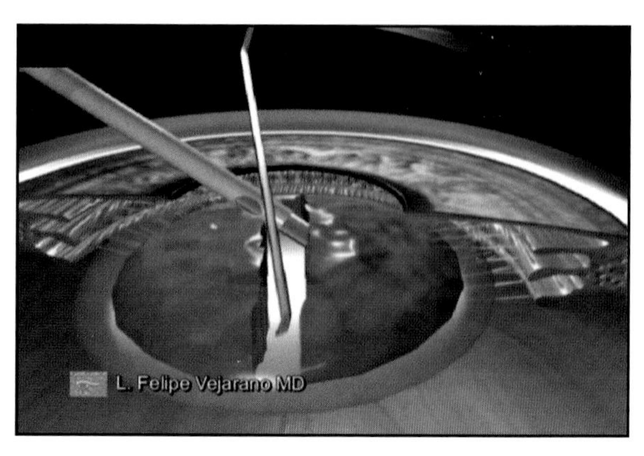

Figure 5-3. After dividing the nucleus in halves, it is rotated and the chopper is inserted into the capsular bag, along the fracture line, up to the equator.

Safe Chop in Phakonit

This chopping technique is very safe and user friendly, and we have found it to be very suitable for microincision phacoemulsification (phakonit). Vejarano's Irrigating Chopper is introduced through the side port in order to maintain adequate space in the anterior chamber. It has an outer diameter of 0.9 mm (approximately 20 gauge) that fits rather tightly in the 1.0 mm side-port incision. A sleeveless Micro Tip or a Micro Flow needle (Bausch & Lomb, Rochester, NY) is introduced into the anterior chamber through the main incision, which is 1.5 mm in length. One of us (LFV) is currently using the 0.7 MST microtip to perform micro-phakonit through 0.9 mm. After aspirating the anterior cortex and epinucleus, the phaco tip, bevel up, is placed in the proximal portion of the nucleus, and ultrasound energy is applied, so that it penetrates deep in the nuclear core. With the Infiniti system, moderate vacuum (250 mmHg), 25 cc/min of flow and phaco energy in pulse or burst mode (set from 20 and to no more than 60%, according to the hardness of the nucleus) are typically used. When the tip is buried into the nucleus, the foot pedal is switched to position 2. Then the irrigating chopper is lightly rotated horizontally, so that the longest length of the tip is not presented toward the space between the CCC edge and the lens material (space that in brunescent cataracts is very small, even absent). The chopper is slid beneath the anterior capsule, opposite the side port, a maneuver that is much easier to perform than trying to slide it under the anterior capsule just in front of the phaco tip (Figure 5-4). It is very important to look through the microscope at the tip of the chopper while the second hand is performing these maneuvers in order to maintain perfect control. Afterward, when reaching the equator of the nucleus, the chopper is rotated vertically and moved inside the bag, to the position in front of the phaco tip, and the chopping maneuvers take place. In hard cataracts, we hold the nucleus between the two instruments for a moment and apply a small amount of additional pulsed ultrasound energy, so that the tip penetrates deeper into the nuclear material (Figure 5-5). This allows us to gain improved control of the whole nucleus during the chopping process, since it doesn't become easily dislodged, as long as the high vacuum and the deep position of the tip maintain a tight occlusion seal around the tip. One very important advantage of this technique is that with this very good purchase of the nucleus, especially in hard cataracts, the chopping process is more effective, and allows us to separate the leather-like posterior layers of those cataracts that often present a challenge to the surgeon.

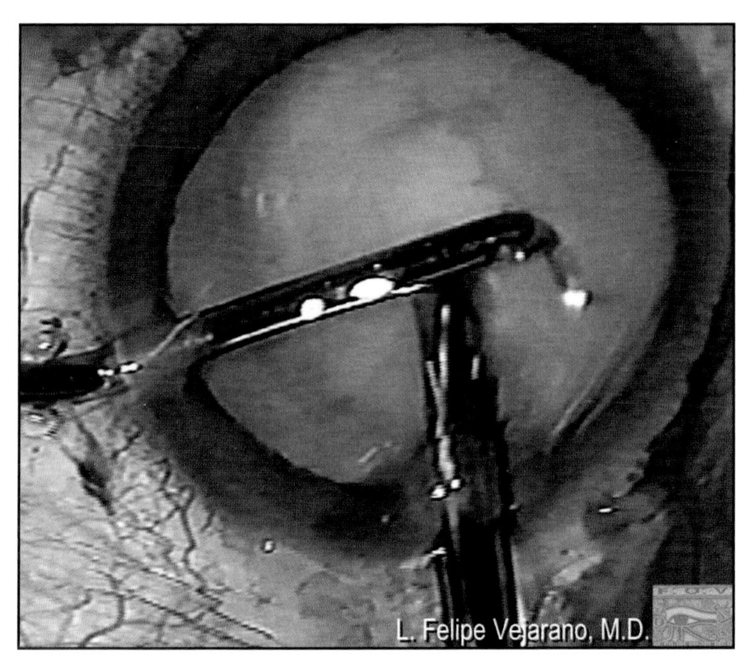

Figure 5-4. The irrigating chopper is inserted beneath the edge of the capsulorrhexis opposite the side-port incision.

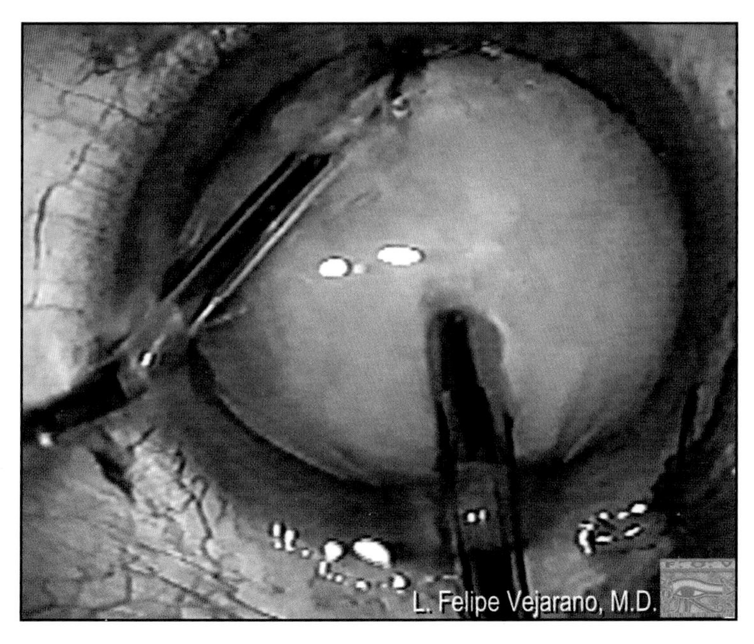

Figure 5-5. The irrigating chopper is moved inside the capsular bag, along the lens equator, and placed in front of the phaco tip. At that moment, additional pulsed ultrasound is applied, so that the tip buries deeper into the nucleus, before the chopping is started.

After dividing the nucleus in halves, we rotate it 45° to get the first piece of the heminucleus. To avoid damaging the CCC while chopping the nuclear fragments, insert the irrigation chopper vertically and always along the fracture lines of the nucleus, where there is more room for the chopper, and move it to reach its chopping position only when it is already at the lens equator (Figures 5-6 and 5-7). The subsequent fragments are managed in the same way. When reaching the nucleus equator, in not too hard

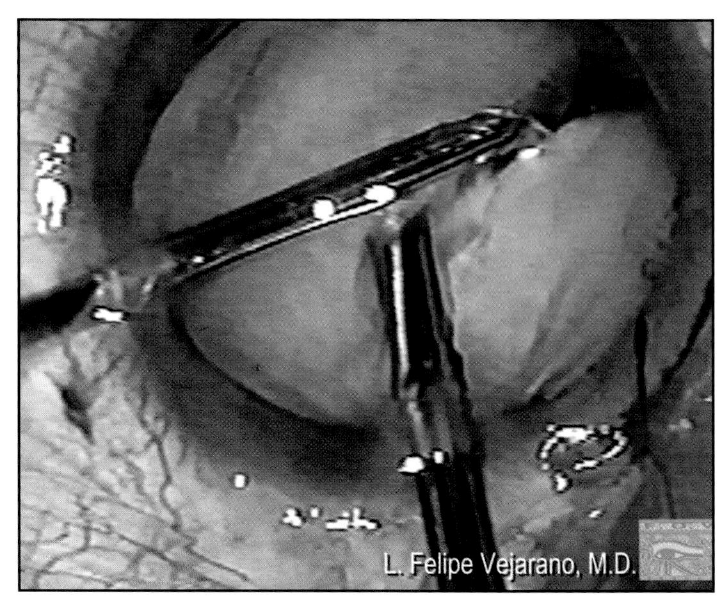

Figure 5-6. After dividing the nucleus in halves, it is rotated and the irrigating chopper is inserted into the capsular bag, along the fracture line, up to the equator.

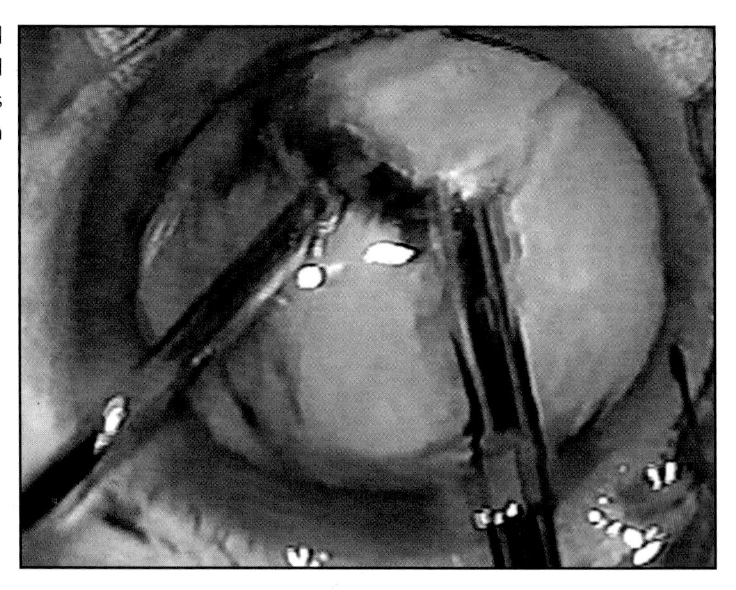

Figure 5-7. The second fracture is performed, and the nuclear fragment is brought to the center in order to be emulsified.

cataracts, it is usually evident that the chopper performs a separation of the epinucleus. This is not a problem at all, and is actually convenient, since we are interested in chopping the nucleus, not the epinucleus. When several nuclear fragments have been emulsified, the amount of remaining nuclear material is less, therefore there is more room in the center and it is not usually necessary to go beneath the anterior CCC in order to chop the remaining nucleus. The epinucleus is aspirated using a flip technique, and protecting the posterior capsule with the irrigating chopper, which is very friendly with the posterior capsule, since its tip has an olive to avoid damaging tissues.

Conclusion

In our opinion, the phaco chop technique will be the future of cataract surgery. However, phaco chop is not for beginners. The surgeon performing the transition should have an experienced surgeon present. This will prevent any phaco nightmares.

Key Points

1. There are two different approaches for making the main incision: a biplanar or a triplanar incision. The surgeons that use the triplanar incision initially make a groove of around 250 to 350 microns before constructing the tunnel with a short dissection using a crescent blade.
2. When the tip is buried, the foot pedal is switched to position 2 and the chopper is slid beneath the anterior capsule, 180° from the side port, with the tip tilted, to occupy less space. This maneuver is much easier to perform than sliding it under the anterior capsule just in front of the phaco tip.
3. When the tip is holding the heminucleus, the foot pedal is switched to position 2, and then the phaco chopper is slid through the space between the two nuclear halves, moved beneath the anterior capsule up to the nucleus equator, and then again displaced inside the bag to the position in front of the phaco tip.
4. The phaco chop technique will be the future of the cataract surgery, though phaco chop is not for beginners.
5. The horizontal chopping technique is suitable even for cases of hard nuclei in which the subcapsular space is very small.

References

1. Nagahara K. Phaco-chop Technique Eliminates Central Sculpting and Allows Faster Safer Phaco. Ocular Surgery News International Edition. 1993, pages 12–13.
2. Wong T, Hingorani M, Lee V. Phacoemulsification time and power requirements in phaco chop and divide and conquer nucleofractis techniques. *J Cataract Refract Surg*. 2000;26:1374–8.
3. DeBry P, Olson RJ, Crandall AS. Comparison of energy required for phaco-chop and divide and conquer phacoemulsification. *J Cataract Refract Surg*. 1998;24:689–92.
4. Mierzejewski A, Kalluzny JJ, Kaluzny B, Eliks I. [Cataract phacoemulsification techniques: "divide and conquer" versus "stop and chop" — comparative evaluation of operation course and early results]. *Klin Oczna*. 2004;106(4–5):612–7.
5. Koch PS, Katzen LE. Stop and chop phacoemulsification. *J Cataract Refract Surg*. 1994;20:566–709.
6. Koch PS . Stop and Chop Phacoemulsification Technique. www.ophthalmic.hyperguides.com
7. Gimbel HV. Divide and conquer nucleofractis phacoemulsification: Development and variations. *J Cataract Refract Surg*. 1991;17:281–291.
8. Gimbel HV, Row PK. Cataract Technique with Divide and Conquer Phaco. www.ophthalmic.hyperguides.com.
9. Shepherd JR. In situ fracture. *J Cataract Refract Surg*. 1990;16(4):436–40.
10. Shepherd JR. The Four Quadrant Divide and Conquer Technique. *www.ophthalmic.hyperguides.com*.
11. Vajpayee RB, Kumar A, Dada T, Titiyal JS, Sharma N, Dada VK. Phaco-chop versus stop-and-chop nucleotomy for phacoemulsification. *J Cataract Refract Surg*. 2000:1638–41.
12. Can I, Takmaz T, Çakici F, Özgül M. Comparison of Nagahara phaco-chop and stop-and-chop phacoemulsification nucleotomy techniques. *J Cataract Refract Surg*. 2004;30:663–668.

13. Chang DF. Making the case for phaco chop. *Review of Ophthalmology*. 2003;10:47–50.
14. Leaming D. Practice styles and preferences of ASCRS member—2003 Survey. *J Cataract Refract Surg*. 2004;30:892–900.
15. Agarwal A, Agarwal S, Agarwal A. Phakonit: lens removal through a 0.9 mm incision. (Letter) *J Cataract Refract Surg*. 2001;27:1531–1532.
16. Tsuneoka H, Takuya S, Takahashi Y. Feasibility of ultrasound cataract surgery with a 1.4 mm incision. *J Cataract Refract Surg*. 2001;27:934–940.
17. Agarwal A, Agarwal S, Agarwal A. Phakonit and laser phakonit: lens removal through a 0.9 mm incision. In: Agarwal S, Agarwal A, Sachdev MS, et al, eds. *Phacoemulsification, Laser Cataract Surgery and Foldable IOLs*. 2nd ed. New Delhi: Jaypee Brothers; 2000:204–216.
18. Alió JL. Microincision Cataract Surgery [MICS] Improves Safety, Surgeon Says. *Ocular Surgery News*. December 1, 2001.
19. Vejarano LF, Tello A, Vejarano A. The safest and most effective technique for cataract surgery. *Highlights of Ophthalmology*. 2004;32(2):13–19.
20. Vejarano LF, Tello A. Outcomes with the ThinOptx IOL. Using the lens as part of Microincisional Cataract Surgery. *Cataract & Refractive Surgery Today*. Sept. 2004, 84.
21. Lane S, Fine H. Perspectives in Lens & IOL Surgery. Getting to the bottom of clear cornea incisions – Part I. *Eye World*. October 2004.
22. Arshinoff SA. Dispersive-cohesive viscoelastic soft shell technique. *J Cataract Refract Surg*. 1999;25:167–173.
23. Horiguchi M, Miyake K, Ohta I, Ito Y. Staining of the lens capsule for circular continuous capsulorrhexis in eyes with white cataract. *Arch Ophthalmol*. 1998;116:535–537.
24. Melles G, de Waard P, Pameyer J, Beekhuis W. Trypan blue capsule staining to visualize the capsulorhexis in cataract surgery. *J Cataract Refract Surg*. 1999;25:7–9.
25. Dada V, Sharma N, Sudan R, Sethi H, Dada T, Pangtey MS. Anterior capsule staining for capsulorhexis in cases of white cataract Comparative clinical study. *J Cataract Refract Surg*. 2004;30:326–33.
26. Arshinoff SA. Using BSS with viscoadaptatives in the ultimate soft-shell technique. *J Cataract Refract Surg*. 2002;28:1509–1514.
27. Fine IH. Choo-choo chop and flip with the soft-shell technique is safer, more efficient. *Ocular Surgery News*. 1998;16(8):23–25.
28. Fine IH. The choo-choo chop and flip phacoemulsification technique. *Operative Tech Cataract Refract Surg*. 1998;1:61–65.
29. Fine IH, Packer M, Hoffman RS.Use of power modulations in phacoemulsification. Choo-choo chop and flip phacoemulsification. *J Cataract Refract Surg*. 2001;27(2):188–97.
30. Chang D. Phaco chop techniques: comparing horizontal vs vertical chop. *Highlights of Ophthalmology*. 2004;32:4:11–13.
31. Chang DF. *Phaco Chop: Mastering Techniques, Optimizing Technology, and Avoiding Complications*. Thorofare, NJ: SLACK Incorporated; 2004.

II
Difficult Cases

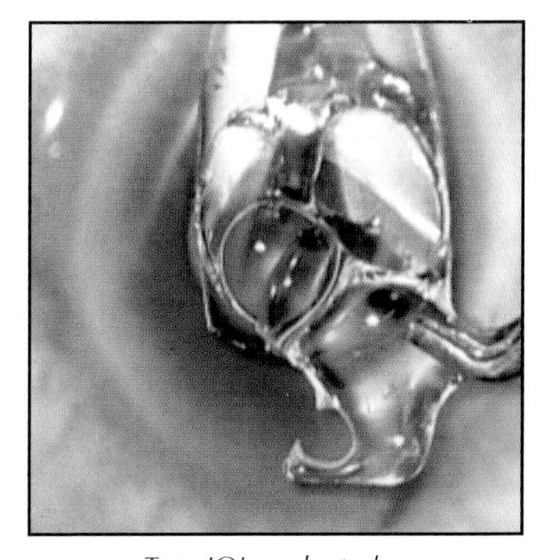

Torn IOL explanted.

Chapter 6

PRINCIPLES AND PARADIGMS OF PEDIATRIC CATARACT SURGERY AND INTRAOCULAR LENS IMPLANTATION

Suresh K. Pandey, MD; M. Edward Wilson, MD

INTRODUCTION

Congenital, early developmental, and traumatic cataracts are common ocular ailments and represent an important cause of visual impairment in childhood.[1–254] Managing cataracts in children remains a challenge; treatment is often difficult, tedious, and requires a dedicated team effort by the parents, pediatrician, surgeon, anesthesiologist, orthoptist, and community health workers. The surgeon plays a significant role in achieving a good visual outcome following the treatment of childhood cataracts.[2]

DIAGNOSIS OF PEDIATRIC CATARACTS

Congenital, developmental, and traumatic cataracts can have different morphological characteristics (Figures 6-1 through 6-3, Table 6-1). These have been reviewed extensively by several authors.[3–5] A thorough ocular and systemic examination is mandatory in every child for the accurate diagnosis of the type of cataract. Ocular examination should include the visual acuity assessment, ocular motility, pupillary response, and posterior segment evaluation. When feasible, biomicroscopic examination of the anterior segment should be performed to evaluate the size, density, and location of the cataract in order to plan the surgical procedure and to determine the visual outcome. Fundus examination should be carried out after pupillary dilatation. A-scan ultrasound helps to measure the axial length for calculating the intraocular lens (IOL) power and monitoring the globe elongation postoperatively. For an eye with total cataract, a B scan evaluation is useful for detection of vitreoretinal pathology. A history from the parents is useful to determine whether the cataract could be congenital, developmental, or traumatic in origin. One must ascertain if there is any history of maternal drug use, infection, or exposure to radiation during pregnancy. Each child should be thoroughly examined by a pediatrician to rule out systemic associations, anomalies, or congenital rubella. This is essential, as the cataract surgery in children is usually performed under general anesthesia.

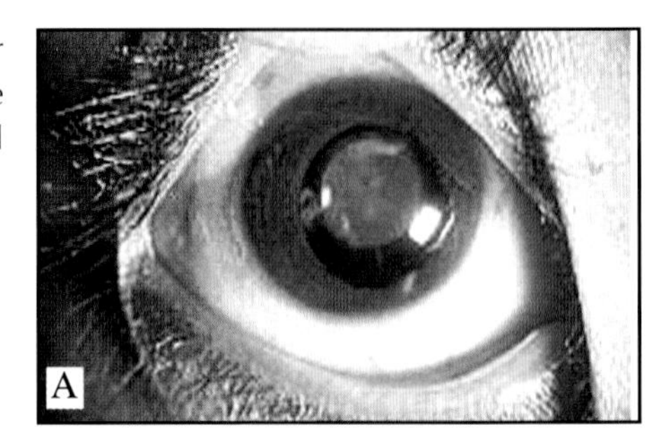

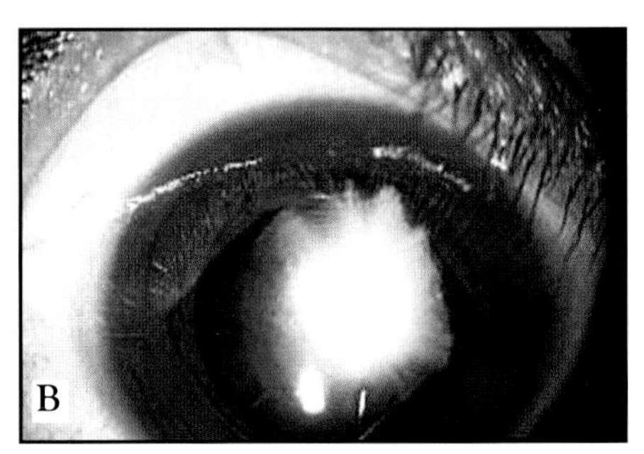

Figure 6-1 A,B. Slit-lamp photographs of zonular cataracts taken from different cases. Note that the lenticular opacity is occupying the central visual axis.

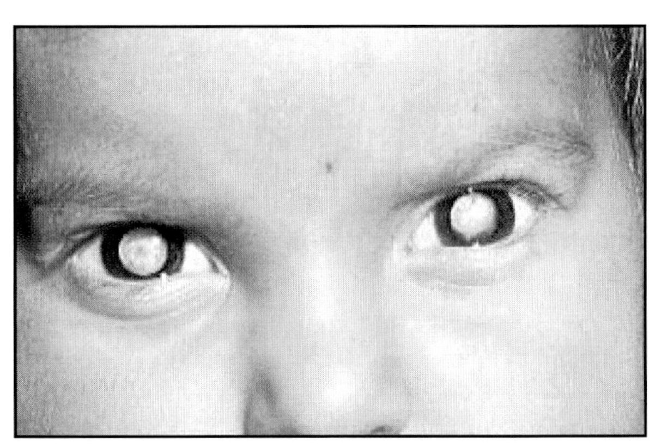

Figure 6-2. Clinical photograph showing bilateral total infantile cataracts in a 9-month-old female child. As opposed to the usual age-related cataract of adults, untreated cataracts of childhood are especially unfortunate since the individual is often doomed to long-term suffering. An early surgical intervention and prompt optical rehabilitation is mandatory in order to prevent irreversible deprivational amblyopia.

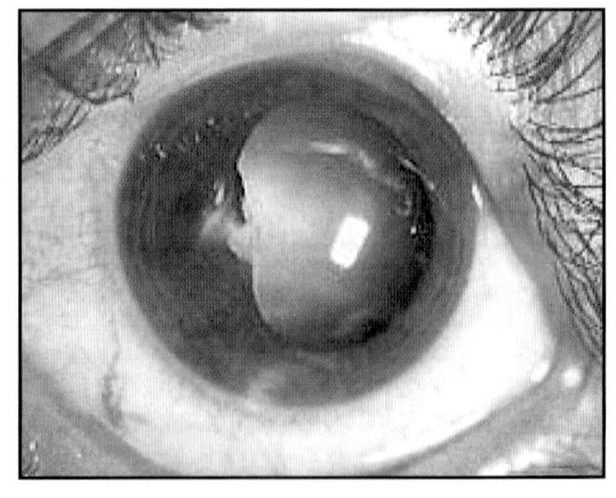

Figure 6-3. Pediatric uniocular cataract following blunt and penetrating trauma. Slit-lamp photograph of the anterior segment of a 6-year-old male child showing traumatic cataract after blunt trauma (firecracker injury). Note the formation of a posterior synechia at 3 o'clock position.

Table 6-1.

Characteristics of Pediatric Cataracts

Congenital/Developmental	*Traumatic*
Total/Diffuse: Uncommon; Rubella cataracts; Bilateral; Variable Visual Prognosis. **Anterior Polar**: Unilateral or bilateral; Sporadic; Opacity <3mm; Usually nonprogressive; Good Visual Prognosis. **Lamellar/Zonular**: Bilateral; Partial; Opacity 5-6mm; Good Visual Prognosis. **Nuclear**: Autosomal Dominant in many; Bilateral (80%); Nonprogressive; Opacity 3.5mm; Moderate visual prognosis. **Posterior Lentiglobus**: Unilateral; Good visual prognosis. **Persistent Hyperplastic Primary Vitreous (PHPV)**: Unilateral; Sporadic and progressive; Poor visual prognosis (when posterior segment involvement present).	**Total/Diffuse** **Anterior Subcapsular** **Posterior Subcapsular** **Intumescent** **Ruptured Anterior Capsule with Flocculent Lens Matter in Anterior Chamber** **Partially Absorbed**
Etiology Idiopathic, Hereditary, Congenital Rubella Syndrome, Galactosemia, Lowe's Syndrome, TORCH Infection. **Associated Ocular Findings**: Strabismus, Amblyopia, Anisometropia, Microphthalmia, Microcornea, Peter's Anomaly, Excessive Elongation of the Globe.	*Etiology* **(Blunt/Penetrating Trauma)** Sports-related Bow and arrow Sticks Firecrackers Thorn **Associated Ocular Findings:** Corneal Lacerations, Hyphema, Angle Recession, Vitreous Hemorrhage, Posterior Capsule Rupture, Retinal Detachment, Berlin's Edema.

Cataract Surgery in Children

How Does Pediatric Cataract Surgery Differ From Adult?

Difficulties are encountered during pre-, intra- and postoperative periods. Preoperative difficulties include late diagnosis, associated conditions like prematurity and systemic disorders. Risk factors for general anesthesia need serious consideration. Intraoperative difficulties are caused as a result of smaller size of the eye, sometimes poorly dilating pupil, highly elastic anterior capsule, low scleral rigidity and dense vitreous giving rise to raised intra vitreal and lenticular pressure. Postoperative examination requires repeated short anesthesia. Propensity for increased postoperative inflammation and capsular opacification, a refractive state that is constantly changing due to growth of the eye, difficulty in documenting anatomic and refractive changes due to poor compliance, and a tendency to develop amblyopia are the factors that make cataract surgery in the child different from that in the adult.[6–11]

In sharp contrast to the treatment of adult cataracts, the timing of cataract surgery in children is of paramount importance. It affects the visual result to a much greater extent than the surgical technique or method of postoperative optical correction utilized by the surgeon. In a young child, a cataract blurs the image received by the retina and disrupts the development of the visual pathways in the central nervous system. In addition to causing amblyopia, visual deprivation can disrupt the process of emmetropization. Abnormal axial growth has been reported even in the absence of amblyopia as a result of the effects of unequal visual inputs to the two eyes.

Despite these differences, improved surgical techniques that are largely a reflection of adult cataract surgery and the advances in postoperative optical rehabilitation have significantly improved the prognosis of cataract surgery in children.[12]

Indications for Treatment

In order to avoid the development of deprivational amblyopia, prompt diagnosis and treatment are necessary for visually significant cataract in neonate, infants, or toddlers.[12] Indications for surgery in these eyes include: cataracts of more than 3 mm in diameter (visually significant), dense nuclear cataracts, cataracts obstructing the examiner's view of fundus or preventing refraction of patient, if the contralateral cataract has been removed, and cataracts associated with strabismus and/or nystagmus.[8,9,13–15]

When children beyond infancy present with dense, central opacities of uncertain duration and Snellen visual acuity cannot be accurately measured, surgery is indicated within a few weeks of detection. Nonsurgical methods such as patching or pharmacological pupillary dilation can be useful to manage partial cataracts.

The threshold for surgical removal of a partial cataract in a child capable of Snellen visual acuity has often been stated to be 20/70 or 20/80. Use of vision charts, eg, Lea Hyvarinen symbol charts, is extremely useful in assessment of the visual status in a young child unable to read. However, individual judgments need to be made (especially in children too young for Snellen visual acuity testing) based on documented progression of the partial cataract and on the child's visual functioning, visual needs, and expected best visual outcome. When possible, low contrast sensitivity testing may provide a helpful guideline for deciding either the need for cataract surgery or treatment for posterior capsule opacification (PCO).

Optical Rehabilitation

Correction of pediatric aphakia can be accomplished with spectacles, contact lenses, epikeratophakia, or IOL implants (Figure 6-4).[16–18] Currently the contact lenses (in infants) and IOLs (in older children) are preferred. In infants, whichever method of optical correction is chosen, it is important to get a reasonably well-focused image on the retinas as early as possible.

Aphakic Glasses

Spectacle correction is safest and their power can be readily changed to compensate for ocular growth. They can be worn at any age and are not unduly expensive. Their magnifying effect may improve the child's acuity and make microphthalmic eyes appear normal size. Spectacles can be the only form of optical correction that is available in a community and most children using contact lenses should have a pair of aphakic glasses as a spare, for when they are not able to use contact lenses. A child wearing contact lenses, or with an IOLs, will need bifocals if his or her acuity is not good enough. Spectacles, however, have the disadvantage of poor cosmesis and inferior optics (Figure 6-4). They cause alteration in the peripheral field of vision by inducing distortion and prismatic effects. An infant's ear and nose are often too insubstantial to support aphakic glasses. In addition, obtaining centration with heavy aphakic glasses is difficult and the optical center of the lens does not move with the eye. Although they provide a satisfactory correction for many children with bilateral aphakia, aphakic spectacles are generally not suitable for children with unilateral aphakia because of marked retinal image size disparity (approximately 30% magnification).

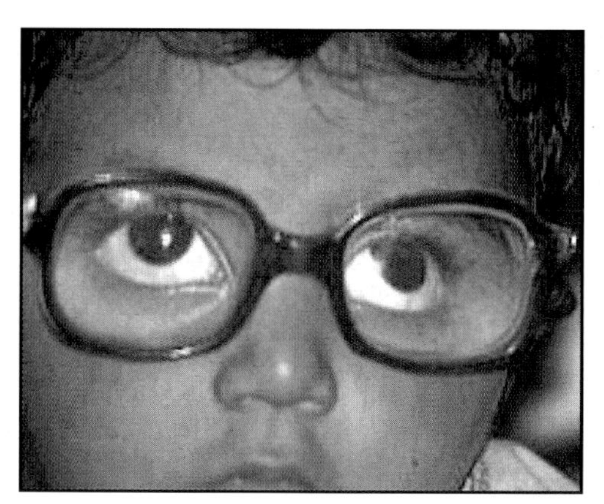

Figure 6-4. Visual rehabilitation in an infant after bilateral cataract surgery using aphakic glasses. Thick and heavy aphakic glasses are not suitable for the infant's nose and facial structure. They are also cosmetically inferior to other modalities (contact lenses/IOLs) of optical corrections.

Contact Lenses

There are three choices of contact lens type for pediatric patients: the hard lens, including polymethylmethacrylate (PMMA) and rigid gas-permeable (RGP) lenses, the hydrogel extended wear or daily wear lens, and the silicone lens. Most of the problems of aphakic spectacles can be overcome by the use of contact lenses. Their power can also be easily adjusted according to the growth of the eye.[19,20]

The RGP contact lenses have the advantage of low cost and can be customized in regards to power and base curve. Their disadvantage is that they must be removed daily and are more difficult for the parents to insert. The hydrogel or soft contact lenses have comfort as their main advantage. These lenses are tolerated in a wide range of base curvatures and thus they are easily fitted. However, insertion difficulties coupled with instability and fragility lead to high damage and lens loss rates. Extended wear poly HEMA lenses have proven to be the lenses of choice for children with unilateral aphakia. They are fairly stable with reduced lens loss rates.

Silicone contact lenses (Silsoft, Bausch & Lomb, Rochester, NY) combine the best features of hard and soft lenses. They are reported to mask up to 2 diopter (D) of astigmatism in the adult. Like the hard lenses, they are easy to handle, have a relatively low loss rate, and can be fitted using either measurement or trial techniques. Most children under the age of 1 year can be fitted with a lens of 7.50 base curve. Older children are most often fit with a base curve of 7.70. A fluorescein pattern may be used during the fitting sequence as needed. Lens movement with blinking is the most critical and important factor to evaluate during fitting. If too much movement is seen, a steeper lens can be tried. If little or no movement is seen, a flatter lens is indicated.

Unique problems facing the fitter of contact lenses in young aphakic children include their small eyes, steep corneas, and high hyperopia. Their continuously changing refraction, primarily related to an increasing axial length and progressive corneal flattening provides an additional challenge. Repeated insertion and removal of a contact lens can be psychologically traumatic to the child. The major disadvantage of contact lenses for the correction of aphakia is the frequency of lens loss.[10] In addition to lens loss, noncompliance is a major problem, particularly in children using contact lenses for correction of monocular aphakia. Assaf and coworkers[21] reported that only 44% of children with unilateral aphakia were wearing their contact lens during their follow-up visits. Loss of lenses, conjunctival erythema, and poor fit were reasons for noncompliance in these cases. With noncompliance comes increased amblyopia and sensory strabismus. Other problems associated with contact lens use, more commonly encountered in patients in developing countries, who often come from rural communities with poor socioeconomic and educational background, include infective keratitis, corneal vascularization, hypoxic corneal ulcerations, and red eye without ulcerations.[22]

Epikeratophakia

Epikeratophakia was introduced in the early 1980s as an alternative means of optically correcting aphakic eyes. It is a refractive corneal surgical technique in which a lathed lamellar corneal disc is sutured to the front surface of the recipient's cornea after removal of the recipient's epithelium. Epikeratophakia corrects the refractive error by changing the anterior curvature of the cornea. Advantages of this technique are that no damage occurs to the recipient's central cornea, it is reversible, entirely extraocular, and may be employed with cataract extraction or as a secondary procedure. Problems like graft failure due to persistent epithelial defects, infections or mechanical trauma are common with this technique. In addition, sutures must be removed after 3 weeks, often necessitating another anesthetic procedure. Amblyopia therapy is generally delayed until 4 to 6 weeks after the initial operation. Epikeratophakia for correcting pediatric aphakia has fallen into disuse due to the difficulty in achieving the target refracting power and the prolonged haziness of the host donor interface.

Intraocular Lens Implantation

Problems such as contact lens intolerance, downward displacement of the lens with induced vertical diplopia, aniseikonia (approximately 6% with contact lenses), and traumatic corneal scars have prompted some investigators to advocate IOL implants for pediatric aphakia.[3–14]

Why Are IOLs Preferred for Pediatric Cataract Surgery?

Several reasons can be cited for the increased use of IOLs in children. The three most important are:

1. First, appropriately sized (11.5 to 12.0 mm), more flexible implants made from PMMA and acrylic foldable materials are now available and can be inserted much more easily into the capsular bag of the child. Despite their increased flexibility, newer lens designs retain enough "memory" to resist the intense equatorial capsular fibrosis seen in children after implantation. In addition, PMMA as an implant material now has a track record of biocompatibility that extends to 30 or more years. Heparin surface modification of PMMA has increased its biocompatibility even more.[44] Also, copolymerization of different acrylate and methacrylate acids has resulted in foldable lenses that have retained the biocompatibility features of PMMA. As an example, foldable acrylic lenses, such as the AcrySof (Alcon) are also being implanted into children's eyes with greater frequency. The biocompatibility of the acrylic lenses may equal or exceed the tried PMMA lenses. The foldable acrylic lenses are easier to insert in a small eye, and the squared edge of the AcrySof IOL optic design result in delayed PCO in young eyes.
2. The second reason for the increased use of IOLs in children is the improved understanding of the surgical principles and refinements in surgical techniques that have ensured capsular fixation of an IOL even over the extended life span of a child. Capsular fixation provides sequestration of the implant away from vascularized tissues. Although ciliary sulcus fixation of the IOL may also be safe with short follow-up, uveal contact for a lifetime is not desirable. In addition, complications such as pupillary capture and IOL decentration are more common with ciliary sulcus fix-

ation. The preference for capsular fixation over ciliary sulcus placement has resulted in more IOLs being implanted in children at the time of cataract extraction, even at very young ages.

3. Finally, customized management of the anterior and posterior capsules for pediatric eyes at the time of implantation has improved outcomes and decreased complications.

How Important Is Intraocular Lens Sizing?

The mean axial length of a newborn's eye is 17.0 mm compared to 23 to 24 mm in an adult. The pediatric eye, especially in the first 1 to 3 years of life, is significantly smaller than the adult. This has led to concerns with implantation of adult-sized IOLs in these patients. Currently available adult-sized IOLs are slightly oversized in relation to capsular bag measurements, but may actually fit into the eye in the first 2 years of life, although possibly not in very small infantile eyes. The small capsular bag may ovalize with these adult sized IOLs. What are the possible consequences of implantation of the adult-sized IOL in the relatively small capsular bag of infants and young children? Firstly, in contrast to adult cataract surgery, dialing of the IOL haptics into the capsular bag can be difficult in infants. Often one of the IOL haptics will dial out of the capsular bag rather than into it, leading to asymmetric (bag-sulcus) fixation, which can lead to decentration of the IOL. Secondly, implantation of an oversized IOL in the capsular bag of an infant may cause marked capsular bag stretching, resulting in posterior capsular folds and striae. The lens epithelial cells may migrate toward the visual axis, through the capsular folds, leading to opacification of the posterior capsule. Thirdly, implantation of an oversized IOL in the capsular bag of an infant may cause zonular stress in the direction parallel to the IOL haptics. The long-term sequelae of the capsular bag stretching (and also the zonular stress) in the axial growth of the globe must be further investigated.

Surgical Techniques

Historical Perspective

Table 6-2 summarizes the major advances influencing the pediatric cataract surgery procedure during the last three decades that considerably popularized the use of IOL implantation in children.[7,156–158]

Anesthesia

Most pediatric cataract surgeries are done under general endotracheal anesthesia. Thus, the occurrence of vomiting in the early postoperative period is not uncommon. This, along with inevitable rubbing of eyes, helps to justify the use of sutures to close the surgical wound even if it appears to be self-sealing. Children also have a very active Bell's phenomenon if they become somewhat light under anesthesia. For this reason, many pediatric surgeons still use a superior rectus traction suture during cataract surgery.

Table 6-2.
Evolution of Pediatric Cataract Surgery

Advances	Year	Authors
First implant in a child for the aphakic correction	1958	Choyce[29]
Manual aspiration of congenital/juvenile cataract	1960	Scheie[30]
Iridocapsular implant	1969	Binkhorst[31]
Binkhorst Intraocular Lenses (IOLs)	1977-82	Hiles[32]
Posterior Chamber IOLs	1982	Hiles[33]
Iris-claw lenses	1983	Singh[34]
Pathophysiology of amblyopia	1977-85	Weisel/Raviola[35]
Posterior Chamber IOLs	1983-93	Sinskey/Hiles[36,37]
Posterior Capsulotomy/Anterior Vitrectomy	1983	Parks[38]
Epikeratophakia	1986	Morgan[39]
Epilenticular IOL/Pars Plana Endocapsular Lensectomy	1988	Tablante[40]
Retropseudophakic vitrectomy via limbus	1991	Mackool/ Chhatiawala[41]
Retropseudophakic vitrectomy + posterior capsulectomy via pars plana	1993	Buckley et al[42]
Primary posterior capsulorrhexis/Optic capture	1994	Gimbel/DeBroff[43]
IOL biomaterials/Designs/Sizing in children	1994	Wilson et al[27]
Primary posterior capsulotomy and anterior vitrectomy	1994-96	BenEzra/Cohen[45] Koch/Kohnen
Anterior capsulotomy for pediatric cataract surgery	1994 (vitrectorhexis),	Wilson et al[46] Auffarth et al[47] (rabbit model)
Heparin in BSS to decrease postoperative inflammation	1995	Brady et al[8]
Dye-enhanced pediatric cataract surgery	2000	Pandey/Werner[56-58]

Wound Construction

Children have thin sclera and markedly decreased scleral rigidity when compared with adults. Scleral collapse results in increased vitreous upthrust (positive vitreous pressure). Collapse of the anterior chamber and prolapse of iris tissue are also much more common when operating on pediatric eyes. Pediatric cataracts can be removed through a relatively small wound, as the lens can be removed in toto because there is usually no formed nucleus. Therefore, wounds should be constructed to provide a snug fit for the instruments that pass into the anterior chamber. When an IOL is not being implanted, two stab incisions are usually made at or near the limbus. These incisions should not be larger than necessary for the instruments being used. For instance, a micro vitreoretinal (MVR) blade creates a 20-gauge opening that is ideal for a 20-gauge vitrector/aspirator to enter the anterior chamber. A 20 gauge blunt-tipped irrigating cannula can also be used through a separate MVR blade stab incision. If the instrument positions need to be reversed, the snug fit is maintained. An anterior chamber entry of 3 mm or less can facilitate manual anterior capsulotomy and cortical aspiration with a phacoemulsification or irrigation/aspiration handpiece. When a rigid IOL is being implanted, a scleral tunnel wound is utilized most often. A half-thickness scleral incision is made initially approximately 2 or 2.5 mm from the limbus and dissected into clear cornea. It is enlarged to the size necessary for IOL insertion. Scleral tunnel wounds decrease the incidence of iris prolapse into the wound during surgery and assist the surgeon in preventing collapse of the anterior chamber, which occurs with greater frequency in the soft eyes of children. Unlike adults, scleral tunnel incisions do not self-seal in children.[173]

According to the study by Basti et al,[174] self-sealing wounds failed to remain watertight in children below 11 years of age, especially when an anterior vitrectomy was combined with cataract extraction. In older (>11 years) children, the wounds remained self-sealing. The authors attributed this to low scleral rigidity resulting in fish mouthing of the wound leading to poor approximation of the internal corneal valve to the overlying stroma. Closure is recommended using a synthetic absorbable suture such as 10-0 Biosorb or Vicryl. When a foldable IOL is being implanted, a corneal tunnel is preferred because it leaves the conjunctiva undisturbed. The corneal tunnel should begin near the limbus (so-called "near clear" incision) for maximum healing and should be sutured with a synthetic absorbable suture.

While the temporal wound presents the same advantages in children as it does in adults, the location is more easily traumatized by children. The superior approach allows the wound to be protected by the brow and the Bell's phenomenon in the trauma-prone childhood years. Both scleral tunnels and corneal tunnels can be easily made from a superior approach because children rarely have deep set orbits or overhanging brows. Locating the site of tunnel according to the pre-existing astigmatism (eg, temporally in against-the-rule astigmatism) can help in reducing the astigmatic component in the postoperative treatment of amblyopia.

Viscoelastic Substances

A high molecular weight viscoelastic substance such as sodium hyaluronate 14 mg/per ml (Healon GV, Pharmacia Corp, Peapack, NJ) is most commonly used in pediatric cataract surgery to effectively resist the increased tendency for anterior chamber collapse due to decreased scleral rigidity and a positive vitreous pressure. This viscoelastic helps to maintain a deep anterior chamber and a lax anterior capsule, facilitating attempts at manual anterior capsulorrhexis. Also, the initially convex posterior capsule is effectively held back during IOL insertion. We have also recently evaluated the use of viscoelastic with even higher viscocity, sodium hyaluronate 23 mg/per ml (Healon 5, Pharmacia Corp) during pediatric cataract surgery. This viscoadaptive appears to be useful during various steps of pediatric cataract surgery. Without a high molecular weight viscoelastic, an IOL inserted in a manner acceptable for an adult eye will result in inadvertent sulcus placement secondary to the posterior vitreous pressure and posterior capsule convexity. The trabecular meshwork of children clears viscoelastic substances more easily, on average, than in adults. However, efforts should still be made to remove all of the viscoelastic material since postoperative intraocular pressure spikes have been documented when Healon GV is inadequately removed.[175]

Anterior Capsule Management

Manual Continuous Curvilinear Capsulorrhexis

Gimbel and Neuhann[176] advocated continuous tear anterior capsulotomy (CCC) technique for small-incision adult cataract surgery in the mid-1990s. During the same time, capsular bag fixation of a posterior chamber IOL placed at the time of cataract surgery became commonplace for children older than age 2. Because manual CCC had become the standard anterior capsulotomy technique in adults, it was naturally also applied to the pediatric age group, but with mixed success.

Clinically, it became evident that the pediatric lens capsule is more elastic than in adults and requires increased force before tearing begins. Laboratory investigations have now verified a markedly higher fracture toughness and extensibility in pediatric anterior capsule as compared to elderly adults. In addition, reduced scleral rigidity results in posterior vitreous upthrust when the eye is entered. This vitreous "pressure" pushes the lens anteriorly and keeps the anterior lens capsule taut. Surgeons found more difficulty completing an intact circular capsulotomy. The so-called "runaway rhexis" became all too common. In addition, a capsulotomy that started out small would end up much larger than intended. This result was also due to the marked elasticity of the child's anterior capsule. Performing an intact CCC is challenging in young children even for an experienced surgeon.

Can-Opener Anterior Capsulotomy

To avoid the difficulties with CCC in children, some surgeons have returned to the can-opener style capsulotomy when operating on children. It is difficult to draw a firm conclusion about can-opener anterior capsulotomy in pediatric eyes, especially in regards to performance and radial tear formation following. However, radial tears have been documented in nearly 100% of adult eyes when the can-opener capsulotomy is used. The radial tear rate may be less with the highly elastic capsules of children but it has not been adequately studied. Decentration has been documented pathologically in up to 50% of adult eyes implanted after a can-opener style anterior capsulotomy. Since children have much greater tissue reactivity and more intense equatorial capsular fibrosis, asymmetric loop fixation would be expected to cause decentration at a higher rate in children than in adults.

Vitrector-Cut Anterior Capsulectomy (Vitrectorhexis)

When creating a vitrectorhexis, the following surgical caveats are offered. Use a vitrector supported by a Venturi pump. Peristaltic pump systems will not cut anterior capsule easily. Use an infusion sleeve or a separate infusion port, but with either approach, maintain a snug fit of the instruments in the incisions through which they are placed. The anterior chamber of these soft eyes will collapse readily if leakage occurs around the instruments, making the vitrectorhexis more difficult to complete.

An MVR blade can be used to enter the eye. The vitrector and the blunt-tip irrigating cannula (Nichamin cannula, Storz, St. Louis, MO) fit snugly into the MVR openings. Do not begin the capsulotomy with a bent-needle cystotome. Merely place the vitrector, with its cutting port positioned posteriorly, in contact with the center of the intact anterior capsule. Turn the cutter on and increase the suction using the foot pedal until the capsule is engaged and opened. A cutting rate of 150 to 300 cuts per minute and an aspiration maximum of 150 to 250 (these settings are for the Alcon Accurus and the Storz Premier—adjustments may be needed for other machines) are recommended. With the cutting port facing down against the capsule, the authors then enlarge the round capsular opening to the desired shape and size. Any lens cortex that escapes into the anterior chamber during the vitrectorhexis is aspirated easily without interrupting the capsulotomy technique. Care should be taken to avoid leaving any right-angle edges, which could predispose to radial tear formation. The completed vitrectorhexis should be slightly smaller than the size of the IOL optic being implanted. The vitrector creates a slightly scalloped edge, but inspection by both the dissecting microscope and the scanning electron microscope has revealed that the scallops roll outward to leave a smooth edge.[182] Any capsular tags or points created at the apex of a scalloped cut from the vitrector are located in an area of low biomechanical stress, much like an irregular outside-in completion of a CCC. These tags do not predispose to radial tear formation as demonstrated by finite element method computer modeling.

Bipolar Radiofrequency Capsulotomy

Radiofrequency diathermy capsulotomy, developed by Kloti et al,[183] has been used as an alternative to CCC for intumescent adult cataracts, and for cataract surgery in children. The Kloti device cuts the anterior capsule with a platinum-alloy-tipped probe using a high frequency current of 500 kHz. The probe tip is heated to about 160° C and produces a thermal capsulotomy as it is moved in a circular path across the anterior capsule. Small gas bubbles are formed while the tip is active, but these do not usually interfere with visibility during the capsulotomy. Gentle pressure must be maintained on the capsule with the tip as it moves either clockwise or counterclockwise. If contact is too light or movement too fast, skipped areas will result. If contact is too firm or movement too slow, the tip will burn through the capsule and enter the lens cortex. Subsequent tip movement drags the capsulotomy edge rather than cutting it, which may cause radial tearing. However, the preferred rate of movement and firmness of capsule contact is quickly learned after a few cases. Even when performed perfectly, a diathermy-cut capsulotomy can be seen to have coagulated capsular debris along the circular edge. In addition, this edge has been shown experimentally to be less elastic than a comparable CCC edge. Since the stretching force needed to break the edge of a diathermy-cut capsulotomy is much reduced compared to a CCC edge, surgical manipulations needed to remove a cataract and place an IOL may result in more radial tears when the diathermy is used. However, the experimental measurements were all made on adult autopsy globes. It is well known that the pediatric capsule responds differently. In fact, Comer et al[184] reported no radial tears when using the diathermy-cut capsulotomy in 14 eyes of 7 children whose mean age was 23 months. Clinically, the diathermy devise is useful in children for both the anterior and posterior capsules. However, the diathermy edge tears more easily than when vitrector or manual CCC techniques are used.

Fugo Plasma Blade Anterior Capsulotomy

The Fugo plasma blade has also been recently introduced as a radiofrequency unit that can be used to perform an anterior capsulectomy (Figure 6-5). The Fugo blade capsulotomy unit is a portable electronic system that operates on rechargeable batteries and provides an alternative to capsulorrhexis. This unit is user friendly and may be clipped to the surgeon's belt or may rest on a countertop. The Fugo blade provides an anterior capsulotomy that requires no red reflex and usually requires less that 10 seconds to perform. The unit also allows the surgeon to easily revise the size of the capsulotomy openings. The instrument developer reports that the Fugo blade is easy to use and does not have a steep learning curve.[255]

The Fugo blade may be particularly suited for the highly elastic capsule of children. Because it cuts the capsule with a "plasma blade", it may not suffer from the tendency for skip areas seen with the Kloti radiofrequency device. However, the edge of a Fugo blade capsulotomy will not likely perform better than the Kloti diathermy edge when stretched.

Lens Substance Removal

Pediatric cataracts are soft. Phacoemulsification is rarely, if ever, needed. Lens cortex and nucleus are usually easily aspirated with an irrigation/aspiration or vitrectomy handpiece. When using the vitrector, bursts of cutting can be used intermittently to facilitate the aspiration of the more "gummy" cortex of young children. The phacoemulsification handpiece can also be very useful when aspirating pediatric lens material. Hydrodissection[185,186] has been thought to be less useful in children than in adults. However, a recent study[103] has shown the intraoperative benefits of performing multi-quadrant hydrodissection. The benefits are overall reduction in the operative time, and the amount of irrigating solution used and facilitation of lens substance removal.[256] A fluid wave can sometimes be generated in older children but not reliably in infants and toddlers. Cortical material strips easily from the pediatric capsule even in the absence of hydrodissection. Attempts at hydrodelineation should be discouraged in children because it does not aid in lens removal and may lead to capsular rupture.

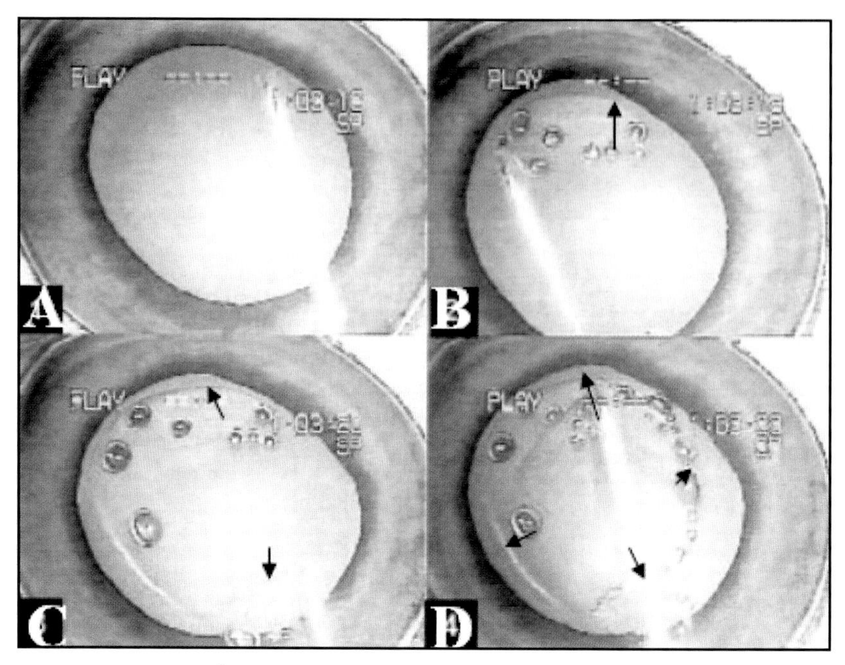

Figure 6-5. Anterior capsulotomy using the Fugo Plasma Blade. **A–D**. Various steps of anterior capsulotomy in a porcine eye model. (Modified from original article: Roy H. Course for Fugo blade is enlightening, surgeon says. *Ocular Surgery News*, September 1, 2001, with permission.)

Primary Intraocular Lens Implantation

Capsular fixation of the IOL is strongly recommended for children.[78,158] Care should be taken to avoid asymmetric fixation with one haptic in the capsular bag and the other in the ciliary sulcus. In contrast to adults, dialing of an IOL into the capsular bag can be difficult in children. An oversized IOL (adult IOL—12 to 12.5 mm) along with the vitreous upthrust often cause the IOL to vault forward, which results in its dialing out of the capsular bag. On the other hand, sulcus fixation of an IOL in a child appears to be easy but the long-term consequences of contact with vascularized uveal tissue is a cause for concern. To minimize the iris-optic contact, lens decentration and to reduce the possibility of erosion into the ciliary body, prolapse of the optic through an intact anterior or posterior capsulotomy is suggested when sulcus fixation of an IOL in a child is necessary.

Secondary Intraocular Lens Implantation

The vast majority of children undergoing secondary IOL implantation have had a primary posterior capsulectomy and anterior vitrectomy. If adequate peripheral capsular support is present, the implant is placed into the ciliary sulcus. Since the sulcus is only 0.5 to 1.0 mm larger than the evacuated capsular bag, most IOLs designed for capsular fixation can also be placed in the ciliary sulcus. Viscodissection is often all that is needed to break synechia between the iris and residual capsule. Both the AcrySof acrylic lens and the all-PMMA lenses have been used by the authors for sulcus fixation in the child.[257] Our current recommendations are to place an all-PMMA heparin-surface-modified IOL rather than an acrylic lens when sulcus placement is required. Prolapsing the IOL optic through the fused anterior and posterior capsule remnants is useful in preventing pupillary capture and assuring lens centration. In some cases, the anterior and posterior capsular remnants can be dissected apart, allowing the IOL to be placed in the capsular bag.[89] An exuberant Soemmering's ring formation will often separate the anterior and posterior capsule leaflets and maintain the peripheral capsular bag. This material can be aspirated cleanly after the anterior capsule edge is lifted off of the posterior capsular edge to which it is usually fused.

When inadequate capsular support is present for sulcus fixation in a child, implantation of an IOL is not recommended unless every contact lens and spectacle option has been fully explored. Although their long-term safety is unknown, modern flexible open loop anterior chamber lenses seem to be well tolerated in children when their anterior segment is developmentally normal. Scleral fixation of posterior chamber IOLs in children have been well tolerated according to some recent studies, but complications such as pupillary capture, suture erosion, and refractive error from lens tilt or anterior/posterior displacement have been reported.[79,90,125] The ab-externo approach is recommended for trans-scleral suture placement in children.

Management of the Posterior Capsule

Management of the pediatric posterior capsule, especially when implanting an IOL at the time of the primary surgery, remains controversial.[187] Several surgical techniques have been used by various surgeons to maintain the long-term clear visual axis.

Primary Posterior Capsulotomy and Anterior Vitrectomy

Primary posterior capsulectomy and anterior vitrectomy during pediatric lensectomy were popularized by Parks in the early 1980s.[83] This led to a dramatic decrease in the need for secondary surgery for congenital cataracts. Pediatric ophthalmologists are accustomed to removing a portion of the posterior capsule and the anterior vitreous at the time of lensectomy. An increase in late complications from primary capsulectomy and vitrectomy has not been reported. Adult cataract surgeons are often more reluctant to perform a primary capsulectomy and vitrectomy for fear that the risk of retinal detachment or cystoid macular edema will be increased. In fact, these complications are exceedingly rare after pediatric cataract surgery with or without a primary capsulectomy and vitrectomy. Neodymium: YAG laser posterior capsulotomy is usually necessary in children when the posterior capsule is left intact. This procedure also carries a risk of retinal detachment and cystoid macular edema. In addition, larger amounts of laser energy are often needed when compared to adults and the posterior capsule opening may close, requiring repeated laser treatments or a secondary pars plana membranectomy.

Posterior Capsulorrhexis with Intraocular Lens Optic Capture

Gimbel and DeBrof[61,188,189] recommend performing a posterior capsulorrhexis with IOL optic capture. This technique is designed to help prevent secondary membrane formation without necessitating a vitrectomy.[190] It also ensures centration of the posterior chamber IOL because the haptics remain in the capsular bag and the optic is captured in the posterior capsular opening opening (Figure 6-6). Vasavada and Trivedi[116] also reported a better centration of the IOL following optic capture. However, they have also expressed concern regarding the resultant increased predisposition to uveal inflammatory sequelae. The same authors,[116] along with other surgeons,[66,67] have reported opacification of the visual axis despite optic capture. Thus, they recommend performing an anterior vitrectomy even when optic capture is utilized through the posterior capsulorrhexis.

Neodymium (Nd): YAG Laser Posterior Capsulotomy

Atkinson and Hiles,[191] on the other hand, recommended leaving the posterior capsule intact even in very young children and performing Neodymium: YAG capsulotomy under a second general anesthesia in the early postoperative period.

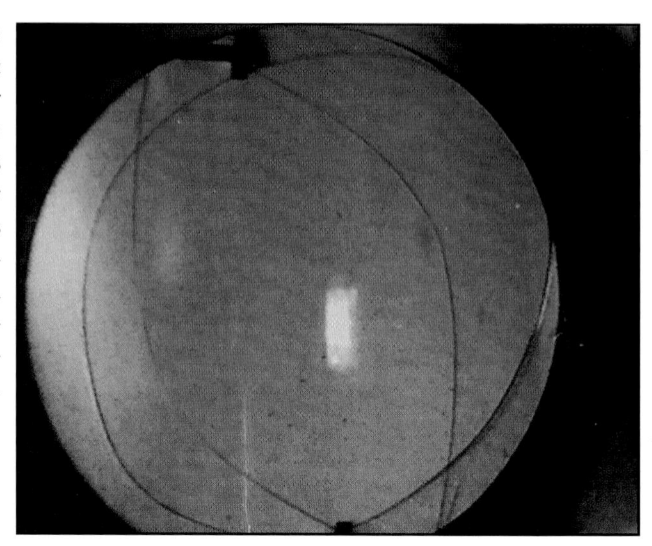

Figure 6-6. Photograph of an eye implanted with an acrylic (AcrySof) IOL in the capsular bag. IOL optic capture through a posterior capsulorrhexis was performed during the primary procedure. This photograph was taken at 1 month postoperatively and shows well-centered IOL and anterior and posterior capsulorrhexis edges. (Photo courtesy of A.R. Vasavada, MD, FRCS, Ahmedabad, India.)

Options for Primary Posterior Capsulotomy

When a decision is made to perform a primary posterior capsulotomy, several options are available.[189,192–194] The posterior capsular opening can be made using a manual posterior continuous curvilinear capsulorrhexis (PCCC) technique or using an automated vitrector or the Kloti radiofrequency bipolar unit. The manual technique and the mechanized vitrector technique can each be performed either before or after the IOL has been placed in the eye. When the vitrector is used after the IOL has been placed, it is usually done via the pars plana. The radiofrequency bipolar unit is not easily manipulated beneath an IOL and is therefore usually performed on the posterior capsule from an anterior approach prior to IOL insertion. In most instances, an anterior vitrectomy is performed simultaneously with the posterior capsulectomy.

Dye-Enhanced Pediatric Cataract Surgery

Use of capsular dyes such as 2% fluorescein sodium, 0.5% indocyanine green (ICG), and 0.1% trypan blue for staining the anterior capsule while performing CCC in white/advanced adult cataract cases is well known. We recently reported our experience of anterior capsule staining for performing CCC in postmortem human eyes with advanced/white cataracts.[80] We also reported the use of capsular dyes to enhance visualization to learn and perform other critical steps of the phacoemulsification procedure, and posterior capsulorrhexis, respectively.[81,195, 258,259] Learning the PCCC procedure (and achieving a consistent size of posterior capsule opening for performing the optic capture) can be difficult for the beginning surgeon due to the thin and transparent nature of the posterior capsule. According to our experimental studies, posterior capsulorrhexis (with or without the optic capture) is relatively easy to perform after staining of the otherwise transparent posterior capsule (Figures 6-7A and 6-7B). The procedure of optic capture with or without anterior vitrectomy can also be accomplished easily after staining the posterior capsule.[81] It is easier to localize an inadvertent tear of the posterior capsule when staining of the posterior capsule has been utilized (Figure 6-7C).

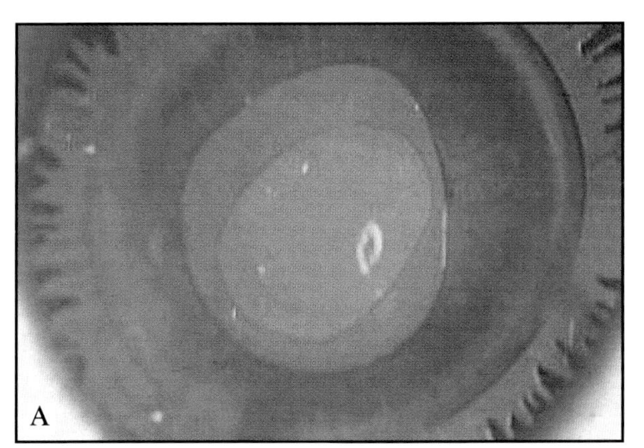

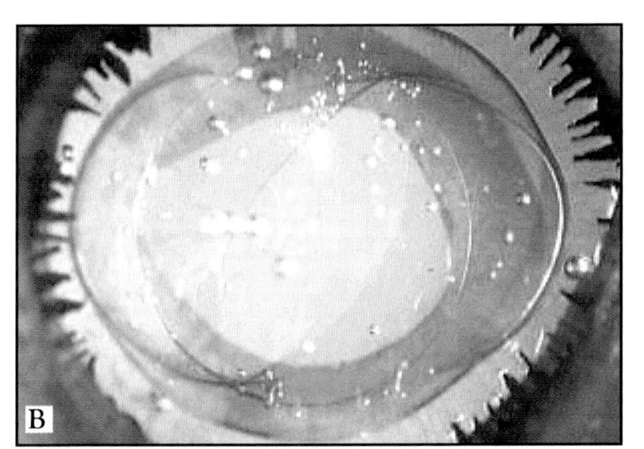

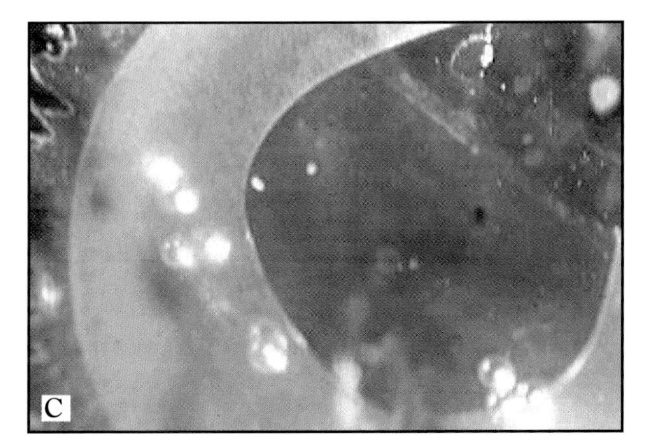

Figure 6-7 A–C. Photographs of a pediatric eye obtained postmortem, taken from anterior (surgeon's view) illustrating the use of the capsular dye to enhance visualization during various steps of the pediatric cataract surgery. **A**. Posterior capsulorrhexis after the staining of the capsular bag with trypan blue. **B**. Posterior capsulorrhexis and optic capture of a foldable IOL after the staining of the capsular bag with trypan blue. **C**. Visualization of a posterior capsule tear after staining of the capsular bag with indocyanine green.

Pediatric Traumatic Cataracts and Their Management

Epidemiology and Etiology

Traumatic cataract in children is a common cause of unilateral loss of vision.[196] Incidence of traumatic cataract in children is reported as high as 29% of all childhood cataracts.[197] Penetrating injuries are usually more common than blunt injuries. Eighty percent of traumatic cataract cases occur in children while playing or when they are involved in sports-related activities. Injuries are also caused by thorns, firecrackers, sticks, or bow and arrows.[198]

Surgical Management

At the time of presentation after the trauma to the eye, primary repair of the corneal or scleral wound is usually preferred. Cataract surgery with IOL implantation is performed later following complete evaluation of damage to the intraocular structures (eg, posterior capsule rupture, vitreous hemorrhage, and retinal detachment) by ancillary methods such as B-scan ultrasonography.[199] Some authors report PC-IOL implantation at the same time as primary repair of corneal lacerations and removal of traumatic cataract.[5] We think repair of corneal or scleral wounds combined with primary IOL implantation should be considered in younger children at the risk of developing amblyopia. Implantation of IOL is preferred in the cases of traumatic cataracts with corneal injuries, because contact lenses may be difficult to fit.[200]

Perioperative and Postoperative Treatment

The perioperative routine includes a drop of 5% povidone iodine at the beginning and at the end of the surgical procedure. It is better to avoid using a miotic at the completion of surgery because this can create increased anterior segment inflammation. Topical steroid/antibiotic and atropine ointment are put in the eye, and a light patch and fox shield placed over the eye. Beginning the next morning, topical steroid drops six times a day and atropine 1% eyedrops once per day for 4 weeks are recommended. A topical antibiotic is added for the first several days. The atropine eyedrops regimen is stopped at 4 weeks and the topical steroid tapered and discontinued. The atropine is sometimes avoided when an IOL is placed in the ciliary sulcus to reduce the chances of pupillary capture. Glasses or an eye shield are worn over the eye continuously for the first week.

Postoperative Complications and Management

Complications associated with pediatric cataract surgery continue to be a major concern for the ophthalmic surgeon. The risk of postoperative complication is higher due to greater inflammatory response after pediatric intraocular surgery.[155] In many cases, these complications may be the primary reason for a poor visual outcome.[205] In some cases, the complications appear to be intrinsically related to associated ocular anomalies that coexist with the developmental cataract. Close follow-up, early detection and management of the complications are mandatory.

Early Onset

Uveitis

Postoperative anterior uveitis (fibrinous or exudative) is a common complication due to increased tissue reactivity in children.

Corneal Edema

Transient corneal edema may occur in pediatric cataract surgery but bullous keratopathy is a rare complication.[209] Cataract surgery does not cause significant endothelial cell loss in children. Reports on corneal endothelial cell count in pediatric aphakia and IOL implantation have shown no significant loss of endothelial cells.[19,114,210] Corneal decompensation may occur if detergents (eg, glutaraldehyde) are used for sterilization of cannulas or instruments and are not rinsed thoroughly before use in the anterior chamber. Indeed, cannulas or tubing should not be sterilized in glutaraldehyde solution because residual chemicals may remain even after thorough rinsing.

Endophthalmitis

Endophthalmitis does occur after cataract extraction in children. It is a rare complication and appears to occur with the same frequency as in adult cataract patients. The prevalence of endophthalmitis reported by Wheeler and associates[211] was 7/10,000 cases, after pediatric cataract surgery. Common organisms are *Staphylococcus aureus, Staphylococcus epidermidis* and *Staphylococcus viridence*. Nasolacrimal duct obstruction, periorbital eczema, and upper respiratory tract infections are important risk factors.[212]

Noninfectious Inflammation

Jameson and colleagues[213] have described a benign syndrome of excessive noninfectious postoperative inflammatory response in young aphakic children. This syndrome presents with excessive photophobia, tearing, and even the inability to open the eyes postoperatively. It may persist for days or even weeks and may preclude the early contact lens fitting that initiates amblyopic therapy. It is not clear whether steroids applied topically or injected into the sub-Tenon's space are efficacious in shortening this benign inflammatory process.

Intermediate/Late Onset

Capsular Bag Opacification

Opacification of the capsular bag universally occurs following pediatric cataract surgery. It includes opacification of the anterior, equatorial and posterior capsules. Excessive anterior capsule fibrosis and shrinkage of the CCC opening can lead to difficulty in examining the retinal periphery and occasionally the decentration of the IOL.[214]

Secondary Membrane Formation

Formation of secondary membranes is a common complication of pediatric cataract surgery, particularly after infantile cataract surgery.[82,216–218] Nd: YAG laser capsulotomy may be sufficient to open them in the early stage. More dense secondary membranes usually need membranectomy and anterior vitrectomy.[219] Pupillary membranes can occur postoperatively in children whether an IOL has been implanted or not. Microphthalmic eyes with microcoria operated in early infancy are at greatest risk, especially when mydriatic/cycloplegic agents have not been used postoperatively. When an IOL is in place, secondary membranes may form over the anterior and/or posterior surface of the implant. The incidence of secondary membranes after neonatal or infantile cataract surgery has been reduced dramat-

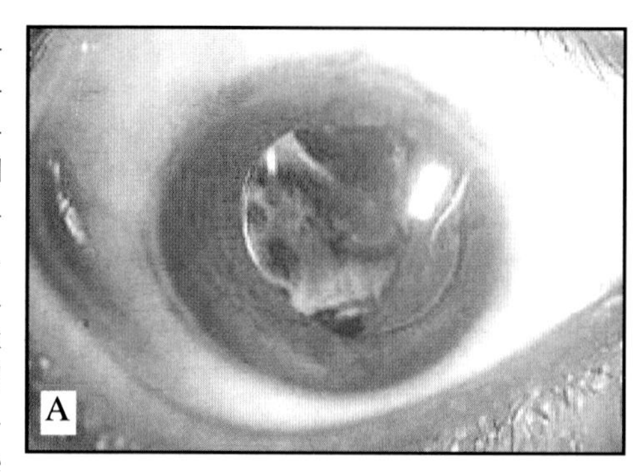

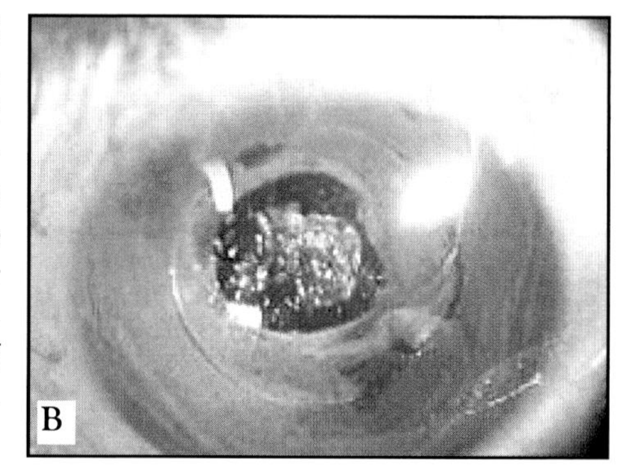

Figure 6-8. Pupillary capture and posterior capsule opacification after pediatric cataract surgery and IOL implantation. **A.** Slit-lamp photograph of the anterior segment of a 12-year-old female child 13 months after ciliary sulcus fixation of a posterior chamber intraocular lens. Note the marked pupillary capture of the IOL optic, extending from 12 o'clock to 5 o'clock associated with pupillo-capsular synechia and marked posterior capsule opacification. Best-corrected visual acuity was 6/24 in this eye due to posterior capsule opacification. It required Nd: YAG laser posterior capsulotomy. **B.** Clinical photograph of the eye of a 10-year-old girl, post PMMA posterior chamber IOL implantation. There is a marked pupillary capture. This is associated with marked posterior capsule opacification. Attempt to perform Nd: YAG laser failed, resulting in multiple pits on the IOL optic. This type of dense PCO is an indication of surgical posterior capsulotomy with anterior vitrectomy.

ically by the "no-iris-touch" aspect of the closed chamber surgery, by applying topical corticosteroids and cycloplegic agents at frequent intervals postoperatively and by performing posterior capsulectomy and an adequate anterior vitrectomy.

Pupillary Capture

Placing the IOL in the capsular bag helps to prevent pupillary capture, a complication that is much more common in children. It is associated with posterior synechia formation and PCO. Incidence of pupillary capture after pediatric cataract surgery varies from 8.5% to 41%. This was reported by several authors: Vasavada and Chouhan[114] in 33% (7 of 21 eyes), Basti et al[192] in 8.5% (7 of 82 eyes), Brady et al[48] in14.2% (3 of 20 eyes), and Bustos et al[52] in 10.5% (2 of 19 eyes). Pupillary capture occurs most often in children younger than 2 years of age, when an optic size less than 6 mm is used and the lens is placed in the ciliary sulcus. In a series of 20 cases of traumatic cataracts with PC-IOL implantation in children, Pandey et al[78] reported an incidence of pupillary capture as high as 40% in ciliary-sulcus fixated IOLs, while none of the eyes with in-the-bag fixation of the PC-IOL had this complication (Figures 6-8A and 6-8B). Pupillary capture can be left untreated if it is not associated with decreased visual acuity, IOL malposition, or glaucoma. However, surgical repair recreates a more round pupil shape and IOL centration. Fixation of PC-IOLs in the capsular bag (whenever possible) is recommended to decrease the incidence of this complication. Prolapsing the optic of a secondary sulcus fixated IOL through the anterior capsulorrhexis opening can also prevent pupillary capture.

Deposits on IOL Surface

Precipitates composed of pigments, inflammatory cells, fibrin, blood breakdown products, and other elements are often seen during the immediate postoperative period on the

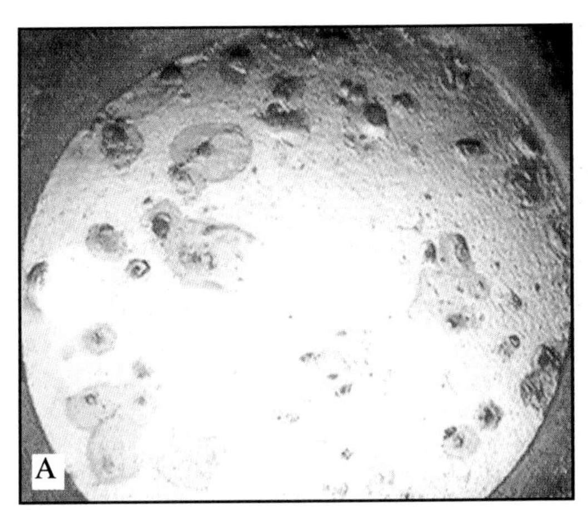

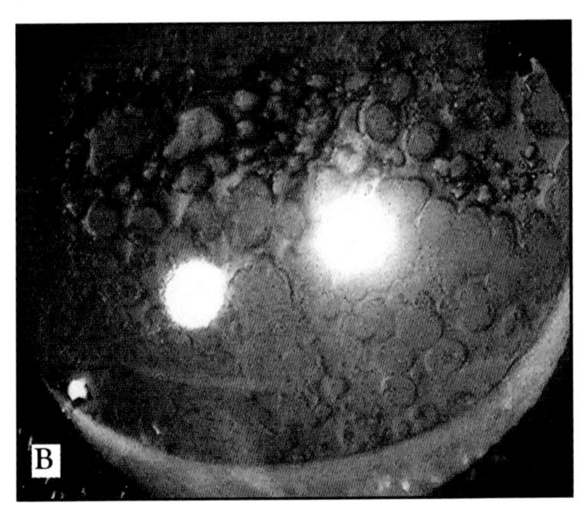

Figure 6-9 A,B. Slit-lamp photographs showing pigment deposition surface of two different IOLs. This complication is not uncommon after pediatric cataract surgery and usually does not cause a decrease in visual acuity. (Photos courtesy of A.R. Vasavada, MD, FRCS, Ahmedabad, India.)

surface of an IOL optic implanted in a child (Figures 6-9A and 6-9B). The deposits can be pigmented or nonpigmented, but are usually not visually significant. They occur much more commonly in children with a dark iris, and when compliance with postoperative medications has been poor. Heparin-surface-modified IOLs have been reported to decrease the incidence of these deposits. The site of IOL implantation can also influence the formation of deposits. Vasavada and Trivedi[116] have found that the incidence of deposits was higher in eyes with the IOL optic captured through the PCCC in comparison with the bag fixated IOLs.

IOL Decentration

Decentration of an IOL can occur because of traumatic zonular loss and/or inadequate capsular support. Capsular bag placement of the IOL is the most successful way to reduce this complication. Posterior capture of the IOL optic also resulted in better centration of the implanted IOL. Incidence of lens malposition in pediatric eyes following posterior chamber IOL implantation was reported as high as 40%.[30] Asymmetric IOL fixation, with one haptic in the capsular bag and the other in the ciliary sulcus, can also lead to decentration and should therefore be avoided. Complete IOL dislocation can occur after trauma. Explantation or repositioning of the IOL may be necessary in some cases presenting with significant decentration/dislocation.

Glaucoma

Pediatric aphakic/pseudophakic glaucoma remains a challenge. Its etiology, pathogenesis, incidence, onset, diagnosis, and successful treatment often confuses the surgeon. The incidence of glaucoma varies from 3% to 32%.[220–225] Although microphthalmic eyes appear to be at the highest risk, cataract surgery before 1 year of age, congenital rubella, and poorly dilated pupils are other important risk factors and should alert the treating ophthalmologist.

Glaucoma occurring soon after surgery is usually due to pupillary block or peripheral anterior synechia formation. This form of glaucoma is rare in children. Vajpayee and coworkers[226] reported the development of pseudophakic pupillary block glaucoma in 16 children after PC-IOL implantation leading to irreversible visual loss in two of their patients. These authors emphasized the necessity of stringent and frequent follow-up for pseudophakic children. Peripheral iridectomy may prevent pupillary block pseudophakic glaucoma. For this reason, some authors recommend that all children having PC-IOLs undergo peripheral iridectomy when there is rupture of the posterior capsule or zonular dehiscence, which may predispose to vitreous plugging. The majority of pediatric cataract surgeons, however, do not routinely perform peripheral iridectomy at the time of cataract surgery.

The most common type of glaucoma that develops after pediatric cataract surgery is open-angle glaucoma. Unlike angle-closure glaucoma, which usually develops soon after surgery, open angle glaucoma is usually seen later, emphasizing the need for life-long follow-up of these children. The reported mean interval from the time of cataract surgery until the detection of glaucoma ranged from 6 years to as long as 56 years.[227] A deep anterior chamber, increased pigmentation of the trabecular meshwork, and the iris inserting into the posterior aspect of the trabecular meshwork are generally seen during the gonioscopic examination. Cataract surgery may accelerate the development of glaucoma in certain eyes that are predisposed to develop open-angle glaucoma.

The diagnosis of glaucoma may be difficult to establish in children after cataract surgery.[228] IOP should be periodically recorded to detect and treat this vision-threatening complication. This may be difficult to measure with the child awake, and view of the optic disc may be compromised by lens remnants, miosis, and nystagmus. Further, it is difficult to assess the visual field until later in childhood. An excessive loss of hyperopia may be the sign of glaucoma in children following cataract surgery as noted by Egbert and Kushner.[223] Asrani and Wilsensky[220] have recommended a screening examination for glaucoma after pediatric cataract surgery every 3 months during the first postoperative year, twice yearly until the tenth year, and annually thereafter. Medical treatment should be tried first to lower the intraocular pressure, but a glaucoma filtering surgery with antimetabolites or a drainage implant are often required to control the intraocular pressure.

Retinal Detachment

The incidence of retinal detachment following pediatric cataract surgery has been reported between 1 to 1.5%. The interval from infantile cataract surgery to retinal detachment ranged from 23 to 34 years according to some authors.[229–231] The significant risk factors for occurrence of retinal detachment are high myopia and repeated surgeries. Retinal detachments following infantile cataract surgery are usually secondary to oval or round holes along the posterior vitreous base. These are difficult to repair in children due to poor visualization and retinal degeneration. Most reported cases have a history of multiple reoperations performed in the years prior to the introduction of automated lensectomy and vitrectomy. The incidence appears to be decreasing as surgical techniques advance and evolve.

Cystoid Macular Edema

Cystoid macular edema (CME) is a rare complication following pediatric cataract surgery, probably due to healthy retinal vasculature.[232,233] Because of the difficulty of performing fluorescein angiography during infancy, surgeons seldom evaluate children for this complication. Hoyt and Nickel[234] in 1982 reported that the development of CME was common in infantile eyes after lensectomy and anterior vitrectomy, but the appearance of the lesions was atypical and they were not documented photographically. The following year, Gilbard and co-workers[235] reported no CME in 25 eyes after pars plicata removal of congenital cataracts. No subsequent paper has documented clinically significant CME after pediatric cataract surgery even when an anterior vitrectomy is performed.

Hemorrhagic Retinopathy

This complication may occur following infantile cataract surgery in up to one-third of eyes as reported by Mets and Del Monte.[236] It presents with flame-shaped retinal hemorrhages and may be associated with concurrent vitreous hemorrhage.[237] The hemorrhages develop during the first 24 hours following surgery, are nonprogressive, and resolve within a few weeks.

Residual Refractive Error

Uncorrected aphakia after pediatric cataract surgery can cause or worsen amblyopia. When a child is left aphakic, every effort should be made to minimize time intervals when the prescribed aphakic glasses or aphakic contact lenses are not worn. Even short intervals of uncorrected aphakia are potentially very damaging to the prognosis.[238–242] When an IOL is implanted, a smaller amount of residual hyperopia may be present. Correction of residual hyperopia and any significant astigmatic error is necessary to optimize visual development and recovery from amblyopia. Some surgeons prefer to correct children to emmetropia with an IOL even at young ages to minimize the amblyogenic effects of residual hyperopia. Since young children's eyes continue to grow axially after cataract surgery and IOL implantation, significant late myopia will be more and more common as the years pass, especially if emmetropia is achieved early in life with an IOL.[243–245] Glasses or contact lenses will be used for correction of secondary myopia in most cases. However, the development of new corneal and intraocular refractive procedures will provide new options for correcting significant late myopia.

Piggyback Foldable Intraocular Lenses in Infants

Polypseudophakia (piggyback IOLs) has been used as a means to provide appropriate optical correction for patients requiring high IOL power or for secondary correction of an undesirable postoperative refraction after cataract surgery. It has been successfully used in adult patients since it was first reported by Gayton and Sanders, and Gills.[246] One of us (MEW), implanted piggyback AcrySof lenses in infantile eyes to manage the changing refractive status of these patients. This procedure, called "temporary polypseudophakia", may help in the prevention and treatment of amblyopia by avoiding residual hyperopia.[247] The posterior lens is implanted in the capsular bag and the anterior lens is placed in the ciliary sulcus. Within 12 to 24 months after the primary surgical procedure, the lens implanted in the ciliary sulcus is explanted/exchanged. To date, 15 infantile eyes have had this procedure successfully.[260] Long-term results would help us to further evaluate this modality of refractive correction after pediatric cataract surgery.

Management of Amblyopia

The postoperative compliant occlusion therapy of the normal eye in cases of unilateral congenital, developmental or traumatic cataract may be needed to reverse or prevent amblyopia in visually immature children.[149,248–254] Pharmacological penalization may be useful in children with amblyopia secondary to unilateral aphakia. Wheeler et al[243] found poor compliance of amblyopia therapy in one-third of the children having PC-IOLs. A best-corrected visual acuity of 20/40 or better was achieved only in 33% of eyes in their series. Noncompliance of occlusion therapy appears to be a major barrier in achieving satisfactory visual outcome during the treatment of amblyopia.

Summary

Pediatric cataracts are common and represent one of the most treatable causes of visual impairment in this population. Management of cataract in children is different from the adult because of increased intraoperative difficulties, propensity of postoperative inflammation, changing refractive state of the eye, difficulty in documenting anatomic and refractive changes due to poor compliance, and a tendency to develop amblyopia. Adoption of different techniques for cataract surgery in children is a must due to a low scleral rigidity, increased elasticity of the anterior capsule, and positive vitreous pressure. Early surgical intervention and adequate visual rehabilitation is necessary to avoid irreversible visual damage secondary to amblyopia. Aphakic glasses are not desirable for the long-term correction of pediatric aphakia because of many disadvantages associated with their use. Although contact lenses offer many advantages over aphakic spectacles, there are problems of infection, lens loss, and a low compliance. Current practice for providing full time correction of pediatric aphakia is shifting toward implantation of intraocular lenses due to refined and perfected microsurgical techniques, as well as the availability of suitable rigid and foldable implant designs. Main postoperative complications noted following pediatric cataract surgery include fibrinous uveitis, pupillary capture, aphakic glaucoma, pigment and cellular deposits on the implants, posterior capsule opacification or secondary membrane formation, and residual refractory error. These side effects may develop after many years. Therefore, it is crucial to follow children closely on a long-term basis after pediatric cataract surgery.

Key Points

1. In sharp contrast to the treatment of adult cataracts, the timing of cataract surgery in children is of paramount importance.
2. In order to avoid the development of deprivational amblyopia, prompt diagnosis and treatment are necessary for visually significant cataract in neonate, infants or toddlers. Indications for surgery in these eyes include: cataracts of more than 3 mm in diameter (visually significant), dense nuclear cataracts, cataracts obstructing the examiner's view of fundus or preventing refraction of patient, if the contralateral cataract has been removed and cataracts associated with strabismus and/or nystagmus.
3. Clinically, it became evident that the pediatric lens capsule is more elastic than in adults and requires increased force before tearing begins.
4. Capsular fixation of the IOL is strongly recommended for children.
5. Prolapsing the IOL optic through the fused anterior and posterior capsule remnants is useful in preventing pupillary capture and assuring lens centration.

REFERENCES

1. Apple DJ, Ram J, Foster A, Peng Q. Elimination of cataract blindness: A global perspective entering the new century. *Surv Ophthalmol.* 2000;45;S1.
2. Astle WF, Gimbel HV, Levin AV: Who should perform pediatric cataract surgery? *Can J Ophthalmol.* 1998;33:132–3.
3. Jain IS, Pillai P, Gangwar DN, et al. Congenital cataract: Etiology and morphology. *J Pediatr Ophthalmol Strabismus.* 1983;20:238–42.
4. Jain IS, Pillai P, Gangwar DN, et al. Congenital cataract: Management and results. *J Pediatr Ophthalmol Strabismus.* 1983;20:242–6.
5. Lambert SR, Drack AV. Infantile cataracts. *Surv Ophthalmol.* 1996;40:427–8.
6. Basti S, Greenwald MJ. Principle and paradigms of pediatric cataract management. *Indian J Ophthalmol.* 1995;43:159–76.
7. Hamill MB, Koch DD. Pediatric cataracts. *Curr Opin Ophthalmol.* 1999;10:4–9.
8. Nelson LB, Wagner RS. Pediatric cataract surgery. *Int Ophthalmol Clin.* 1994;34:165–9.
9. Nelson LB. Diagnosis and management of cataracts in infancy and childhood. *Ophthalmic Surg.* 1984;15:688–97.
10. Neumann D, Weissman BA, Isenberg SJ, et al. The effectiveness of daily wear contact lenses for the correction of infantile aphakia. *Arch Ophthalmol.* 1993;111:927–30.
11. Obstbaum SA. Cataract surgery and intraocular lens implantation in the pediatric patient. *J Cataract Refract Surg.* 1994;20:577.
12. Linebarger EJ, Hardten DR, Shah GK, Lindstrom RL. Phacoemulsification and modern cataract surgery. *Surv Ophthalmol.* 1999;44:123–47.
13. France TD, Frank JW. The association of strabismus and aphakia in children. *J Pediatr Ophthalmol Strabismus.* 1984;21:223–6.
14. Gelbart SS, Hoyt CS, Jastrebeski G, Marg E. Long-term results in bilateral congenital cataract. *Am J Ophthalmol.* 1982;93:615–21.
15. Helveston EM. Infantile cataract surgery. *Int Ophthalmol Clin.* 1977;17:75–82.
16. Ainsworth JR, Cohen S, Levin AV, Rootman DS. Pediatric cataract management with variations in surgical technique and aphakic optical correction. *Ophthalmology.* 1997;104:1096–1101.
17. Amaya LG, Speedwell L, Taylor D. Contact lenses for infant aphakia. *Br J Ophthalmol.* 1990;74:150–4.
18. Kaufman HE. The correction of aphakia. XXXVI Edward Jackson Memorial Lecture. *Am J Ophthalmol.* 1980;89:1–10.
19. Baker JD. Visual rehabilitation of aphakic children. *Surv Ophthalmol.* 1990;34:366–71.
20. Lorenz B, Worle J. Visual results in congenital cataract with the use of contact lenses. *Graefes Arch Clin Exp Ophthalmol.* 1991;229:123–32.
21. Assaf AA, Wiggins R, Engle K, et al. Compliance with prescribed optical correction in cases of monocular aphakia in children. *Saudi J Ophthalmol.* 1994;8:15–22.
22. Ram J, Pandey SK, Jain A, Gupta A. Intraocular lens implantation in infantile cataract. In: Pasricha JK, ed. *Indian Ophthalmology: Yearbook.* New Delhi, India: Aravali Publishers;1998:123–5.
23. Dahan E. Lens implantation in microphthalmic eyes of infants. *Eur J Implant Refract Surg.* 1989;1:9–11.
24. Dahan E, Salmenson BD, Levin J. Ciliary sulcus reconstruction for posterior implantation in the absence of an intact posterior capsule. *Ophthalmic Surg.* 1989;20:776–80.
25. Davies PD, Tarbuck DT. Management of cataracts in infancy and childhood. *Trans Ophthalmol Soc UK.* 1977;97:148–52.
26. Drummond GT, Scott WE, Keech RV. Management of monocular congenital cataract. *Arch Ophthalmol.* 1989;107:45–51.

27. Gieser SC, Apple DJ, Loftfield K, et al. Phthisis bulbi after intraocular lens implantation in a child. *Can J Ophthalmol.* 1985;20:184–5.
28. Hiles DA, Watson BA. Complications of implant surgery in children. *J Am Intra-Ocular Implant Soc.* 1979;5:24–32.
29. Hiles DA. Implant surgery in children. *Int Ophthalmol Clin.* 1979;19:95–123.
30. Hiles DA. Intraocular lens implantation in children with monocular cataracts. 1974–1983. *Ophthalmology.* 1984;91:1231–7.
31. Hiles DA. Intraocular lens implantation in children. *Ann Ophthalmol.* 1977;9:789–97.
32. Hiles DA. Intraocular lenses in children. *Int Ophthalmol Clin.* 1977;17:221–42.
33. Hiles DA. Peripheral iris erosions associated with pediatric intraocular lens implants. *J Am Intra-Ocular Implant Soc.* 1979;5:210.
34. Hiles DA. The need for intraocular lens implantation in children. *Ophthalmic Surg.* 1977;8:162–9.
35. Hiles DA. Visual acuities of monocular IOL and non-IOL aphakic children. *Ophthalmology.* 1980;87:1296–1300.
36. Hiles DA. Visual rehabilitation of aphakic children. III. Intraocular lenses. *Surv Ophthalmol.* 1990;34:371–79.
37. Hing S, Speedwell L, Taylor D. Lens surgery in infancy and childhood. *Br J Ophthalmol.* 1990;74:73–7.
38. Keech RV, Toungue AC, Scott WE. Complications after surgery for congenital and infantile cataracts. *Am J Ophthalmol.* 1989;108:136–41.
39. Menezo JL, Esteve JT, Perez-Torregrosa VT. IOL implantation in children—17 years' experience. *Eur J implant Refract Surg.* 1994;6:251–6.
40. Menezo JL, Taboada JF, Ferrer E. Complications of intraocular lenses in children. *Trans Ophthalmol Soc UK.* 1985;104:546–52.
41. Wilson-Holt N, Hing S, Taylor DS. Intraocular lens implantation for unilateral congenital cataract. *J Pediatr Ophthalmol Strabismus.* 1991;28:116–8.
42. Wilson ME, Bluestein EC, Wang XH. Current trends in the use of intraocular lenses in children. *J Cataract Refract Surg.* 1994;20:579–83.
43. Balyeat HD, Richard JM, Scott MH, Weir KD: Cataract surgery and intraocular lens implantation in children. *Am J Ophthalmol.* 1996;121:226–7.
44. Basti S, Aasuri MK, Reddy MK, et al. Heparin-surface-modified intraocular lenses in pediatric cataract surgery: prospective randomized study. *J Cataract Refract Surg.* 1999;25:782.
45. Biglan AW, Cheng KP, Davis JS, Gerontis CC. Results following secondary intraocular lens implantation in children. *Trans Am Ophthalmol Soc.* 1996;94:353–373.
46. Biglan AW, Cheng KP, Davis JS, Gerontis CC. Secondary intraocular lens implantation after cataract surgery in children. *Am J Ophthalmol.* 1997;123:224–34.
47. Blumenthal M, Yalon M, Treister G. Intraocular lens implantation in traumatic cataract in children. *J Am Intra-Ocular Implant Soc.* 1983;9:40.
48. Brady KM, Atkinson CS, Kilty LA, et al. Cataract surgery and intraocular lens implantation in children. *Am J Ophthalmol.* 1995;120:1–9.
49. Brar GS, Ram J, Pandav SS, et al. Postoperative complications and visual results in uniocular pediatric traumatic cataract. *Ophthalmic Surg Lasers.* 2001;32(3):233-8.
50. Buckley EG, Klombers LA, Seaber JH, et al. Management of the posterior capsule during pediatric intraocular lens implantation. *Am J Ophthalmol.* 1993;115:722.
51. Burke JP, Willshaw HE, Young JD. Intraocular lens implants for uniocular cataracts in childhood. *Br J Ophthalmol.* 1989;73:860.
52. Bustos FR, Zepeda LC, Cota DM. Intraocular lens implantation in children with traumatic cataract. *Ann Ophthalmol.* 1996;28:153.

53. Crouch, Jr. ER, Pressman SH, Crouch ER. Posterior chamber intraocular lenses: long-term results in pediatric cataract patients. *J Pediatr Ophthalmol Strabismus*. 1995;32:210–18.
54. Dahan E, Salmenson BD. Pseudophakia in children: precautions, techniques, and feasibility. *J Cataract Refract Surg*. 1990;16:75–82.
55. Devaro JM, Buckley EG, Awner S, Seaber J. Secondary posterior chamber intraocular lens implantation in pediatric patients. *Am J Ophthalmol*. 1997;123:24–30.
56. Eckstein M, Vijayalakshmi P, Killedar M, et al. Use of intraocular lens in children with traumatic cataract in south India. *Br J Ophthalmol*. 1998;82:911.
57. Ellis FD. Intraocular lenses in children. *J Pediatr Ophthalmol Strabismus*. 1992;29:71.
58. Ghosh B, Gupta AK, Taneja S, et al. Epilenticular lens implantation versus extracapsular cataract extraction and lens implantation in children. *J Cataract Refract Surg*. 1997;23(Suppl):612.
59. Gimbel HV, Basti S, Ferensowicz M, DeBroff BM. Results of bilateral cataract extraction with posterior chamber intraocular lens implantation in children. *Ophthalmology*. 1997;104:1737–43.
60. Churchill AJ, Noble BA, Etchells DE, George NJ. Factors affecting visual outcome in children following uniocular traumatic cataract. *Eye*. 1995;9:285–91.
61. Gimbel HV. Posterior continuous curvilinear capsulorrhexis and optic capture of the intraocular lens to prevent secondary opacification in pediatric cataract surgery. *J Cataract Refract Surg*. 1997;23(Suppl):652.
62. Greenwald MJ, Glaser SR. Visual outcomes after surgery for unilateral cataract in children more than two years old; posterior chamber intraocular lens implantation versus contact lens correction of aphakia. *J Am Assoc Pediatric Ophthalmol Strabismus*. 1998;2:168.
63. Gupta AK, Grover AK, Gurha N. Traumatic cataract surgery with intraocular lens implantation in children. *J Pediatr Ophthalmol Strabismus*. 1992;29:73.
64. Hutchinson AK, Wilson ME, Saunders RA. Outcomes and ocular growth rates after intraocular lens implantation in the first 2 years of life. *J Cataract Refract Surg*. 1998;24:846.
65. Knight-Nanan D, O'Keefe M, Bowell R. Outcome and complications of intraocular lenses in children with cataract. *J Cataract Refract Surg*. 1996;2:730.
66. Koch DD, Kohnen T. A retrospective comparison of techniques to prevent secondary cataract formation following posterior chamber intraocular lens implantation in infants and children. *Trans Am Ophthalmol Soc*. 1997;95:351.
67. Koch DD, Kohnen T. Retrospective comparison of techniques to prevent secondary cataract formation following posterior chamber intraocular lens implantation in infants and children. *J Cataract Refract Surg*. 1997;23(Suppl):657.
68. Koenig SB, Ruttum MS, Lewandowski MF, et al. Pseudophakia for traumatic cataracts in children. *Ophthalmology*. 1993;100:1218.
69. Koenig SB, Ruttum MS. Management of posterior capsule during pediatric intraocular lens implantation. *Am J Ophthalmol*. 1993;116:656.
70. Kora Y, Inatomi M, Fukado Y, et al. Long-term study of children with implanted intraocular lenses. *J Cataract Refract Surg*. 1992;18:485.
71. Kora Y, Shimizu K, Inatomi M, et al. Eye growth after cataract extraction and intraocular lens implantation in children. *Ophthalmic Surg*. 1993;24:467.
72. Lam DS, Ng JS, Fant DS, et al: Short-term results of scleral intraocular lens fixation in children. *J Cataract Refract Surg*. 1998;24:1474.
73. Mackool RJ, Chhatiawala H. Pediatric cataract surgery and intraocular lens implantation: a new technique for preventing or excising postoperative secondary membranes. *J Cataract Refract Surg*. 1991;17:62.
74. Malukiewicz-Wisniewska G, Kaluzny J, Lesiewska-Junk H, Eliks I. Intraocular lens implantation in children and youth. *J Pediatr Ophthalmol Strabismus*. 1999;36:129.
75. Markham RHS, Bloom PA, Chandna A, Newcomb EH. Results of intraocular lens implantation in pediatric aphakia. *Eye*. 1992;6:493.

76. Metge P, Cohen H, Chemila JF. Intercapsular implantation in children. *Eur J Cataract Refract Surg.* 1990;2:319.
77. Pandey SK, Ram J, Jain AK, Gupta A. Visual results and postoperative complications of capsular bag versus sulcus fixation of PC IOL implantation in traumatic cataracts in children. In: Pasricha JK, ed. *Indian Ophthalmology: Year book.* New Delhi, India: Aravali Publishers, 1998:135.
78. Pandey SK, Ram J, Werner L, et al. Visual results and postoperative complications of capsular bag versus ciliary sulcus fixation of posterior chamber intraocular lenses for traumatic cataract in children. *J Cataract Refract Surg.* 1999;25:1576.
79. Pandey SK, Wilson ME, Trivedi RH, et al. Pediatric cataract surgery and intraocular lens implantation: current techniques, complications and management. *Int Ophthalmol Clin.* 2001; 41:175.
80. Pandey SK, Werner L, Escobar-Gomez M, et al. Dye-enhanced cataract surgery. Part I. Anterior capsule staining for capsulorrhexis in advanced/white cataracts. *J Cataract Refract Surg.* 2000;26:1052.
81. Pandey SK, Werner L, Escobar-Gomez M, et al. Dye-enhanced cataract surgery. Part III. Staining of the posterior capsule to learn and perform posterior continuous curvilinear capsulorrhexis. *J Cataract Refract Surg.* 2000;26:1066.
82. Parks MM, Johnson DA, Reed GW. Long term visual results and complications in children with aphakia: a function of cataract type. *Ophthalmology.* 1993;100:826.
83. Parks MM. Posterior lens capsulectomy during primary cataract surgery in children. *Ophthalmology.* 1983;90:344.
84. Parks MM. Visual results in aphakic children. *Am J Ophthalmol.* 1982;94:441.
85. Pavlovic S, Jacobi FK, Graef M, Jacobi KW. Silicone intraocular lens implantation in children: preliminary results. *J Cataract Refract Surg.* 2000;26:88.
86. Peterseim MW, Wilson ME. Bilateral intraocular lens implantation in pediatric population. *Ophthalmology.* 2000;107:1261.
87. Rosenbaum AL, Masket S. Intraocular lens implantation in children. *Am J Ophthalmol.* 1995;120:105.
88. Rosenbaum AL, Masket S. Cataract surgery and intraocular lens implantation in children. *Am J Ophthalmol.* 1996;121:225.
89. Sharma A, Basti S, Gupta S. Secondary capsule-supported intraocular lens implantation in children. *J Cataract Refract Surg.* 1997;23:675.
90. Sharpe MR, Biglan AW, Gerontis CC. Scleral fixation of posterior chamber intraocular lenses in children. *Ophthalmic Surg Lasers.* 1996;27:337.
91. Simons BD, Siatkowski RM, Schiffman JC, et al. Surgical technique, visual outcome, and complications of pediatric intraocular lens implantation. *J Pediatr Ophthalmol Strabismus.* 1999;36:118.
92. Singh D. Intraocular lenses in children. *Indian J Ophthalmol.* 1984;32:499.
93. Singh D. Intraocular lenses in children. *Indian J Ophthalmol.* 1987;35:249.
94. Sinskey RM, Amin PA, Stoppel J. Intraocular lens implantation in microphthalmic patients. *J Cataract Refract Surg.* 18:480–4,1992
95. Sinskey RM, Karel F, Dal Ri E. Management of cataracts in children. *J Cataract Refract Surg.* 1989;15:196.
96. Sinskey RM, Patel J. Posterior chamber intraocular lens implants in children: report of a series. *J Am Intra-Ocular Implant Soc.* 1983;9:157.
97. Sinskey RM, Stoppel JO, Amin PA. Long-term results of intraocular lens implantation in pediatric patients. *J Cataract Refract Surg.* 1993;19:405.
98. Sinskey RM, Stoppel JO, Amin PA. Ocular axial length changes in a pediatric patient with aphakia and pseudophakia. *J Cataract Refract Surg.* 1993;19:787.
99. Spierer A, Desantik H. Refractive status in children after long-term follow-up of cataract surgery with intraocular lens implantation. *J Pediatr Ophthalmol Strabismus.* 1999;36:25.

100. Swinger CA. Comparison of results obtained with keratophakia, hypermetropic keratomileusis, intraocular lens implantation and extended wear contact lenses. *Int Ophthalmol Clin.* 1983;23:59.
101. Mullner-Eidenbock A, Amon M, et al. Morphological and functional results of AcrySof intraocular lens implantation in children: prospective randomized study of age-related surgical management. *J Cataract Refract Surg.* 200329:285.
102. Wilson ME, Pandey SK, Thakur J. Paediatric cataract blindness in the developing world: surgical techniques and intraocular lenses in the new millennium. *Br J Ophthalmol.* 2003;87:14–9.
103. Vasavada AR, Trivedi RH, Apple DJ, Ram J, Werner L. Randomized, clinical trial of multiquadrant hydrodissection in pediatric cataract surgery. *Am J Ophthalmol.* 2003;135:84–8.
104. Raina UK, Gupta V, Arora R, Mehta DK. Posterior continuous curvilinear capsulorrhexis with and without optic capture of the posterior chamber intraocular lens in the absence of vitrectomy. *J Pediatr Ophthalmol Strabismus.* 2002;39:278–87.
105. Jensen AA, Basti S, Greenwald MJ, Mets MB. When may the posterior capsule be preserved in pediatric intraocular lens surgery? *Ophthalmology.* 2002;109:324–7, discussion 328.
106. Jacobi PC, Dietlein TS, Konen W. Multifocal intraocular lens implantation in pediatric cataract surgery. *Ophthalmology.* 2001;108:1375–80.
107. O'Keefe M, Mulvihill A, Yeoh PL. Visual outcome and complications of bilateral intraocular lens implantation in children. *J Cataract Refract Surg.* 2000;26:1758–64.
108. Ahmadieh H, Javadi MA. Intra-ocular lens implantation in children. *Curr Opin Ophthalmol.* 2001;12:30–34.
109. Pandey SK, Wilson ME, Werner L, Apple DJ. Pediatric cataract-intraocular lens surgery: past, present and future. In: Garg A, Pandey SK, Sharma V, Apple DJ, eds. *Advances in Ophthalmology.* New Delhi, India: Jaypee Brothers; 2003:238–244.
110. Wilson ME. The challenge of pediatric cataract surgery. *JAAPOS.* 2001;5:265–6.
111. Tablante RT, Cruz EDG, Lapus JV, Santos AM. A new technique of congenital cataract surgery with primary posterior chamber intraocular lens implantation. *J Cataract Refract Surg.* 1988;14:149–157.
112. Thouvenin D, Arne JL, Lesueur L. Comparison of fluorine-surface-modified and unmodified lenses for implantation in pediatric aphakia. *J Cataract Refract Surg.* 1996;22:1226–31.
113. van der Pol BA, Worst JG. Iris-claw intraocular lenses in children. *Doc Ophthalmol.* 1996;92:29–35.
114. Vasavada A, Chauhan H. Intraocular lens implantation in infants with congenital cataracts. *J Cataract Refract Surg.* 1994;20:592–7.
115. Vasavada A, Desai J. Primary posterior capsulorrhexis with and without anterior vitrectomy in congenital cataracts. *J Cataract Refract Surg.* 1997;23(suppl):647–51.
116. Vasavada A, Trivedi R. Role of optic capture in congenital cataract and intraocular lens surgery in children. *J Cataract Refract Surg.* 2000;26:824–9.
117. Vasavada AR, Trivedi RH, Singh R. Necessity of vitrectomy when optic capture is performed in children older than 5 years. *J Cataract Refract Surg.* 2001;27:1185–93.
118. Vasavada A. Posterior capsule management in congenital cataract surgery. In: Crandall A, Masket S. *An Atlas of Cataract Surgery.* Philadelphia, PA: Taylor & Francis; 1999:281–90.
119. Wagners RS, Nelson LB. Problems in pediatric cataract–intraocular lens implantation. *J Pediatr Ophthalmol Strabismus.* 1997;34:332.
120. Wheeler DT, Mullaney PB, Awad A, et al. Pediatric IOL implantation. The KKESH experience. *J Pediatr Ophthalmol Strabismus.* 1997;34:341–6.
121. Wilson ME, Englert JA, Greenwald MJ. In-the-bag secondary intraocular lens implantation in children. *J Pediatr Ophthalmol Strabismus.* 1999;3:350–5.
122. Wilson ME. Intraocular lens implantation: has it become the standard of care for children? (Editorial). *Ophthalmology.* 1996;103:1719–20.
123. Wisniewska GM, Kaluzny J, Junk HL, Elicks I. Intraocular lens implantation in children and youth. *J Pediatr Ophthalmol Strabismus.* 1999;36:129–33.

124. Zetterstrom C, Kugelberg U, Oscarson C. Cataract surgery in children with capsulorrhexis of anterior and posterior capsules and heparin-surface-modified intraocular lenses. *J Cataract Refract Surg*. 1994;20:599–601.
125. Zetterstrom C, Lundvall A, Weeber H Jr, Jeeves M. Sulcus fixation without capsular support in children. *J Cataract Refract Surg*. 1999;25:776–81.
126. Zwaan J. Simultaneous surgery for bilateral pediatric cataracts. *Ophthalmic Surg Lasers*. 1996;27:15–20.
127. Buckley E, Lambert SR, Wilson ME. IOLs in the first year of life. *J Pediatr Ophthalmol Strabismus*. 1999;36:281–6.
128. Rush DP, Bazarian RA. Intraocular lenses in children. *Adv Clinical Ophthalmol*. 1994;1:263–74.
129. Oliver M, Milstein A, Pollack A. Posterior chamber lens implantation in infants and juveniles. *Eur J Implant Ref Surg*. 1990;2:309–14.
130. Dahan E, Drusedau MUH. Choice of lens and dioptric power in pediatric pseudophakia. *J Cataract Refract Surg*. 1997;23:618–23.
131. Gordon RA, Donzis PB. Refractive development of the human eye. *Arch Ophthalmol*. 1985;103:785–9.
132. McClatchey SK, Dahan E, Maselli E, et al. A comparison of the rate of refractive growth in pediatric aphakic and pseudophakic eyes. *Ophthalmology*. 2000;107:118–22.
133. McClatchey SK, Parks MM. Myopic shift after cataract removal in childhood. *J Pediatr Ophthalmol Strabismus*. 1997;34:88–95.
134. McClatchey SK, Parks MM. Theoretic refractive changes after lens implantation in childhood. *Ophthalmology*. 1997;104:1744–51.
135. Plager DA, Lipsky SN, Snyder SK, et al. Capsular management and refractive error in pediatric intraocular lenses. *Ophthalmology*. 1997;104:600–7.
136. Wilson ME. Clinician's Corner. In Ruttum MS. *Childhood Cataracts*. American Academy of Ophthalmology, Focal Points, Clinical Modules for Ophthalmologists, Volume 14/1, March 1996.
137. Awner S, Buckley EG, DeVaro JM, et al. Unilateral pseudophakia in children under 4 years. *J Pediatr Ophthalmol Strabismus*. 1996;33:230–6.
138. Andreo LK, Wilson ME, Saunders RA. Predictive value of regression and theoretical IOL formulas in pediatric intraocular lens implantation. *J Pediatr Ophthalmol Strabismus*. 1997;34:240–3.
139. Bluestein EC, Wilson ME, Wang XH, et al. Dimensions of the pediatric crystalline lens: implications for intraocular lenses in children. *J Pediatr Ophthalmol Strabismus*. 1996;33:18–20.
140. Pandey SK, Werner L, Wilson ME, Izak AM, Apple DJ. Capsulorhexis ovaling and capsular bag stretch after rigid and foldable intraocular lens implantation: experimental study in pediatric human eyes. *J Cataract Refract Surg*. 2004;30:2183-91.
141. Wilson ME, Apple DJ, Bluestein EC, Wang XH. Intraocular lenses for pediatric implantation: biomaterials, designs and sizing. *J Cataract Refract Surg*. 1994;20:584–91.
142. Gerding H. Does the refractive shift in pseudophakic eyes of children develop slower than expected? *Invest Ophthalmol Vis Sci*. 1996;37:1935–6.
143. Griener ED, Dahan E, Lambert SR. Effect of age at time of cataract surgery on subsequent axial length growth in infant eyes. *J Cataract Refract Surg*. 1999;25:1209–13.
144. Lambert SR, Fernandes A, Drewa-Botsch C, Tigges M. Pseudophakia retards axial elongation in neonatal monkeys. *Invest Ophthalmol Vis Sci*. 1996;37:451–8.
145. Lambert SR, Fernandes A, Grossniklaus H, et al. Neonatal lensectomy and intraocular lens implantation: effects in rhesus monkeys. *Invest Ophthalmol Vis Sci*. 1995;36:300–10.
146. Lambert SR, Grossniklaus HE. Intraocular lens implantation in monkeys: Clinical and histopathological finding. *J Cataract Refract Surg*. 1997;23:605–11.
147. Lorenz B, Worle J, Friedl N, et al. Ocular growth in infant aphakia. Bilateral versus unilateral congenital cataracts. *Ophthalmic Paediatr Genetics*. 1993;14:177–88.

148. Rasooly R, BenEzra D. Congenital and traumatic cataract: the effect on ocular axial length. *Arch Ophthalmol.* 1988;106:1066–8.
149. Weisel TN, Raviola E. Myopia and eye enlargement after neonatal lid fusion in monkeys. *Nature.* 1977;266:66–8.
150. Wilson JR, Fernandes A, Chandler CV, et al. Abnormal development of the axial length of aphakic monkey eyes. *Invest Ophthalmol Vis Sci.* 1987;28:2096–9.
151. Kugelberg U, Zetterström C, Lundgren B, et al. After-cataract and ocular growth in newborn rabbit eyes implanted with a capsule tension ring. *J Cataract Refract Surg.* 1997;23:635–40.
152. Kugelberg U, Zetterström C, Lundgren B, Syren-Nordqvist S. Eye growth in aphakic newborn rabbit. *J Cataract Refract Surg.* 1996;22:337–41.
153. Kugelberg U, Zetterström C, Lundgren B, Syren-Nordqvist S. Ocular growth in newborn rabbit eyes implanted with a poly(methyl methacrylate) or silicone intraocular lens. *J Cataract Refract Surg.* 1997;23:629–34.
154. Kugelberg U, Zetterström C, Syren-Nordqvist S. Ocular axial length in children with unilateral congenital cataract. *Acta Ophthalmol Scand.* 1996;74:220–3.
155. Lambert SR, Buckley EG, Plager DA, et al. Unilateral intraocular lens implantation during the first six months of life. *J Pediatr Ophthalmol Strabismus.* 1999;3:344–9.
156. Hiles DA, Hered RW. Modern intraocular lens implants in children with new age limitations. *J Cataract Refract Surg.* 1987;13:493–7.
157. Hiles DA, Wallar PH. Visual results following infantile cataract surgery. *Int Ophthalmol Clin.* 1977;17:265–82.
158. Wilson ME, Pandey SK, Werner L, et al. Pediatric cataract surgery: current techniques, complications and management. In: Agarwal A, Agarwal S, Apple DJ, Buratto L, Agarwal A, eds. *Textbook of Ophthalmology*. Thorofare, NJ: SLACK Incorporated; 2000:370–378.
159. Scheie HG. Aspiration of congenital or soft cataracts: a new technique. *Am J Ophthalmol.* 1960;50:1048–56.
160. Ridley H. Artificial intraocular lenses after cataract extraction. St. Thomas' Hospital Reports 7(Series):12–4,1952.
161. Choyce DP. Correction of uniocular aphakia by means of anterior chamber acrylic implants. *Trans Ophthalmol Soc UK.* 1958;78:459–70.
162. Binkhorst CD, Gobin MH, Leonard PA. Post-traumatic artificial lens implants (pseudophakoi) in children. *Br J Ophthalmol.* 1969;53:518–29.
163. Binkhorst CD, Gobin MH, Leonard PA. Post-traumatic pseudophakia in children. *Ophthalmologica.* 1969;158(Suppl):284–91.
164. Binkhorst CD, Gobin MH. Injuries to the eye with lens opacity in young children. *Ophthalmologica.* 1964;148:169–83.
165. Binkhorst CD, Greaves B, Kats A, Bermingham AK. Lens injury in children treated with irido-capsular supported intra-ocular lenses. *J Am Intraocular Implant Soc.* 1978;4:34–49.
166. Binkhorst CD, Greaves B, Kats A, Bermingham AK. Lens injury in children treated with irido-capsular supported intra-ocular lenses. *Doc Ophthalmol.* 1979;46:241–77.
167. Binkhorst CD. Iris-clip and irido-capsular implants (pseudophakoi); personal techniques of pseudophakia. *Br J Ophthalmol.* 1967;51:767–71.
168. BenEzra D. Cataract surgery and intraocular lens implantation in children. *Am J Ophthalmol.* 1996;121:224–6.
169. BenEzra D, Cohen E, Rose L. Traumatic cataract in children: correction of aphakia by contact lens or intraocular lens. Am J Ophthalmol. 1997;123:773–82.
170. BenEzra D, Cohen E. Cataract surgery in children with chronic uveitis. *Ophthalmology.* 2000;107:1255–60.
171. BenEzra D, Cohen E. Posterior capsulectomy in pediatric cataract surgery: the necessity of a choice. *Ophthalmology.* 1997;104:2168–74.

172. BenEzra D, Paez JH. Congenital cataract and intraocular lenses. *Am J Ophthalmol.* 1983;96:311–4.
173. Gimbel HV, Sun R, DeBrouff BM. Recognition and management of internal wound gape. *J Cataract Refract Surg.* 1995;21:121–124.
174. Basti S, Krishnamachary M, Gupta S. Results of sutureless wound construction in children undergoing cataract extraction. *J Pediatr Ophthalmol Strabismus.* 1996;33:52–4.
175. Englert JA, Wilson ME: Postoperative intraocular pressure elevation after the use of Healon GV in pediatric cataract surgery. *J Pediatr Ophthalmol Strabismus.* 2000;4:60–1.
176. Gimbel HV, Neuhann T. Development, advantages, methods of the continuous circular capsulorrhexis technique. *J Cataract Refract Surg.* 1990;16:31–7.
177. Auffarth GU, Wesendahl TA, Newland TJ, Apple DJ. Capsulorrhexis in the rabbit eye as a model for pediatric capsulectomy. *J Cataract Refract Surg.* 1994;20:188–91.
177b. Tahi H, Fantes F, Hamaoui M, Parel JM. Small peripheral anterior continuous curvilinear capsulorrhexis. *J Cataract Refract Surg.* 1999;25:744–7.
178. Anwar M, Bleik JH, von Noorden GK, et al. Posterior chamber lens implantation for primary repair of corneal lacerations and traumatic cataracts in children. *J Pediatr Ophthalmol Strabismus.* 1994;31:157–61.
179. Krag S, Thim K, Corybon L, et al. Biomechanical aspects of the anterior capsulotomy. *J Cataract Refract Surg.* 1994;20:410–6.
180. Wilson ME, Bluestein EC, Wang XH, et al. Comparison of mechanized anterior capsulectomy and manual continuous capsulorrhexis in pediatric eyes. *J Cataract Refract Surg.* 20:602–6,1994
181. Wilson ME. Anterior capsule management for pediatric intraocular lens implantation. *J Pediatr Ophthalmol Strabismus.* 1999;36:1–6.
182. Wilson ME, Saunders RA, Robert EL, Apple DJ. Mechanized anterior capsulectomy as an alternative to manual capsulorrhexis in children undergoing intraocular lens implantation. *J Pediatr Ophthalmol Strabismus.* 1996;33:237–40.
183. Kloti R. Anterior high frequency capsulotomy. Part I: experimental study. *Klin Monatsbl Augenheilkd.* 1992;200:507–10.
184. Comer RM, Abdulla N, O'Keefe M. Radiofrequency diathermy capsulorrhexis of the anterior and posterior capsules in pediatric cataract surgery: preliminary results. *J Cataract Refract Surg.* 1997;23(suppl)1:641–4.
185. Faust KJ. Hydrodissection of soft nuclei. *J Am Intraocular Implant Soc.* 1984;10:75–7.
186. Fine IH. Cortical cleaving hydrodissection. *J Cataract Refract Surg.* 1992;18:508–12.
187. Mackool RJ. Management of posterior capsule during intraocular lens implantation. *Am J Ophthalmol.* 1994;117:121–3.
188. Gimbel HV, DeBroff DM. Posterior capsulorrhexis with optic capture: maintaining a clear visual axis after pediatric cataract surgery. *J Cataract Refract Surg.* 1994;20:658–64.
189. Gimbel HV. Posterior capsulorrhexis with optic capture in pediatric cataract and intraocular lens surgery. *Ophthalmology.* 1996;103:1871–5.
190. Fenton S, O'Keefe M. Primary posterior capsulorrhexis without anterior vitrectomy in pediatric cataract. *J Cataract Refract Surg.* 1999;25:763–7.
191. Atkinson CS, Hiles DA. Treatment of secondary posterior capsular membrane Nd:YAG laser in a pediatric population. *Am J Ophthalmol.* 1994;118:496–501.
192. Basti S, Ravishankar V, Gupta S. Results of a prospective evaluation of three methods of management of pediatric cataracts. *Ophthalmology.* 1996;103:713–20.
193. Wang XH, Wilson ME, Bluestein EC, et al. Pediatric cataract surgery and IOL implantation techniques: a laboratory study. *J Cataract Refract Surg.* 1994;20:607–9.
194. Pandey SK, Werner L, Apple DJ. Posterior capsule opacification: etiopathogenesis, clinical manifestations, and management. In: Garg A, Pandey SK, eds. *Textbook of Ocular Therapeutics.* New Delhi, India: Jaypee Brothers; 2002:408–425.

195. Werner L, Pandey SK, Escobar-Gomez M, Hoddinott DSM, Apple DJ. Dye-enhanced cataract surgery. Part II. An experimental study to learn and perform critical steps of phacoemulsification in human eyes obtained post-mortem. *J Cataract Refract Surg*. 2000;26:1060–1065..
196. Pandey SK, Wilson ME, Apple DJ, Werner L, Ram J. Childhood cataract surgical technique, complications and management. In: Garg A, Pandey SK, eds. *Textbook of Ocular Therapeutics*. New Delhi, India: Jaypee Brothers; 2002:457–486.
197. Eckstein M, Vijayalakshmi P, Killedar M, et al. Aetiology of childhood cataract in south India. *Br J Ophthalmol*. 1996;80:628–32.
198. Krishnamachary M, Rathi V, Gupta S. Management of traumatic cataract in children. *J Cataract Refract Surg*. 1997;23:681–7.
199. Hemo Y, BenEzra D. Traumatic cataracts in young children: correction of aphakia by intraocular lens implantation. *Ophthalmic Paediatr Genetics*. 1987;8:203–7.
200. Jain IS, Mohan K, Gupta A. Unilateral traumatic aphakia in children: role of corneal contact lenses. *J Pediatr Ophthalmol Strabismus*. 1985;224:137–9.
201. Bienfait MF, Pameijer JH, Wildervanck de Blecourt-Devilee M. Intraocular lens implantation in children with unilateral traumatic cataract. *Int Ophthalmol*. 1990;14:271–276.
202. Hiles DA, Wallar PH, Biglan AW. The surgery and results following traumatic cataracts in children. *J Pediatr Ophthalmol*. 1976;13:319–25.
203. Jain IS, Bansal SL, Dhir SP, et al. Prognosis in traumatic cataract surgery. *J Pediatr Ophthalmol Strabismus*. 1979;16:301–5.
204. Sharma N, Pushker N, Dada T, et al. Complications of pediatric cataract surgery and intraocular lens implantation. *J Cataract Refract Surg*. 1999;25:1585–8.
205. Ram J, Pandey SK. Infantile cataract surgery: techniques, complications and their management. In: Dutta LC, ed. *Modern Ophthalmology*. New Delhi, India: Jaypee Brothers; 2000:378–84.
206. Mullaney PB, Wheeler DT, al-Nahdi T. Dissolution of pseudophakic fibrinous exudate with intraocular streptokinase. *Eye*. 1996;10:362–6.
207. Klais CM, Hattenbach LO, Steinkamp GW, et al. Intraocular recombinant tissue-plasminogen activator fibrinolysis of fibrin formation after cataract surgery in children. *J Cataract Refract Surg*. 1999;25:357–62.
208. Leung TSA, Lam DSC, Rao SK. Fibrinolysis of postcataract fibrin membranes in children. *J Cataract Refract Surg*. 2000;26:4–5.
209. Rozenman Y, Folberg R, Nelson LB, Cohen EJ. Painful bullous keratopathy following pediatric cataract surgery with intraocular lens implantation. *Ophthalmic Surg*. 1985;16:372–4.
210. Hiles DA, Biglan AW, Fetherolf EC. Central corneal endothelial cell counts in children. *J Am Intra-Ocular Implant Soc*. 1979;5:292–300.
211. Wheeler DT, Stagger DR, Weakley DR, Jr. Endophthalmitis following pediatric intraocular surgery for congenital cataracts and congenital glaucoma. *J Pediatr Ophthalmol Strabismus*. 1992;29:139–41.
212. Good WV, Hing S, Irvine AR, et al. Postoperative endophthalmitis in children following cataract surgery. *J Pediatr Ophthalmol Strabismus*. 1990;27:283–5.
213. Jameson NA, Good WV, Hoyt CS. Inflammation after cataract surgery in children. *Ophthalmic Surg*. 1992;23:99–102.
214. Werner L, Pandey SK, Escobar-Gomez M, et al. Anterior capsule opacification: a histopathological study comparing different IOL styles. *Ophthalmology*. 2000;107:463–71.
215. Apple DJ, Solomon KD, Tetz MR, et al. Posterior capsule opacification. *Surv Ophthalmol*. 1992;37:73–116.
216. Kugelberg U. Visual acuity following treatment of bilateral congenital cataracts. *Doc Ophthalmol*. 1992;82:211–5.
217. Morgan KS, Karcioglu ZA. Secondary cataracts in infants after lensectomies. *J Pediatr Ophthalmol Strabismus*. 1987;24:45–8.

218. Zetterstrom C, Kugelberg U, Lundgren B, Syren-Nordqvist S. After cataract formation in newborn rabbits implanted with intraocular lenses. *J Cataract Refract Surg.* 1996;22:85-8.
219. Menezo JL, Taboada JF, Ferrer E. Managing dense retro-pseudosphakos membranes with a pars plana vitrectomy. *J Am Intra-Ocular Implant Soc.* 1985;11:24–7.
220. Asrani SG, Wilensky JT. Glaucoma after congenital cataract surgery. *Ophthalmology.* 1995;102:863–7.
221. Brady KM, Atkinson CS, Kilty LA, Hiles DA. Glaucoma after cataract extraction and posterior chamber lens implantation in children. *J Cataract Refract Surg.* 1997;23(suppl):669–74.
222. Chrousos GA, Parks MM, O'Neill JF. Incidence of chronic glaucoma, retinal detachment and secondary membrane surgery in pediatric aphakic patients. *Ophthalmology.* 1984;91:1238–41.
223. Egbert JE, Kushner BJ. Excessive lodd of hyperopia: presenting sign of juvenile aphakic glaucoma. *Arch Ophthalmol.* 1990;108:1257–9.
224. Simon JW, Metge P, Simmons ST, et al. Glaucoma after pediatric lensectomy/vitrectomy. *Ophthalmology.* 1991;98:670–4.
225. Walton DS. Pediatric aphakic glaucoma: a study of 65 patients. *Trans Am Ophthalmol Soc.* 1995;93:403–20.
226. Vajpayee RB, Angra SK, Titiyal JS, et al. Pseudophakic pupillary block glaucoma in children. *Am J Ophthalmol.* 1991;11:715–8.
227. Phelps CD, Arafat NI. Open-angle glaucoma following surgery for congenital cataracts. *Arch Ophthalmol.* 1977;95:1985–7.
228. Wallace DK, Plager DA. Corneal diameter in childhood aphakic glaucoma. *J Pediatr Ophthalmol Strabismus.* 1996;33:230–4.
229. Jagger JD, Cooling RJ, Fison LG, et al. Management of retinal detachment following congenital cataract surgery. *Trans Ophthalmol Soc UK.* 1983;103:103–7.
230. Kanski JJ, Elkington AR, Daniel R. Retinal detachment after congenital cataract surgery. *Br J Ophthalmol.* 1974;58:92–5.
231. Toyofuku H, Hirose T, Schepens CL. Retinal detachment following congenital cataract surgery. *Arch Ophthalmol.* 1980;98:669–75.
232. Morgan KS, Franklin RM. Oral fluorescein angioscopy in aphakic children. *J Pediatr Ophthalmol Strabismus.* 1984;21:33–6.
233. Pinchoff BS, Ellis FD, Helveston EM, Sato SE. Cystoid macular edema in pediatric aphakia. *J Pediatr Ophthalmol Strabismus.* 1988;25:240–3.
234. Hoyt CS, Nickel B. Aphakic cystoid macular edema: occurrence in infants and children after transpupillary lensectomy and anterior vitrectomy. *Arch Ophthalmol.* 1982;100:746–9.
235. Gilbard SM, Peyman GA, Goldberg MF. Evaluation for cystoid maculopathy after pars plicata lensectomy-vitrectomy for congenital cataracts. *Ophthalmology.* 1983;90:1201–6.
236. Mets MB, Del Monte M. Hemorrhagic retinopathy following uncomplicated pediatric cataract extraction. *Arch Ophthalmol.* 1986;104:975–9.
237. Christiansen SP, Munoz M, Capo H. Retinal hemorrhage following lensectomy and anterior vitrectomy in children. *J Pediatr Ophthalmol Strabismus.* 1993;30:24–7.
238. Birch EE, Stager DR. Prevalence of good visual acuity following surgery for congenital unilateral cataract. *Arch Ophthalmol.* 1988;106:40–2.
239. Birch EE, Stager DR. The critical period for surgical treatment of dense, congenital, unilateral cataracts. *Invest Ophthalmol Vis Sci.* 1996;37:1532–8.
240. Birch EE, Swanson WH, Stager DR, et al. Outcome after very early treatment of dense congenital unilateral cataract. *Invest Ophthalmol Vis Sci.* 1993;34:3687–99.
241. Bradford GM, Keech RV, Scott WE. Factors affecting visual outcome after surgery for bilateral congenital cataracts. *Am J Ophthalmol.* 1994;117:58–64.
242. Catalano RA, Simon JW, Jenkins PL, Kandel GL. Preferential looking as a guide for amblyopia therapy in monocular infantile cataracts. *J Pediatr Ophthalmol Strabismus.* 1987;24:56–63.

243. Enyedi LB, Peterseim MW, Freedman SF, Buckley EG. Refractive changes after pediatric intraocular lens implantation. *Am J Ophthalmol.* 1998;126:772–81.
244. Huber C. Increasing myopia in children with intraocular lenses: An experiment in form deprivation myopia? *Eur J Implant Ref Surg.* 1993;5:154–8.
245. Hutchinson AK, Drews-Botsch C, Lambert SR. Myopic shift after intraocular lens implantation during childhood. *Ophthalmology.* 1997;104:1752–7.
246. Gayton JL, Apple DJ, Peng Q, et al. Interlenticular opacification: clinicopathological correlation of a new complication of piggyback posterior chamber intraocular lenses. *J Cataract Refract Surg.* 2000;20:330–36.
247. Wilson ME, Peterseim MW, Englert JA, Lall-Trail JK, Elliott LA. Pseudophakia and polypseudophakia in the first year of life. *J AAPOS.* 2001;5:238-45.
248. Gregg FM, Parks MM. Stereopsis after congenital monocular cataract extraction. *Am J Ophthalmol.* 1992;114:314–7.
249. Keech RV, Mutschke PJ. Upper age limit for the development of amblyopia. *J Pediatr Ophthalmol Strabismus.* 1995;32:89–95.
250. Lloyd IC, Dowler JG, Kriss A, et al. Modulation of amblyopia therapy following early surgery for unilateral congenital cataracts. *Br J Ophthalmol.* 1995;79:802–6.
251. Taylor D. Monocular infantile cataract, intraocular lenses and amblyopia (Editorial). *Br J Ophthalmol.* 1989;73:857–8.
252. Taylor D. The Doyne Lecture Congenital Cataract: the history, the nature, and the practice. *Eye.* 1998;12:9–36.
253. Tytla ME, Lewis TL, Maurer D, Brent HP. Stereopsis after congenital cataract. *Invest Ophthalmol Vis Sci.* 1993;34:1767–73.
254. Verma A, Singh D. Active vision therapy for pseudophakic amblyopia. *J Cataract Refract Surg.* 1997;23:1089–94.
255. Fugo RJ, Coccio D, McGrann D, Becht L, DelCampo D. The Fugo Blade . . . the next step after capsulorrhexis. Presented at the ASCRS Symposium on Cataract, IOL and Refractive Surgery, Congress on Ophthalmic Practice Management; May 23, 2001; Boston, Mass.
256. Trivedi R, Vasavada AR, Apple DJ, et al. Cortical cleaving hydrodissection in congenital cataract surgery. Presented at the ASCRS Symposium on Cataract, IOL and Refractive Surgery; May 2001; San Diego, Calif.
257. Wilson ME, Holland DR. In-the-bag Secondary Intraocular Lens Implantation in Children. Presented at the ASCRS Symposium on Cataract, IOL, and Refractive Surgery; April 1998; San Diego, Calif.
258. Pandey SK, Werner L, Apple DJ, et al. Anterior Capsule Staining in Advanced Cataracts: A Laboratory Study using Postmortem Human Eyes. Presented at the annual meeting of the American Academy of Ophthalmology, October 1999; Orlando, Fla.
259. Pandey SK, Werner L, Apple DJ, et al. Dye-Enhanced Cataract Surgery in Human Eyes Obtained Post-mortem: A Laboratory Study to Learn and Perform Critical Steps of Phacoemulsification. Prize winning video (second place, Scientific Value). Presented at the ESCRS Symposium on Cataract, IOL, and Refractive Surgery; September 1999; Vienna, Austria.
260. Wilson ME. Pseudophakia and polypseudophakia in first year of life. Presented at the ASCRS Symposium on Cataract, IOL and Refractive Surgery; May 2000; Boston, Mass.

The authors have no financial or proprietary interest in any product mentioned in this chapter.

Chapter 7

Subluxated Cataracts and Endocapsular Rings

Athiya Agarwal, MD, FRSH, DO

Introduction

The surgical management of cataract associated with zonular dialysis is a real challenge for the ophthalmic surgeon. Due to recent advances in equipment and instrumentation, better surgical techniques and understanding of the fluidics, the surgeon is able to perform relatively safe cataract surgery in the presence of compromised zonules. Implantation of a capsular tension ring can stabilize a loose lens and allow the surgeon to complete phacoemulsification and intraocular lens (IOL) implantation.

History

Insertion of a ring into the capsular bag fornix (equator) to support the zonular apparatus was first described by Hara and coauthors in 1991.[1] Hara et al introduced the concept of "equator ring", "endocapsular ring", or "capsular tension ring (CTR)". In 1993, the first CTR for use in humans was designed.[2] In 1994, Nagamoto and Bissen-Miyajima[3] suggested using an open polymethylmethacrylate (PMMA) ring to provide adaptability.

Advantages

This technique offers four main advantages:

1. The capsular zonular anatomical barrier is partially reformed, so that vitreous herniation to the anterior chamber during surgery is reduced or even avoided.
2. A taut capsular equator offers counter traction for all traction maneuvers, making them easier to perform and decreasing the risk of extending the zonular dialysis. The great advantage of using the capsular ring during the phacoemulsification rather than after, just to center the lens is a great deal safer. Any force that is transmitted to the capsule is not applied directly to the adjacent zonules, but rather distributed circumferentially to the entire zonular apparatus.

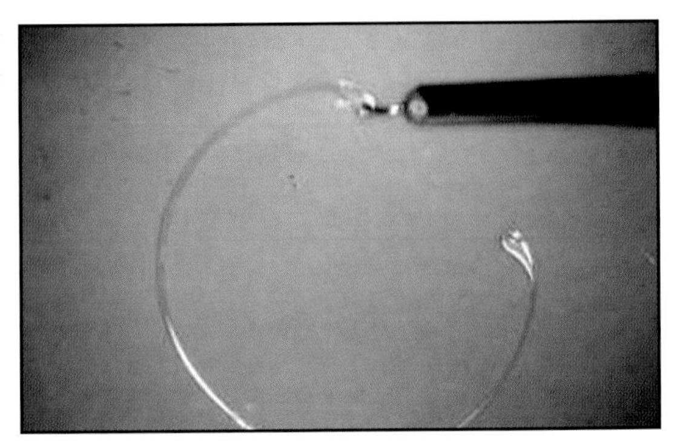

Figure 7-1. Capsular tension ring or endocapsular ring. Note the injector for the capsular tension ring.

3. The necessary capsular support for an in-the-bag, centered implant is obtained.
4. The capsular bag maintains its shape and does not collapse, which can lead to proliferation and migration of epithelial cells, development of capsular fibrosis syndrome, and late intraocular pressure (IOP) decentration.

Designs and Descriptions

The capsular tension ring (Figure 7-1) is made of one piece PMMA and is available in different sizes, depending on their use in patients with emmetropia, low or high myopia. An injector is also present for loading the ring. The original capsular tension ring with characteristic eyelets on both ends is marketed by Morcher GmbH (Stuttgart, Germany) in cooperation with Dr. Mitchel Morcher. Meanwhile, various similar products are being marketed (eg, by Ophtec Physiol, corneal, IOL Tech, Acrimed, Rayner, Hanita, Lens Tec). As a standard capsular tension ring, the 12.0/10.0 mm diameter ring (Morcher type 14) and the 13.0/11.0mm diameter ring (Ophtec 13/11) are the most commonly used by surgeons. Morcher type 14 is for normal axial length eyes, while types 14A and 14C are for myopic eyes.

The modifications used by Morcher include two types of capsular tension rings with iris shields (Type L and G, with integrated iris shields of 60° and 90°, respectively) and two types of capsular bending rings (CBRs) designed to prevent capsule opacification (types E and F).These modified versions incorporate fixation elements that allow the surgeon to suture the ring to the scleral wall through the ciliary sulcus without violating the capsular ring.[4]

Special Designs for Suturing in Severe Zonular Dehiscence

In cases where severe or progressive zonular dehiscence is present, implantation of the CTR alone may not be adequate. This may lead to severe postoperative capsular bag shrinkage as well as IOL decentration and pseudophakodonesis.[5] Also, complete luxation of the bag along with the CTR and the IOL cannot be excluded (Figure 7-2).

A modified design developed by Cionni with a fixation hook for severe or progressive cases of zonular deficiency[6] solves this problem (Figure 7-3). The hook is kept opposite to the meridian of decentration and is pulled peripherally using a transscleral fixation suture, to counteract capsular bag decentration and tilt. In severe cases, two such rings or the two-hooked model can be used. However, the Cionni ring has its limitations. It is difficult to

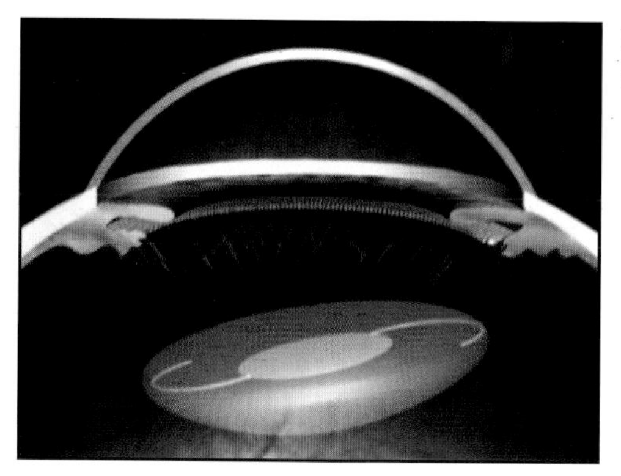

Figure 7-2. Luxation of the bag with the IOL can occur.

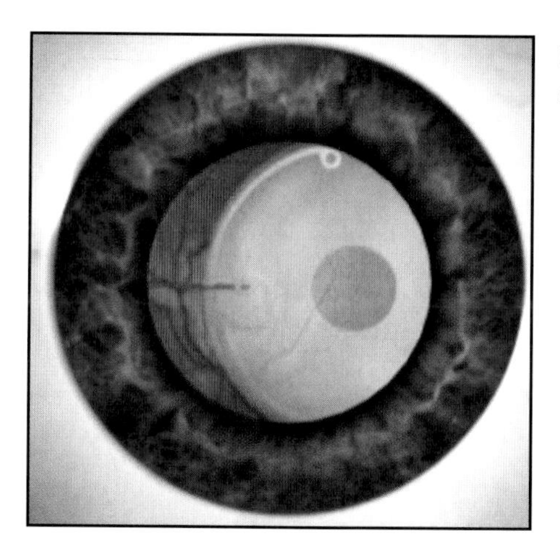

Figure 7-3. Cionni ring being sutured onto the sclera.

implant if the capsulorrhexis is small, and in such cases the hook may even drag on the edge of the anterior capsule, and as the fixation plane is anterior to the anterior capsule, it may lead to iris chafing, pigment dispersion, and chronic uveitis.

An alternative is to fix the ring by guiding the needle of the scleral suture through the equator of the capsular bag, just inside the capsular tension ring.[7] This technique has to be completed as a one-step procedure because the suture may cheese-wire through both capsules leaving along the equator.

Another alternative in cases of severe decentration is to make a small equatorial capsulorrhexis through which a standard capsular tension ring can be inserted. A scleral suture can then be passed around the exposed capsular tension ring, which is then used to center the lens before capsulorrhexis.

INDICATIONS

The capsular tension ring is indicated in all cases of subluxation of lens (Table 7-1), ranging from the common ones like traumatic displacement (mechanical or surgical), Marfan's syndrome, pseudoexfoliation syndrome, and hypermature cataract to the rare ones like aniridia and intraocular tumors.

Table 7-1.

Etiology of Subluxated Lenses

A. *Isolated Ocular Abnormality*

- Simple ectopia lentis
- Simple microsherophakia
- Spontaneous late subluxation of lens

B. *Associated With Other Ocular Abnormality*

- Aniridia
- Ectopia lentis et pupillae
- Uveal coloboma
- Cornea plana

C. *Associated With Heritable Systemic Syndromes*

- Marfan's syndrome
- Homocystinuria
- Weil Marchesani syndrome
- Ehler Danlos syndrome
- Reiger's syndrome
- Hyperlysinemia
- Sulfite oxide deficiency
- Sturge Weber syndrome
- Pflander's syndrome
- Crouzen's syndrome
- Sprengel's anomaly
- Oxycephaly

D. *Associated With Other Ocular Conditions*

- Mature or Hypermature cataract
- Mechanical stretching of zonules
  —Buphthalmos
  —Staphylomas
  —Ectasias of globe
  —High myopia
  —Perforation of large central corneal ulcer
- Pull on zonules
  —Cyclytic inflammatory adhesions
  —Eales' disease
  —Persistent hyperplastic primary vitreous
  —Intraocular tumors
  —Retinal detachment

continued

Table 7-1, continued

Etiology of Subluxated Lenses

- Degeneration of zonules
  - —Uveitis
  - —Retinitis pigmentosa
  - —Chalcosis
  - —Prolonged silicone oil tamponade
  - —High myopia
  - —Hypermature cataract

E. Traumatic Subluxation/Dislocation and Surgical Trauma

APPLICATIONS

Zonular Dehiscence

The efficacy of the capsular tension ring in managing zonular dialysis has been demonstrated in vitro[8,9] depending on where the zonular defect presents. The CTR may be inserted at any stage of cataract procedure. By reestablishing the contour of the capsule, the CTR protects the capsular fornix from being aspirated, avoiding consecutive zonular dialysis extension, irrigation fluid running behind the capsular diaphragm with the posterior capsule bulging, and vitreous prolapse into the anterior chamber with possible aspiration. With preexisting zonular defects such as those caused by blunt trauma, the CTR is inserted before phacoemulsification is started.

Zonular Weakness

Ocular and systemic conditions may result in a zonular weakness that may be profound and progressive. Pseudoexfoliation syndrome with or without glaucoma and Marfan's syndrome are the most common causes. If zonular weakness is profound, the CTR is implanted before the cataract is emulsified and a 10–0 nylon anchoring suture may be temporarily threaded through the eyelets to remove the CTR if the zonules fail during surgery.

In pseudoexfoliation syndrome, the anterior capsule may contract excessively after in-the-bag IOL placement (capsular phimosis). This can be prevented by providing a locking mechanism that would prevent the eyelets from overlapping, suturing together the two eyelets or by using two larger implants. This can be supplemented by meticulously polishing the anterior capsule leaf overlapping the implant.

In case of Marfan's syndrome, the zonules may be disintegrated or elongated while the remaining may be still functional, giving rise to lens decentration, which may be progressive. In case of Weil-Marchesani syndrome, microsherophakia and zonular degeneration may occur. Secondary scleral suturing to remedy IOL decentration and tilt may be useful in such cases.[7]

Use of prolonged silicone oil tamponade may lead to progressive zonular atrophy and emulsified oil or oil bubble gaining access into the anterior chamber spontaneously or dur-

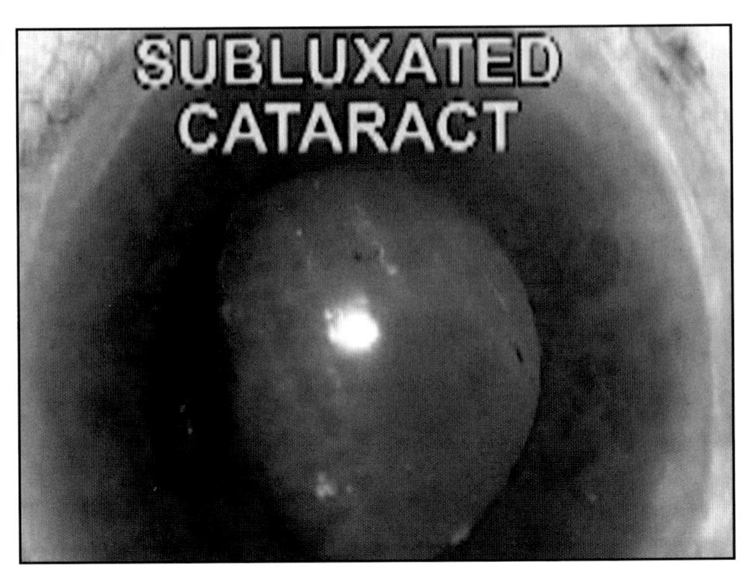

Figure 7-4. Eye with subluxated cataract.

ing the cataract surgery. In such cases, a large capsular tension ring should be implanted before phacoemulsification is done.

TECHNIQUE

Anesthesia

Both general and peribulbar anesthesia are suitable for creation of scleral windows and transscleral suturing of the capsular ring or of the IOL if necessary. Special mention is required about 1% intracameral lidocaine. There is a risk of its passage through the zones lacking zonular fibers, and transitory loss of sight resulting from retinal toxicity, as described in cases of capsular ruptures.[10]

Incisions

The first step is to make an incision in the eye that has a subluxated cataract (Figure 7-4). A needle with viscoelastic is injected inside the eye in the area where the second site is made. This will distend the eye so that when you make a clear corneal incision, the eye will be tense and you can create a good valve. Now use a straight rod to stabilize the eye with the left hand. With the right hand make the clear corneal incision.

Capsulorrhexis

Commencing capsulorrhexis (Figure 7-5) is difficult because of capsular instability. It is better to begin the capsulorrhexis in the area where the zonules are whole and where the capsule offers sufficient resistance. If vitreous is present in the anterior chamber, the gel must be first isolated and vitrectomy should be performed if required. After the vitreous has been removed from the anterior chamber, a viscoelastic preferably dispersive is inserted by first covering the zone. Capsulorrhexis can be performed after the zone of zonular dehiscence and iridocrystalline diaphragm have been stabilized. Do not use trypan blue in such cases, as it will go into the vitreous cavity through the zonular dehiscence and make the

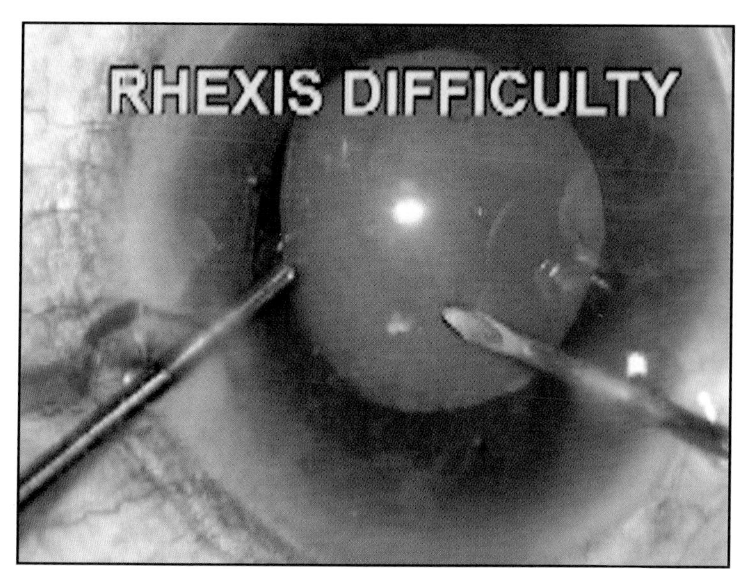

Figure 7-5. Rhexis with a needle. Note no forceps holds the eye. Note also the subluxation seen.

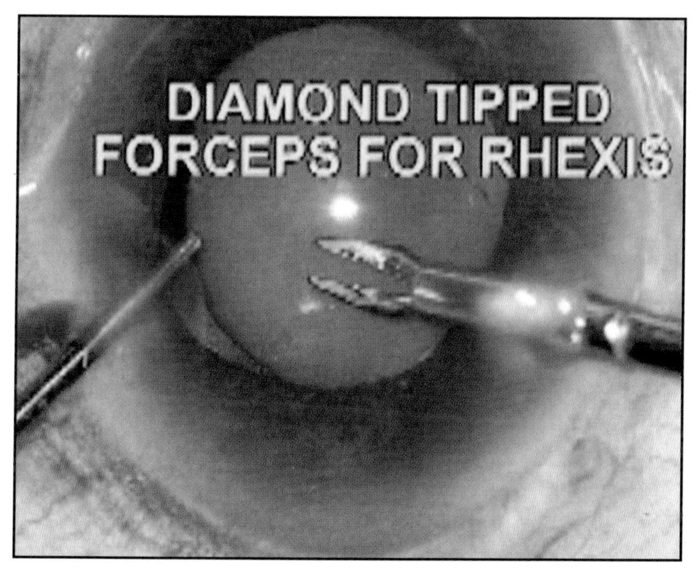

Figure 7-6. Intraocular rhexis forceps used to complete the rhexis.

whole vitreous cavity blue. This will make visualization difficult in surgery. Completion of rhexis can be done using an intraocular rhexis forceps (Figure 7-6).

Hydrodissection—Hydrodelineation

Hydromaneuvers should be performed meticulously to ensure correct freeing of the lens nucleus. The hydrodissection cannula should be inserted in the direction of the zone of disinsertion rather than in the opposite direction, which would enlarge the disinsertion. Viscoelastic may be required to separate the nucleus and cortical material and also to separate the cortex from the lens capsule.

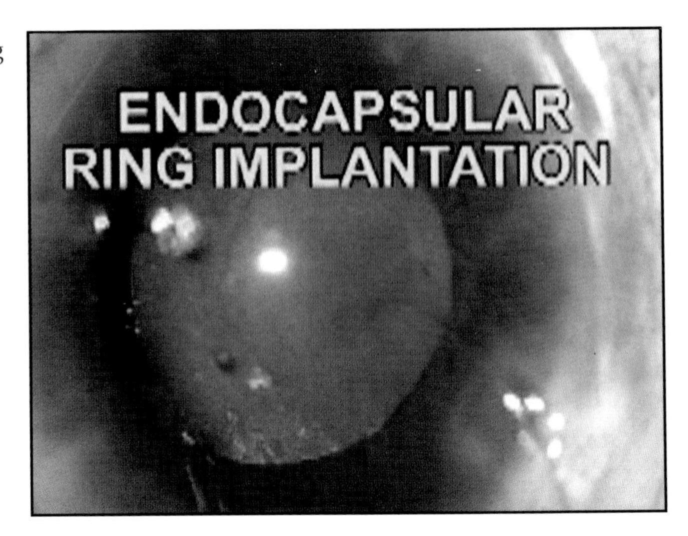

Figure 7-7. Endocapsular ring being implanted.

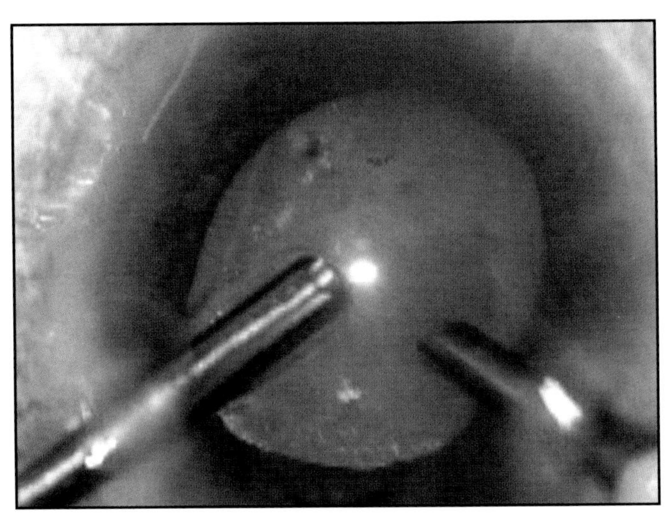

Figure 7-8. Bimanual phaco (Phakonit) being performed.

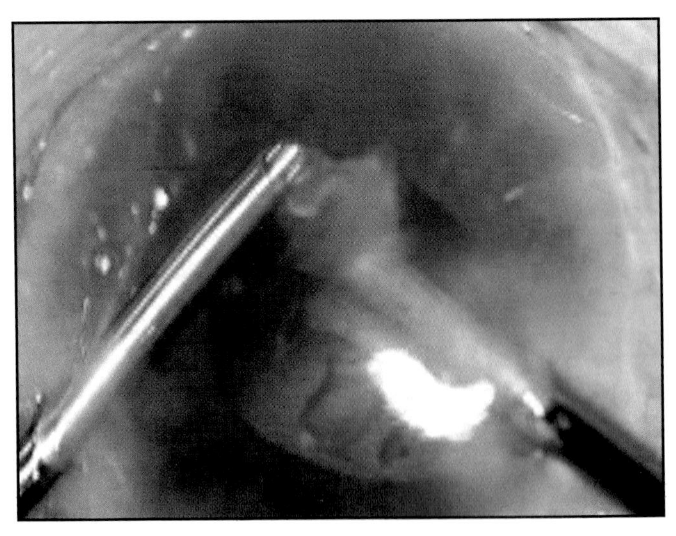

Figure 7-9. Nucleus removal nearly complete.

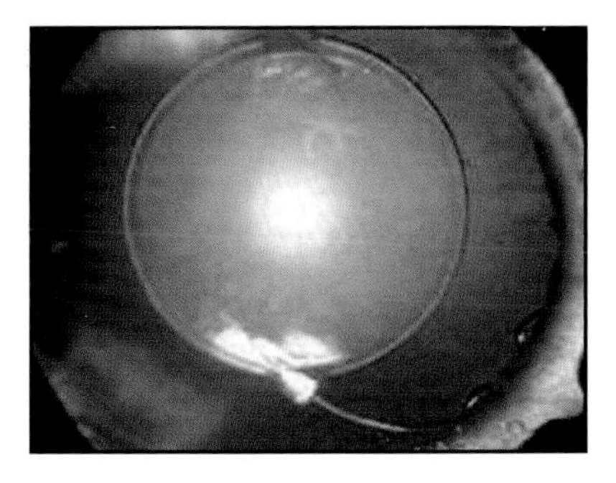

Figure 7-10. Capsular tension ring and foldable IOL in the bag. One day postoperative photo.

Implantation of Capsular Ring

Capsular tension rings can be easily inserted in the capsular bag if it is well expanded with viscoelastic. The instruments used to implant a CTR include Kelman-McPherson type forceps (Figure 7-7), special injectors (marketed by Ophtec and Geuder) suitable for both Ophtec and Morcher CTRs (see Figure 7-1) and the one developed by Menapace and Nishi for use with CBR, and last but not least, a guiding suture.

Phacoemulsification

Nuclear phacoemulsification can be performed using coaxial phaco or bimanual phaco/phakonit (Figures 7-8 and 7-9) in the bag or out of the bag, depending on the surgeon's preference. In general, phacoemulsification in these situations may be considered a safe proposition if performed in a proper way.

Cortical Aspiration

When performing automated aspiration, movements of the tip should not be radial because of the risk of traction on the ring and the capsular bag.

Implantation of the Intraocular Lens

It is desirable to implant a larger diameter lens to minimize symptoms if lens decentration were to occur. The foldable lens is loaded and implanted in the capsular bag (Figure 7-10) followed by viscoelastic removal. In either case, rotational maneuvers must be avoided or minimized.[11]

Key Points With the Use of Capsular Tension Rings

1. Use a high viscosity viscoelastic.
2. Make the incision at a meridian with no zonular dialysis, in order to avoid damage to zonular fibers with the movement of the phaco tip.
3. Perform slow-motion phaco, with low flow rate, low vacuum, and low infusion bottle height.
4. Emulsification can be done in the bag when the nucleus is soft and in the anterior chamber if the nucleus is hard thereby avoiding as much stress as possible to the already damaged zonular apparatus.
5. Perform a careful two port anterior vitrectomy with lax infusion bottle and low aspiration pressure when necessary.

Figure 7-11. Aniridia rings being implanted.

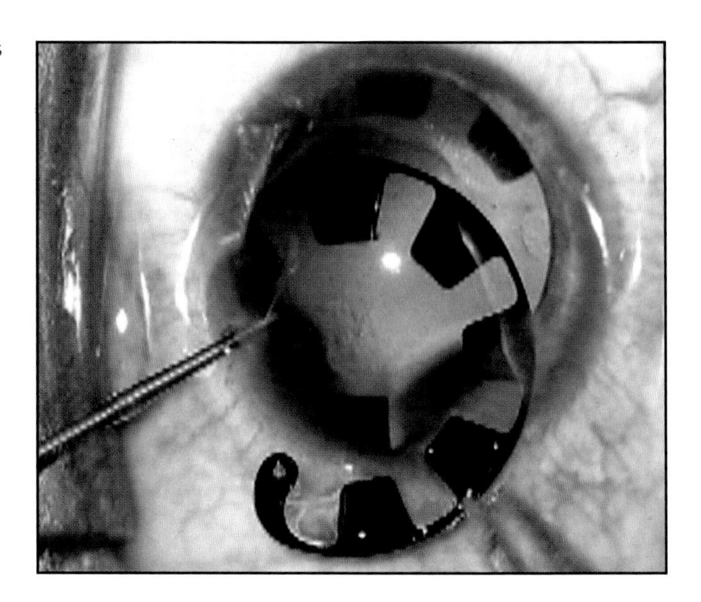

6. Try to place IOL haptics in the meridian of the zonular disinsertion.
7. IOL stability must be checked at the end of the surgery, both in the frontal and sagittal plane in order to consider if suturing one haptic to the sulcus is necessary.[6]

Special Conditions

1. *Coloboma shield for large sector iris defects or iridodialysis*: Tinted capsular tension ring with an integrated 60 to 90° sector shield designed by Rasch can be used to protect against glare and/or monocular diplopia (Morcher L and G). The capsular tension ring can be placed to cover sector iris defects and /or coloboma. If more than 90° of defect is present, then more than one CTR can be used.[4]
2. *Multisegmented coloboma ring for aniridia*: This multisegmented ring designed by Rasch (Morcher type 50 C) is used in combination with the one of the same kind so that the interspaces of the first ring are covered by the sector shields of the second forming a contiguous artificial iris (Figure 7-11).
3. *Anterior eye wall resection for uveal melanoma or other intraocular malignancy*: A combined use of a standard and coloboma capsular tension ring is advocated in cataract surgery after anterior eye wall resection for intraocular malignancy like uveal melanoma. Uveal tumors involving the anterior segment of the eye may need uveal resection, resulting in large iris coloboma and zonular dehiscence. The crystalline lens may be cataractous or may become opaque after the surgery of the tumor requiring its removal sooner or later. For technical approach, intracapsular cataract extraction was considered previously, but the combined use of a standard and coloboma CTR may help preserve the capsular bag and cover the iris defects.
4. *Along with primary posterior capsulorrhexis*: For preexisting central capsule fibrosis or as a general preventive measure against capsule opacification.[12] As the capsular tension ring is in place, vector forces during primary posterior capsulorrhexis can be controlled better as the ring stretches the posterior capsule, giving uniform radi-

al vector forces. As the CTR is in place, distortion in shape of the primary posterior capsulorrhexis can be avoided and folds on the capsule caused by traction due to oversized and rigid lens loop can be prevented. This allows closer and perfect apposition of the posterior capsule with the optic of the IOL. This prevents lens epithelial cells (LECs) from entering the retrolental space in the posterior capsulorrhexis margin, and the secondary primary posterior capsulorrhexis closure.

5. *In combined cataract and vitreous surgery*: When the capsular tension ring is in place, the posterior capsule remains uniformly distended and a perfect peripheral view is possible. Also, as the CTR is in place, silicone oil can be removed through the same phaco incision from the primary posterior capsulorrhexis, which can be performed in a controlled manner with the capsular tension ring in place.
6. *As a tool to measure capsular bag circumference*: The CTR in vivo can be visualized gonioscopically from a well-dilated pupil.The distance between the eyelets can be determined by adjusting the width of the slitbeam of the slit lamp to fill in the space between the eyelets, which can be read out on the slit lamp directly. This capsular bag biometry can be used for quantifying in vivo capsular bag circumference[13] and capsular bag shrinkage dynamics.[14]
7. *For prevention of posterior capsular opacification*: Theoretically, the lesser the space in between the lens optic and the posterior capsule, the lesser the chances of lens epithelial cells migrating behind the optic, ie, no space, no cells. When the capsular bending ring is in place, this interspace is less. Also, by keeping the anterior capsule away from the posterior capsule, myofibroblastic transdifferentiation of lens epithelial cells on the anterior capsule edge and back surface can be prevented. The capsular bending ring is an open, band-shaped PMMA ring measuring 11 mm in diameter with pretension (13 mm diameter when open), 0.2 mm in thickness, and 0.7 mm in thickness. The ring is minimally polished to keep the edges sharp and rectangular, facilitating the creation of a sharp, discontinuous band in the equatorial capsule. A crooked islet is located at both the ring ends to prevent spearing of the capsular fornix and to facilitate manipulation during insertion. The capsular bending ring reduces anterior capsular fibrosis and shrinkage as well as posterior capsular opacification. The ring may be useful in patients who are at high risk of developing eye complications from opacification that require Nd:YAG laser capsulotomy, in those expected to have vitreoretinal surgery and photocoagulation, and in cases of pediatric cataract.[15]

Dropped Endocapsular Ring

An endocapsular ring can get dislocated during surgery if there are complications (Figure 7-12 A-B). In such a case, one should remove it by vitrectomy. It is better to use the chandelier illumination system for this, because with this light source fixed onto the infusion cannula, an endoilluminator is not necessary. The advantage of this is that we can do proper bimanual vitrectomy and use two forceps to remove the endocapsular ring (Figure 7-12 C-E). Visualization is done using the contact wide field lens system.

Summary

Capsular tension rings or endocapsular rings have solved the problems of phaco in subluxated cataracts. They have made life much easier for the cataract surgeon.

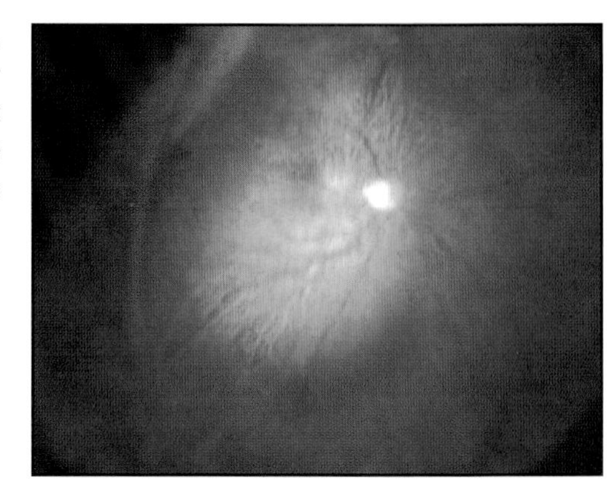

Figure 7-12A. Dropped endocapsular ring. Note the illumination through the chandelier illumination system seen in the upper right corner. The left hand is depressing the eye from outside so that the endocapsular ring is visualized.

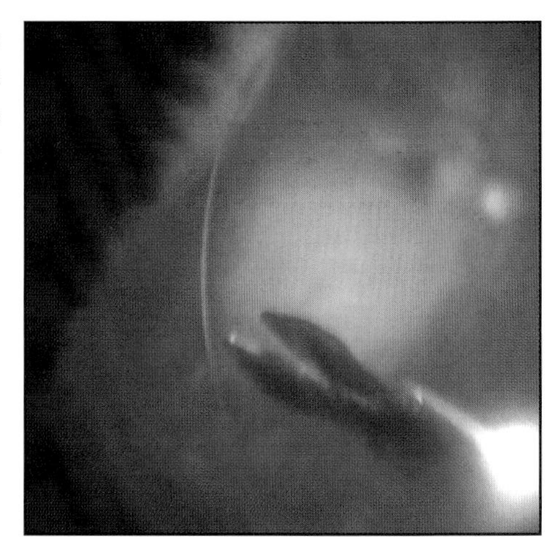

Figure 7-12B. Diamond-tipped forceps about to pick up the ring. Left hand is depressing the eye from outside. Note no endoilluminator in the hand. A wide field contact lens is used for visualization so that the entire retina is seen.

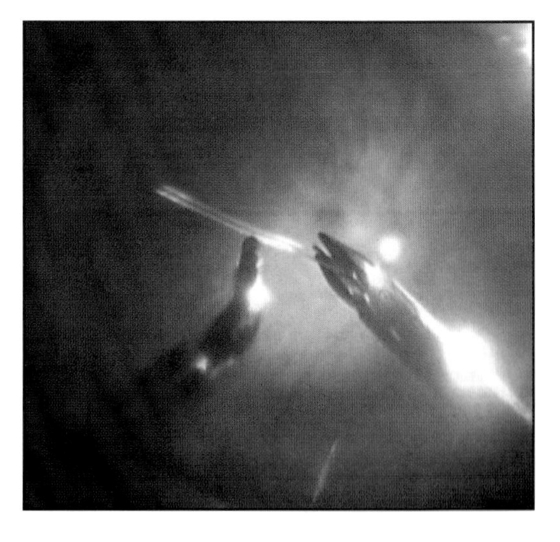

Figure 7-12C. Two intraocular vitrectomy forceps holding the endocapsular ring.

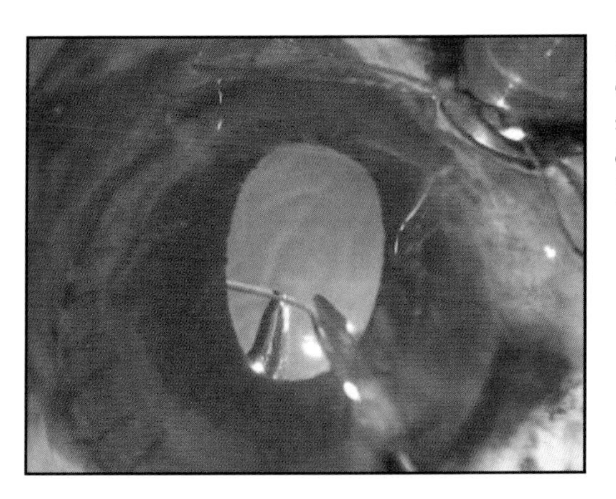

Figure 7-12D. Endocapsular ring brought out through a limbal section. Note the infusion metal cannula in the upper right hand corner. This has the chandelier illumination in it.

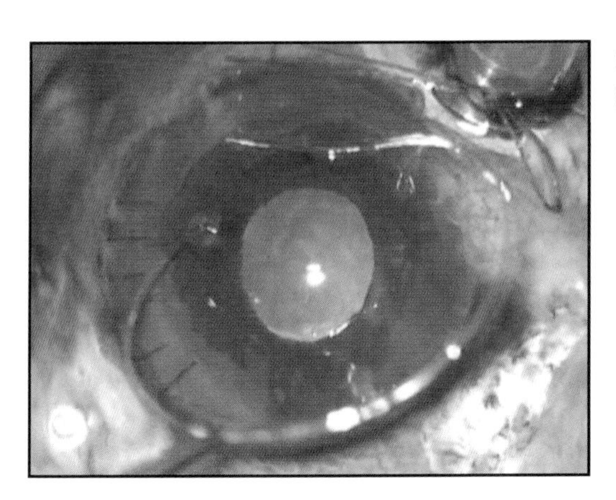

Figure 7-12E. Entire endocapsular ring is brought out.

Key Points

1. The capsular tension ring is made of one piece PMMA and is available in different sizes, depending on their use in patients with emmetropia, low or high myopia.
2. The capsular tension ring may be inserted at any stage of cataract procedure.
3. Ocular and systemic conditions may result in a zonular weakness that may be profound and progressive. Pseudoexfoliation syndrome with or without glaucoma and Marfan's syndrome are the most common causes.
4. Do not use trypan blue in subluxated cataracts, as it will go into the vitreous cavity through the zonular dehiscence and make the whole vitreous cavity blue.
5. The instruments used to implant a capsular tension ring include Kelman-McPherson type forceps and special injectors.

REFERENCES

1. Hara T, Hara T, Yamada Y. "Equatorial ring" for maintenance of the completely circular contour of the capsular bag equator after cataract removal. *Ophthalmic Surg.* 1991;22:358–359.
2. Hara T, Hara T, Sakanishi K, Yamada Y. Efficacy of equator rings in a experimental rabbit study. *Arch Ophthalmol.* 1995;113:1060-1065.
3. Nagamoto T, Bissen-Miyajima H. A ring to support the capsular bag after continuous curvilinear capsulorrhexis. *Cataract Refract Surg.* 1994;20:417–420.
4. Menapace R, Findl O, Georgopoulos M, Rainer G, Vass C, Schmetter K. The capsular tension ring: designs, applications, and techniques. *J Cataract Refract Surg.* 2000;898–912.
5. Nishi O, Hishi K, Sakanishi K, Yamada Y. Explantation of endocapsular posterior chamber lens after spontaneous posterior dislocation. *J Cataract Refract Surg.* 1996;22:272–275.
6. Groessl SA, Anderson CJ. Capsular tension ring in a patient with Weill-Marchesani syndrome. *J Cataract and Refract Surg.* 1998;24:1164–1165.
7. Fischel JD, Wishart MS. Spontaneous complete dislocation of the lens in pseudoexfoliation syndrome. *Eur J Implant Refract Surg.* 1995;7:31–33.
8. Sun R, Gimbel HV. In vitroevaluation of the efficacy of the capsular tension ring for managing zonular dialysis in cataract surgery. *Ophthalmic Surg Lasers.* 1998;29:502–505.
9. Gimble HV, Sun R, Heston JP.Management of zonular dialysis in phacoemulsification and IOL implantation using the capsular tension ring. *Ophthalmic Surg Lasers.* 1997;28:273–281.
10. Gills J, Fenzil R. Intraocular lidocaine causes transient loss of vision in small number of cases. *Ocular Surgery News.* 1996.
11. Agarwal S, Agarwal A, Sachdev MS, Mehta KR, Fine IH, Agarwal A. *Phacoemulsification, Laser Cataract Surgery & Foldable IOLs.* 2nd ed. Delhi, India: Jaypee Brothers; 2000.
12. Van Cauwenberge F, Rakic J-M, Galand A. Complicated posterior capsulorhexis: etiology, management, and outcome. *Br J Ophthalmol.* 1997;81:195–198.
13. Vass C, Menapace R, Schametter K, et al. Prediction of pseudophakic capsular bag diameter on biometric variables. *J Cataract Refract Surg.* 1999;25:1376–1381.
14. Strenn K, Menapace R, Vass C. Capsular bag shrinkage after implantation of an open loop silicone lens and a polymethyl methacrylate capsule tension ring. *J Cataract Refract Surg.* 1997;23:1543-547.
15. Nishi O, Nishi K, Menapace R, Akura J. Capsular bending ring to prevent posterior capsule opacification: 2 year follow up. *J Cataract Refract Surg.* 2001;27:1359–1365.

Please see Subluxated Cataract video on enclosed CD-ROM.

Chapter 8

Mature Cataracts and Dyes

Amar Agarwal, MS, FRCS, FRCOphth

Introduction

One of the biggest problems for a phaco surgeon is to perform a rhexis in a mature cataract (Figure 8-1). Once one performs rhexis in mature and hypermature cataracts, then phaco can be done in these cases and a foldable intraocular lens (IOL) implanted.[1,2]

Rhexis in Mature Cataracts

Various techniques can help one perform rhexis in mature cataracts.

1. Use a good operating microscope. If the operating microscope is good, one can faintly see the outline of the rhexis.
2. Use an endoilluminator. While one is performing the rhexis with the right hand (dominant hand), in the left hand (nondominant hand) one can hold an endoilluminator. By adjusting the endoilluminator in various positions, one can complete the rhexis because the edge of the rhexis can be seen.
3. Use forceps. A forceps is easier to use than a needle, especially in mature cataracts. One can use a good rhexis forceps to complete the rhexis.
4. Use paraxial light.

Even with all these techniques, one is still not very sure of completing a rhexis in all cases. Many times if the rhexis is incomplete, one might have to convert to an extracapsular cataract extraction (ECCE) to prevent a posterior capsular rupture or nucleus drop.

Trypan Blue

The solution to this problem is to use a dye that stains the anterior capsule. This dye is trypan blue. It is marketed as Blurhex by Dr. Agarwal's Pharma. Each ml of Blurhex contains 0.6 mg trypan blue, 1.9 mg of sodium mono-hydrogen orthophosphate, 0.3 mg of sodium di-

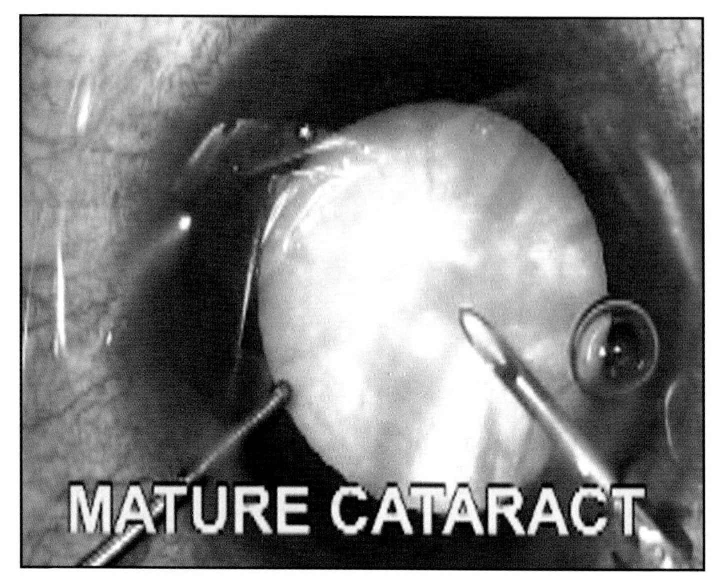

Figure 8-1. Mature cataract. It is difficult to visualize the rhexis in such cases, so we need to stain the anterior capsule with a dye.

hydrogen orthophosphate, 8.2 mg of sodium chloride, sodium hydroxide for adjusting the pH and water for injection. There are many other companies making this dye as well.

Indocyanine Green

Indocyanine green (ICG) is available in the United States. It comes as a lyophilized compound, which must first be dissolved in 0.5 cc of sterile diluent supplied by the manufacturer. It is then further diluted with 4.5 cc of BSS Plus (Alcon) immediately prior to use. This creates a 270 mOsm, 0.5% concentration. ICG creates a pale green staining of the capsule, which is gone by the conclusion of the case. One slight disadvantage is that the dye is lyophilized and larger particles often remain suspended in the mixture.

Technique

We always tend to perform a temporal clear corneal incision. If the astigmatism is plus at 90° then the incision is made superiorly. Trypan blue can be injected under air or directly into the anterior chamber. Trypan blue is withdrawn from the vial into a syringe. This is then injected by a cannula into the anterior chamber between the air bubble and the lens capsule. It is kept like that for a minute or two for staining of the anterior capsule to occur. Next viscoelastic is injected into the anterior chamber to remove the air bubble and the Trypan blue.

Now, rhexis is started with a needle (Figure 8-2). One can use a forceps also. We prefer to use a needle as it gives better control on the size of the rhexis. Note the left hand holding a rod stabilizing the eye while the rhexis is being performed. The rhexis is continued with the needle. Note the contrast between the capsule, which has been stained, and the cortex, which is not stained. The rhexis is continued and finally completed.

Hydrodissection is then done. One will not be able to see the fluid wave in such cases as the cataract is very dense. In such cases, a simple way is to see if the lens comes up

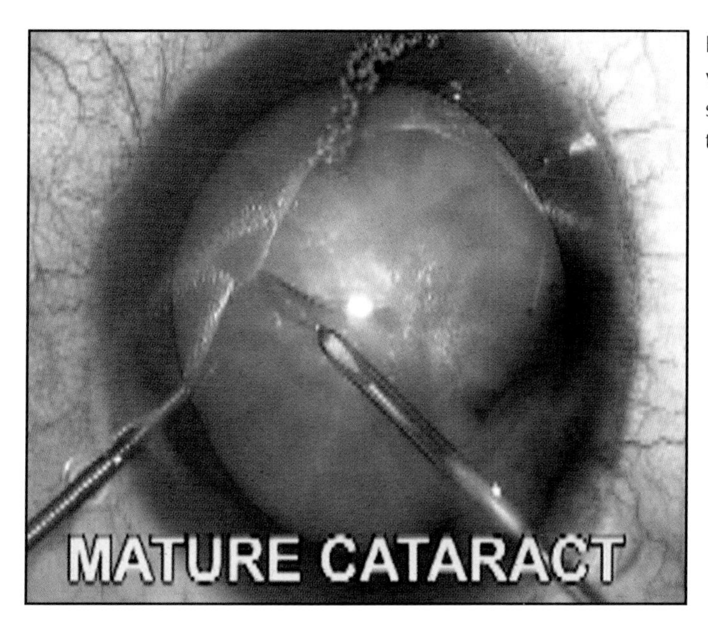

Figure 8-2. Rhexis started with the needle. Note a straight rod in the left hand to stabilize the eye.

anteriorly a little bit. This will indicate hydrodissection being completed. One can also test this by rotating the nucleus before starting phaco.

We then insert the phaco probe through the incision slightly superior to the center of the nucleus. At that point, apply ultrasound and see that the phaco tip gets embedded in the nucleus. The direction of the phaco probe should be obliquely downwards toward the vitreous and not horizontally towards the iris. Then only the nucleus will get embedded. The settings at this stage are 70% phaco power, 24 ml/minute flow rate, and 101 mm Hg suction. We always use the air pump or gas-forced infusion in our cases. By the time the phaco tip gets embedded in the nucleus, the tip has reached the middle of the nucleus. Now, with the chopper cut the nucleus with a straight downward motion and then move the chopper to the left when you reach the center of the nucleus. In other words, your left hand moves the chopper like an inverted L. Do not go to the periphery for chopping but do it at the center. Once you have created a crack, split the nucleus till the center. Then rotate the nucleus 180° and crack again so that you get two halves of the nucleus.

Now that you have two halves, you have a shelf to embed the probe. Place the probe with ultrasound into one half of the nucleus and chop. In this way, create three quadrants in one half of the nucleus. Then make another three halves with the second half of the nucleus. Thus, you now have six quadrants or pie-shaped fragments.

Once all the pieces have been chopped, take out each piece one by one and in pulse phaco mode aspirate the pieces at the level of the iris. Do not work in the bag unless the cornea is preoperatively bad or the patient is very elderly.

The next step is to do cortical washing. Always try to remove the subincisional cortex first, as that is the most difficult. Note that the left hand has the straight rod controlling the movements of the eye every time. If necessary, use a bimanual irrigation aspiration technique. Then inject viscoelastic and implant the IOL. At the end of the procedure, inject the BSS inside the lips of the clear corneal incision. This will create a stromal hydration at the wound. This will create a whiteness, which will disappear after 4–5 hours. The advantage of this is that the wound gets sealed better.

Adverse Effects

1. We are still not sure if extended contact between trypan blue and the corneal endothelium produces corneal damage. At present, no cases have been reported because the trypan blue is washed off with the viscoelastic and the BSS fluid.
2. Postsurgical inflammatory reactions and some bullous keratopathy have been known to occur after using vital staining agents.
3. Extreme care must be taken when using trypan blue on patients who are hypersensitive to any of its components.
4. During animal experiments, a teratogenic and/or mutagenic effect has been reported after repeated and/or high dose intraperitoneal or intravenous injections with trypan blue. It should not be used in pregnant women.

Summary

Trypan blue or ICG can make life much easier for the phaco surgeon, especially in cases of mature and hypermature cataracts by staining the anterior capsule.

Key Points

1. One of the biggest problems for a phaco surgeon is to perform a rhexis in a mature cataract. The solution to this problem is to use a dye, like trypan blue, to stain the anterior capsule.
2. Indocyanine green (ICG) is available in the United States. It comes as a lyophilized compound, which must first be dissolved in 0.5 cc of sterile diluent supplied by the manufacturer.
3. One will not be able to see the fluid wave during hydrodissection in mature cataracts because the cataract is very dense. In such cases, if the lens comes up anteriorly a little bit, this will indicate hydrodissection being completed.
4. Postsurgical inflammatory reactions and some bullous keratopathy have been known to occur after using vital staining agents.

References

1. Agarwal A, Agarwal A, Agarwal S. Phakonit and laser phakonit. In: Agarwal S, Agarwal A, Sachdev M, et al, eds. *Phacoemulsification, Laser Cataract Surgery and Foldable IOLs*. 2nd ed. New Delhi: Jaypee Brothers; 2000:204-216.
2. Agarwal A. No anaesthesia cataract surgery with karate chop. In: Agarwal S, Agarwal A, Sachdev M, et al, eds. *Phacoemulsification, Laser Cataract Surgery and Foldable IOLs*. 2nd ed. New Delhi: Jaypee Brothers; 2000:217-226.

Chapter 9

Small Pupil Phacoemulsification

Amar Agarwal, MS, FRCOphth, FRCS;
Soosan Jacob, MS, DNB, FRCS, MNAMS, FERC

Introduction

The pupil size has always played a very important role in performing any type of cataract surgery, be it an intracapsular cataract extraction, extracapsular cataract extraction, phacoemulsification, bimanual phacoemulsification, or microphakonit. A large sized, well-dilated pupil increases the ease of surgery dramatically, but unfortunately a miotic pupil (less than 4.0 mm), is a common problem that every surgeon faces at some time. Miotic, nondilating pupil (Figure 9-1A and B) may be secondary to a variety of reasons (Table 9-1). Phacoemulsification is especially difficult in these cases because it affects all steps, from capsulorrhexis to emulsification of the nucleus, cortical removal, and in-the-bag intraocular lens (IOL) insertion. The surgeon is forced to perform a small capsulorrhexis, which further adds to the difficulty in performing surgery. A small pupil may cause damage to the patient's eye by emulsification of the iris or cause complications such as sphincter tears, intraoperative bleeding, zonular dialysis, posterior capsular rent, or nucleus drop. Prolonged surgical time and increased maneuvering may result in postoperative complications such as striate keratopathy; uveitis; secondary glaucoma; floppy, torn or atrophic iris; irregular pupil; endophthalmitis; or cystoid macular edema, all resulting in a suboptimal surgical outcome and an unhappy patient. A study of 1,000 consecutive extracapsular cataract extractions (ECCE) showed that a small pupil was the most common factor associated with vitreous loss and capsular rupture.[1]

A hypotonic, mid-dilated, irregular pupil postoperatively can also be aesthetically bad, especially noticeable in light colored irides. Such a pupil can also have significant effect on the pupillary function, leading to iatrogenic glare dysfunction. Masket reported that an enlarged pupil can be responsible for postoperative glare disability in eyes that were anatomically normal except for having pseudophakia.[2] All these factors makes it mandatory for a phaco surgeon to know how to tackle a miotic pupil.

There are a variety of techniques for the management of the small pupil, including iris hooks, iris rings, and pupillary stretching with or without the use of multiple half-width sphincterotomies.[3]

Table 9-1.

Causes for Miotic Pupil

Causes for Miotic Pupil
Age-related dilator atrophy
Diabetes mellitus
Synechiae
Previous trauma
Previous surgery
Uveitis
Iridoschisis
Pseudoexfoliation syndrome
Chronic miotic therapy
Congenital
Idiopathic
Marfan's syndrome
Chronic lues

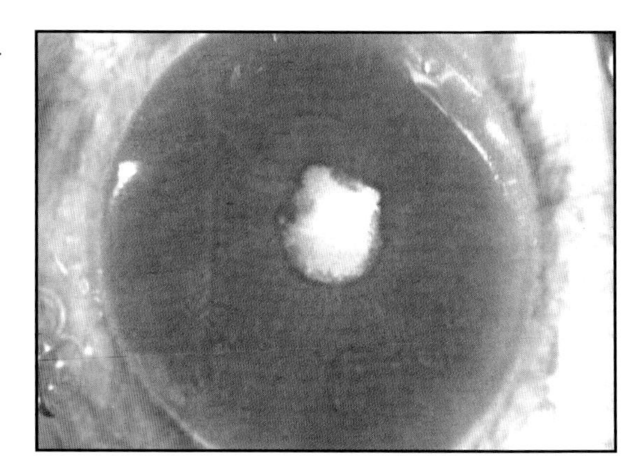

Figure 9-1A. Miotic nondilating pupil.

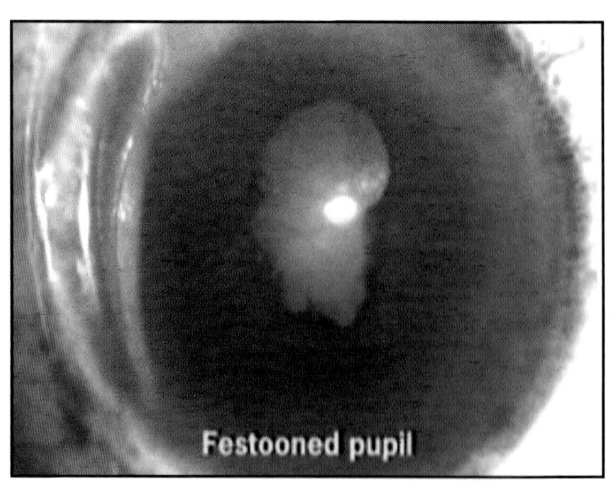

Figure 9-1B. Festooned pupil.

Preoperative Evaluation

A dilated preoperative examination is mandatory for every patient, not just for assessing the posterior segment, but also to detect cases of suboptimal pupillary dilatation. Appropriate history is important for detecting any underlying etiology for the miotic pupil. One should check for intraoperative floppy iris syndrome and usage of tamsulosin (Flomax, Boehringer-Ingelheim Pharmaceuticals, Inc., Ridgefield, CT) as suggested by David Chang (see Chapter 10). A careful slit lamp examination is mandatory for detecting the cause as well as any associated complicating conditions that may coexist, such as zonular weakness in a case of pseudoexfoliation. Proper planning of the surgical steps should be done preoperatively. Synechiolysis or membranectomy may be required in cases of chronic uveitis. For patients on chronic miotic therapy, these drugs should be stopped preoperatively and replaced if necessary with other suitable medications.

Pharmacological Mydriasis

The topical agents used preoperatively for dilating the patient's eye should include a cycloplegic, a mydriatic, and a nonsteroidal anti-inflammatory drug (NSAID).[4]

Cycloplegics

The most commonly used cycloplegic agent is cyclopentolate hydrochloride 1%, which provides good cycloplegia and pupillary dilatation. The pupillary dilatation can last up to 36 hours. Tropicamide hydrochloride 1% is also a good pupillary dilator, though shorter acting and with slightly lesser degree of cycloplegia. Atropine sulfate 1% is a longer lasting mydriatic and can be considered in cases of chronic uveitis, long-standing diabetics, etc.

Mydriatics

Phenylephrine hydrochloride 2.5% is a good pupil dilator, especially when combined with a cycloplegic. The 10% solution gives stronger dilatation, especially in resistant cases, but the disadvantage is that it may increase the blood pressure in some patients and can also result in corneal punctate keratopathy. Mydricaine, a product which contains atropine, procaine, and adrenaline, can also be used as subconjunctival injections preoperatively.

Nonsteroidal Anti-Inflammatory Drugs

NSAIDs decrease the incidence of intraoperative constriction of the pupil. This is especially important in case of prolonged surgeries and surgery with increased intraoperative manipulation. Suprofen, diclofenac Ketorolac, flurbiprofen, etc are commonly used for this purpose.[5–10]

Pharmacological mydriasis may not be effective in all cases, especially in cases with posterior synechiae and scarred pupils. Such pupils have to be dealt with appropriately during surgery to avoid a cascade of complications (Table 9-2).

Table 9-2.
Methods for Enlarging the Pupil

Sphincter-sparing techniques:
• Synechiolysis
• Pupillary membranectomy
• Viscomydriasis
Sphincter-involving techniques:
• Mini sphincterotomies
• Pupil stretch
• Iris hooks
• Pupil ring expanders

Intraoperative Procedures not Involving the Sphincter

Viscomydriasis

A new ophthalmic viscosurgical device (OVD), 2.4% Hyaluronate can be used for mechanically dilating the pupil in certain cases.[4,11] It is injected into the center of the pupil to mechanically dissect any synechiae and to stretch the sphincter. It should be completely removed at the end of the procedure to avoid postoperative intraocular pressure increase.

Synechiolysis

A blunt spatula is passed through the side-port incision after injecting viscoelastic into the eye[4]. A second side-port incision may be required in case of extensive synechiae. This is followed by utilizing one of the other techniques to maintain the pupil in a dilated stage, eg, viscomydriasis, iris hooks, or pupil expanders. A blunt rod can also be used to sweep any posterior synechiae free, without any stretch motions (Figure 9-2).

Pupillary Membranectomy

Pupillary membranes can cause small pupils. These membranes can be taken care of with a combination of preoperative pharmacotherapy and intraoperative surgical removal by stripping the fine fibrin pupillary membrane using Utrata forceps.

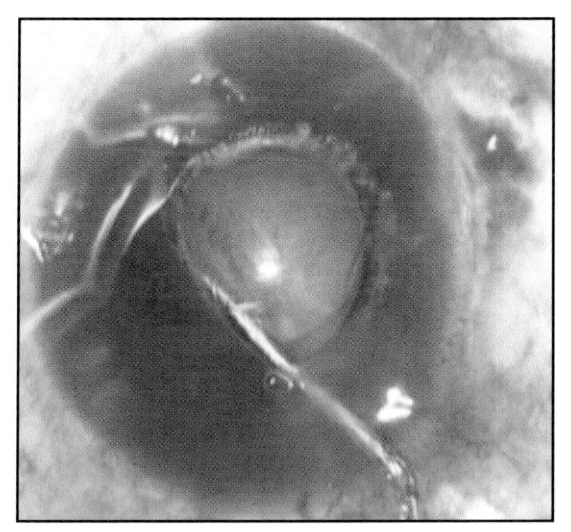

Figure 9-2. A blunt rod being used for synechiolysis.

Intraoperative Procedures Involving the Sphincter

Mini Sphincterotomies

Mini sphincterotomies[4,11] can be done with either Vanass scissors through the main port incision or with vitreoretinal scissors placed through the paracentesis. Very small partial cuts, no larger than 0.75 mm in radial length, are made limited to the sphincter tissue. As long as the incisions are kept very small, postoperatively the pupil should be normal both functionally and aesthetically. The disadvantage is that regardless of the wound position, the incision is more difficult to create in the clock hour of the wound.

Pupil Stretch

Pupil stretch[12] can be done either using push-pull instruments or pronged instruments that stretch the pupillary sphincter. Pupillary stretching generally causes multiple fine partial sphincter tears. If combined with preplaced mini sphincterotomies, the effect can be increased.[3] It generally results in a functionally and aesthetically acceptable pupil postoperatively. The disadvantage is that the iris sometimes becomes flaccid and may either move into an undesirable location or may prolapse through the incision during surgery. Rarely, it may cause complications like hematoma or larger sphincter tears, pigment dispersion, postoperative uveitis, pressure spike, and an abnormal and nonfunctional pupil postoperatively.

Bimanual Push-Pull Instruments

Using viscoelastic cover, two hooks are used in a slow, controlled fashion to stretch the pupil in one or more axes.[2] One hook is used for pushing the pupillary margin and the other one for pulling. The push-pull should be done simultaneously, in a controlled manner, to avoid large sphincter tears. This technique usually achieves an adequately sized pupil for effective phacoemulsification. A two-handed, two-instrument bimanual stretch technique with an angled Kuglen hook and Lindstrom star nucleus rotator is very effective.

Pronged Instruments

Instruments available[12] are the Keuch two-pronged pupil stretcher (Katena) or the four-pronged pupil stretcher (Rhein Medical's Beehler pupil dilator). Postoperatively, the pupil continues to react normally. This technique, popularized by Luther Fry,[4] is an efficient and cost-effective method. The prongs (Figure 9-3) should be maintained parallel to the iris plane and should not slip out into the pupil margin, especially on starting to depress the plunger to create the pupil stretch.

Iris Hooks

Commercially available iris hooks (Grieshaber, Schaffhausen, Switzerland) were originally used for posterior segment surgeries.[13] They can also be utilized for phacoemulsification[14] (Figures 9-4 through 9-7), but the disadvantage is that unless properly placed (Figure 9-8A and B), they can pull the iris diaphragm forward, resulting in chaffing (Figure 9-9) and thermal damage during phacoemulsification.[15,16] To avoid this, the hooks should be placed parallel to the iris plane through small, short tract, peripheral paracenteses or by releasing the hooks after creating the capsulorrhexis but before phacoemulsification. Gradual enlargement of the pupil should be done and a pupil size just enough for the surgical procedure created to avoid postoperative pupillary atony. The other disadvantage is that it adds to the time and cost of surgery. Iris hooks have also been used in cases of zonular dialysis to stabilize the capsular bag by hooking it around the capsulorrhexis margin.

Iris Retainer Methods

Pupil Ring Expanders

Pupil ring expanders (Figure 9-10) enlarge the pupil without sphincter damage. Here, incomplete pupil ring expanders are used to stretch the pupil.[17] They are inserted through the main port and manipulated into the pupil space. They can create the largest diameter pupil, creating a uniform expanding force around approximately 300° of the pupil. Thus they have the least tendency for sphincter tears, as they do not produce point pressure on the pupillary margin. The disadvantages with these devices are that they are rigid, cumbersome, and slightly difficult to insert into the eye through a small incision. They require manipulation to engage the sphincter. They may also hamper entry, exit, and maneuvering of additional instruments through the incisions. It also adds to the time and cost of surgery. The one-piece retaining rings are often difficult to position and even more difficult to remove.

Three expanders are the Grather, Siepser and Morcher.[4] They are made of solid PMMA, silicone, or expandable hydrogel material.

The Graether's pupil expander consists of a silicone ring with an indentation, which fits all along the edge of the pupil.[18] The iris fits like a tire around the ring, which is like an iron wheel. The disadvantage is that it can loosen easily with intraocular maneuvers.

Perfect Pupil Device

Developed by John Milverton, MD of Sydney, Australia, the Perfect Pupil device is a sterile, disposable, flexible polyurethane ring with an integrated arm (Figure 9-11) that allows for easy insertion and removal.[11] It is inserted with a forceps or injected (Figures 9-12 and 9-13) with an injector through the main port. The integrated arm remains outside the eye to aid in easy removal. It can be inserted through an incision less than 100 microns. Because of the open ring design of the Perfect Pupil, there is no interference with other instrumentation.

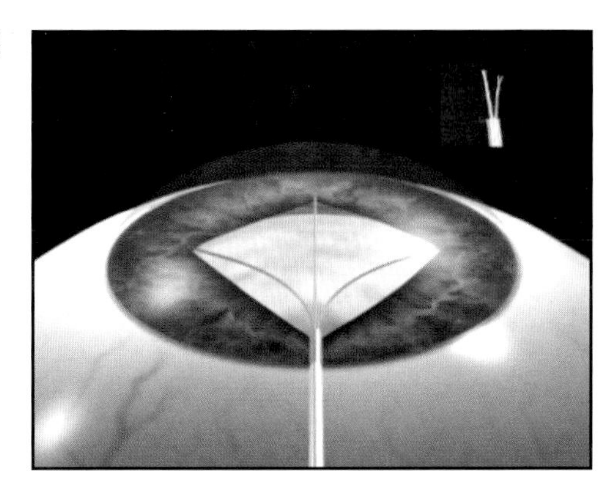

Figure 9-3. Pupil stretch using pronged pupil stretcher.

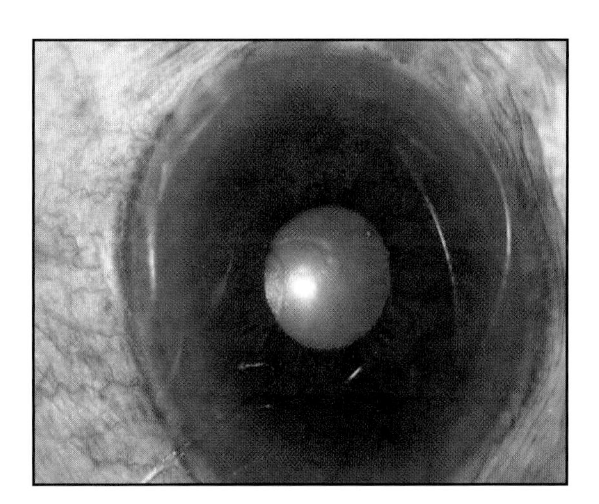

Figure 9-4. Miotic pupil.

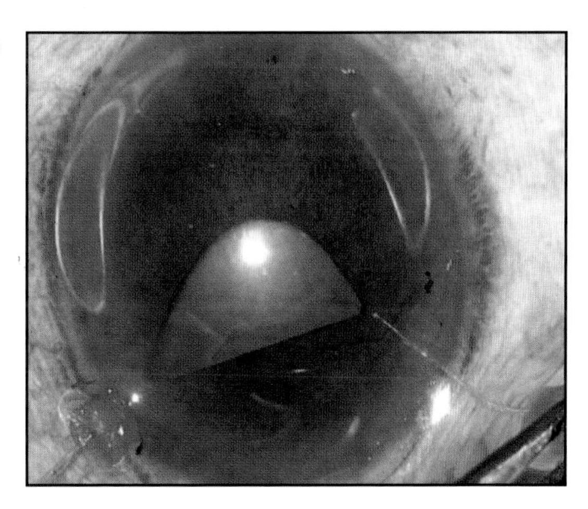

Figure 9-5. Iris hooks inserted to enlarge the pupil.

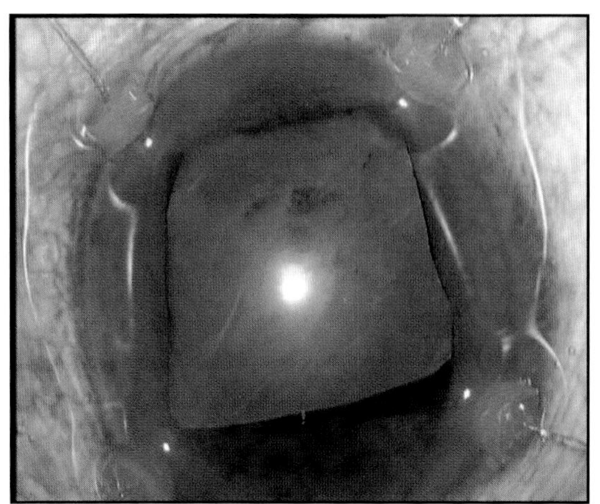

Figure 9-6. All four iris hooks in place.

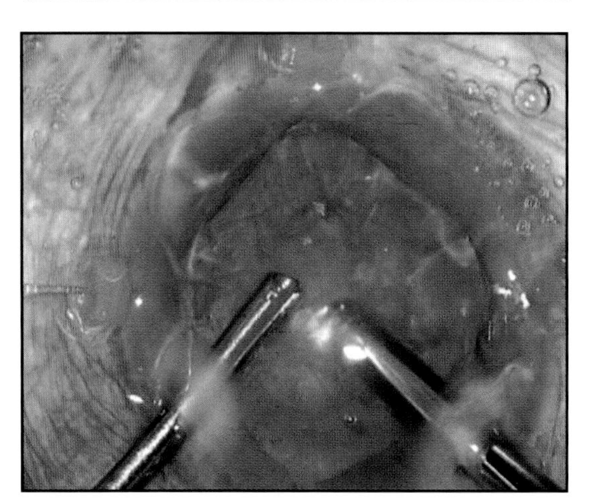

Figure 9-7. Phakonit being performed with the iris hooks in place.

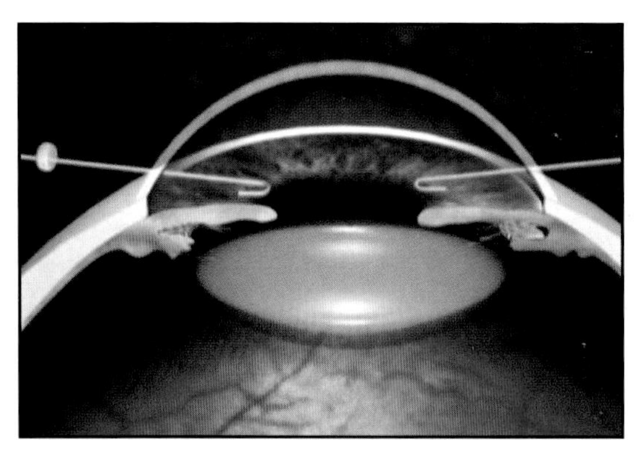

Figure 9-8A. Iris hooks being placed.

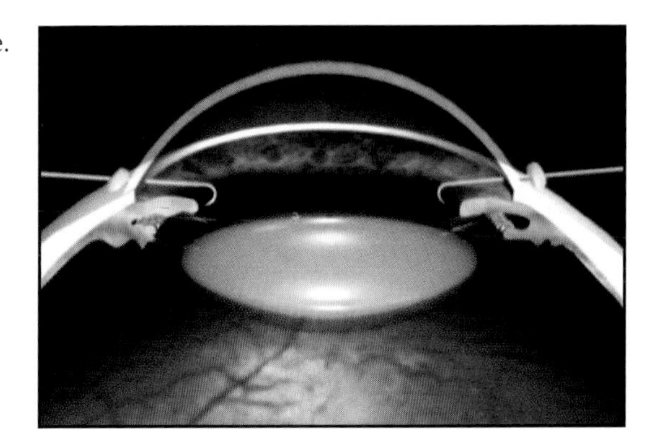

Figure 9-8B. Iris hooks properly in place.

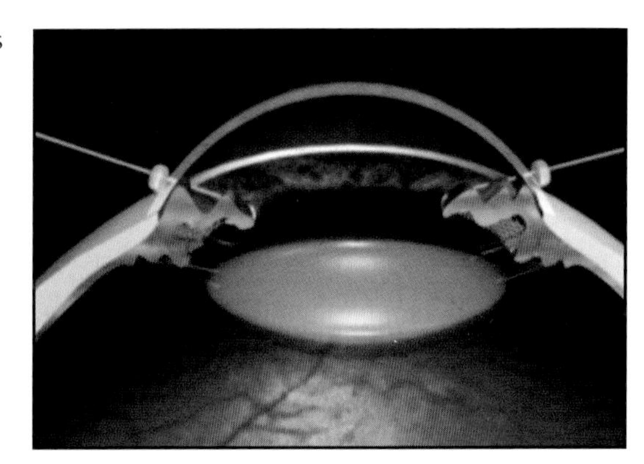

Figure 9-9. If not placed properly, iris hooks can lead to chafing of the iris.

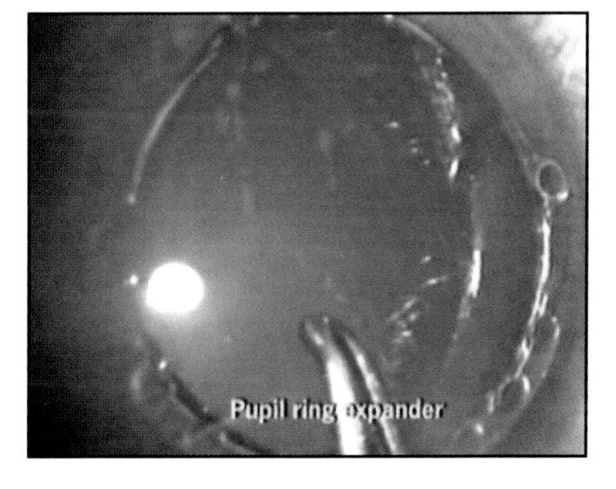

Figure 9-10. Pupil ring expander. (Photo courtesy of Dr. Lincoln L. Freitas.)

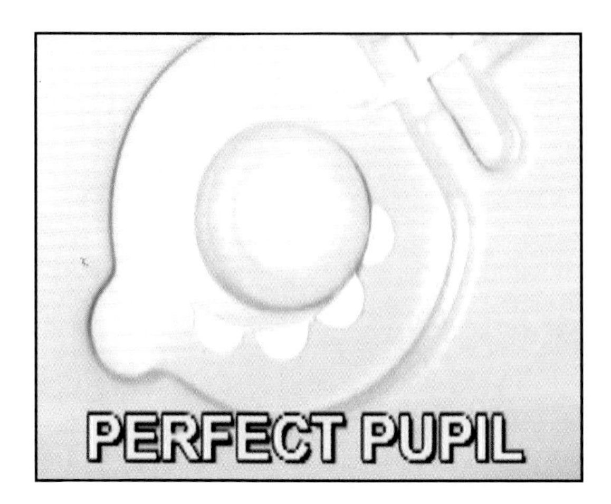

Figure 9-11. Perfect Pupil device.

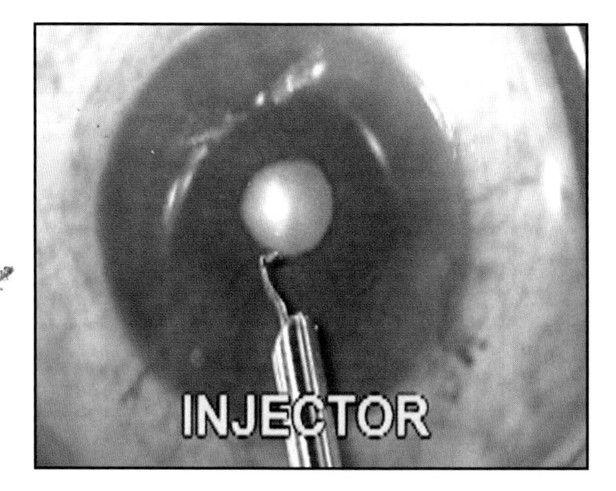

Figure 9-12. Perfect Pupil injector.

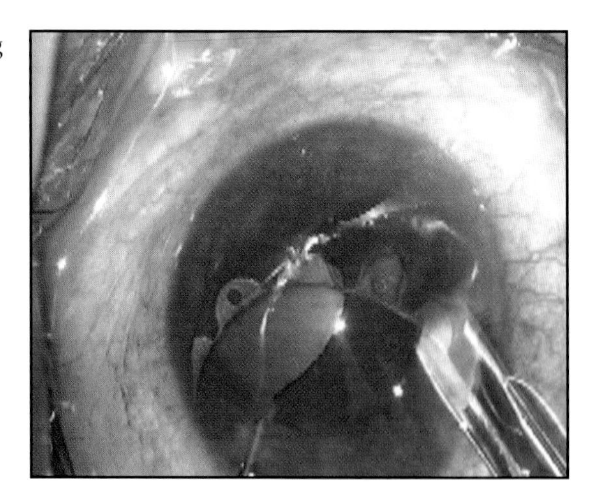

Figure 9-13. Perfect Pupil device being injected into the eye with the injector.

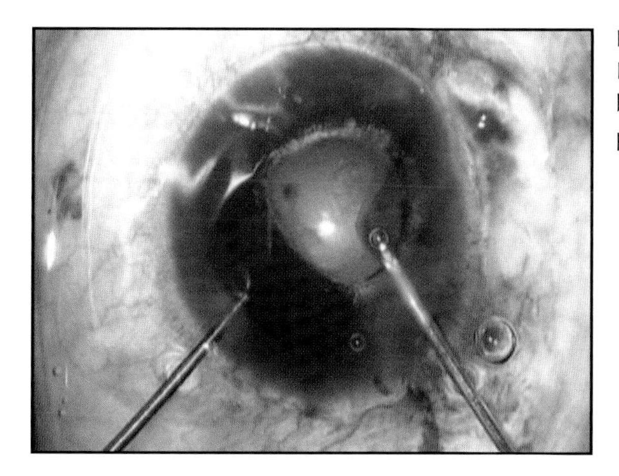

Figure 9-14. Dye (trypan blue, Blurhex) enhanced capsulorrhexis being performed in a miotic, fibrotic pupil.

Surgical Complications

Bleeding may occur with these techniques.[4] It generally subsides on its own and any postoperative hyphema gets absorbed spontaneously. In case of significant bleeding intraoperatively, the IOP should be increased by elevating the bottle height, or by injecting a viscoelastic agent or air to the eye. In case of a major, unresponsive bleed within the eye, one can add fibrin. Instrument-related damages that can occur include corneal endothelial damage,[4] iridodialysis, bleeding, and iris pigment dispersion. Postoperatively, the patient may have an atonic, distorted pupil. Large tears to the iris sphincter can result in this. Pupillary dilatation should be done gradually to minimize sphincter tears and only the minimum amount of stretching that is required for the surgical steps should be done.[4] A forcibly, maximally dilated pupil can result in postoperative atonic pupil. Other postoperative complications include uveitis, increased IOP, and pigments on the IOL. These can be avoided by careful, gentle instrumentation and as little manipulation as possible within the eye.

Phacoemulsification Pearls

- The experience of the surgeon and the nature of the cataract dictate the minimum pupil diameter for a case.
- Generally, if the pupil is large enough to perform an adequate capsulorrhexis, it is large enough for the remainder of the surgical procedure.
- In cases with small pupil, the corneal incision must be made anteriorly to avoid the risk of iris prolapse with posterior corneal incisions.
- Capsular dyes such as indocyanine green (ICG) or trypan blue (Figure 9-14) should be injected under the iris to aid in making the rhexis as well as to visualize the capsule as the pupil later enlarges.
- Hydrodissection should be gentle, as an excessive fluid wave can cause iris prolapse.

- A retentive viscoelastic such as Healon 5 should be used, as it pressurizes the anterior chamber. As the IOP increases, the viscoelastic remains in the eye and pushes down on the lens-iris diaphragm, thus mechanically enlarging the pupil. A cohesive type of viscoelastic is not as effective because it evacuates easily from the eye when IOP increases.
- Mini sphincterotomies or the bimanual stretching technique of Luther Fry work well with fibrotic pupils such as those in patients on chronic miotic therapy. They are not as effective when the iris is elastic and floppy because the sphincter does not readily tear and the iris snaps back following stretching.
- A Sinskey or Kuglen hook can be inserted through the side-port incision to move the pupil away while doing capsulorrhexis to achieve a larger sized rhexis.
- Sculpting is more difficult with small pupils because visualization is poor. The peripheral lens cannot be seen and the red reflex, which is required to visualize the depth of sculpting, is reduced by the smaller pupil diameter. These problems are overcome to a large extent using phaco chop techniques.
- For nucleus removal, phaco chop, particularly vertical chop, is the ideal technique in a miotic pupil, as it does not require a large pupil. Here, the phaco tip stays in the center of the pupil for the majority of the time, and the chances of capturing the iris or capsular edge are much lower. The second instrument can be used to move the pupil away to get a perfect position and then phaco chop can be performed.
- An injector is preferred over the folding forceps for inserting the IOL. The tip of the folder may catch the iris in the presence of iris prolapse or a flaccid iris and cause a dialysis. The injector tip immediately plugs the incision and there will be a net influx of viscoelastic instead.
- An injector separates the IOL from the surrounding tissues, keeping it sterile. It also helps in exact positioning of the IOL, which is an advantage in a small pupil or a flaccid iris.
- As long as the tip of the injector fits into the capsulorrhexis, the IOL can be delivered into the bag without stretching or tearing the capsulorrhexis.
- The second instrument or viscoelastic can be used to push the iris back and away from the bevel of the injector where it might otherwise be caught.
- For the trailing haptic, two instruments can be used—one to hold the iris and the other to dial in the trailing haptic.
- With plate haptic IOLs, anterior capsular contracture is greater and there is also more giant cell reaction, hence older silicone IOLs should be avoided in eyes that are likely to be inflamed.
- Latest generation silicone IOLs, such as Clariflex (AMO), have no difference in long-term inflammatory profiles between hydrophobic acrylic and second generation silicone. The latest generation silicone achieved statistically significantly less inflammation than the AcrySof IOL in the long term. The second- and higher-generation silicone IOLs are also more chemically pure and have a better overall design with a higher refractive index and thinner profile. Silicone IOLs also have a greater ease of implantation and reduced incision size as compared to acrylic IOLs.
- The Unfolder Emerald injector allows the surgeon to use a full size 6-mm optic acrylic IOL in a three-piece model through a 3-mm incision.
- A Lester hook (Katena Products, Inc.) can be used in the second hand to retract the pupil to re-tear and enlarge a small capsulorrhexis.

- Regardless of the method chosen for enlarging the pupil during phacoemulsification, the pupil should be constricted at the end of surgery with an intraocular miotic. If necessary, the pupil should be stroked with a blunt, gentle instrument to reduce its size. This prevents optic capture, capsular adhesion, or other manner of pupillary deformity.
- Postoperatively, topical anti-inflammatory agents should be used to take care of the increased inflammatory activity secondary to increased maneuvering and longer and more difficult surgery.

Key Points

1. A small pupil may cause damage to the patient's eye by emulsification of the iris or cause complications such as sphincter tears, intraoperative bleeding, zonular dialysis, posterior capsular rent, or nucleus drop.
2. There are a variety of techniques for the management of the small pupil, including iris hooks, iris rings, and pupillary stretching with or without the use of multiple half-width sphincterotomies.
3. The topical agents used preoperatively for dilating the patient's eye should include a cycloplegic, a mydriatic, and a nonsteroidal anti-inflammatory drug.
4. The Perfect Pupil is a sterile, disposable, flexible polyurethane ring with an integrated arm that allows for easy insertion and removal.
5. Capsular dyes such as indocyanine green (ICG) or trypan blue should be injected under the iris to aid in making the rhexis, as well as to visualize the capsule as the pupil later enlarges.

References

1. Guzek JP, Holm M, Cotter JB, et al. Risk factors for intraoperative complications in 1000 extracapsular cataract cases. *Ophthalmology*. 1987;94:46–466.
2. Masket S. Relationship between postoperative pupil size and disability glare. *J Cataract Refract Surg*. 1992;(18):506–507.
3. Fine IH. Phacoemulsification in the presence of a small pupil. In: Steinert RF, ed. Cataract Surgery: Technique, Complications, & Management. Philadelphia, PA: WB Saunders; 1995: 199–208.
4. Masket S. Cataract surgery complicated by the miotic pupil. In: Buratto L, Osher RH, Masket S, eds. *Cataract Surgery in Complicated Cases*. Thorofare, NJ: SLACK Incorporated; 2000:131–137.
5. Thaller VT, Kulshrestha MK, Bell K. The effect of pre-operative topical flurbiprofen or diclofenac on pupil dilatation. *Eye*. 2000;Aug14(Pt4):642.
6. Snyder RW, Siekert RW, Schwiegerling J, Donnenfeld E, Thompson P. Acular as a single agent for use as an antimiotic and anti-inflammatory in cataract surgery. *J Cataract Refract Surg*. 2000; 26(8):1225.
7. Gupta VP, Dhaliwal U, Prasad N. Ketorolac tromethamine in the maintenance of intraoperative mydriasis. Ophthalmic Surg Lasers. 1997;28(9):731.
8. Solomon KD, Turkalj JW, Whiteside SB, Stewart JA, Apple DJ.Topical 0.5% ketorolac vs 0.03% flurbiprofen for inhibition of miosis during cataract surgery. *Arch Ophthalmol*. 1997;115(9):1119.
9. Gimbel H, Van Westenbrugge J, Cheetham JK, DeGryse R, Garcia CG. Intraocular availability and pupillary effect of flurbiprofen and indomethacin during cataract surgery. *J Cataract Refract Surg*. 1996;22(4):474.

10. Brown RM, Roberts CW. Preoperative and postoperative use of nonsteroidal antiinflammatory drugs in cataract surgery. *Insight*. 1996;21(1):13.
11. Kershner RM. Management of the small pupil in clear corneal cataract surgery. *J Cataract Refract Surg*. 2002;28.
12. Shephard DM. The pupil stretch technique for miotic pupils in cataract surgery. *Ophthalmic Surg*. 1994;24:851.
13. De Juan Jr E, Hickingbotham D. Flexible iris retractors. *Am J Ophthalmol*. 1991;111:766.
14. Smith GT, Liu CSC. Flexible iris hooks for phacoemulsification in patients with iridoschisis. *J Cataract Refract Surg*. 2000;26:1277.
15. Nichamin LD. Enlarging the pupil for cataract extraction using flexible nylon iris retractors. *J Cataract Refract Surg*. 1993;19:793.
16. Masket S. Avoiding complications associated with iris retractor use in small pupil cataract extraction. *J Cataract Refract Surg*. 1996;22:168.
17. Graether JM. Graether pupil expander for managing the small pupil during surgery. J Cataract Refract Surg. 1996;22:530.
18. Benjamin Boyd. *The Art and Science of Cataract Surgery*. Panama: Highlights of Ophthalmology; 2001.

Please see Small Pupil video on enclosed CD-ROM.

Chapter 10

Intraoperative Floppy Iris Syndrome

David F. Chang, MD

In January 2005, John R. Campbell, MD and I reported on two companion studies that we undertook to study the characteristics, incidence, surgical outcomes, and etiology of floppy irides during cataract surgery[1]. We named this condition the intraoperative floppy iris syndrome (IFIS) (Figure 10-1). Based upon retrospective observations by Dr. Campbell regarding a possible association with tamsulosin (Flomax, Boehringer-Ingelheim Pharmaceuticals, Inc., Ridgefield, CT), we attempted to evaluate IFIS with both a retrospective and a prospective study. Because there is no mention of any such syndrome in the literature, we were not even sure how to define this syndrome at first.

From a prospective study of 900 consecutive cases in which the surgeon (DFC) was masked as to the patient's medication history, approximately 2% of the eyes (21/900) and 2% of the total patients (16/741) were deemed to have a floppy iris. Fifteen out of sixteen of these patients were either on Flomax or had taken Flomax in the past. This systemic alpha 1-antagonist drug is the most commonly prescribed medication for benign prostatic hyperplasia (BPH). None of the 725 non-IFIS patients were taking Flomax.

The retrospective study evaluated every cataract surgery performed in a two-surgeon (JRC) practice during the prior calendar year (2003). A "floppy iris" was noted in the operative report in approximately 2% of the total cases (16/706) and patients (10/511). Every one of the IFIS patients was on Flomax. Six patients taking Flomax did not have a floppy iris noted in the operative report. An additional 1.5% (11/706) of the patients were taking other systemic alpha-blockers (Hytrin, Cardura, or Minipres). None of these patients demonstrated a floppy iris. The rate of IFIS in the two combined studies, totaling more than 1600 eyes and 1250 patients, was 2%.

Pharmacology of Systemic Alpha-1 Blockers

Tamsulosin (Flomax) is one of several systemic alpha-1 blockers used to treat the urinary symptoms of BPH. Other drugs in this group include terazosin (Hytrin), doxazosin

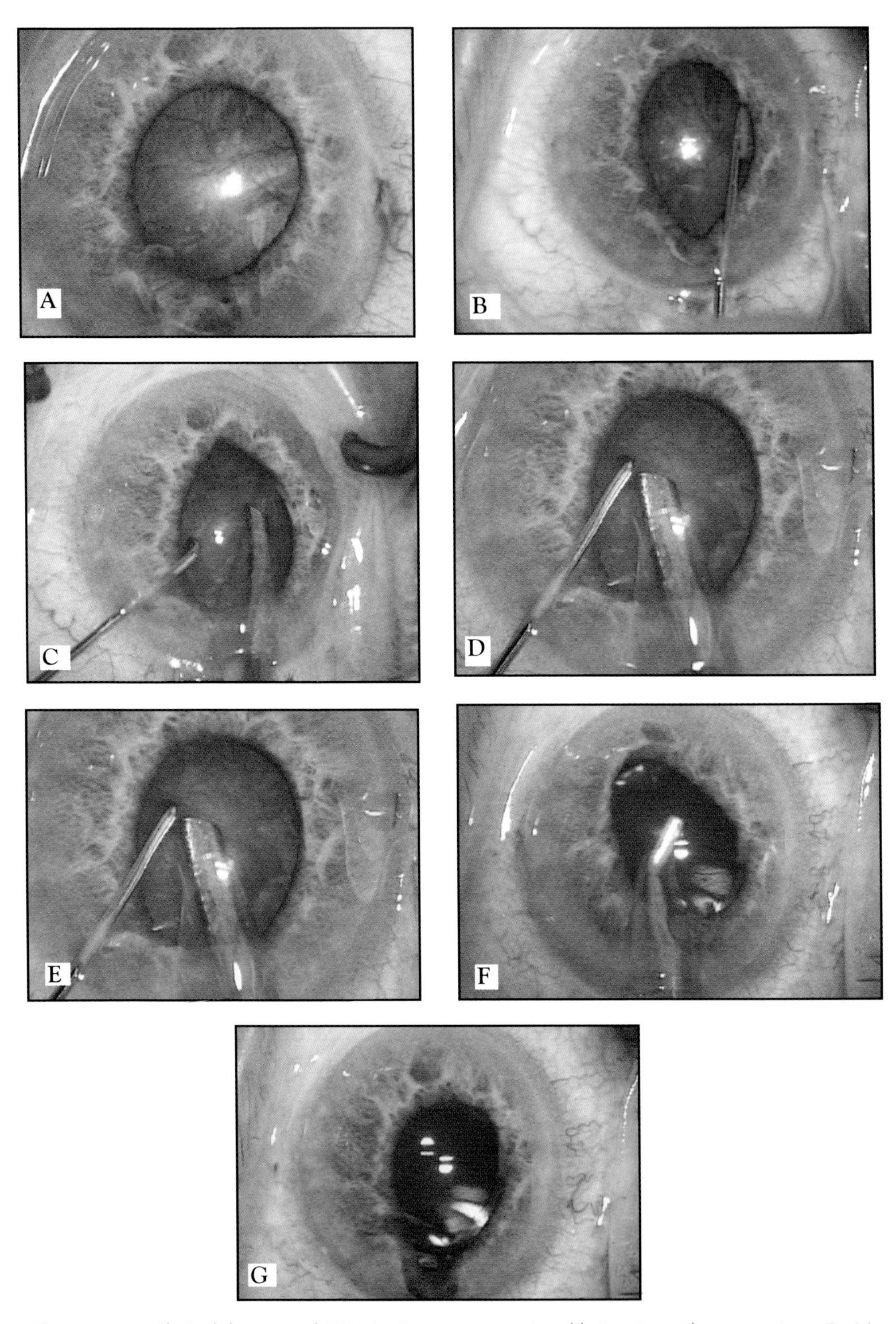

Figure 10-1. Clinical features of IFIS. **A.** Poor preoperative dilation in a Flomax patient. **B.** Iris prolapses during hydrodissection. **C.** Iris billows with normal irrigation currents. **D.** Iris prolapses to phaco and side port incisions. **E.** Pupil constricts intraoperatively following prolapse. **F.** Iris billows during irrigation-aspiration maneuver. **G.** Iris prolapses after withdrawing instrument.

(Cardura), and alfuzosin (Uroxatral). These drugs improve urinary outflow by relaxing the smooth muscle in the prostate and bladder neck. However, side effects can include postural hypotension due to alpha-1 blockade of the vascular wall smooth muscle. Recently, urologists have begun to treat urinary retention symptoms in women with Flomax.[2] Predictably, anecdotal reports are emerging that these women demonstrate IFIS as well.

Molecular studies have demonstrated the presence of three different alpha-1 receptor subtypes—A, B, and D. Flomax exhibits extremely high affinity and specificity for the alpha-1A receptor subtype, which is the predominant receptor found in the prostatic and bladder smooth muscle. Being the only drug in this class that is specific to one receptor subtype, Flomax is much more uroselective than Hytrin and Cardura, and is preferred over these two agents because of a much lower incidence of postural hypotension. Alfuzosin (Uroxatral) is a newer alpha-1 blocker that is also not subtype specific, but has a much lower incidence of postural hypotension. It is therefore also considered "uroselective". It did not become available in the United States until 2004.

We reviewed the pharmacologic literature to find which alpha-1 receptor subtype mediates contraction of the iris dilator smooth muscle. Indeed, based upon a number of animal studies, it appears that alpha-1A is the predominant receptor subtype in the iris dilator muscle as well[3] While these drugs differ in their receptor subtype affinities, it is not clear why IFIS was not seen in our patients taking Hytrin and Cardura. Because Flomax accounts for almost 80% of the alpha-blocker market for BPH treatment in the United States, it may be that other alpha-1 antagonists are associated with IFIS, but that not enough of these patients have undergone cataract surgery for this to be apparent. Another possibility is that Flomax is not only alpha-1A specific, but also has a much higher affinity for this receptor than the other non-subtype specific agents. A higher affinity may result in more complete and prolonged shutdown of the iris dilator muscle, which could then result in permanent atrophic changes in the muscle. We are undertaking a prospective study to evaluate whether IFIS is also associated with alfuzosin.

Clinical Features

Based upon features common to all of our cases, we defined IFIS according to a triad of signs:

- A floppy iris that billows in response to normal irrigation currents in the anterior chamber (see Figure 10-1c, f).
- A marked propensity for the iris to prolapse to the phaco and side-port incisions (see Figure 10-1b, d, g).
- Progressive pupil constriction during surgery (see Figure 10-1e).

While there are other possible causes of either iris prolapse or intraoperative miosis, it is the combined presence of all three features that defines and characterizes IFIS. The pupil frequently dilates poorly or suboptimally, but this variable feature was not uniform to all cases in our study (Figure 10-1a). Mechanical pupil stretching or partial thickness sphincterotomies are among the most commonly used techniques for small pupils.[4] A surprising and disappointing feature of IFIS was the ineffectiveness of these techniques for achieving or maintaining adequate pupil expansion during surgery.

In the retrospective series, 2/16 (12.5%) IFIS cases incurred posterior capsule rupture with vitreous loss. We also encountered several IFIS fellow eyes that had vitreous loss during prior surgery performed elsewhere and outside of the study period. There were no instances of capsular rupture in the prospective IFIS series, but iris transillumination defects of varying severity resulted from iris prolapse in a number of eyes.

One Northern California surgeon reviewed the charts of every posterior capsule rupture case since 2000, and noted that 5/6 of these patients was on Flomax (R. Beller, 2005, personal communication). At the Massachusetts Eye and Ear Infirmary, a retrospective review of the resident cataract database was undertaken for the most recent 2-year period. They found seven charts in which the patient was listed as taking Flomax, and that vitreous loss had occurred in five of these patients (B. Henderson, 2005, personal communication).

We believe that two features of IFIS, in particular, increase the risk of posterior capsular rupture. The first is the relative ineffectiveness of mechanical pupil stretching, with or without partial thickness sphincterotomies, for expanding the IFIS pupil. Mechanical stretching in patients with posterior synechiae or taking chronic miotics creates microscopic tears in the fibrotic edge of the inelastic pupil. This is not the case in IFIS where, like an elastic waistband, the pupil simply snaps back to its original size. The IFIS pupil does expand following viscoelastic injection, particularly with Healon 5 (Advanced Medical Optics). The surgeon may develop a false sense of safety as the capsulorrhexis is easily completed, and is unprepared for the iris prolapse and unexpected pupil constriction that occurs during phaco. By this point, inserting iris hooks or a pupil expansion ring is more difficult, and can tear the capsulorrhexis edge.

IFIS Is Semi-Permanent

Another surprising feature is the occurrence of IFIS even after stopping the drug for 1 to 2 weeks. Although this seemed to improve the preoperative dilation and iris floppiness in several patients, there were others in whom full-blown IFIS still occurred. Even more interesting has been the observation of IFIS in several patients who had stopped Flomax for more than 1 year prior to surgery. I have observed iris billowing without prolapse and constriction in both eyes of a patient who had discontinued Flomax 3 years prior to his surgery. Another surgeon has reported detecting iris floppiness in both eyes of a patient who was not on Flomax at the time of surgery. Further questioning revealed that the patient had stopped taking Flomax 5 years prior to his cataract surgery (S. Lane, 2005, personal communication).

One interesting case addresses the question of over what length of time Flomax must be used in order to produce IFIS. A patient who was not taking Flomax had unremarkable cataract surgery performed in the first eye, only to manifest IFIS in the second eye 1 month later. At that point, further questioning revealed that he had been started on Flomax two weeks prior to the second eye surgery (M. Daniels, 2005, personal communication). This would indicate that the onset of IFIS can be surprisingly soon after initiating the drug.

We postulate that the iris billowing and propensity to prolapse result from a lack of dilator smooth muscle tone. While the dilator muscle accounts for only a small fraction of the overall iris stromal thickness, the usual intraoperative rigidity of the iris must be the result of normal muscle tone. The persistence of IFIS long after discontinuing Flomax suggests a semi-permanent muscle atrophy and loss of tone. We do not know how long one must be on Flomax before these chronic muscle changes occur.

Surgical Recommendations

IFIS is best managed by using devices or viscoelastic agents that mechanically hold the pupil open and restrain the iris from prolapsing. Of all the different viscoelastics, Healon 5 is best able to viscodilate the pupil, and it is uniquely able to block the iris from prolapsing to the incisions (Figure10-2). However, low aspiration flow and vacuum settings (eg, ≤22 cc/min; ≤200 mmHg) must be used to delay its evacuation from the anterior chamber. As the pupil constricts during phaco, Healon 5 can be repeatedly reinjected. Robert Osher, MD, Douglas Koch, MD, and others have described this IFIS strategy. Steven Arshinoff, MD has described using his "ultimate soft shell technique" for IFIS, in which he combines Viscoat and Healon 5. Compared to expansion devices, this Healon 5 method is

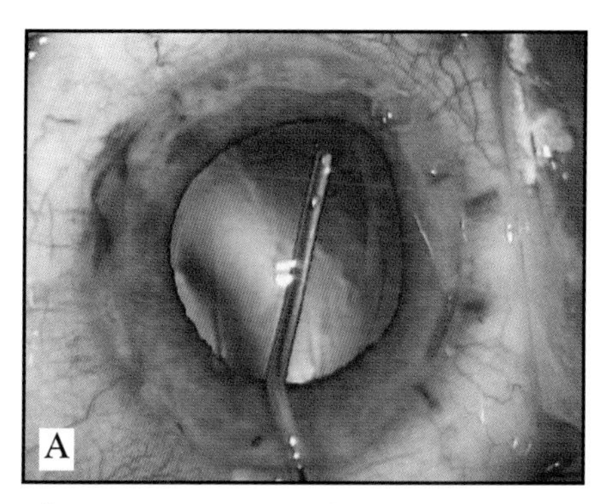

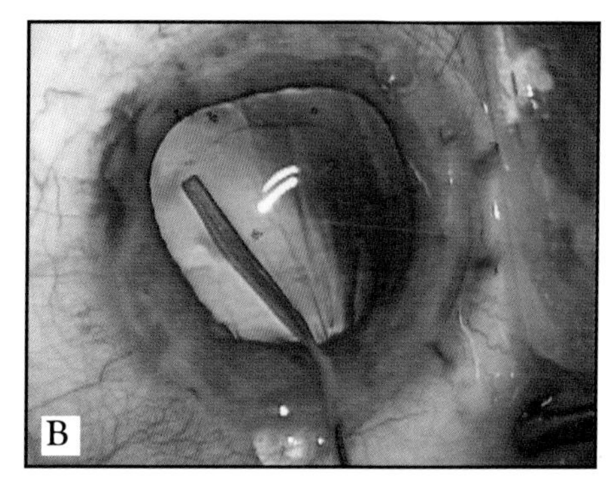

Figure 10-2 A, B. Healon 5 viscomydriasis.

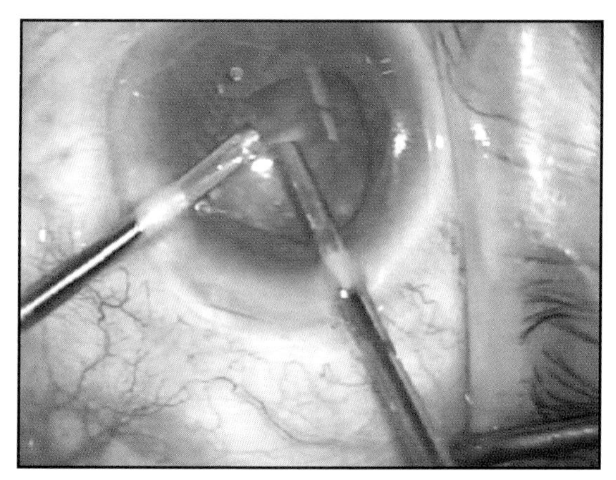

Figure 10-3. Iris prolapse in IFIS despite bimanual MICS instrumentation.

more dependent upon surgical technique and fluidic parameters, and is most effective when the preoperative pupil diameter is reasonably large. Temporarily stopping Flomax for 1 to 2 weeks prior to surgery can be considered if one intends to use this technique. Alternative pharmacologic dilating approaches may help in managing IFIS. Sam Masket, MD has proposed using atropine preoperatively. Richard Packard, MD has reported using intracameral phenylephrine if IFIS is noted. Joel Shugar, MD has reported similar success using intracameral epinephrine.

Bimanual microincisional phaco may have some inherent advantages. The incisions are generally sized more tightly, and this can lessen the tendency for the iris to prolapse. The ability to aim the irrigation currents more consistently anterior to the iris may also be of help. This technique is more effective if the pupil has dilated reasonably well to begin with. However, if the pupil dilates poorly, then IFIS will still occur despite using this technique (Figure 10-3).

Iris retractors or a pupil expansion ring are the most reliable means of maintaining a safe pupil diameter during surgery. These devices are more costly and time-consuming to insert, and placement of expansion rings is difficult if the pupil is small or the anterior chamber is shallow. It is safer to insert these devices before, rather than after capsulorrhexis initiation. As suggested by Thomas Oetting MD, one should place iris retractors in a diamond configuration[9] (Figure 10-4). This requires a separate stab incision just posterior to the clear corneal incision, but maximizes surgical exposure immediately in front of the incision

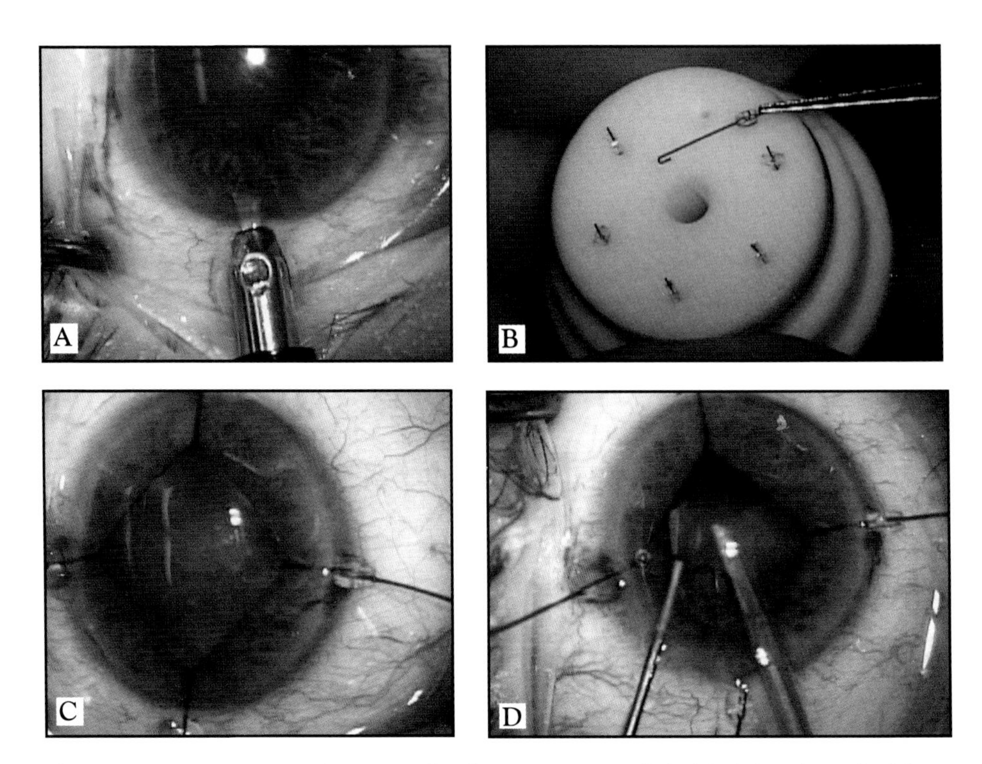

Figure 10-4. A. Separate subincisional stab incision is made behind the phaco incision. **B.** Reusable iris retractors (Katena). **C,D.** Iris retractors in diamond configuration.

(Figure 10-4A). This also retracts the iris posteriorly, as compared to laterally situated iris hooks (square configuration), which tent the iris up anteriorly in front of the phaco incision. I recommend using iris retractors in Flomax patients if the pupil is small, if the nucleus is dense (requiring high vacuum), if the anterior chamber is shallow, or if the surgeon is not experienced with using Healon 5. Stopping Flomax preoperatively should not be necessary if one plans to use iris hooks.

Like all conditions, I believe that there is a spectrum of severity with IFIS. How well the iris dilates preoperatively will often indicate the extent of dilator muscle dysfunction. In my experience, if the pupil dilates well, the alternative pharmacologic measures, Healon 5 techniques, and bimanual microincisional phaco frequently allow surgery to proceed quite normally. However, a poorly dilating pupil usually indicates more advanced dilator muscle dysfunction, and predicts a more refractory degree of IFIS. Mechanical retractors or expansion rings may be necessary in these eyes.

Is Flomax Safe?

As urologists and patients learn that Flomax causes IFIS, the question of whether this drug is safe to use in the cataract population will arise. In our two companion studies, the surgeons had no way to foresee the occurrence of IFIS. Being able to elicit a prior history of Flomax use now enables cataract surgeons to anticipate IFIS, and to employ alternative methods of small pupil management prior to starting the capsulorrhexis. Educating ophthalmologists about IFIS is paramount for this reason, and led the American Society of

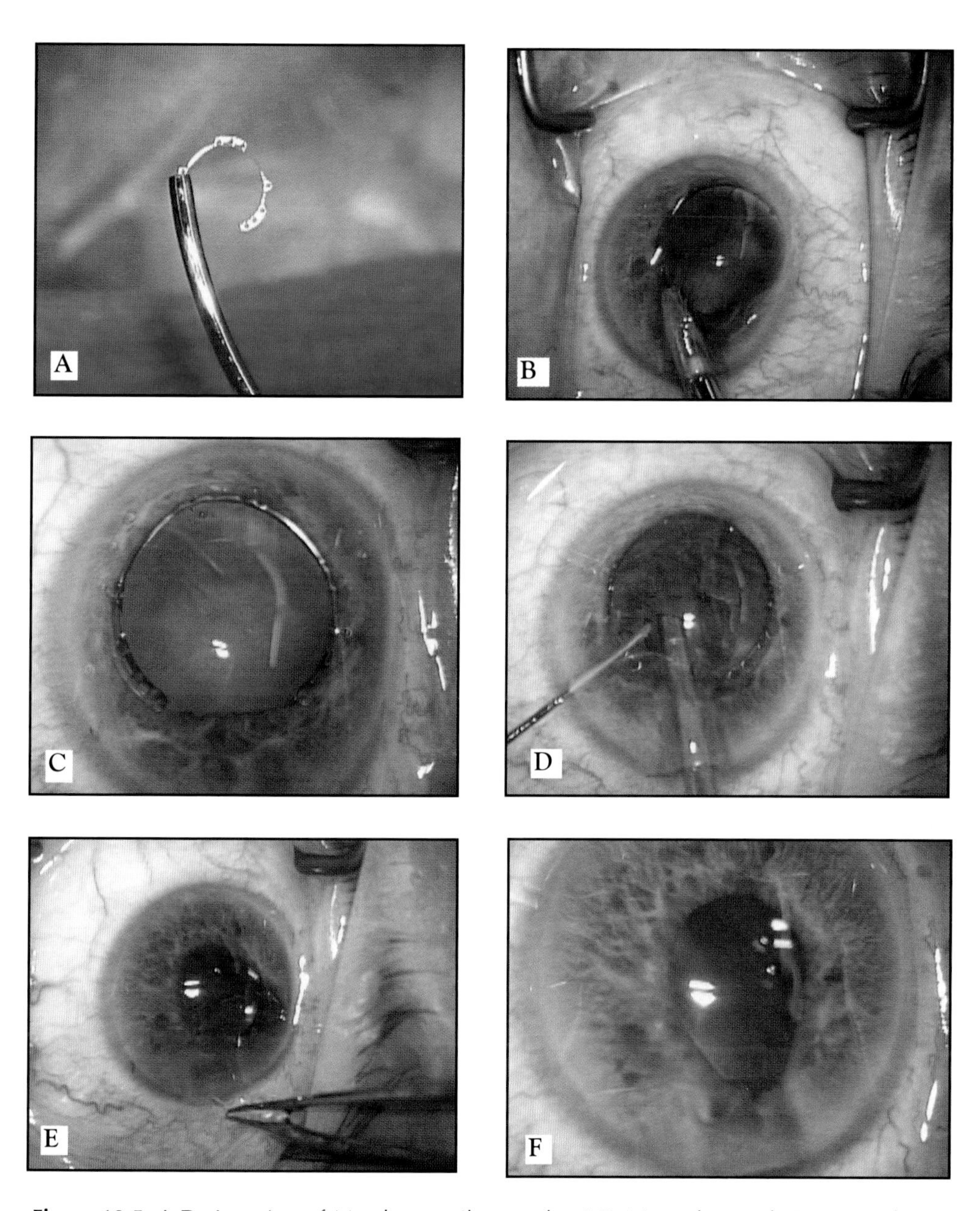

Figure 10-5. A-D. Insertion of Morcher pupil expander. **E,F.** Iris prolapses during viscoelastic removal following removal of the pupil expansion ring.

Cataract and Refractive Surgery (ASCRS) to issue a member advisory alert regarding Flomax in January 2005. I believe that using iris retractors, a pupil expansion ring, or the Healon 5 technique should result in cataract surgical outcomes comparable to non-IFIS eyes. We organized a multicenter trial to prospectively determine the complication rate and surgical outcomes in Flomax patients when one of these three pupil-expanding strategies is used. During a 7-month period, 169 consecutive patients taking Flomax were enrolled, with a resulting posterior capsule rupture rate of less than 1%.

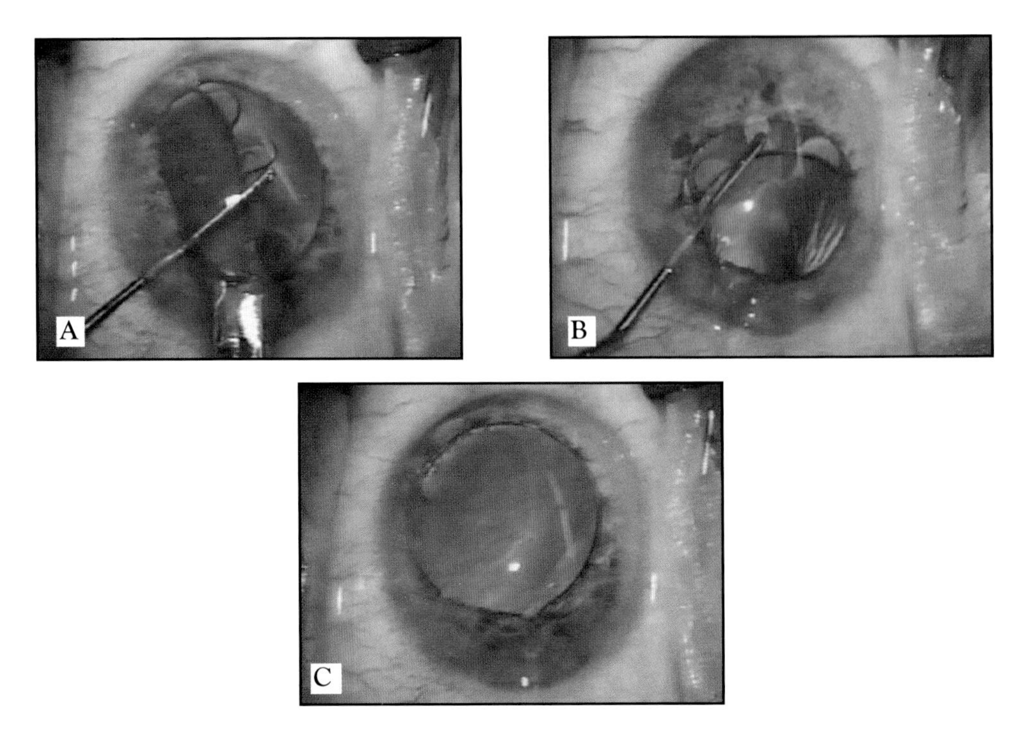

Figure 10-6. A–C. Insertion of Milvella Perfect Pupil expansion device.

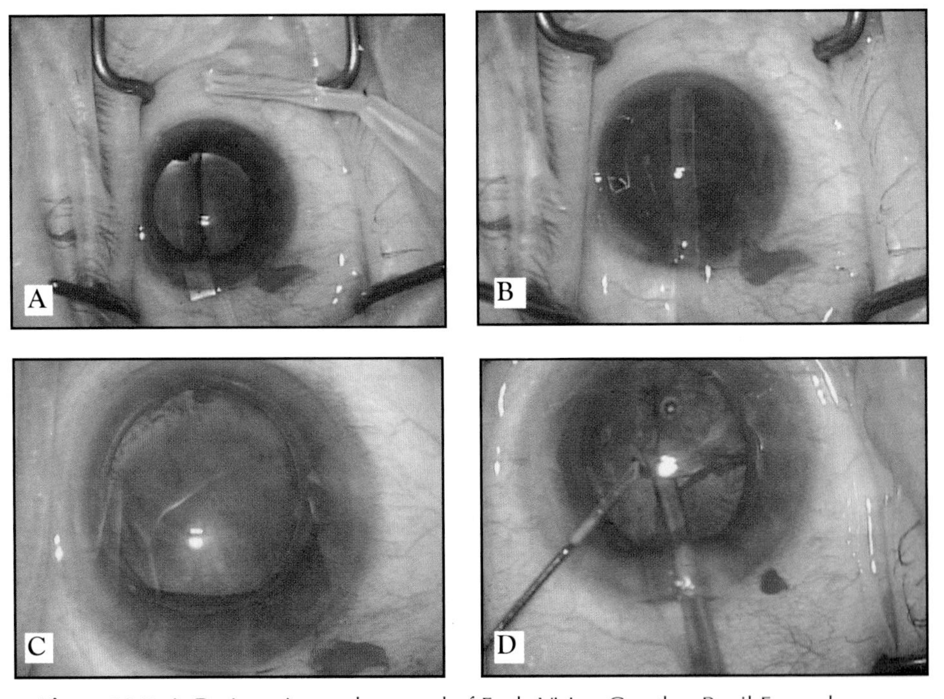

Figure 10-7. A–D. Insertion and removal of Eagle Vision Graether Pupil Expander.

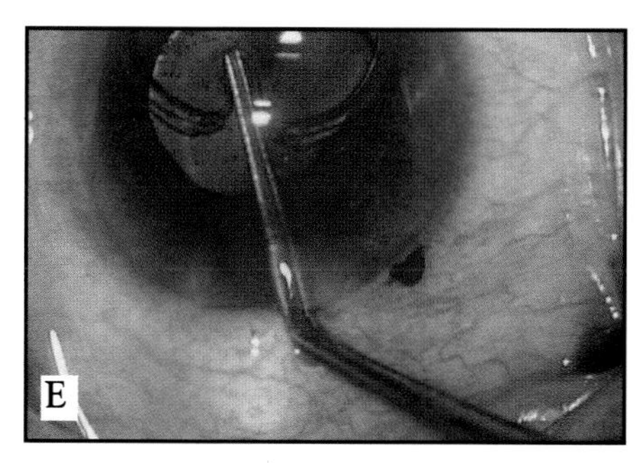

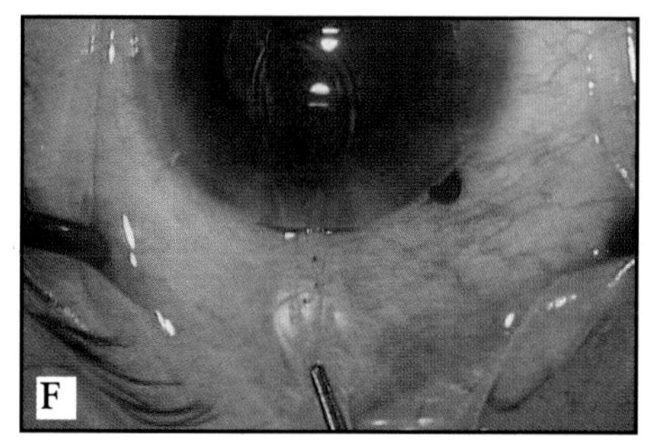

Figure 10-7. E,F. Insertion and removal of Eagle Vision Graether Pupil Expander.

Key Points

1. Tamsulosin (Flomax) is one of several systemic alpha 1 blockers used to treat the urinary symptoms of benign prostatic hypertrophy. Other drugs in this group include terazosin (Hytrin), doxazosin (Cardura), and alfuzosin (Uroxatral). These drugs improve urinary output by relaxing the smooth muscle in the prostate and bladder neck.
2. Alpha-1A is the redominant receptor subtype in the iris dilator muscle as well.
3. The intraoperative floppy iris syndrome (IFIS) has a triad of signs: A floppy iris that billows in response to normal irrigation currents in the anterior chamber, a marked propensity for the iris to prolapse to the phaco and side-port incisions, and progressive pupil constriction during surgery.
4. IFIS is best managed by using devices or viscoelastic agents that mechanically hold the pupil open and restrain the iris from prolapsing. Of all the different viscoelastics, Healon 5 is best able to viscodilate the pupil, and it is uniquely able to block the iris from prolapsing to the incisions.
5. Bimanual microincisional phaco may have some inherent advantages. The incisions are generally sized more tightly, and this can lessen the tendency for the iris to prolapse.

References

1. Chang DF, Campbell JR. Intraoperative floppy iris syndrome associated with tamsulosin (Flomax). *J Cataract Refract Surg*. 2005;31:664–673.
2. Reitz A, Haferkamp A, Kyburz T, et al. The effect of tamsulosin on the resting tone and the contractile behaviour of the female urethra: a functional urodynamic study in healthy women. *Eur Urol*. 2004;46:235–240.
3. Yu Y, Koss MC. Studies of a-Adrenoceptor antagonists on sympathetic mydriasis in rabbits. *J Ocul Pharmacol Ther*. 2003;19:255–263.
4. Akman A, Yilmaz G, Oto S, Akova Y. Comparison of various pupil dilatation methods for phacoemulsification in eyes with a small pupil secondary to pseudoexfolication. *Ophthalmology*. 2004;111:1693–1698.
5. Oetting TA, Omphroy LC. Modified technique using flexible iris retractors in clear corneal surgery. *J Cataract Refract Surg*. 2002;28:596–598.

Chapter 11

Surgical Approach to Iris Reconstruction for Iris Diaphragm Deficiency or Dysfunction

Christopher Khng, MD; Robert H. Osher, MD;
Michael E. Snyder, MD; Scott E. Burk, MD, PhD

Introduction

Iris reconstructive surgery is among the most difficult operations performed by the anterior segment surgeon, especially in cases following ocular trauma. Patients in need of such reconstructive efforts, either in cases of congenital, traumatic, or other causes of iris loss often are significantly debilitated by glare and other visual disturbances resulting from a compromised iris diaphragm. Surgical options and techniques of iris reconstruction are reviewed with emphasis on severity and type of iris dysfunction or loss. The anatomic and functional outcomes from a repaired iris diaphragm often are excellent, and can be extremely gratifying, both for the patient and the surgeon.

Iris Loss

Patients with partial or total iris loss, whether from congenital, traumatic, or other causes, suffer from varying amounts of visual disability. The visual dysfunction may vary from mild to severe and includes glare, photophobia, reduced visual acuity, and contrast sensitivity loss. In addition, significant cosmetic issues may also be present, especially when the patient has a light colored iris. Abnormalities of pupil size, shape and location may also be reasons for pupil reconstruction. This chapter discusses the approach to the surgical management in cases where iris repair or an iris prosthesis is required.

The following considerations for loss of iris tissue have been suggested by us:

1. Suture repair is preferable to the use of an iris prosthesis whenever possible, although poor quality iris stroma may not be repairable.
2. Create and maintain a pupil size to alleviate symptoms, yet allow adequate visualization of the fundus.
3. Small incision surgery is desirable whenever possible.
4. Detailed informed consent and observation of regulatory protocol is necessary because the iris devices are not FDA approved in the United States.

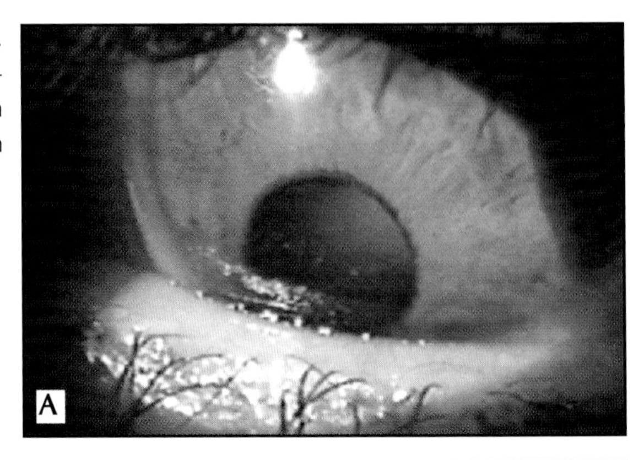

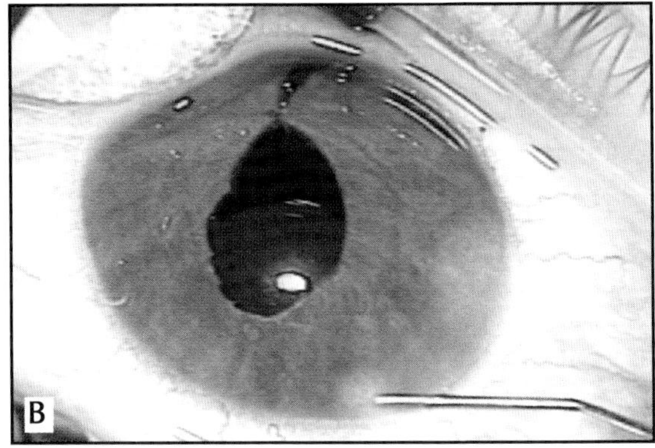

Figure 11-1. Congenital iris coloboma. **A**. Iris coloboma with inferior pupil displacement. **B**. Coloboma closed with iris imbrication sutures. Pupil margin excised superiorly to recenter pupil.

Classification

The various situations in which iris repair and reconstruction might be considered in patients who are symptomatic may be classified into the following:

1. Iris stromal loss.
2. Iris root disinsertion (iridodialysis).
3. Abnormalities of pupil size, position, and shape.
4. Iris functional loss.

Iris Stromal Loss

The repair options available to the surgeon depend upon the extent of iris tissue loss. This can conveniently be described in terms of clock hours, or quadrants of loss.

One Quadrant or Less

With less than 3 clock hours of loss (Figure 11-1A), the management options are straightforward. Examples of such an iris defect are iatrogenic iris atrophy with a transillumination defect adjacent to the corneal tunnel post-phaco in which iris prolapse has occurred repeatedly, a congenital iris coloboma, or an excessively large surgical iridectomy. The primary repair option is with imbricating sutures to the iris leaflets, or edges of the defect using Prolene 10/0 sutures with a modification of the Siepser[1] or McCannel[2] technique (Figure 11-1B). If the operation is going to be combined with cataract surgery, implantation of both a single sector iris prosthesis such as the Morcher 96 (or single fin Ophtec IPS element) and a foldable IOL, each placed into the capsular bag, may be chosen if the remaining iris stroma cannot be adequately closed primarily. Although the sector implant affords good functional results, the cosmetic result may be suboptimal since the 96 series of implants are only available in black polymethylmethacrylate (PMMA) and the Ophtec device colors may not be an exact match at the present time. Therefore, in addition to the implant, we will often place an imbricating suture through the iris defect for cosmesis.

Between One and Two Quadrants

Between 3 and 6 clock hours, for example in a case following iridocyclectomy for an iris tumor or post-traumatic iris loss, two pieces of either the partial aniridia ring (Model 96, Morcher) or the Ophtec single-element Iris Prosthetic System (IPS, Ophtec BV, Groningen, Netherlands) may be placed into the capsular bag. If the capsular bag is absent, a full-sized prosthetic iris device may be sutured with scleral fixation. Alternately, if the iris defect is only marginally beyond 3 clock hours, imbricating sutures may be attempted depending on the elasticity or friability of the iris tissue. In the situation with iris sutures, an additional McCannel type suture may need to be placed to attach the newly created iris root to the sclera in the area of the repair.

Beyond Two Quadrants

Beyond 6 clock hours of iris loss, there are several good surgical options. If a small incision is possible, two multiple-fin (Figure 11-2) endocapsular rings (Morcher type 50C, D, or E with respective apertures of 6, 4, or 3.5 mm, respectively) may be placed in the capsular bag combined with phacoemulsification and implantation of a foldable intraocular lens (IOL). While the 50C aniridia rings from Morcher give good functional results, they are less suitable from a cosmetic point of view in patients with light colored irides, as it is currently only available in black (colored options to be available soon). Another alternative is implantation of the IPS, which is available in a variety of colors including light blue, light green, mid brown, and black. The IPS is unsuitable in cases when a compromised bag is present because of the significant manipulation required during insertion. By contrast, the Morcher type 50C and type 96 simulate the function of a capsular tension ring and may prove to be a useful endocapsular option when weak zonules are present. A tear through either the anterior or posterior capsule necessitates a sulcus sutured diaphragm implant (Morcher 67 series or Ophtec 311) with or without lens power depending upon whether cataract extraction is also indicated. The best choice of suture material is not yet determined, although either Gore-Tex 8/0 or Prolene 9/0 provides greater strength and durability than 10/0 Prolene. If some remnant iris tissue is present, it should be gently grasped with Utrata forceps and stretched out of the angles in an attempt to cover as much of the prosthesis as possible for a better cosmetic result. It is occasionally surprising how much iris tissue can be recovered by this approach.

In cases of congenital aniridia, a different approach has to be taken because of the very thin and fragile anterior lens capsule.[3] When the rhexis is intact, it may be possible to implant paired Morcher 50C rings or Ophtec IPS elements, although a tear in the anterior capsule will necessitate a sutured or sulcus fixated iris diaphragm IOL. The capsular diaphragm should be preserved in these cases whenever possible as it affords additional stability to the IOL while restraining vitreous from entering the anterior segment. It should also be emphasized that there may be a greater risk of glaucomatous complications when a full-size diaphragm IOL is used, especially if inadvertently placed in the angle.[4–6]

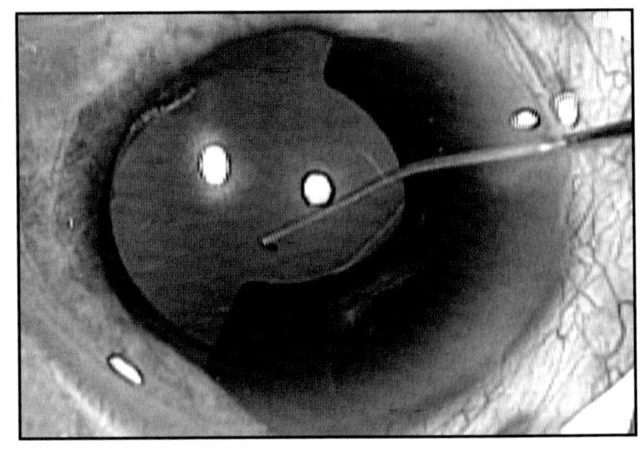

Figure 11-2. Previous iridocyclectomy with 120° of iris loss. Two Morcher 96G segments reestablishing a complete iris diaphragm.

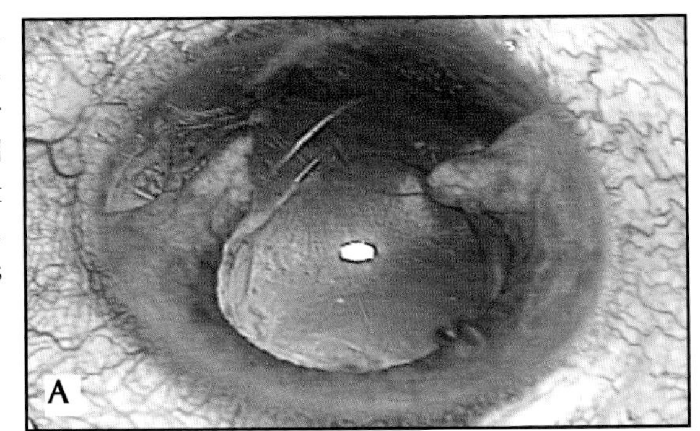

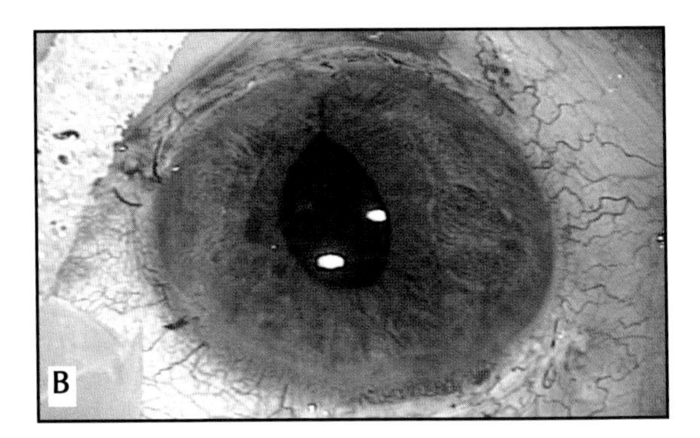

Figure 11-3. Traumatic iridodialysis with iris loss and aphakia. **A**. Iris loss between 2:00 and 7:00 and zonular dialysis between 4:00 and 5:00 and intact posterior capsule. **B**. Final result after lens implantation into the sulcus, pupilloplasty and repair of iridodialysis with mattress sutures.

Iris Root Disinsertion

The surgical options for repair of iridodialysis (Figure 11-3A) are relatively straightforward. Mattress sutures are used to reattach the iris to the sclera, the number and placement of which would depend on the extent and location of disinsertion (Figure 11-3B). For convenience, the iridodialysis may be classified as mild, moderate, or severe as defined by the number of clock hours of disinsertion. One to 2 clock hours may be considered mild, 3 to 4 clock hours moderate, while 5 or more clock hours would constitute a severe dialysis.

Mild disinsertion may require just a single horizontal mattress suture tied externally suture to close, while severe cases may need more. At the present time, Prolene 10/0 sutures, double-armed on CIF-4 needles are our preference. The sutures may either be placed under previously dissected scleral flaps, or tied at the scleral surface and the knot rotated into the sclera. In massively disinserted irides, it is prudent to fix the iris segment opposite the attached segment first, so as to equally distribute iris on each side of that initial attachment, provided that the anatomy allows recognition of the median of the disinserted section. When this is not clear, it may be necessary to start near the normal anatomy and work serially circumferentially. We wish to emphasize that even massively disinserted irides may be successfully repaired, so iris tissue should not be indiscriminately excised at the time of the initial traumatic or surgical event.

Abnormalities of Pupil Size, Position, and Shape

Abnormalities of pupil size range from an absent pupil to a large unresponsive pupil. Pupils obliterated by posterior synechiae may be abnormal in position (eccentric, corectopia) as well as in size. In this situation, synechiolysis alone or the peeling of the peripupillary membrane may restore adequate pupil size and centration.[7] A severely displaced pupil may require the creation of a new central pupil with either a vitrector or a fine intraocular scissors, followed by imbricating sutures to close the previous pupil.

A pupil may be either too small or too large. Bound-down pupils from previous anterior uveitis or long-standing pilocarpine usage may be the cause of fixed miosis. Our approach is to first attempt to lyse the posterior synechiae with a cohesive viscoelastic agent injected at the pupil edge. Any separation of tissue will allow insertion of the injection cannula as viscodissection is highly effective. If the membrane cannot be penetrated, a flat blunt instrument such as a cyclodialysis spatula may prove more helpful in dissecting the iris edge off the lens capsule followed by viscoelastic injection. While sharp dissection is possible, care must be taken to avoid inadvertent puncture of the anterior lens capsule. A safer option is to create a small iridectomy midway between the pupil edge and the iris root through which the viscoelastic agent is injected, which by itself may lyse the posterior synechiae. Recalcitrant synechiae can be severed by either blunt or sharp dissection using the iridectomy for entry. Alternatively, a 20 or 25 gauge vitreoretinal scissors can be helpful instrumentation. The iris defect can be closed by sutures as previously described if the surgeon desires. Once the pupil edge has been elevated off the lens capsule, a peripupillary membranectomy (Figure 11-4A-C) may prove successful in peeling the discrete ribbon-like membrane off the iris border. This often permits a significant enlargement of the pupil, once the restrictive membrane is removed. If however, the pupil is still not an adequate size, a pupil stretching technique may be performed with two blunt manipulating instruments[8] followed by viscomydriasis. Other options include multiple sphincterotomies[9] or pupil "sculpting" with either a vitrector or an intraocular scissors.

At the other end of the spectrum is the dilated atonic pupil. Common causes include previous traumatic mydriasis or herpetic iris atrophy. The easiest surgical approach, described by Osher, is to use a McCannel-like imbricating suture of 10/0 Prolene passed in each quadrant.[10] Another more elegant solution, although it is more technically demanding is to use the Ogawa pupil cerclage (Figure 11-5A-C) suture.[11] We prefer to use Prolene 10/0 on a CTC-6L needle, and the suture is placed with needle passes just inside the pupil margin. With this technique, the more bites of the iris the better, as too few bites causes scalloping of the pupil margin. Typically, around 20 to 24 bites are taken before the suture is tied to itself. The pupil size may be adjusted by tightening the cerclage. Once an adequate pupil size is attained, the suture is locked. The final option in a case with a fixed dilated pupil is to use two Morcher 50 series prosthetic iris rings placed into the capsular bag, an Ophtec

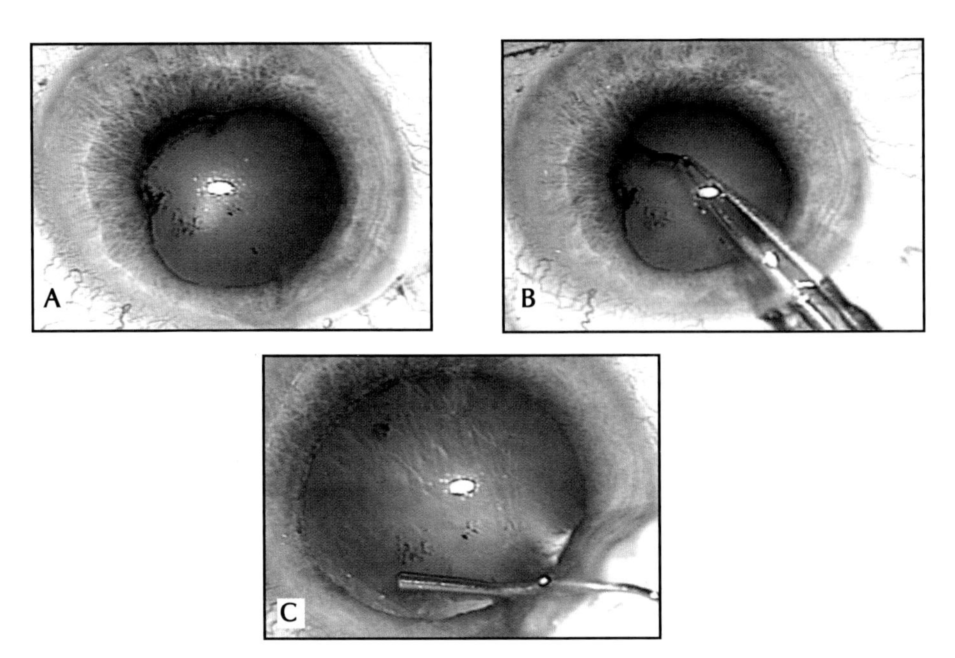

Figure 11-4. Peripupillary membranectomy. **A**. Poor pupil dilation despite lysis of posterior synechiae. **B**. Peeling of the peripupillary membrane. **C**. Good pupil dilation achieved.

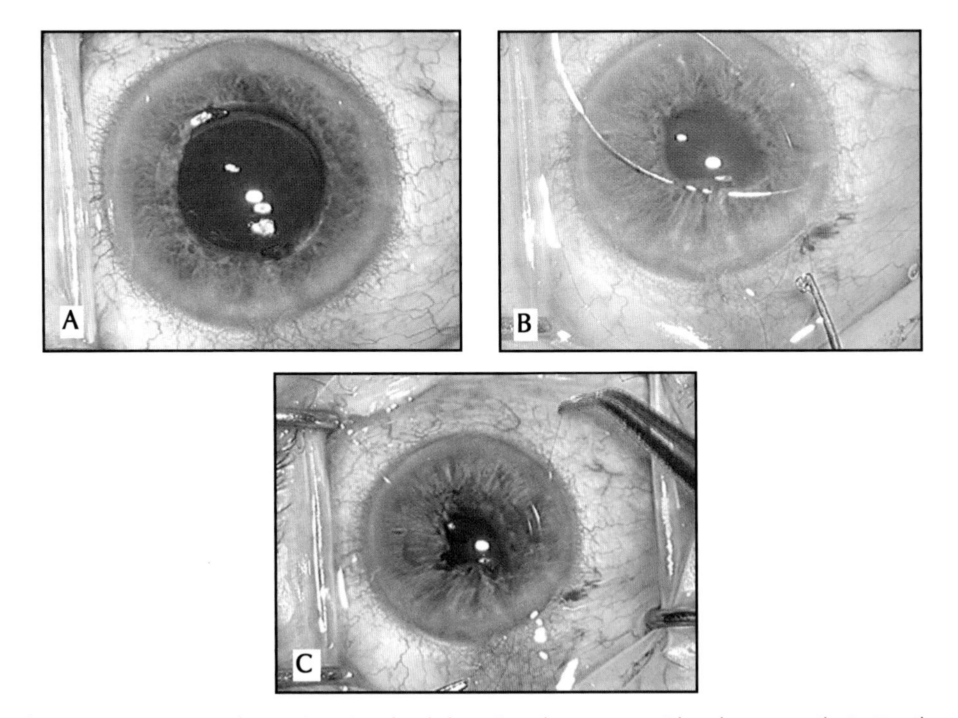

Figure 11-5. Captured anterior piggyback lens in a hyperope with a large pupil. **A**. Pupil capture of anterior sulcus-fixated optic. **B**. Cerclage suture being placed using a long curved needle on a Prolene 10/O suture. **C**. Cerclage being tightened with reducing pupil size and elimination of potential for recurrent pupil capture.

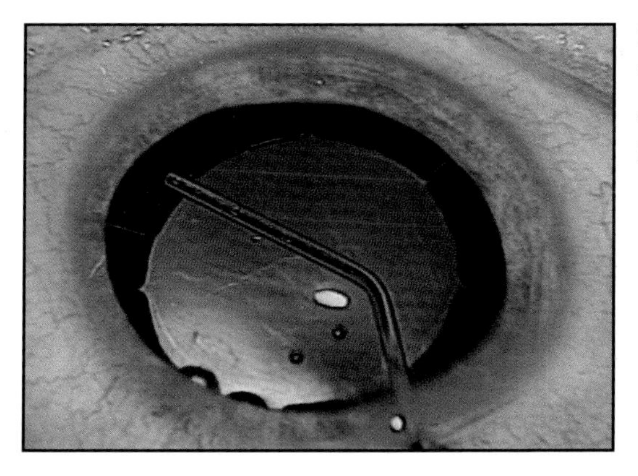

Figure 11-6. Oculocutaneous albinism with cataract and disabling glare. Appearance after paired Morcher 50C prosthetic iris rings after rotation.

IPS prosthesis, a model 311 diaphragm prosthesis (fixated or not fixated), or a model 67 sulcus-fixated prosthetic iris device. However, in view of the small incision, the cosmetic benefit, and the regulatory availability issues, suture repair is our first choice before considering an artificial iris. A pupil that is either eccentric or severely oval can be improved by either extending the pupil into the visual axis or by creating a new centered pupil. The previous eccentric pupil can be closed by placing imbricating iris sutures.

Iris Functional Loss

This group of iris conditions has neither lost nor missing iris tissue, but the iris present is poorly functional. Examples include the diaphanous irides of the albino, which has missing pigment within the iris pigment epithelium, cases of chronic uveitis where the iris tissue is poorly or nonfunctional from inflammation, and the iridocorneal endothelial (ICE) syndromes where spontaneous iris holes develop as the iris tissue pulls apart, even though no actual tissue is lost. With severe transillumination defects in the albino, the functional loss may be little better than congenital aniridics. Fortunately, the same capsular fragility problems that are associated with congenital aniridia are absent. We have had mixed responses in terms of glare reduction in albinoid patients undergoing phacoemulsification and foldable lens implantation with placement of paired Morcher 50C or 50E rings, or an IPS prosthesis into the capsular bag (Figure 11-6). In the absence of adequate capsular support, an iris diaphragm IOL prosthesis such as the Morcher 67 or Ophtec 311 may be sutured to the sclera. For both the uveitic iris and cases of ICE syndrome, repair of the iris using sutures may be unsuccessful because of the poor quality of iris tissue. Our patients with either uveitis or ICE syndrome have enjoyed a significant reduction in glare with a prosthetic iris device.

Conclusion

Iris diaphragm deficiency is a collection of protean conditions that share in common iris dysfunction, which often brings patients to their eye care providers. Glare, photosensitivity, visual disability, and cosmetic issues have varying degrees of importance to each individual patient. This series of representative cases is intended to stimulate discussion and thought, though it is neither intended to be exhaustive, nor imply only a single "right" way to manage these complex problems. Certainly, for each case the surgeon must consider the options and skill sets that are available in a given patient's situation. Fortunately, with better surgical techniques and iris prosthetic devices, we are able to help these patients and the future can, perhaps, look "less bright" for these individuals who would otherwise have remained incapacitated by light.

Acknowledgment

The authors would like to acknowledge the assistance of Linda Jaakobovitch from the Cincinnati Eye Institute Audiovisual department in obtaining the video captures.

Key Points

1. Patients with partial or total iris loss, whether from congenital, traumatic, or other causes, suffer from varying amounts of visual disability. The visual dysfunction may vary from mild to severe and includes glare, photophobia, reduced visual acuity, and contrast sensitivity loss. In addition, significant cosmetic issues may also be present, especially when the patient has a light colored iris.
2. With less than 3 clock hours of loss, the primary repair option is with imbricating sutures to the iris leaflets, or edges of the defect using Prolene 10/0 sutures with a modification of the McCannel or Siepser technique.
3. Between 3 and 6 clock hours, for example in a case following iridocyclectomy for an iris tumor or post-traumatic iris loss, two pieces of either the partial aniridia ring (Model 96, Morcher) or the Ophtec single-element Iris Prosthetic System (IPS) may be placed into the capsular bag. If the capsular bag is absent, a full-sized prosthetic iris device may be sutured with scleral fixation.
4. The surgical options for repair of iridodialysis are more limited and straightforward. Mattress sutures are used to reattach the iris to the sclera, the number and placement of which would depend on the extent and location of disinsertion.
5. Pupils obliterated by posterior synechiae may be abnormal in position (eccentric, corectopia) as well as in size. In this situation, synechiolysis alone or the peeling of the peripupillary membrane may restore adequate pupil size and centration. A severely displaced pupil may require the creation of a new central pupil with either a vitrector or a fine intraocular scissors, followed by imbricating sutures to close the previous pupil.

References

1. Siepser SB. The closed chamber slipping suture technique for iris repair. *Ann Ophthalmol.* 1994;26(3):71–72.
2. McCannel MA. A retrievable suture idea for anterior uveal problems. *Ophthalmic Surg.* 1976;7(2):98–103.
3. Schneider S, Osher RH, Burk SE, et al. Thinning of the anterior capsule associated with congenital aniridia. *J Cataract Refract Surg.* 2003;29(3):523–525.
4. Beltrame G, Salvetat ML, Chizzolini M, et al. Implantation of a black diaphragm intraocular lens in ten cases of post-traumatic aniridia. *Eur J Ophthalmol.* 2003;13(1):62–68.
5. Thompson CG, Fawzy K, Bryce IG, Noble BA. Implantation of a black diaphragm intraocular lens for traumatic aniridia. *J Cataract Refract Surg.* 1999;25:808–813.
6. Sundmacher R, Reinhard T, Althaus C. Black-diaphragm intraocular lens for correction of aniridia. *Ophthalmic Surg.* 1994;25(3):180–185.

7. Osher RH. Peripupillary membranectomy. *Video Journal of Cataract and Refractive Surgery*. 1991;VII:3.
8. Fry L. Pupil stretching. *Video Journal of Cataract and Refractive Surgery*. 1995;XI:1.
9. Fine IH. The pupil-sphincterotomies. *Video Journal of Cataract and Refractive Surgery*. 1991; VII:3.
10. Osher RH. Consultation section. *J Cataract Refract Surg*. 1994;20(1):101–102.
11. Ogawa GS. The iris cerclage suture for permanent mydriasis: a running suture technique. *Ophthalmic Surg Lasers*. 1998;29(12):1001–1009.

The authors have no financial interest in any of the products mentioned in this article. This study received no financial support.

Chapter 12

Posterior Polar Cataract

Abhay R. Vasavada, MS, FRCS; Shetal M. Raj, MS

Introduction

Posterior polar cataract (PPC) is a clinically distinctive entity consisting of a dense white, well-demarcated, disk-shaped opacity located in the posterior cortex or subcapsular region (Figure 12-1A, B). Two types of PPC have been described in literature: stationary and progressive.[1] The stationary type consists of concentric rings around the central plaque opacity that looks like a bull's eye (Figure 12-2). This type is compatible with good vision. Normally the patient seeks help in the third or fourth decade of life. The common symptom is intolerance to light. Glare is most severe when the source of light is close to the object of vision. In the progressive type, changes take place in the posterior cortex in the form of radiating rider opacities (Figure 12-3). Patients with progressive opacity become more symptomatic as the peripheral extensions enlarge.

The inheritance pattern of this cataract is reported to be autosomal dominant.[2–7] Osher and colleagues had mentioned a positive family history for congenital cataracts in 55% (12/22) of patients.[8] The gene for PPC has been linked with the haptoglobin locus on chromosome 16.[9] A recent study reported that mutations in the PITX3 gene in humans result in PPC and variable anterior segment mesenchymal dysgenesis (ASMD).[10] Studies have indicated that a majority of these patients present with bilateral cataracts, the incidence being 80% in our earlier study,[11] and 70% in a study conducted by Gavris and colleagues.[12] There is no gender predilection in PPC. The polar opacity consists of abnormal lens fiber cells and an accumulation of extracellular materials.[13–15]

PPC presents a special challenge to the phacoemulsification surgeon as it is known to be predisposed to posterior-capsule dehiscence during surgery.[8,11] In 1990, Osher and coauthors reported a 26% (8/31 eyes) incidence of posterior capsule rupture (PCR) during surgery in eyes with PPC.[8] We have earlier reported 36% (9/25 eyes) in 1999,[11] while in 2003, Hayashi and coauthors,[16] and Lee and coauthors,[17] reported 7.1% (2/28 eyes) and 11% (4/36 eyes), respectively. Liu and coauthors reported 16.4% (10/61 eyes).[18] A study by Gavris and colleagues in 2004 reported an incidence of 40% (4/10 eyes).[12] Our study

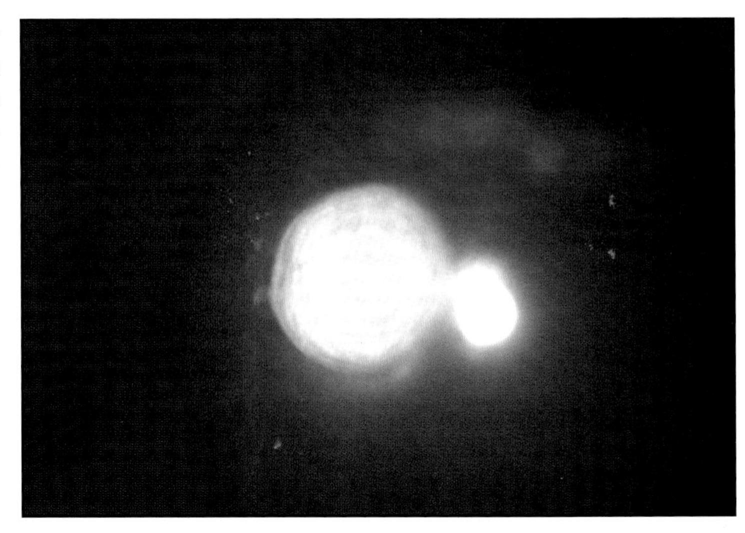

Figure 12-1A. Posterior polar cataract (PPC) characterized by dense white, well-demarcated, disk-shaped opacity.

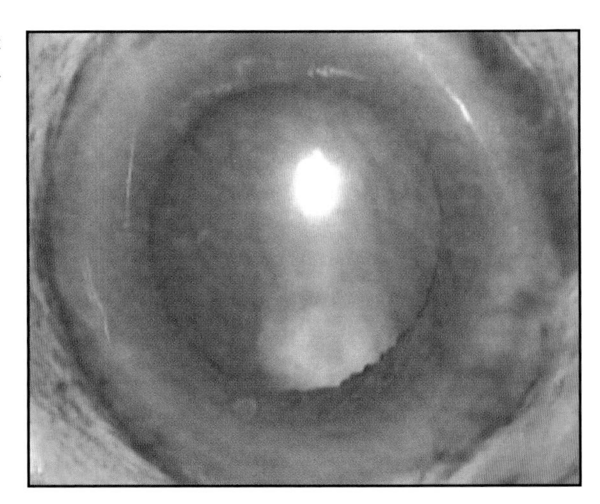

Figure 12-1B. Rare case of eccentric posterior polar cataract. (Photo courtesy of Dr. Agarwal's Eye Hospital.)

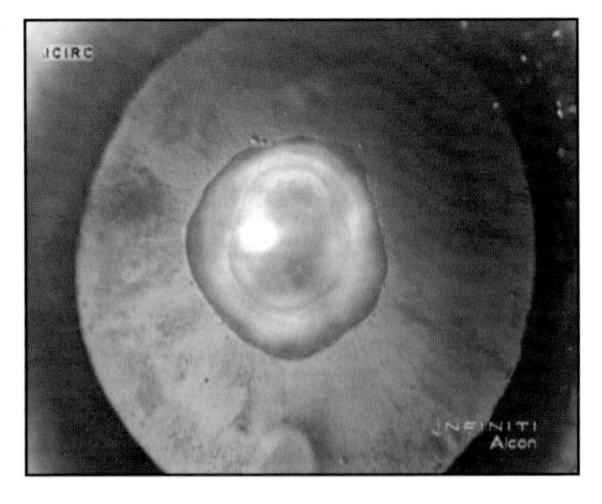

Figure 12-2. In the stationary type of PPC, concentric rings are seen around the central plaque opacity resembling a bull's eye.

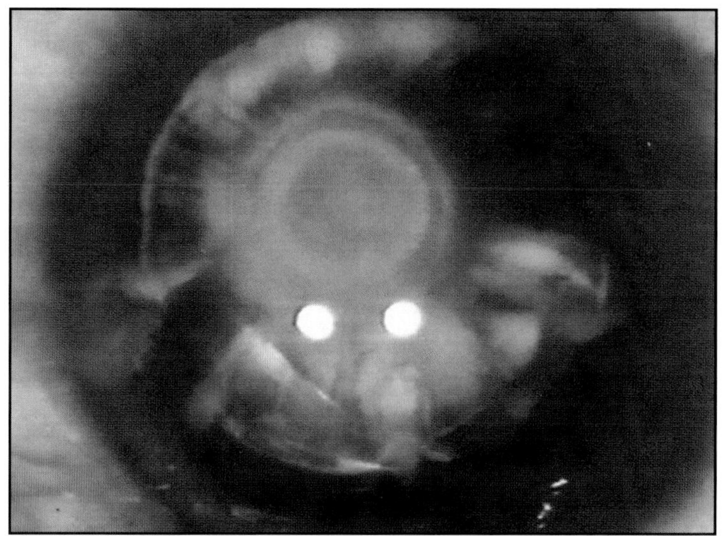

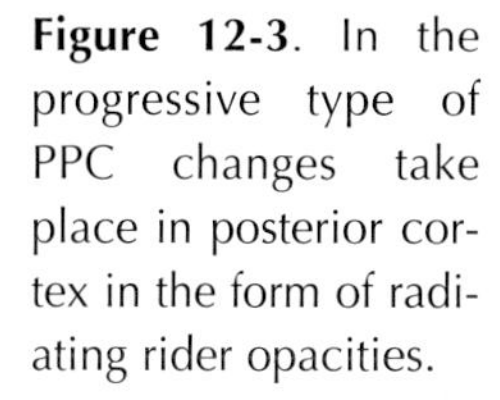

Figure 12-3. In the progressive type of PPC changes take place in posterior cortex in the form of radiating rider opacities.

reports that the antero-posterior dimensions of the lens in eyes with PPC is significantly thinner compared to the posterior subcapsular cataracts (in review).

To prevent PCR, Osher and colleagues recommend slow-motion phacoemulsification with low aspiration flow rate, vacuum and infusion pressure.[8] Fine and coauthors avoid overpressurization of the anterior chamber with viscodissection to mobilize epinucleus and cortex,[19] Allen and Wood also perform viscodissection,[20] and Lee and Lee prefer a lamda technique with dry aspiration.[17] We prefer inside-out delineation.[21] This technique, along with modern instrumentation, refined surgical strategies, better understanding of phacodynamics and cumulative surgical experience has enabled us to reduce PCR to 8% (2/25 eyes).[21]

Diagnosis

The bull's eye appearance is pathognomonic of PPC (see Figure 12-1A). However, this entity could be camouflaged under a dense nuclear sclerosis or a total white cataract. In our opinion, surgery should be delayed as long as possible and undertaken only if the patient finds it difficult to perform his routine activities.

Surgical Technique

Counseling

During preoperative examination, the patient should be informed of the possibility of intraoperative PCR dropped nucleus, relatively longer operative time, secondary posterior segment intervention, and likely delayed visual recovery. The need to perform Nd: YAG capsulotomy for residual plaque[8,11,16] and possibility of preexisting amblyopia especially in unilateral PPC should be envisaged at the preliminary stage.[16]

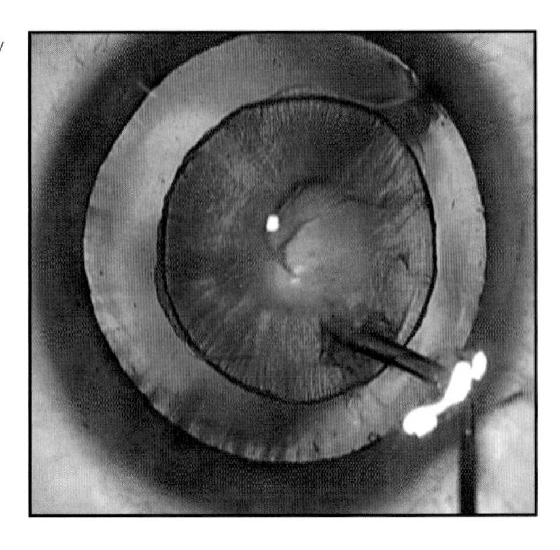

Figure 12-4A. Hydrodelineation. (Photo courtesy of Dr. Agarwal's Eye Hospital.)

Anesthesia

Peribulbar anaesthesia with oculopressure to soften the globe diminishes intraoperative posterior pressure.[8] With increasing experience, one may use topical anaesthesia in a selective manner.

Surgical Technique

We prefer to use a closed chamber technique. The contours of the cornea and the globe should be maintained through the procedure.

Hayashi and coauthors perform either phacoemulsification, pars plana lensectomy or intracapsular cataract extraction depending on the size of opacity and density of nuclear sclerosis.[16]

Incision

A paracentesis is performed with 15° Ophthalmic knife (Alcon Surgical, Fort Worth, Texas). The aqueous is exchanged with Sodium Hyaluronate (Provisc, Alcon Laboratories). A temporal corneal single plane valvular incision of 2.6 mm is performed. A cohesive viscoelastic in the anterior chamber prevents chamber collapse and forward movement of iris-lens diaphragm during entry into the eye. Fine and coauthors caution against increasing the pressure in the anterior chamber.[19]

Capsulorrhexis

The optimal size is approximately 5 mm. While a rhexis size of 4 mm could be detrimental in the event of necessity to prolapse the nucleus into the anterior chamber, a larger opening may not leave adequate support for a sulcus-fixated intraocular lens (IOL) in case the posterior chamber is compromised.[11,19]

Hydro Procedures

Cortico-cleaving hydrodissection[22] can lead to hydraulic rupture and should be avoided.[8,11] It would be logical to perform hydrodelineation (Figure 12-4A, B) to create a mechanical cushion of epinucleus.[11,16,20,23] Masket,[24] Hayashi and colleagues,[16] Allen and Wood,[20] and Lee and Lee[17] recommend hydrodelineation. In addition to hydrodelineation, Fine and coauthors also perform hydrodissection in multiple quadrants, injecting tiny amounts of fluid gently, so that the fluid wave is not allowed to spread/extend across the posterior capsule.[19]

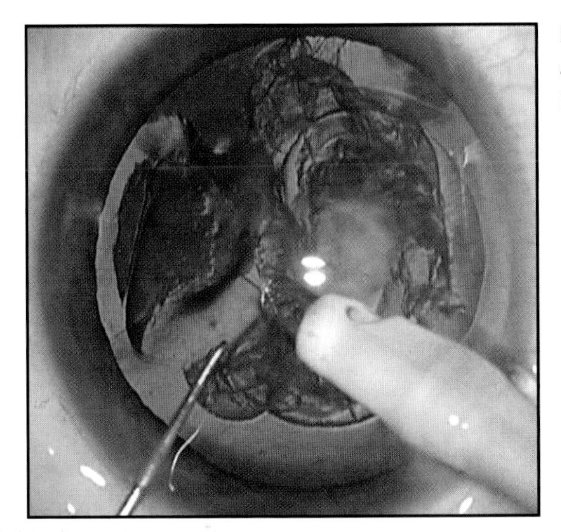

Figure 12-4B. Phaco removal of the nucleus after hydrodelineation. (Photo courtesy of Dr. Agarwal's Eye Hospital.)

We propose inside-out delineation to precisely delineate the central core of nucleus.[21]

Inside-Out Delineation

A central trench is sculpted the slow motion technique (Infinity Phacoemulsifier, Alcon Laboratories). In nuclear sclerosis < grade 3 (grading system from grade 1 to 5),[25] preset parameters are: ultrasound energy (U/S) 30–60% (supra-optimal power), vacuum 60 mmHg, aspiration flow rate (AFR) 18 cc/min, and bottle height (BH) 70 cm. Care should be taken not to mechanically rock the lens. Dispersive viscoelastic (Viscoat, Alcon Laboratories) is injected through the side port before retracting the probe to avoid forward movement of iris-lens diaphragm. A specially designed right-angled cannula mounted on a 2 cc syringe filled with fluid is introduced through the main incision and the tip is placed adjacent to the right wall of the trench at an appropriate depth, depending on the density of the cataract. It then penetrates the central lens substance and fluid is injected through the right wall of the trench (Figure 12-5A). Delineation is produced by the fluid traversing inside-out. A golden ring within the lens is evidence of successful delineation (Figure 12-5B). Fluid injection may be repeated in the left wall of the trench with another right-angled cannula (Figure 12-6). The trench allows the surgeon to reach the central core of the nucleus. As fluid is injected at a desired depth, under direct vision, a desired thickness of epinucleus cushion can be achieved (Figure 12-7). It provides a precise epinucleus bowl that acts as a mechanical cushion to protect the posterior capsule during subsequent maneuvers.

With conventional hydrodelineation, the cannula is penetrated within the lens substance, causing the fluid to traverse from outside to inside. It is sometimes difficult to introduce the cannula within a firm nucleus, leading to rocking and stress to the capsular bag and zonules. There is also a possibility of fluid being injected inadvertently in the subcapsular plane, leading to unwarranted hydrodissection. Inside-out delineation is easy to perform, provides superior control, reduces stress to zonules and precisely demarcates the central core of nucleus.

Rotation

An attempt to rotate the nucleus can lead to posterior capsule rupture and is therefore avoided.[11]

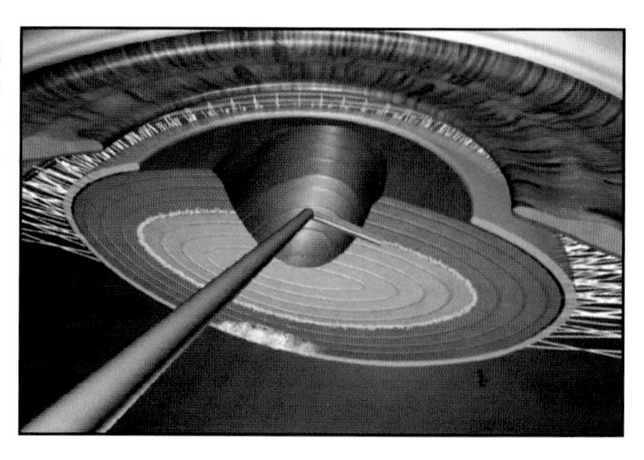

Figure 12-5A. Sketch demonstrating technique of inside-out delineation. The cannula penetrates the central lens substance and fluid is injected through right wall of the trench.

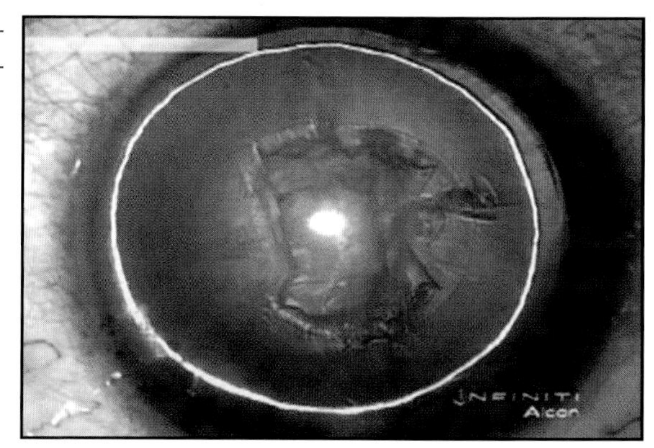

Figure 12-5B. The golden ring indicates end point of inside-out delineation.

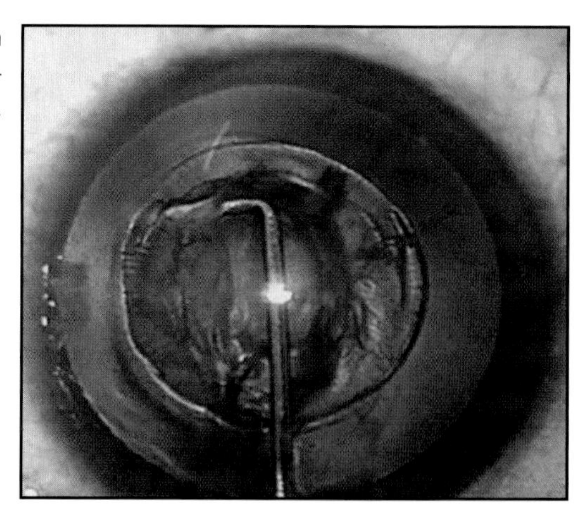

Figure 12-6. Fluid injection is repeated in the left wall of the trench with another right-angled cannula, if delineation is incomplete.

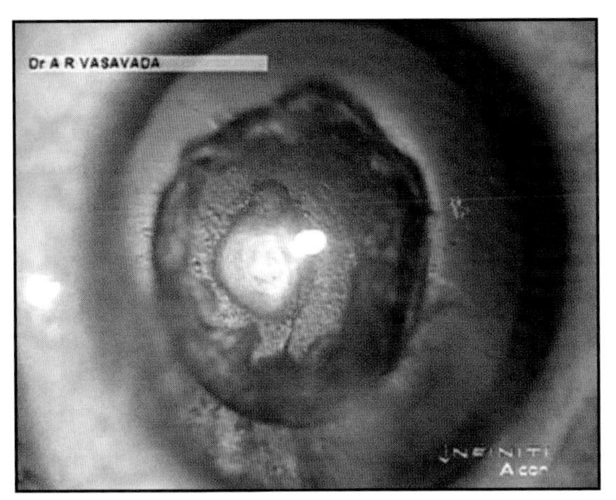

Figure 12-7. Mechanical cushion consisting of epinucleus—nucleus protects the posterior capsule.

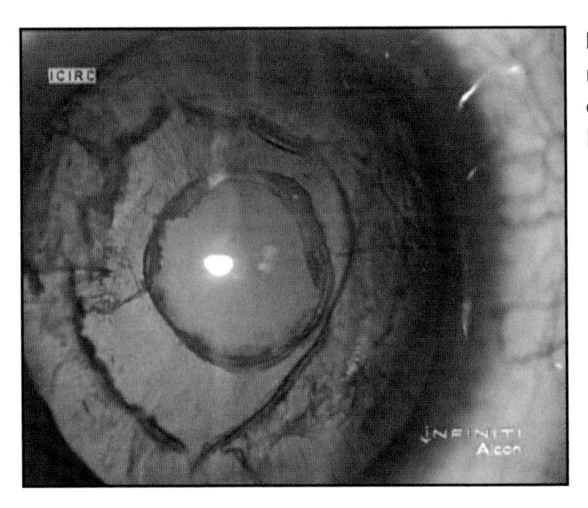

Figure 12-8. Capsular bag after nucleus removal showing a central breach in continuity of epinucleus at the site of PPC.

Division and Fragment Removal

All techniques are geared to facilitate the removal of nucleus within the cushion effect of the epinucleus. Bimanual cracking and division of the nucleus involve outward movements and can result in distortion of the capsular bag. In nuclear sclerosis >2 we use the step-by-step chop in situ and lateral separation technique,[26] for chopping using U/S 40 to 50%, vacuum 150 to 250 mmHg, AFR 18 cc/min, and BH 70 to 90 cm. The resultant fragments are removed with stop, chop, chop and stuff technique.[27] In nuclear sclerosis >2, the entire nucleus is aspirated within the epinucleus shell using AFR 16 cc/min and vacuum 100 to 120 mmHg. Figure 12-8 shows the capsular bag after the nucleus removal showing a central breach in the continuity of the epinucleus at the site of the PPC. Traction of posterior lens fibers and posterior polar opacity during surgery are enough to break the weak posterior capsule. Thus the slow motion technique is recommended to reduce turbulence in the anterior capsule.[28] Collapse of the anterior capsule and forward bulge of the posterior capsule is prevented throughout the procedure by injecting viscoelastic before the instrument is withdrawn.[11,29]

Lee and coauthors use the lambda technique to sculpt the nucleus, followed by cracking along both arms and removal of central piece.[17]

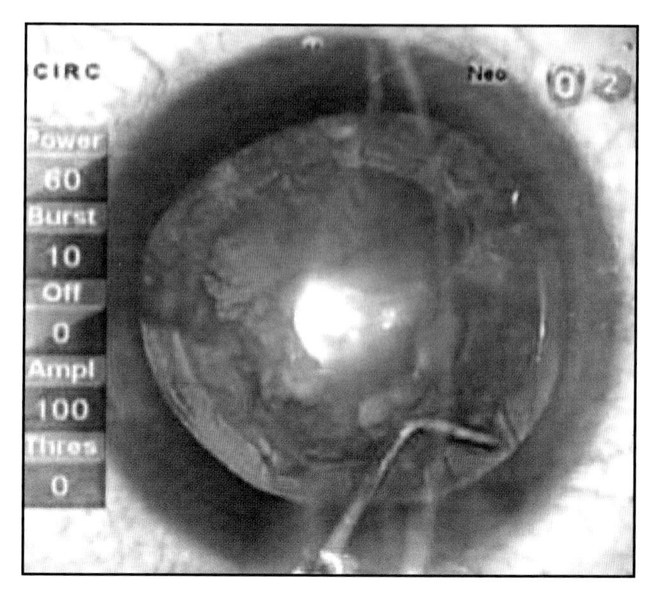

Figure 12-9. Removal of upper half of epinucleus using focal and multiquadrant hydrodissection.

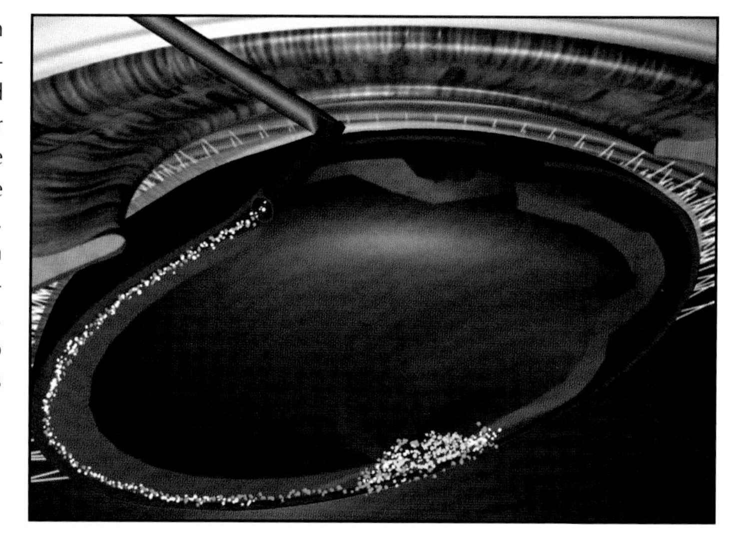

Figure 12-10. Sketch demonstrating the technique of injecting fluid in the subcapsular region to cleave the cortex from the capsule proximal to incision. The nucleus has been emulsified and the capsular bag is empty. Therefore, it is safe to hydrodissect at this stage.

Epinucleus Removal

First, only the peripheral lower half of epinucleus is stripped off using U/S 30%, vacuum 80 to 100 mmHg, AFR 16 cc/minute, and BH 80 to 90 cm. The central area is left attached.[11,19,24] Then the peripheral upper epinucleus (subincisional epinucleus) is mobilized with a gentle focal and multiquadrant hydrodissection with a right-angled cannula facing right and left (Figures 12-9 and 12-10). The fluid wave travels along the cleavage formed between the capsule and lower epinucleus, which does not threaten the integrity of the posterior capsule. Also, it is safe to hydrodissect because the capsular bag is not fully occupied. Therefore, the hydraulic pressure built up is not sufficient to rupture the posterior capsule. The entire epinucleus is then aspirated, finally detaching the central area.

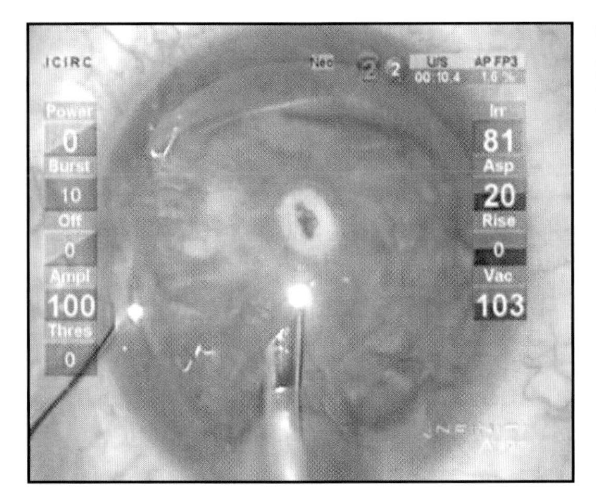

Figure 12-11. A pseudohole suggestive of a defect is observed in posterior cortex, but the posterior capsule remains intact.

Allen[20] and Fine[19] suggest viscodissection of the epinucleus performed by injecting viscoelastic (Healon 5 or GV and Viscoat, respectively) under the capsular edge to mobilize the rim of epinucleus. It is removed with a coaxial irrigation-aspiration (I/A) handpiece. Lee and colleagues perform manual dry aspiration with Simcoe cannula.[17]

At times the classic appearance suggestive of a defect is observed in the posterior cortex, but the posterior capsule remains intact. This is a "pseudohole" (Figure 12-11).

Cortex Removal

Bimanual automated I/A using AFR 20 cc/min, vacuum 400 mmHg optimizes control, ensures anterior chamber maintenance, and aids in complete removal of the cortex. Fine and colleagues using coaxial protect the posterior chamber with viscoelastics during cortex removal.[19]

Posterior Capsule Vacuum Polishing

This is avoided even if the posterior chamber is not open because of its potential fragility.[8,11,16,19,24] The traction on an excessively adhered plaque to an otherwise normal posterior capsule could eventually rupture the posterior capsule. Postoperative neodymium-yttrium-aluminum-garnet (Nd:YAG) laser posterior capsulotomy is preferable.

Posterior Capsule Dehiscence

If a defect is present in the posterior chamber, Viscoat is injected over the area of posterior chamber defect before the phaco or I/A probe is withdrawn from the eye,[29] and two-port limbal anterior vitrectomy is performed using cut rate 800 cuts/min, vacuum 300 mmHg, and AFR 25 cc/min. Once the anterior chamber is free from vitreous, the cortex is aspirated by bimanual I/A. A posterior capsulorrhexis (PCCC) may be performed if the rupture is confined to a small central area.

Intraocular Lens Implantation

In eyes with the posterior chamber defect, an IOL is implanted in the bag only if PCCC can be achieved. In eyes with a large posterior capsule defect, the IOL is placed over the anterior capsule in ciliary sulcus. Fine and colleagues have suggested capture of the optic through the anterior capsulorrhexis.[19,30] We believe optic capture induces more inflammation.[31]

After IOL implantation, viscoelastic is removed by two-port vitrectomy rather than I/A because vitrectomy aspirates in a piecemeal and gradual manner and reduces the chances of rapid aspiration of vitreous.

We do not suture the main valvular incision, but suture paracentesis in eyes with posterior capsule defect. In these eyes, a periodic evaluation for retinal break, cystoid macular edema, and raised intraocular pressure is necessary.

Surgical Pearls

- Thorough counseling.
- Avoid cortico-cleaving hydrodissection.
- Inside-out delineation.
- Closed chamber technique.
- Slow-motion technique for lens removal.
- Focal and multiquadrant hydrodissection for cleavage of subincisional epinucleus.

Key Points

1. Posterior polar cataract (PPC) is a clinically distinctive entity consisting of a dense white, well-demarcated, disk-shaped opacity located in the posterior cortex or subcapsular region. Two types of PPC have been described in literature: stationary and progressive.
2. The inheritance pattern of this cataract is reported to be autosomal dominant.
3. The bull's eye appearance is pathognomonic of posterior polar cataracts.
4. Cortico-cleaving hydrodissection can lead to hydraulic rupture and should be avoided. It would be logical to perform hydrodelineation to create a mechanical cushion of epinucleus.
5. At times the classic appearance suggestive of a defect is observed in the posterior cortex, but the posterior capsule remains intact. This is a pseudohole.

The authors do not have any financial interest or commercial connection in marketing any product, instrument or piece of equipment discussed in this chapter.

References

1. Duke-Elder S. posterior polar cataract. In: Duke-Elder S, ed. *System of Ophthalmology, Vol 3, pt 2: Normal and Abnormal Development, Congenital Deformities*. St Louis, MO: CV Mosby; 1964:723–726.
2. Tulloh CG. Hereditary posterior polar cataract with report of a pedigree. *Br J Ophthalmol.* 1955;39(6):374.
3. Tulloh CG. Hereditary posterior polar cataract. *Br J Ophthalmol.* 1956;40(9):566.
4. Nettleship E, Ogilvie FM. A peculiar form of hereditary congenital cataract. *Trans Ophthalmol Soc UK*. 1906;26:191–207.
5. Harman NB. New pedigree of cataract – posterior polar, anterior polar and microphthalmia, and lamellar. *Trans Ophthalmol Soc UK*. 1909;29:296–306.
6. Yamada K, Tomita HA, Kanazawa S, Mera A, Amemiya T, Niikawa N.Genetically distinct autosomal dominant posterior polar cataract in a four-generation Japanese family. *Am J Ophthalmol.* 2000;129(2):159–65.
7. Berry V, Francis P, Reddy MA, eta al. Alpha-B crystallin gene (CRYAB) mutation causes dominant congenital posterior polar cataract in humans. *Am J Hum Genet*. 2001;69(5):1141.
8. Osher RH, Yu BC, Koch DD. Posterior polar cataracts: a predisposition to intraoperative posterior capsular rupture. *J Cataract Refract Surg*. 1990;16:157–162.
9. Maumenee IH. Classification of hereditary cataracts in children by linkage analysis. *Ophthalmology*. 1979;86:1554–1558.
10. Addison PK, Berry V, Ionides AC, Francis PJ, Bhattacharya SS, Moore AT. Posterior polar cataract is the predominant consequence of a recurrent mutation in the PITX3 gene. *Br J Ophthalmol.* 2005;89(2):138–41.
11. Vasavada AR, Singh R. Phacoemulsification with posterior polar cataract. *J Cataract Refract Surg*. 1999;25:238–245.
12. Gavris M, Popa D, Caraus C, Gusho E, Clocotan D, Horvath K, Ardelean A, Sangeorzan D. Phacoemulsification in posterior polar cataract. *Oftalmologia*. 2004;48(4):36–40.
13. Eshaghian J, Streeten BW. Human posterior subcapsular cataract; an ultrastructural study of the posteriorly migranting cells. *Arch Ophthalmol.* 1980;98:134–143.
14. Eshagian J. Human posterior subcapsular cataracts. *Trans Ophthalmol Soc UK*. 1982;102:364–368.
15. Nagata M, Marsuura H, Fujinaga Y. Ultrastructure of posterior subcapsular cataract in human lens. *Ophthalmic Res*. 1986;18:180.
16. Hayashi K, Hayashi H, Nakao F, et al. Outcomes of surgery for posterior polar cataract. *J Cataract Refract Surg*. 2003;29:45.
17. Lee MW, Lee YC. Phacoemulsification of posterior polar cataracts—a surgical challenge. *Br J Ophthalmol*. 2003,87:1426–1427.
18. Liu Y, Liu Y, Wu M, Zhang X. Phacoemulsification in eyes with posterior polar cataract and foldable intraocular lens implantation. *Yan Ke Xue Bao*. 2003;19(2):92.
19. Fine IH, Packer M, Hoffman RS. Management of posterior polar cataract. *J Cataract Refract Surg*. 2003;29:16–19.
20. Allen D, Wood C. Minimizing risk to the capsule during surgery for posterior polar cataract. *J Cataract Refract Surg*. 2002;28:742–744.
21. Vasavada AR, Raj SM. Inside-out delineation. *J Cataract Refract Surg*. 2004;30: 1167.
22. Fine IH. Cortico-cleaving hydrodissection. *J Cataract Refract Surg*. 1992;18:508.
23. Anis AY. Understanding hydrodelineation: the term and procedure. *Doc Ophthalmol.* 1994;87(2):123–137.
24. Masket S. Consultation section. *J Cataract Refract Surg*. 1997;23:819.

25. Emery JM, Little JH. Phacoemulsification and aspiration of cataracts, surgical technique, complications and results. St Louis, MO: CV Mosby; 1979:45–49.
26. Vasavada AR, Singh R. Step-by-step chop in situ and separation of very dense cataracts. *J Cataract Refract Surg.* 1998;24:156.
27. Vasavada AR, Desai JP. Stop, chop, chop and stuff. *J Cataract Refract Surg.* 1996;22:526.
28. Osher RH. Slow motion phacoemulsification approach (letter). *J Cataract Refract Surg.* 1993;19(5):667.
29. Cionni RJ, Osher RH. Intraoperative complications of phacoemulsification surgery. In: Steinert RF, ed. *Cataract Surgery, Technique, Complications, and Management.* 1st ed. Philadelphia, PA: WB Saunders; 1995:336.
30. Gimbel HV, DeBroff BM. Posterior capsulorhexis with optic capture: maintaining a clear visual axis after pediatric cataract surgery. *J Cataract Refract Surg.* 1994;20:658.
31. Vasavada AR, Trivedi R. Role of optic capture in congenital cataract and IOL surgery in children. *J Cataract Refract Surg.* 2000;26:824.

Please see Posterior Polar Cataract video on enclosed CD-ROM.

Chapter 13

Combined Cataract and Glaucoma Surgery

Amar Agarwal, MS, FRCS, FRCOphth, FRCS;
Soosan Jacob, MS, DNB, FRCS, MNAMS, FERC

Introduction

Cataract is the foremost cause of blindness worldwide and continues to remain an important cause of visual impairment in the United States.[1–4] In the Baltimore Eye Survey, cataract was found to be the leading cause of blindness among the population over 40 years of age, and unoperated cataract was found to be four times more common among African Americans than Caucasian Americans.[3] The Salisbury Eye Evaluation Study (n = 2,520) found that after refractive error, cataract was the leading cause of visual impairment in African Americans and Caucasian Americans.[4]

Cataract and glaucoma often coexist in the elderly, especially so with increasing longevity of the human race. It is especially important to be able to appropriately manage this patient subgroup in whom central vision is compromised due to cataract and peripheral vision due to glaucoma.

Surgical Options

When a patient with cataract has glaucoma, surgical options are cataract surgery alone, glaucoma surgery first followed later by cataract surgery, cataract surgery first followed later by glaucoma surgery, or cataract surgery combined with filtering surgery. The decision is based on the degree of visual field damage, optic nerve head damage and retinal nerve fibre layer loss, the patient's response to medical or laser therapy, grade of cataract, and the surgeon's experience and personal preferences. The factors favoring a combined procedure are many. While cataract surgery with intraocular lens (IOL) implantation lowers intraocular pressure (IOP) by 2 to 4 mmHg in long-term studies,[5,6] a glaucoma procedure combined with cataract surgery lowers IOP more effectively (6 to 8 mmHg).[7–9] Following either extracapsular cataract extraction (ECCE) or phacoemulsification, many of the glaucomatous eyes suffer an IOP spike to 30 mmHg or more, which may lead to anterior ischemic optic neuropathy or progressive glaucomatous damage. It is essential to avoid IOP spikes in eyes with severe optic disc damage and visual field loss close to fixation. Combining drainage surgery with cataract extraction can significantly reduce the frequency of these spikes. The disadvantages of performing filtration surgery first followed by cataract surgery 3 to 6 months after a mature bleb has formed include delayed visual recovery, all attendant anesthetic as well as perioperative risks of having to undergo two intraocular surgical procedures, decreased cost efficiency, and the possibility of inducing bleb failure.

In a patient who requires both cataract extraction and glaucoma surgery for IOP control, a combined surgery would be preferred. The advantages of a combined procedure (cataract extraction with IOL implantation and trabeculectomy) are avoiding the IOP rise that may occur following cataract surgery alone, rapid visual recovery, and long-term glaucoma control with a single operation. Phacoemulsification combined with trabeculectomy results in good IOP control as well as an improvement in the visual acuity.[7,10,11] The disadvantage of combined procedures is that they are technically slightly more difficult and time consuming.

In a patient for whom only glaucoma surgery is definitely indicated, the decision to combine it with a cataract extraction as well depends on the patient's age, visual acuity, visual requirements, grade of cataract, and associated ocular comorbidity such as subluxated lens, pseudoexfoliation syndrome, etc. Trabeculectomy hastens the onset and progression of cataract, which will make optic nerve head and field evaluation difficult and also result in an unhappy patient who then requires a second surgery for the cataract soon after. The second step cataract surgery may also result in failure of a previously functioning bleb, all of which lead to an extremely unhappy patient and a difficult situation for the surgeon. All these factors favor a combined surgery for these patients.[12]

One may also consider combining glaucoma surgery in a patient who is going to undergo a cataract extraction depending on the IOP control, number of drugs required for IOP control, and patient's intolerance or noncompliance with drugs.[12]

Preoperative Preparation

Apart from the usual preoperative preparations, it is extremely important to control the IOP prior to surgery to avoid choroidal effusion, choroidal hemorrhage, or expulsive hemorrhage. Phacoemulsification is especially advantageous here, as it is a closed chamber procedure; nevertheless, IOP may suddenly drop to values close to zero even with phaco.[13] Preoperative control of IOP can be done with topical medications, systemic carbonic anhydrase inhibitors, oral glycerol, or intravenous mannitol.

Surgical Techniques

Peripheral Iridectomy With Phacoemulsification

A simple peripheral iridectomy can be done with a vitrectomy probe at the time of phacoemulsification in some cases of angle-closure glaucoma. Care should be taken that the iridectomy is in a position that is covered by the lids in order to avoid intractable monocular diplopia for the patient.

Single Site Trabeculectomy With Phacoemulsification

Either a limbus-based or fornix-based conjunctival flap is created followed by a scleral flap that will be large enough to allow implantation of the IOL (Figure 13-1). Anterior chamber is entered under the scleral flap and phacoemulsification is performed as usual. After IOL implantation, sclerectomy and iridectomy are made and the scleral and conjunctival flaps are sutured.

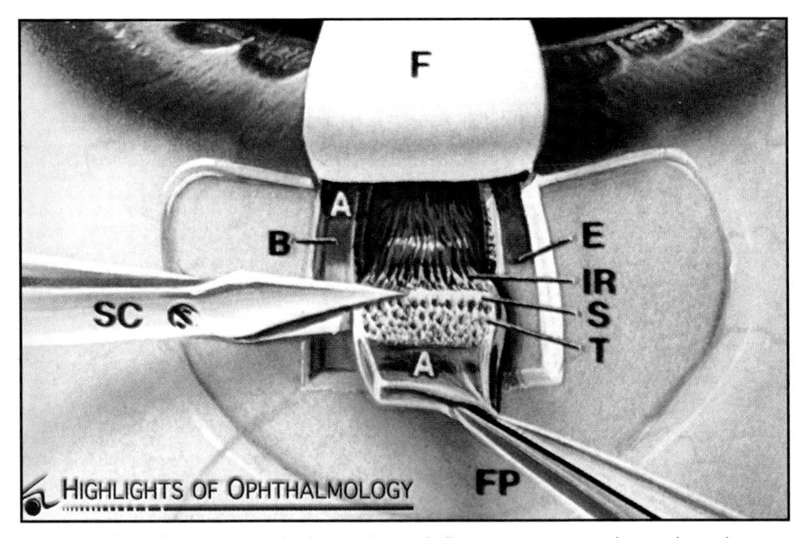

Figure 13-1. Trabeculectomy with fornix-based flap—removing the trabecular window—surgeon's view. This is a surgeon's view of the final incision to remove the trabecular window. It also reveals the surgeon's view of the structures most important to proper trabeculectomy. The trabeculectomy flap, which is being excised, has been hinged backwards, exposing its deep surface to the surgeon's view. The Vannas scissors (SC), make the final cut just in front of the scleral spur (S), on the trabecular tissue, which is here being reflected back with forceps (FP). The scleral spur is localized externally (E) by the junction of white sclera and gray band (B). Scleral flap (F). Clear cornea (A). Iris (I). Iris root (IR). Trabeculum (T). (Courtesy of Benjamin F. Boyd, Maurice H. Luntz, Samuel Boyd, Eds. *Innovations in the Glaucomas—Etiology, Diagnosis and Management*. Highlights of Ophthalmology. English Edition, 2002.)

Two Site Trabeculectomy With Phacoemulsification

Conjunctival and scleral flaps are made at the beginning of the surgery. Clear corneal phacoemulsification is then carried out in another quadrant. Filtering surgery is then completed at the end of the surgery (Figure 13-2).

Trabeculectomy With Microphakonit

Here, a 0.7 mm gauge phaco probe, irrigating chopper, and irrigation/aspiration (I/A) instruments are used for performing bimanual micro incision cataract surgery. Trabeculectomy is performed as previously mentioned (Figure 13-3).

Trabeculotomy With Phacoemulsification (Single Site and Two Site)

In trabeculotomy,[14] a direct communication is created between the anterior chamber and the Schlemm's canal (see Figure 13-1). The conjunctival and scleral flaps are raised. In single site surgery, the scleral flap is then incised from its backside with a shallow incision, from which a sclerocorneal pocket is dissected with a keratome for the phaco probe. In two site surgery, the phacoemulsification is done from a different quadrant. Next, the Schlemm's canal is identified by its pigmentation and by the blood refluxed into the canal during phacoemulsification. In case of difficulty in identification because of too thick scleral bed

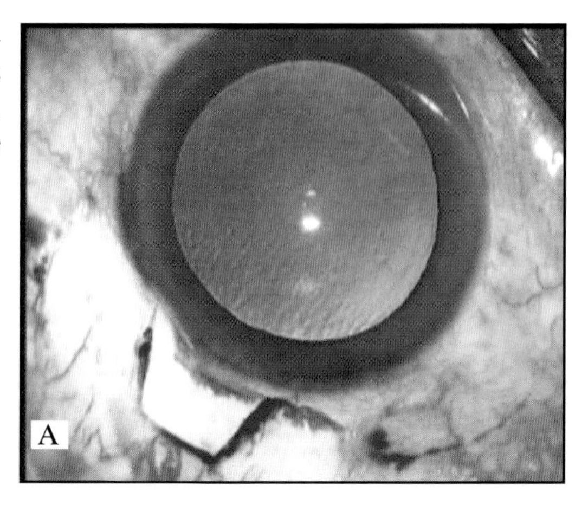

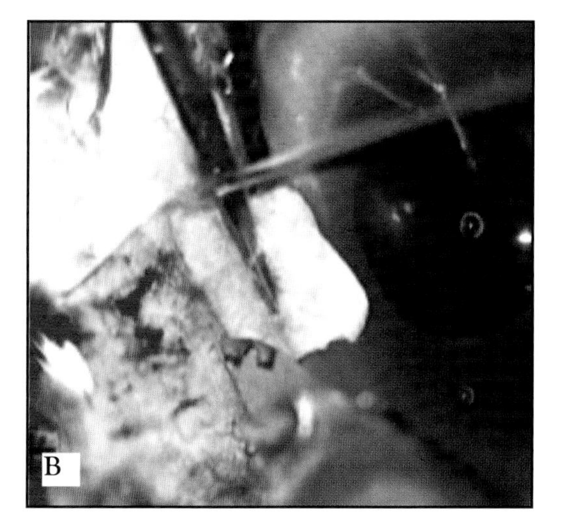

Figure 13-2. A. Superficial scleral flap dissected out, then phacoemulsification is done in another site and the IOL implanted. **B**. Inner scleral window about to be made after IOL insertion.

remaining, a second inner scleral flap is raised. Once the overlying sclera is thick enough, the Schlemm's canal can be easily identified. The scleral lamellae over Schlemm's canal are then incised parallel to the canal taking care to avoid entering the anterior chamber. This can be facilitated by lifting the incised roof of Schlemm's canal with a fine forceps and widening the incision after an initial puncture in the roof with fine Vannas scissors. A specially curved canalicular probe is then inserted into the Schlemm's canal, and the trabecular meshwork ruptured with a forward and inward motion. This is then repeated on the opposite side as well through the same entry site. The scleral flap and conjunctiva are closed in a water-tight manner. One can do microphakonit (700 micron cataract surgery) with trabeculectomy too (Figure 13-3).

Nonpenetrating Glaucoma Surgery With Phacoemulsification

VISCOCANALOSTOMY AND PHACOEMULSIFICATION

This is a nonperforating technique described by Stegman in 1991. It is aimed at avoiding fibrosis-related bleb failure. It works by facilitating outflow of aqueous through the physiological pathway, viz. canal of Schlemm and the collector channels. This is done by creating a Descemetic window, which is composed of the innermost layers of the trabecu-

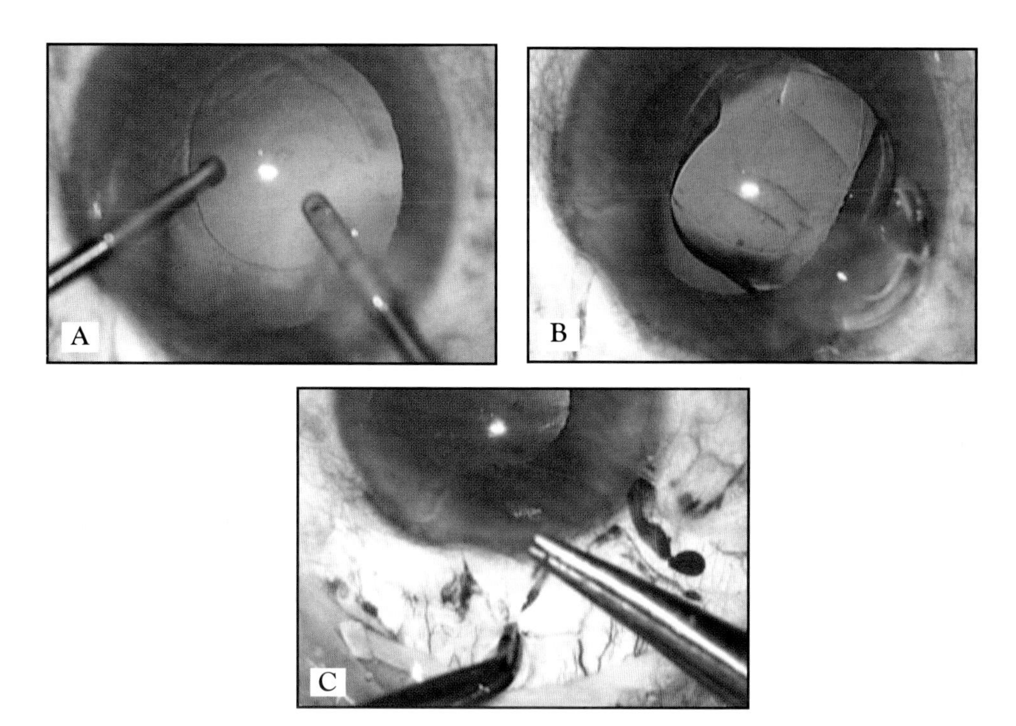

Figure 13-3. A. Microphakonit being performed using 0.7 mm gauge instruments after making superficial scleral flap. Cortex has been removed with 0.7 mm gauge instruments in microphakonit. **B**. IOL inserted after enlarging the microphakonit incision. **C**. The superficial scleral flap being sutured after taking the inner scleral punch and performing the iridectomy.

lar meshwork and the Descemet's membrane.[15] Aqueous flows out through these layers and collects in an intrascleral space, through which it flows into the cut ends of the Schlemm's canal, which has been dilated previously by injecting high viscosity viscoelastic. It has also been postulated that there may be increased uveoscleral outflow after the surgery. Because viscocanalostomy is a nonpenetrating procedure, postoperative complications such as hypotony, shallow anterior chamber, uveitis, endophthalmitis, and cataract formation are avoided. Also, the lack of external filtration avoids all bleb-related complications such as bleb failure due to scarring, blebitis, discomfort, etc.

Under retrobulbar or peribulbar anaesthesia, a fornix-based conjunctival flap is made. As little cautery as possible is used to avoid damage to Schlemm's canal and the collector channels. An outer parabolic flap, sized 5 x5 mm, approximately 200 mm thick, is then dissected, followed by an inner 4 x4 mm scleral flap. One should be able to see the dark reflex from the underlying choroid after dissecting the inner flap. The cut is advanced towards the limbus and the Schlemm's canal is deroofed. The two openings of the canal remain patent at the lateral edges of the cut. The inner flap is then extended into the clear cornea by approximately 1 mm using blunt dissection with a cotton tipped applicator. The inner scleral flap is then excised and the ostia of Schlemm's canal are cannulated with a specific cannula through which high-molecular-weight sodium hyaluronate (Healon GV, Pharmacia & Upjohn, Sweden) is injected to distend it. This is done to prevent collapse and scarring in the early postoperative period. If adequate percolation is not seen through the Descemetic window, the juxtacanalicular meshwork along with the inner wall of the Schlemm's canal can be stripped with a fine forceps. The outer scleral flap is then tightly sutured and Healon GV is injected beneath the flap to prevent the intrascleral lake from collapsing and scarring in the early postoperative period. Two lateral stitches hold the conjunctiva in place. The conjunctiva is then closed. In case of perforation of the Descemetic window, one can convert to a trabeculectomy. Viscocanalostomy can be combined with phacoemulsification[15] using the same site or a different site. In single site, phacoemulsification is done via a superior scleral tunnel and a block of deep sclera is excised at the end and viscocanalostomy is completed as usual. In case of two site surgery, viscocanalostomy is done after phaco has been completed through the temporal approach. When viscocanalostomy is combined with phaco, aqueous leakage from the tunnel can be differentiated from a perforation of the Descemetic membrane by drying the window surface with a sponge.

Deep Sclerectomy and Phacoemulsification

This is also a nonpenetrating surgery, which differs from viscocanalostomy by producing sub-Tenon filtration.

Under retrobulbar or peribulbar anaesthesia, a 4 x4 mm, 200 to 250 microns square superficial scleral flap is made, followed by a deep scleral flap similar to that in viscocanalostomy. The dissection is extended anteriorly to deroof the Schlemm's canal and a Descemetic window is created. The deep flap is excised and the superficial flap is closed less tightly to allow percolation into the sub-Tenon space. The conjunctiva is then closed.[15]

Collagen or reticulated hyaluronic acid implants[15] can be inserted into the scleral lake for improving long-term filtration. These devices are slowly absorbed, thus maintaining the intrascleral lake and preventing its closure by fibrosis. A high-molecular-weight viscoelastic[15] (Healon 5) may also be injected into the intrascleral lake to decrease wound healing. Deep sclerectomy can also be combined with the application of antimetabolites.[15] The hypotensive effect may also be increased even after surgery by perforating the Descemetic window ab interno with a YAG laser.

Deep sclerectomy can be combined with phacoemulsification just as in viscocanalostomy.

Laser Sclerotomy With Phacoemulsification

Here, the laser fiber optic of the Nd YAG laser is passed through the clear corneal incision and a short burst of laser is given directly opposite the planned site of sclerotomy.[16] The aiming beam is used as a guide and hence a goniolens is not required. When the aiming beam is seen around 1.5 mm from the limbus, a short burst of laser brings the laser fiber optic out of the sclera and under the conjunctiva. The laser fiber optic has a Helium Neon aiming beam and the diameter of the optic end is 380 microns. The fiber optic is encased in a silicone sleeve. The remaining phacoemulsification is carried out as usual. Excimer laser can also be used.

Seton Procedure

This can be done in cases that do not respond to conventional surgeries (Figure 13-4).

Antimetabolites

The use of antifibrotics (mitomycin-C[17] and 5-fluorouracil[18] to reduce the potential for bleb failure in combined phacotrabeculectomy is controversial. Mitomycin-C may result in lower long-term IOPs when used with combined procedures[9,17] but 5-fluorouracil does not

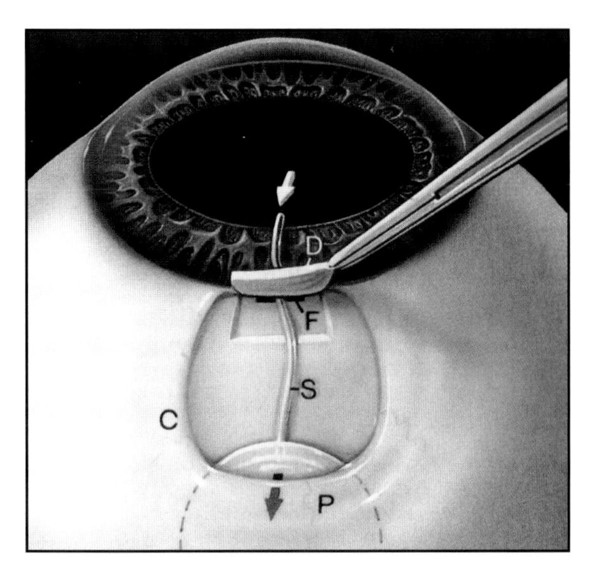

Figure 13-4. Seton implantation procedure. A fornix-based conjunctival flap (C) is raised and the methylmethacrylate baseplate (P) of the Seton is pushed under the conjunctival flap posteriorly and sutured to the scleral surface. The implant has a biconcave shape with the inferior surface shaped to fit the sclera. A small 3 mm square half-thickness lamellar scleral flap (D) is raised just as in a trabeculectomy. An incision (F) is made into the anterior chamber under this scleral flap and the long silicone tube (S) of the Seton is placed into the anterior chamber (the end of the silicone tube can be seen in the anterior chamber near the tip of the white arrow). Next, the scleral flap (D) is sutured down around the tube (S) of the Seton. Finally, the conjunctiva is sutured back in place. Aqueous then drains from the anterior chamber (white arrow) down through the tube (S) to the baseplate (P) (black arrow), where a bleb forms. (Courtesy of Benjamin F. Boyd, Maurice H. Luntz, Samuel Boyd, Eds. *Innovations in the Glaucomas—Etiology, Diagnosis and Management*. Highlights of Ophthalmology. English Edition, 2002.)

seem to.[9,18] The potential vision-threatening complications of antimetabolites such as bleb-related endophthalmitis,[19,20] hypotonic maculopathy,[21,22] and late-onset bleb leaks[23] should be considered while deciding to use these agents.

Type of Intraocular Lens

Friedrich et al found that foldable silicone IOLs may induce late postoperative inflammatory membranes with pigment precipitates, especially after combined surgery.[24]

Complications

Postoperative uveitis or rise in IOP can usually be tackled with appropriate medications. Hyphema, if small, usually resolves by itself. If very large, it may need to be evacuated. Excessive filtration may occur leading to choroidal detachment. When associated with a flat anterior chamber or other severe complications, it may require fluid drainage and bleb revision. Shallow anterior chamber may also be due to bleb leak. Hypotonic maculopathy may rarely be seen, especially in a young myopic patient. Other postoperative complications that may occur after routine phacoemulsification may occur in this setting too. Late post-operative complications include cystoid macular edema, capsular phimosis syndrome, IOL decentration, posterior capsular opacification, bleb failure, and bleb-related endophthalmitis.

KEY POINTS

1. The summary of the Evidence on Intraocular Pressure Control with Surgical Treatment of Coexisting Cataract and Glaucoma on Long-term Intraocular Pressure Control states that there is good evidence that long-term IOP control is greater with combined procedures than with cataract extraction alone and fair evidence that trabeculectomy alone lowers long-term IOP more than combined ECCE and trabeculectomy. There is weak evidence that cataract extraction in glaucoma patients lowers IOP on average by 2 to 4 mmHg, trabeculectomy alone appears to lower IOP more than combined phaco and trabeculectomy, phaco and trabeculectomy lowers IOP by approximately 8 mmHg in individuals followed up for a mean of 1 to 2 years, ECCE and trabeculectomy lowers IOP by approximately 6 to 8 mmHg in individuals followed up for a mean of 1 to 2 years. The evidence was insufficient to determine the impact of cataract extraction on preexisting filtering blebs, to determine if other combined techniques (eg, cyclodialysis and endolaser) work as well as cataract extraction and trabeculectomy and to determine if combined phaco and trabeculectomy lowers IOP on the first postoperative day more than phaco alone.
2. An Evidence-Based Practice Center sponsored by the Agency for Healthcare Research and Quality reviewed 131 studies on the treatment of adults with coexisting cataract and glaucoma, assessed the study quality and data, and reported it in evidence tables. The investigators concluded that the findings that glaucoma surgery was associated with an increased risk of postoperative cataract and that a glaucoma procedure added to cataract surgery lowers IOP more than cataract surgery alone were strongly supported by the literature.
3. The other findings that were found to be moderately supported by the literature[9] were that limbus- and fornix-based conjunctival incisions provided the same degree of long-term IOP lowering in combined surgery; in combined surgery using phacoemulsification, the size of the cataract incision did not affect long-term IOP control; when used with combined procedures, 5-fluorouracil was not beneficial in further lowering IOP, whereas mitomycin-C was efficacious in producing lower long-term IOPs when used with combined procedures.
4. Findings weakly supported by literature are that combined procedures resulted in lower IOP at 24 hours than cataract extraction alone; ECCE alone appears to increase IOP at 24 hours; in the long term, cataract surgery alone lowered IOP by 2 to 4 mm Hg, combined cataract and glaucoma surgery lowered IOP by 6 to 8 mm Hg, and the performance of a glaucoma procedure alone provided even greater long-term IOP lowering than combined cataract and glaucoma surgery; combined surgery in which the incisions for the cataract extraction and glaucoma procedure are separate provided slightly lower long-term IOP than a one-site approach and that combined surgery in which phacoemulsification is used provided slightly lower long-term IOP than nuclear expression.

References

1. Age-Related Eye Disease Study Research Group. A randomized, placebo-controlled clinical trial of high-dose supplementation with vitamins C and E and beta carotene for age-related cataract and vision loss: AREDS Report No. 9. *Arch Ophthalmol.* 2001;119:1439–52.
2. Sperduto RD, Hu TS, Milton RC, et al. The Linxian cataract studies. Two nutrition intervention trials. *Arch Ophthalmol.* 1993;111:1246–53.
3. Mares-Perlman JA, Klein BE, Klein R, Ritter LL. Relation between lens opacities and vitamin and mineral supplement use. *Ophthalmology.* 1994;101:315–25.
4. Leske MC, Wu SY, Connell AM, et al. Lens opacities, demographic factors and nutritional supplements in the Barbados Eye Study. *Int J Epidemiol.* 1997;26:1314–22.
5. Shingleton BJ, Gamell LS, O'Donoghue MW, et al. Long-term changes in intraocular pressure after clear corneal phacoemulsification: normal patients versus glaucoma suspect and glaucoma patients. *J Cataract Refract Surg.* 1999;25:885–90.
6. Tennen DG, Masket S. Short-and long-term effect of clear corneal incisions on intraocular pressure. *J Cataract Refract Surg.* 1996;22:568–70.
7. Wedrich A, Menapace R, Radax U, Papapanos P. Long-term results of combined trabeculectomy and small incision cataract surgery. *J Cataract Refract Surg.* 1995;21:49–54.
8. Gimbel HV, Meyer D, DeBroff BM, et al. Intraocular pressure response to combined phacoemulsification and trabeculotomy ab externo versus phacoemulsification alone in primary open-angle glaucoma. *J Cataract Refract Surg.* 1995;21:653–60.
9. Agency for Healthcare Research and Quality. Evidence Report/Technology Assessment. Number 38. Treatment of coexisting cataract and glaucoma. Washington, DC: AHRQ Publication No. 01-E049; 2001.
10. Wyse T, Meyer M, Ruderman JM, et al. Combined trabeculectomy and phacoemulsification: a one-site vs a two-site approach. *Am J Ophthalmol.* 1998;125:334–9.
11. Park HJ, Weitzman M, Caprioli J. Temporal corneal phacoemulsification combined with superior trabeculectomy. A retrospective case-control study. *Arch Ophthalmol.* 1997;115:318–23.
12. Guillermo L, Urcelay-Segura JL, Ortega-Usobiaga J, et al. Combined cataract extraction and filtering surgery. In: Agarwal S, Agarwal A, Agarwal A, eds. *Phacoemulsification.* 3rd ed. Vol 2. Thorofare, NJ: SLACK Incorporated; 2004: 596–608.
13. Buratto L, Zanini M. Phacoemulsification in glaucomatous eyes. In: Buratto L, Osher RH, Masket S, eds. *Cataract Surgery in Complicated Cases.* Thorofare, NJ: SLACK Incorporated; 2000.
14. Neuhann T, Ernest PH. Combined phacoemulsification with trabeculectomy. In: Buratto L, Osher RH, Masket S, eds. *Cataract Surgery in Complicated Cases.* Thorofare, NJ: SLACK Incorporated; 2000.
15. Obstbaum S, Zanini M. Combined cataract and glaucoma surgery. In: Buratto L, Osher RH, Masket S, eds. *Cataract Surgery in Complicated Cases.* Thorofare, NJ: SLACK Incorporated; 2000.
16. Agarwal S, Sundaram, AB. Laser sclerotomy, laser phakonit and IOL implantation. In: Agarwal S, Agarwal A, Agarwal A, eds. *Phacoemulsification.* 3rd ed. Vol 2. Thorofare, NJ: SLACK Incorporated; 2004:596–608.
17. Shin DH, Simone PA, Song MS, et al. Adjunctive subconjunctival mitomycin C in glaucoma triple procedure. *Ophthalmology.* 1995;102:1550–8.
18. Wong PC, Ruderman JM, Krupin T, et al. 5-Fluorouracil after primary combined filtration surgery. *Am J Ophthalmol.* 1994;117:149–54.
19. Higginbotham EJ, Stevens RK, Musch DC, et al. Bleb-related endophthalmitis after trabeculectomy with mitomycin C. *Ophthalmology.* 1996;103:650–6.
20. Greenfield DS, Suñer IJ, Miller MP, et al. Endophthalmitis after filtering surgery with mitomycin. *Arch Ophthalmol.* 1996;114:943–9.

21. Zacharia PT, Deppermann SR, Schuman JS. Ocular hypotony after trabeculectomy with mitomycin C. *Am J Ophthalmol*. 1993;16:314–26.
22. Costa VP, Wilson RP, Moster MR, et al. Hypotony maculopathy following the use of topical mitomycin C in glaucoma filtration surgery. *Ophthalmic Surg*. 1993;24:389–94.
23. Greenfield DS, Liebmann JM, Jee J, Ritch R. Late-onset bleb leaks after glaucoma filtering surgery. *Arch Ophthalmol*. 1998;116:443–7.
24. Friedrich Y, Raniel Y, Lubovsky E, Friedman Z. Late pigmented-membrane formation on silicone intraocular lenses after phacoemulsification with or without trabeculectomy. *J Cataract Refract Surg*. 1999;25:1220–1225.
25. Jampel HD, Lubomski LH, Friedman DS, et al. Treatment of Coexisting Cataract and Glaucoma. Baltimore: Evidence-Based Practice Center, Johns Hopkins University, 6 Oct 2000. Contract No. 290–097–0006, Task Order 3.

Chapter 14

PHACOEMULSIFICATION AND KERATOPLASTY

Javier Mendicute, MD; Yolanda Gallego, MD; Aritz Bidaguren, MD; Marta Ubeda, MD; Cristina Irigoyen, MD

INTRODUCTION

In certain circumstances, and despite the existence of a cataract, lens surgery may not be sufficient to achieve correct visual recovery. This is particularly true when associated with corneal pathology. In cases of this kind, the only way to restore the visual function is by associating cataract surgery with keratoplasty.

There are several classic ways of dealing with this problem: 1) Firstly, performing cataract or cornea surgery and subsequently implementing a keratoplasty or cataract surgery where necessary; 2) The simultaneous carrying out of both procedures (keratoplasty and cataract surgery); and 3) Triple procedures (keratoplasty, cataract surgery, and intraocular lens [IOL] implantation).

Given problems of infrastructure and the cornea donor requirements of keratoplasty, it used to be common practice to start by performing lens surgery, then potentially considering a keratoplasty[1-4] depending on the visual recovery achieved. Performing a keratoplasty and subsequently cataract surgery where necessary was less common. This latter option had the following drawbacks: firstly, a new incision, either corneal or scleral, had to be made. This incision usually had to be long in the case of both intracapsular and extracapsular extraction. Secondly, endothelial damage to the transplanted cornea sometimes threatened its viability. It was also true that cataracts often developed following the keratoplasty, whether due to the surgical intervention itself or to the required postoperative medication.

Combined procedures were therefore considered. These first of all took the shape of double procedures combining intracapsular or extracapsular cataract extraction (ECCE) with keratoplasty. When the procedure implemented was intracapsular extraction, vitreous contact with the corneal endothelium was described as the cause of keratoplasty rejection, whether or not the anterior hyaloid was intact. Although vitreous-endothelium contact was avoided during ECCE, the potential appearance of secondary posterior capsule opacification, and the absence of Yag laser, meant that another surgical procedure was required to solve the problem at hand. In any case, double procedures were, at least in theory, highly attractive.

Table 14-1.

Triple Procedure With Extracapsular Extraction: Drawbacks

- Necessary pupil dilatation can complicate centering of the keratoplasty.
- Most of the procedure is performed with open-sky surgery.
- Difficult extraction of the nucleus in hypotonic eyes.
- Difficult aspiration of the cortical mass.
- In the case of capsular rupture, vitreous loss may be problematic.
- In the case of choroidal or expulsive hemorrhage, the consequences can be devastating.

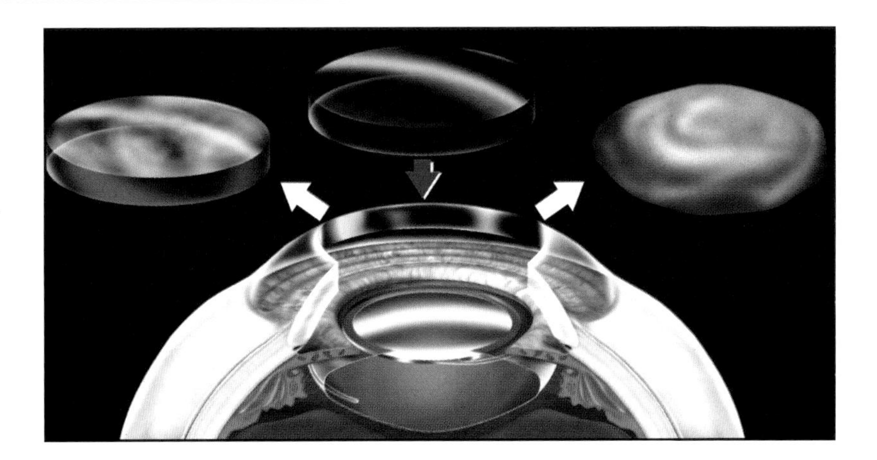

Figure 14-1. Triple procedure: keratoplasty, ECCE, and IOL implantation.

With the modern development of extracapsular lens extraction, plus introduction of the IOL and Yag laser, triple procedures seemed to offer the best possible surgical option: an operation, an incision, three procedures (keratoplasty, extracapsular extraction, and IOL implantation) (Figure 14-1) in one surgical operation and the possibility of good visual recovery in a relatively short time. The drawbacks in triple procedure are shown in Table 14-1.

The following question has therefore emerged in recent years: Why not perform phacoemulsification in triple procedures?

We believe that this procedure would have certain advantages (Table 14-2) and perhaps certain limitations rather than drawbacks.

INDICATIONS

When considering a combined procedure (keratoplasty and cataract surgery), we have to evaluate not only the condition of the lens but also the state of the cornea and the degree of visual incapacity potentially justifying corneal and lens alteration. When considering keratoplasty, and based on its level of complexity, we must also evaluate the potential visual acuity of the affected eye.

Table 14-2.
Triple Procedure With Phacoemulsification: Advantages

• Most of the triple procedure is performed with closed-system surgery.
• Cortical aspiration is simpler.
• If the IOL is implanted prior to the keratoplasty, the pupil may contract, thus facilitating centering of the keratoplasty.
• The zonule-capsular barrier, reinforced by implantation of the IOL, maintains its ocular compartmentalization.
• Potential capsular rupture or choroidal hemorrhage is more controllable.

Cataract Evaluation in Patients With Corneal Opacification

Having diagnosed the corneal problem, we must evaluate/interpret the degree of lens opacification in order to establish whether or not a simultaneous procedure is advisable.

It is useful to evaluate the thickness of the affected cornea:

1. If opacification is superficial, we can consider either phototherapeutic excimer laser or superficial lamellar keratectomy. Phototherapeutic keratectomy can be useful if the opacification covers no more than the most superficial 140 µm of the cornea. This technique can cause hyperopia, which is more pronounced if the area treated is deeper and smaller in diameter.[5] Superficial keratectomy with microkeratome is useful if opacification of the anterior stroma only involves the anterior 180 µm of the cornea.[6] In none of these cases is it necessary to substitute eliminated anterior corneal tissue with donor tissue.
2. In cases where the corneal pathology lies in deeper anterior stromal layers, we can consider an anterior lamellar keratoplasty (ALK) associated with phacoemulsification as an alternative to penetrating keratoplasty.
3. If almost all of the corneal thickness is opacified but the deepest membrane and endothelial-Descemet complex are normal, we can perform a deep anterior lamellar keratoplasty together with a phacoemulsification.[7,8]

Corneal Evaluation in Patients With Cataracts

We occasionally have to consider the inverse situation: that of having to evaluate the state of the cornea in a patient with cataract, given that it is not unusual to come across cornea guttata, Fuchs' dystrophy, or other corneal pathologies that tend to increase considerably in frequency and seriousness with age. When alterations in the corneal endothelium membrane exist, it could be useful to study the membrane in question with endothelial specular microscopy. Another examination which provides important information, is ultrasound pachymetry (Table 14-3).

However, practically speaking, the decision of whether to simply operate on the cataract or to perform a combined procedure (keratoplasty and cataract extraction) initially depends on two factors: 1) the corneal stromal edema, and 2) the central corneal pachymetry. If the pachymetric readings are higher than 640–650 µm and a stromal edema exists, a combined procedure is advisable. If there is no edema, and the reading is lower than 640 µm, an isolated phacoemulsification technique implies no great risk of endothelial decompensation given that the latest cataract surgery advances and the appropriate use of viscoelastics has reduced the risk of corneal decompensation in pathologies like Fuchs' dystrophy.[9]

Table 14-3. Corneal Evaluation in Patients With Cataracts
• Endothelial specular microscopy
• Corneal edema
• Central corneal thickness by pachymetry
• Corneal topography

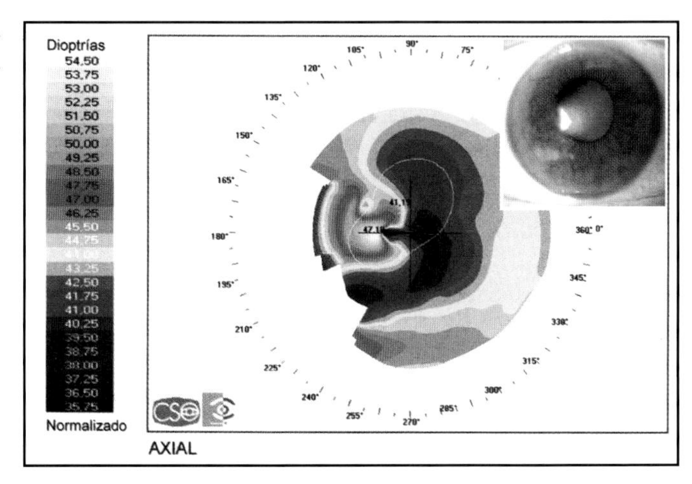

Figure 14-2. Corneal topography demonstrating anterior corneal surface damage.

However, we have to use a viscoelastic providing maximum endothelial protection in order to reduce this risk. In this respect, hyaluronate sodium and chondroitin sulphate seem to provide maximum intraoperative endothelial protection, causing a lower postsurgical loss of endothelial cells.[10,11]

Corneal topography may well be extremely useful when evaluating corneal status in these situations. This procedure helps to establish whether corneal opacity exists on the anterior surface of the cornea (Figure 14-2), in which case it would become obvious, or inside the stroma (eg, interstitial keratitis), where the topography would suffer no alteration. This differentiation is crucial and we must not forget that the anterior corneal surface is responsible for greater refractive power of the eye and that its alteration strongly compromises visual acuity. On the contrary, a relatively dense stromal scar may not cause obvious impairment to the visual function. Attempting to adapt a contact lens with a view to reducing irregular astigmatism can be useful in evaluating potential visual acuity and can even improve the sight.

When to Operate?

Surgery must be considered when the corneal opacity and cataract are sufficiently dense to justify the visual limitations indicated by the patient and when optical and medical alternatives are not sufficient to recover the sight or to satisfy the patient's needs. On the other hand, recourse should be taken to nonsurgical treatment when the visual function, aesthetics, and discomfort or pain can be improved and eased by other methods.

We must occasionally consider surgery when pain or ugliness justifies the decision without waiting for the recovery of sight; this said, it will probably not be necessary to perform a triple procedure in these cases given that a keratoplasty may be sufficient.

COMBINED OR TWO-STAGE PROCEDURE?

Having made the decision to remove the cataract and perform a keratoplasty, we must ask ourselves whether to do so in two separate stages or in one single procedure.

Combined Procedures

The advantages of performing cataract surgery and a keratoplasty in one single operation, as part of a combined procedure, are:

1. A single operation.
2. The use of a standard, well-known technique.
3. Lower financial cost.
4. Less risk for the corneal endothelium than performing cataract surgery at a future time following penetrating keratoplasty;[12,13] this said, certain authors[14] find no particular difference in endothelial readings among patients on whom a combined procedure was performed and those on whom a second phacoemulsification was performed following keratoplasty, probably due to advances in phacoemulsification technology and the rational use of new viscoelastics.
5. Not having to repeat cataract surgery, a procedure which has almost become standard postkeratoplasty[15] due to the cataractogenic nature of corneal transplant surgery, in general, and to the use of steroids at the postoperative stage, in particular.
6. Evidence that posterior capsular opacification occurs less frequently (9.8% vs. 36.2%) and at a later stage (45.6 vs. 24.3 months) with combined procedures than with isolated cataract extraction.[16]
7. The higher tendency for the cataract to progress in patients previously treated with keratoplasty.

The advantages of ECCE are obvious given the knowledge that intracapsular lens surgery is recognized as one of the risk factors behind the development of corneal failure in combined procedures. The risk of intracapsular extraction could be the result of the vitreous/corneal endothelium contact arising with this technique due to the nonexistence of anatomical barriers.[17] The differences between conventional extracapsular surgery and phacoemulsification are not yet well defined.

Two-Stage Procedure

Among the advantages of performing keratoplasty and cataract surgery in two stages, as independent procedures, are:

1. Improved refractive predictability when the cataract surgery is performed following keratoplasty, given the possibility of obtaining true keratometric readings. Numerous articles have been published in the past indicating the results obtained with the triple procedure; these studies describe refractive errors varying between -14.7 to +8.0 diopters, with the percentage of patients showing a final refraction of ±2.0 diopters standing at between 26% and 68%.[14]
2. Technically speaking, independent keratoplasty is safer due to the fact that it can be carried out with the patient in miosis; hence the pupil becomes a useful reference for centering the keratoplasty.
3. Sequential cataract surgery, although complicated by the keratoplasty interface and occasionally by the presence of suturing, may be simpler, given that performing an open-sky capsulorrhexis or cortical aspiration, as opposed to a combined procedure, is more complex.

IOL Calculation

One of the greatest drawbacks of the combined procedure, an advantage therefore of the two-stage technique (keratoplasty followed by cataract surgery), is the difficulty of correctly calculating the power of the lens to be implanted during a triple procedure of cataract extraction, IOL implantation, and keratoplasty. One of the reasons for residual refractive error following triple procedures is not having preoperative knowledge of the keratometric reading resulting from the keratoplasty. Calculating the power of the lens to be implanted seems to be more predictable if we consider the refractive results obtained on carrying out the procedures separately, with up to 95% of patients showing readings of ±2.0 diopters.[21]

Whatever the case, when performing two-stage surgery, we must wait for a minimum of 3 months between the keratoplasty and cataract extraction for the keratometric readings to offer minimum reliability for lens calculation. Even so, the central corneal curvature will not be totally stable until the corneal sutures have been removed (a year after the keratoplasty). And even then, calculating the power of the lens can bring more postoperative refractive surprises than using the postoperative K, generally more curved than the physiological preoperative version, especially if we use donor grafts of a larger diameter than the recipient beds. Using this K can cause defects in the effective lens position (ELP) calculation if based on the SRK/T formula. Given the above, in the case of keratoplasty followed by cataract surgery, we use the double K method recommended for cataract surgery following corneal refractive surgery,[22] using the K of the contralateral eye, if it is normal, in the first part of the formula to calculate the ELP and the true keratometry following the keratoplasty in the second part of the formula serving to calculate the lens power for a specific keratometry and axial length. If the contralateral eye is not normal, we recommend that a normal average keratometry (43 to 44 diopters) be used in the first part of the formula serving to calculate the ELP.

What Technique Should We Use?

We have selected some of the above-mentioned alternatives based on our observations regarding the grade of corneal opacification and its depth (Table 14-4):

1. The appropriate alternative in the case of superficial opacification (0 to 140 μm) is phototherapeutic keratectomy (PTK). One drawback of this option is that it has to be performed with an excimer laser, which is not always available in the same operating theater, meaning that the patient has to be moved. It can be performed at the same time as or prior to phacoemulsification. We must remember that this process will modify the corneal curvature, a factor that could affect the IOL power calculation. If performed previously, this change can be considered in the biometric calculation; however, if performed simultaneously, we will not know the correct keratometry, a factor affecting the refractive result.
2. If opacification is somewhat deeper (0 to 180 μm), a free superficial keratectomy with microkeratome and no corneal substitution could be the solution in certain cases.[6] Here we would be faced with the same limitation as indicated above when calculating the IOL. This said, free superficial keratectomy can be performed in the operating theater itself. Although the corneal surface following operation becomes irregular and can complicate the visualization of intraocular structures, the effect is not as great as corneal opacification. In this case, the given optical aids can be useful, the best of which is application of viscoelastic to the cornea.

Table 14-4.
Phacokeratoplasty: Selection of Techniques

0 to 140 μm corneal opacity	Phototherapeutic keratectomy (PTK)
0 to 180 μm corneal opacity	Free superficial keratectomy
0 to 300 μm corneal opacity	Automated lamellar keratoplasty (ALK)
0 to 500 μm corneal opacity	Deep anterior lamellar keratoplasty
Full thickness corneal opacity	Transitory keratoprosthesis or graft

3. If the corneal pathology is located in deeper anterior stromal layers (0 to 300 μm), we can consider an ALK associated with phacoemulsification as an alternative to penetrating keratoplasty. Here we would start by performing a free-running anterior keratectomy at the desired depth, followed by a phacoemulsification, and finally transplantation of the anterior corneal tissue.
4. The chosen technique for deep opacities (0 to 500 μm) is ALK.[7] First we eliminate the anterior corneal stroma, performing a phacoemulsification after having applied viscoelastic to the deep corneal stroma to favor visualization, finally substituting the anterior corneal stroma at the end of the procedure.
5. If the entire thickness of the cornea is compromised, complete trephination may be necessary. In this case, if we do not want to renounce phacoemulsification, we will have to use a transitory keratoprosthesis[20] or a transitory corneal graft[21] for substitution at a later date by the definitive cornea.

Nine Optical Aids for Improving Visualization

The basic key for completion of phacoemulsification on a cornea with obvious opacification is visualization of the anterior segment structures (Table 14-5).

The following procedures, listed from simple to complex, may be useful:[22]

1. Switching off the main lights in the operating theater.
2. Applying viscoelastics to the cornea, which, once in place, magnify the anterior chamber structures, thus potentially facilitating the different phacoemulsification stages.
3. Using a light optic fiber from outside the eye or introducing it to the anterior chamber by paracentesis.
4. It is sometimes possible to focus the microscope beneath the cornea and obtain suitable visualization for proceeding with the phacoemulsification. Doing this can serve to modify the microscope angle of inclination and to move the ocular globe into different positions in the attempt to find the areas of best visualization.
5. In the case of epithelial edemas or highly irregular corneal epithelial surfaces, it is useful to deepithelialize the cornea before starting the procedure.
6. When the above measures are insufficient, performing lamellar keratoplasties of sufficient thickness to include the corneal opacity and smoothing the resulting surface with viscoelastic material facilitates lens visualization. This kind of keratectomy can be performed manually or automatically with a microkeratome. Using a microkeratome shortens surgical time.

Table 14-5. Optical and Visual Aids for Phacoemulsification With Corneal Opacification
• Switching off the main lights in the operating theater.
• Applying viscoelastics to the cornea.
• Using a light optic fiber.
• Focussing the microscope beneath the cornea for adequate visualization during phacoemulsification.
• Deepithelializing in the case of epithelial edemas or irregular corneal epithelial surfaces.
• Lamellar keratectomies of sufficient thickness to include corneal opacification.
• Deep anterior lamellar keratoplasties in the case of corneal opacifications located in deep stromal layers.
• Using trypan blue for capsular tincture.
• Transitory corneal prosthesis.

7. If the above measures are insufficient, deep ALK will make it possible to overcome the visualization problems caused by deep corneal opacification.[7]
8. As a last option for dense corneal opacification when wishing to proceed with a phacoemulsification, we can perform a complete trephination, followed by a transitory corneal prosthesis, phacoemulsification, removal of the transitory prosthesis, and transplant.
9. Another interesting option is to apply trypan blue for improved capsule visibility,[23] thus increasing contrast and potentially facilitating the capsulorrhexis.

Phacoemulsification and Penetrating Keratoplasty

The conventional combined procedure (cataract surgery and keratoplasty) consists of performing a corneal trephination, open-sky extracapsular lens extraction, IOL implantation, and suturing of the donor corneal button to the recipient bed. Nowadays, with phacoemulsification as the generally preferred method for cataract extraction, another triple procedure has come to light: lens phacoemulsification, IOL implantation, and performing a keratoplasty as if we were dealing with a phakic eye. The only circumstance affecting the performing of phacokeratoplasty is the degree of corneal opacity. The only cases where this technique cannot be performed is when the cornea is sufficiently opaque to prevent visualization of the anterior segment structures, as is the case with Schnyder's dystrophy.

Incision

We believe that making the incision in a clear cornea is not advisable when the phacoemulsification is to be associated with a keratoplasty. Although certain authors[24] do use this technique, we believe that it can have a number of drawbacks: proximity of the incision in the clear cornea to the donor-recipient interface means that mutual tractions threat-

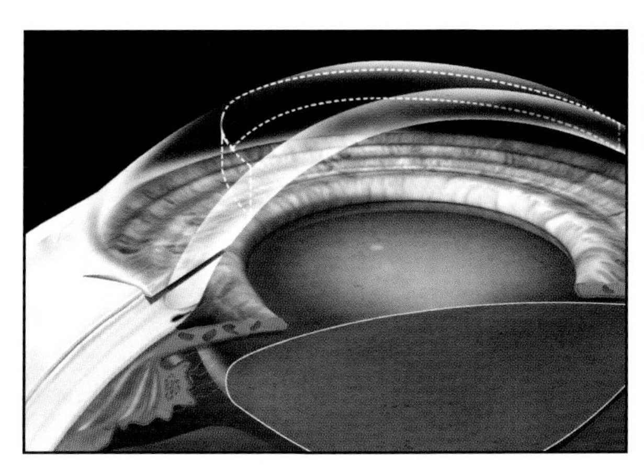

Figure 14-3. The entrance to the anterior chamber must not be too advanced given that it could damage the limits of the keratoplasty.

en their watertightness once both have been sutured. In our opinion, making a frown-type incision in the superior sclera is the best option. Once the conjunctiva has been dissected, we coagulate the scleral bed and mark a frown incision measuring 2.75 to 3.2 mm in width. We then tunnel the scleral incision, performing an ancillary puncture (for right-handed surgeons) to the left of the frown, filling the anterior chamber via this puncture with viscoelastic liquid and proceeding to approach the anterior chamber through the sclera tunnel with a 2.75 to 3.2 mm scalpel. Here it is extremely important not to advance excessively on the cornea at the entrance to the anterior chamber because this could interfere with the borders of the corneal transplant (Figure 14-3). It is precisely now, and at no other time, that we must apply viscoelastic to the cornea in the case of suspected visualization problems. Prior to this, it is not appropriate because it would complicate control of the entrance incision to the anterior chamber, and later it may no longer be necessary and would oblige us to suspend the procedure during the time it takes for the viscoelastic to spread over the corneal convexity.

Capsulorrhexis

Having filled the anterior chamber with viscoelastic, the next step is to perform the capsulorrhexis. Here we must attempt to apply the options considered in Table 14-5. Having started the capsulorrhexis in the desired area with either a cystotome or forceps, it will be simpler to continue with forceps alone in the case of poor visibility. It is a good idea to control the anterior capsule, not by its line of progress, but by its radius (Figure 14-4), an area in which visualization may be simpler given the formation of reflections at this level.

Hydrodissection

This must be no different from the procedure employed in any other phacoemulsification process. Here we would only point out that it must be sufficiently meticulous to ensure correct liberation of the crystalline lens nucleus without endangering capsular integrity, a risk which is greater in these cases due to deficient visualization of the different surgical steps.

Figure 14-4. Controlling the capsulorhexis by visualizing its radius through a corneal opacification.

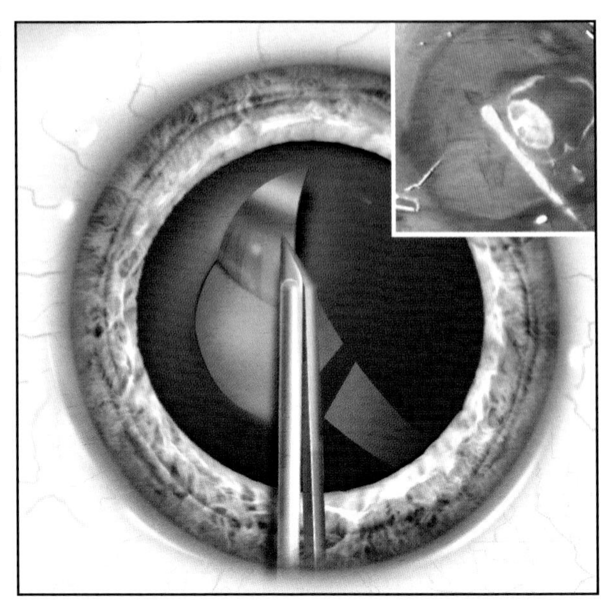

Nuclear Phacoemulsification

Nuclear phacoemulsification can be performed inside or outside the capsular bag. Personally, we are more familiar with phacoemulsification inside the bag, and perform it in combined procedures. Other authors[24–30] suggest that the phacoemulsification be performed outside the bag, in the anterior chamber, assuring that there is a lower risk of capsular rupture, a claim which may be true, while defending the fact that the greater loss of endothelial cells is of scant importance given that the cornea is being transplanted immediately. However, we would say that not the whole cornea is transplanted, only the central button, and that a phacoemulsification in the anterior chamber may decrease endothelial density of the recipient cornea, even though we only conserve its rim. We would add that being able to luxate the nucleus into the anterior chamber, either by hydrodissection or viscoexpression, requires having performed an extensive capsulorrhexis.

Aspiration of the Cortex

As far as parameters and strategies are concerned, irrigation-aspiration of the cortex is identical to that performed in other situations. We use an aspiration rate of 25 cc/min, vacuum of 500 mm Hg (linear mode) and bottle height at 65 to 80 cm. On occasions when visibility is exceedingly poor, we can use an aspiration rate of 18 to 20 cc/min, hence stressing safety over rapidity, while moving the globe toward areas in which the aspiration point is more visible.

Intraocular Lens Implantation

Having completed aspiration of the cortex, we proceed to fill the capsular bag with viscoelastic liquid and subsequently enlarge the scleral incision according to the lens to be implanted.

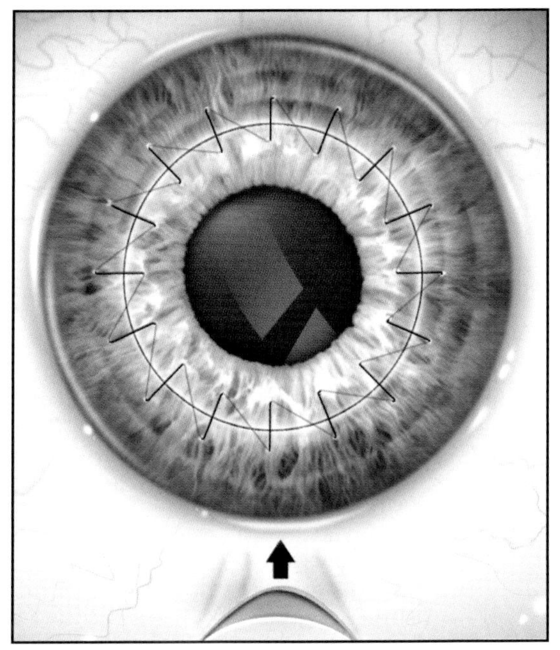

Figure 14-5. Closing the scleral incision. Incision incorrectly sutured.

Closing the Scleral Incision

The situation described (frown incision when performing a phacokeratoplasty) is the only occasion in which we use systematic suturing in a phacoemulsification with scleral incision; not in order to maintain watertightness of the globe during the keratoplasty, but to ensure that, once the donor button has been sutured, there is no traction on the anterior lip of the scleral incision. Although a traction of this kind could half-open the incision (Figure 14-5), this is not our greatest concern, but rather the fact that it could provide poor support to the corneal rim of the bed receiving the keratoplasty at the phacoemulsification incision level. We normally use two radial sutures (Figure 14-6) or one horizontal Nylon 10/0 suture, subsequently burying the knot.

Corneal Trephination

Before performing this operation, we fill the anterior chamber with acetylcholine to achieve a good miosis, facilitating centering of the trephination. Before starting the corneal trephination, we prepare the trephines and donor button, storing the latter in viscoelastic liquid on an ancillary table. Our technique is as follows: we always trephine the donor button on its endothelial face (we work with preserved corneal buttons) and similarly always do so with Hessburg-Barron trephines.

Suturing the Keratoplasty

The suturing of the graft is, together with the quality of the donor cornea, the main factor conditioning the final result of the operation. Correctly suturing the graft (see Figure 14-6) to the host will determine its proper healing and can have a decisive influence on an ideal, or at least acceptable, refractive result permitting visual rehabilitation of the eye.

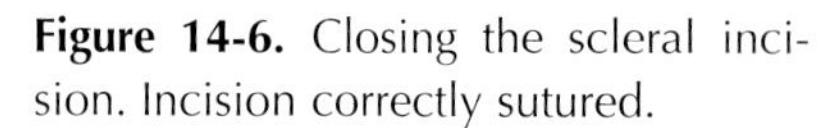

Figure 14-6. Closing the scleral incision. Incision correctly sutured.

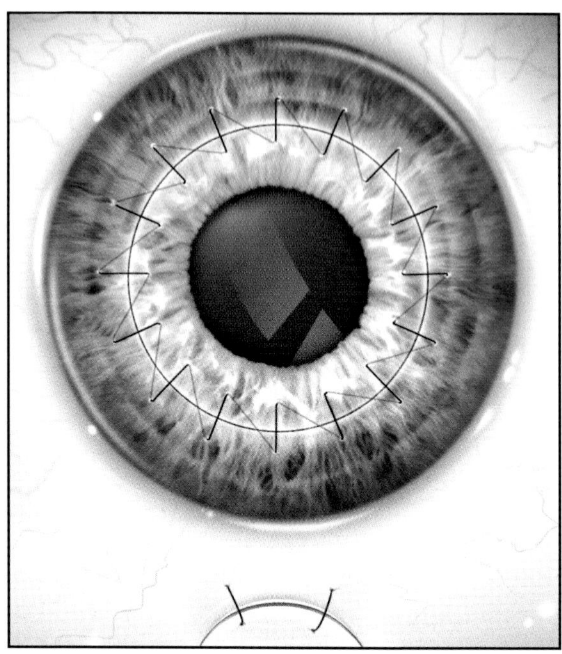

Phacoemulsification and Lamellar Techniques

The introduction in recent years of lamellar techniques means that we can use their surgical principles either to facilitate phacoemulsification and simultaneously perform a penetrating keratoplasty or to replace these with other lamellar keratoplasty techniques.

Complete Thickness Corneal Opacity

In this situation, if we wish to perform a phacoemulsification, we have to take recourse to complete trephination of the cornea, its substitution with a transitory keratoprosthesis (Figure 14-7), then perform phacoemulsification, and finally replace the transitory prosthesis with the donor cornea. Our choice of transitory prosthesis is Eckhardt, the diameter of which obliges us to perform trephinations of 7 mm.

Summary

Despite varying opinions, we believe that phacoemulsification as a cataract extraction technique within a triple procedure can offer certain advantages. In addition to the security offered by working in a closed system, in our experience it is obvious that extraction of the nucleus and of the cortex, despite poor corneal transparency, is much simpler than when working open-sky. The amount of time of ocular exposure without a corneal button is also shorter and complications of a capsular rupture or expulsive hemorrhage, if they occur, have less consequence.

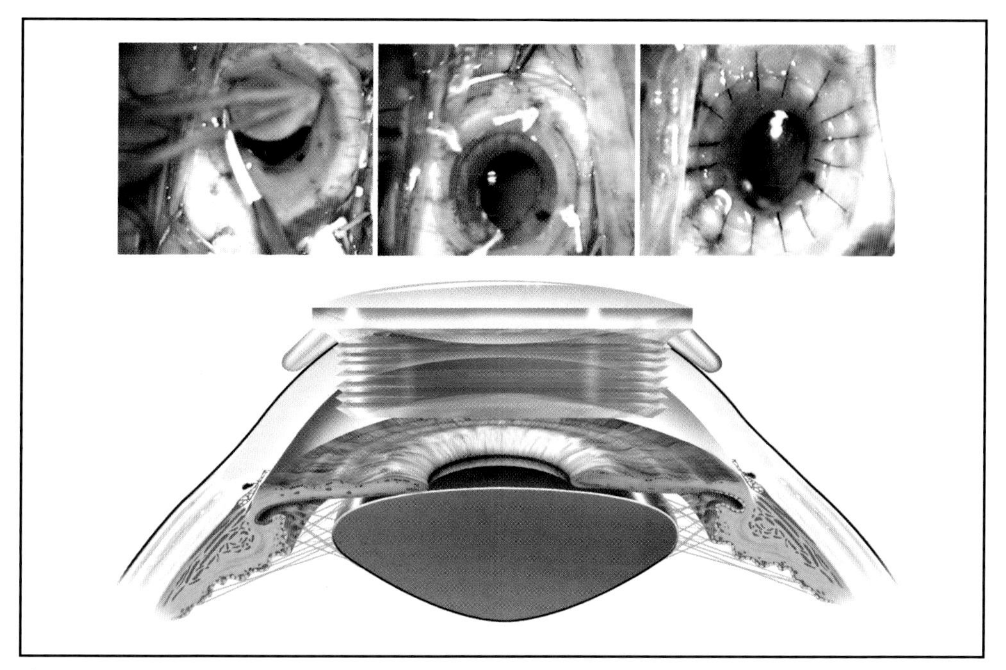

Figure 14-7. Keratoprosthesis and phacoemulsification.

Key Points

1. When considering a combined procedure (keratoplasty and cataract surgery) we have to evaluate not only the condition of the lens but also the state of the cornea and the degree of visual incapacity potentially justifying corneal and lens alteration.
2. The decision of whether to simply operate on the cataract or to perform a combined procedure (keratoplasty and cataract extraction) initially depends on two factors: the corneal stromal edema, and the central corneal pachymetry.
3. One of the greatest drawbacks of the combined procedure, an advantage therefore of the two-stage technique (keratoplasty followed by cataract surgery), is the difficulty of correctly calculating the power of the lens to be implanted during a triple procedure of cataract extraction, IOL implantation and keratoplasty.
4. The conventional combined procedure (cataract surgery and keratoplasty) consists of performing a corneal trephination, open-sky extracapsular lens extraction, IOL implantation, and suturing of the donor corneal button to the recipient bed.
5. With the spread of phacoemulsification as the generally preferred method for cataract extraction, another triple procedure has come to light: lens phacoemulsification, IOL implantation, and performing keratoplasty as if we were dealing with a phakic eye.

References

1. Malbran ES, Malbran E, Buonsanti J, Adrogué E. Closed-system phacoemulsification and posterior chamber implant combined with penetrating keratoplasty. *Ophth Surg.* 1993; 24:403–406.
2. Baca SL, Epstein RJ. Closed chamber capsulorhexis for cataract extraction combined with penetrating keratoplasty. *J Cataract Refract Surg.* 1998;24:581–584.
3. Caporossi A, Traversi C, Simi C, Tosi GM. Closed-system and open-sky capsulorhexis for combined cataract extraction and corneal transplantation. *J Cataract Refract Surg.* 2001;27:990–993.
4. Chu TG, Green RL. Suprachoroidal hemorrhage. *Surv Ophthalmol.* 1999;43:471–486.
5. Dogru M, Katakami C, Yamanaka A. Refractive changes after excimer laser phototherapeutic keratectomy. *J Cataract Refract Surg.* 2001;27:686–692.
6. Pérez-Santonja JJ, Galal A, Muñoz G. Queratectomía lamelar superficial. En: Villarrubia A, Mendicute J, Pérez-Santonja JJ, Jiménez I, Güell JL, eds. *Queratoplastia lamelar: técnicas quirúrgicas.* Madrid: Mac Line S.L.; 2005:36–43.
7. Muraine MC, Collet A, Brasseur G. Deep lamellar keratoplasty combined with cataract surgery. *Arch Ophthalmol.* 2002;120:812–815.
8. Alldredge CD, Alldredge OC Jr. Penetrating keratoplasty and cataract extraction. En: Krachmer JH, Mannis MJ, Holland EJ, eds. *Cornea.* 3 vols. St. Louis: Mosby, 1997;II:1593–1601.
9. Seitzman GD, Gottsch JD, Stark WJ. Cataract surgery in patients with Fuchs´s corneal dystrophy: expanding recomendations for cataract surgery without simultaneous keratoplasty. *Ophthalmology.* 2005;112:441–446.
10. Craig MT, Olson RJ, Mamalis N. Air bubble endothelial damage during phacoemulsification in human eye bank eyes: the protective effects of Healon and Viscoat. *J Cataract Refract Surg.* 1990; 16:597–602.
11. Koch DD, Liu JF, Glasser DB, Merin LM, Haft E. A comparison of corneal endothelial changes after use of Healon or Viscoat during phacoemulsification. *Am J Ophthalmol.* 1993;115:188–201.
12. Zacks CM, Abbott RL, Fine M. Long-term changes in corneal endothelium after keratoplasty. A follow-up study. *Cornea.* 1990;9:92–97.
13. Binder PS. Intraocular lens implantation after penetrating keratoplasty. *Refract Corneal Surg.* 1989;5:224–230.
14. Shimmura S, Ohashi Y, Shiroma H, Shimazaki J, Tsubota K. Corneal opacity and cataract: triple procedure versus secondary approach. *Cornea.* 2003;22:234–238.
15. Martin TP, Reed JW, Legault C, et al. Cataract formation and cataract extraction after penetrating keratoplasty. *Ophthalmology.* 1994;101:113–119.
16. Dangel ME, Kirkham SM, Phipps MJ. Posterior capsule opacification in extracapsular cataract extraction and the triple procedure: a comparative study. *Ophth Surg* 1994;25:82–87.
17. Bersudsky V, Rehany U, Rumelt S. Risk factors for failure of simultaneous penetrating keratoplasty and cataract extraction. *J Cataract Refract Surg.* 2004;30:1940–1947.
18. Geggel HS. Intraocular lens implantation after penetrating keratoplasty: improved unaided visual acuity, astigmatism, and safety in patients with combined corneal disease and cataract. *Ophthalmology.* 1990;97:1470–1477.
19. Aramberri J. Intraocular lens power calculation after corneal refractive surgery: double-K method. *J Cataract Refract Surg.* 2003;29:2063–2068.
20. Menapace R, Skorpik C, Grasl M. Modified triple procedure using a temporary keratoprothesis for closed system, small-incision cataract surgery. *J Cataract Refract Surg.* 1990;16:230–234.
21. Nardi M, Giudice V, Marabotti A, Alfieri E, Rizzo S. Temporary graft for closed-system cataract surgery during corneal triple procedures. *J Cataract Refract Surg.* 2001;27:1172–1175.
22. Mendicute J. Facoemulsificación y queratoplastia penetrante. En: Mendicute J, Cadarso L, Lorente R, Orbegozo J, Soler JR, eds. *Facoemulsificación.* Madrid: CF Comunicación; 1999: 325–338.

23. Bhartiya P, Sharma N, Ray M, Vajpayee RB. Trypan blue assisted phacoemulsification in corneal opacities. *Br J Ophthalmol.* 2002;86:857–859.
24. Malbrán ES. Facoemulsificación, lente intraocular y queratoplastia. *An Inst Barraquer.* 1996;25:599–604.
25. Lesiewska-Junk H, Kaluzny J, Malukiewicz-Wisniewska G. Long-term evaluation of endothelial cell loss after phacoemulsification. *Eur J Ophthalmol.* 2002;12:30–33.
26. Millá E, Vergés C, Ciprés MC. Corneal endothelium evaluation after phacoemulsification with continuous anterior chamber infusion. *Cornea.* 2005;24:278–282.
27. Melles GRJ, Eggink FAGJ, Lander F, et al. A surgical technique for posterior lamellar keratoplasty. *Cornea.* 1998;17:618–626.
28. Melles GRJ, Lander F, van Dooren BTH, Pels E, Beekhuis WH. Preliminary clinical results of posterior lamellar keratoplasty through a sclerocorneal pocket incision. *Ophthalmology.* 2000;107: 1850–1857.
29. Melles GRJ, Rietveld FJR, Beekhuis WH, Binder PS. A technique to visualize corneal incision and lamellar dissection depth during surgery. *Cornea.* 1999;18:80–86.
30. Mendicute J. Queratoplastia y ciru-gía de la catarata. En: Mendicute J, Aramberri J, Cadarso L, Ruiz M, eds. *Biometría, fórmulas y manejo de la sorpresa refractiva.* Madrid: Mac Line S.L.; 2000: 197–210.

Chapter 15

Phacoemulsification for Hyperopia and Nanophthalmos

Amar Agarwal, MS, FRCS, FRCOphth; R. Sujatha, DO, FERC

Introduction

Hyperopia is a form of refractive error in which parallel rays of light are brought to focus at some distance behind the sentient layer of the retina when the eye is at rest. The image formed is therefore made up of circles of diffusion of considerable size and consequently blurred.[1] The hyperopic eye is small, and the anterior chamber is shallow and predisposed to angle-closure glaucoma. Patients with hyperopia, depending on their age and magnitude of refractive error, are unable to see clearly both at distance and near. This problem worsens as they approach the presbyopic age. The increase in plus lenses leads to spherical aberrations.

Alternate Treatments

Various surgical procedures were developed over the years to correct hyperopia including keratophakia, hexagonal keratotomy, automated lamellar keratoplasty (ALK), thermal keratoplasty, photorefractive keratectomy (PRK), and laser in situ keratomileusis (LASIK).[2] Significant regression, poor predictability, and instability have been the problems of hyperopic refractive surgeries. Hexagonal keratotomy was fraught with poor wound healing, corneal edema, and irregular astigmatism.[3] Thermal keratoplasty causes regression to pretreatment steepness of the central cornea.[2,4] Fyodorov's radial thermokeratoplasty causes damage to corneal endothelium. Holmium:YAG laser thermokeratoplasty causes regression.[5,6] Lamellar procedures include keratophakia, cryolathe keratomileusis, epikeratophakia, ALK, and excimer laser PRK and LASIK.[2] Keratophakia caused induced keratometric astigmatism.[7] Epikeratophakia led to regression and problems with the cryolathe.[8,9] PRK for hyperopia used large optical zones with attendant adverse effects.[10] ALK has been found to be unpredictable and caused ectasia in a few cases. LASIK has been tried for hyperopia with better predictability, less regression, and less corneal haze than PRK. Posterior chamber phakic IOLs have been tried to treat hyperopia. The results support short-term safety, efficacy, and stability with surgical implantable contact lens.[11] Iris-claw lens has been used in phakic eyes, but observation with specular microscopy is mandatory.[12] Clear lens extraction with posterior chamber IOL implantation for hyperopia has been proposed as an alternative treatment.

Surgical Procedure

The eye is prepared for surgery with cyclopentolate hydrochloride 1% and phenylephrine 5% eye drops, 1 drop every 10 minutes 1 hour before surgery. Routine cleaning and draping of the eyes is done. The approach used is temporal clear corneal. If the axis is plus at 90 degrees then a superior incision is made. The anterior chamber is entered through the side port through clear cornea with a 26 G needle and viscoelastic Hydroxypropylmethyl cellulose 2% injected. A temporal clear corneal incision is made of 3.2 mm width with a sapphire knife. A continuous curvilinear capsulorrhexis is made with a bent 26 G needle mounted on a viscoelastic syringe. Hydrodissection is then done. Nucleus is emulsified and the remaining cortex aspirated. Peripheral iridectomy is done if the angles are found to be occludable. One 10–0 nylon suture can be used to close the tunnel if there is shallowing of the anterior chamber. This can be removed after a week.

Tips

1. It is essential to use the air pump (see Chapter 2) because gas-forced infusion helps deepen the anterior chamber. This will prevent endothelial damage.
2. It is better to do these complex cases under a peribulbar block, because once again the pressure might be high, and if operating under a block the vitreous pressure will not be that high.
3. Use a suture to close the wound if necessary.
4. Do an iridectomy by using a vitrectomy probe.
5. Be careful of biometry. Whatever the reading in a high hyperope, implant an IOL at least 2 diopters higher. If it reads okay postoperatively, fine, otherwise if it comes myopic then when you are doing the other eye adjust the IOL power accordingly to make the other eye emmetropic. This way patient will be able to read and see distance without glasses.

Lenses

Various lenses can be implanted in the eye. Alcon (Fort Worth, Texas) has their multifocal IOL, which is a single-piece acrylic lens under the name ReStor (Figure 15-1). Pharmacia/Pfizer (New York, NY) has also designed a diffractive multifocal IOL, the Ceeon 811E, that has been combined with the wavefront adjusted optics of the Technis Z9000 with the expectation of improved quality of vision in addition to multifocal optics (Figure 15-2). The two accommodative IOLs that have received the most investigation to date are the Model AT-45 CrystaLens (Figure 15-3) (Eyeonics, Aliso Viejo, California) and the 1 CU (Humanoptics, Mannheim, Germany).

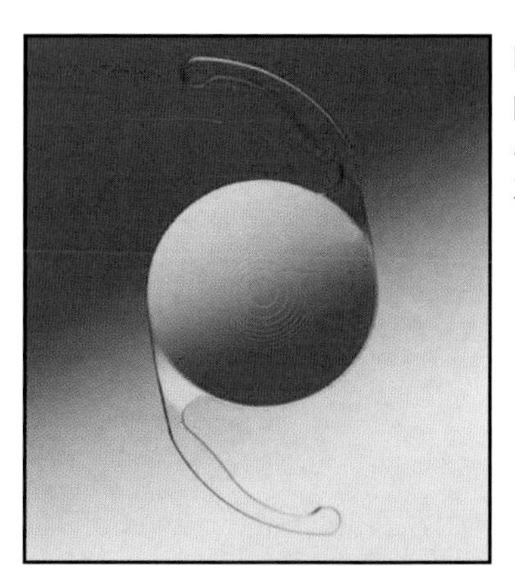

Figure 15-1. The Alcon ReStor multifocal IOL. (Reprinted with permission from Agarwal A. *Bimanual Phaco: Mastering the Phakonit/MICS Technique*. Thorofare, NJ: SLACK Incorporated; 2005.)

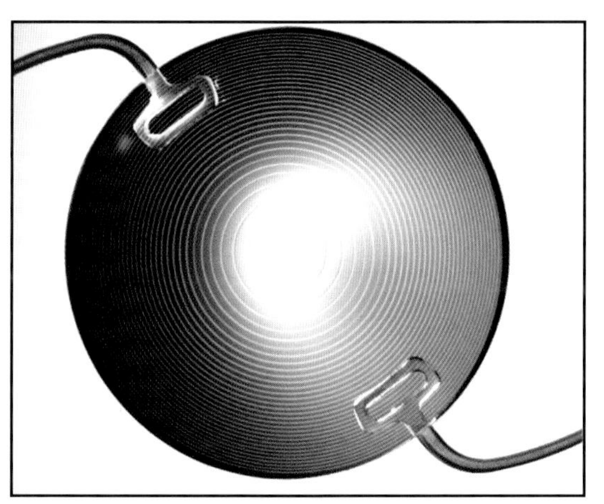

Figure 15-2. The Tecnis ZM001 multifocal IOL. (Reprinted with permission from Agarwal A. *Bimanual Phaco: Mastering the Phakonit/ MICS Technique*. Thorofare, NJ: SLACK Incorporated; 2005.)

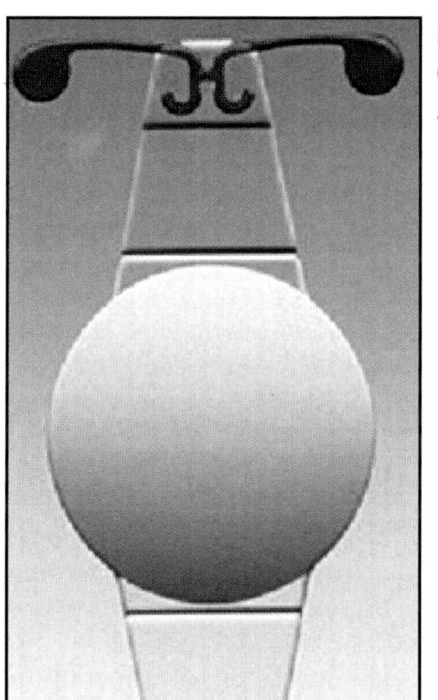

Figure 15-3. The Eyeonics CrystaLens accommodating IOL. (Reprinted with permission from Agarwal A. *Bimanual Phaco: Mastering the Phakonit/MICS Technique*. Thorofare, NJ: SLACK Incorporated; 2005.)

One of the most exciting technologies is the light adjustable lens (LAL) (Calhoun Vision, Pasadena, California). The LAL is designed to allow for postoperative refinements of lens power in situ. The current design of the LAL is a foldable three-piece IOL with a cross-linked silicone polymer matrix and a homogeneously embedded photosensitive macromer. The application of near-ultraviolet light to a portion of the lens optic results in polymerization of the photosensitive macromers and precise changes in lens power through a mechanism of macromer migration into polymerized regions and subsequent changes in lens thickness (Figure 15-4).

Results

A prospective study was conducted in our center in which 20 hyperopic eyes of 12 patients aged between 19 to 50 years were included. Clear lens extraction with posterior chamber IOL implantation was done. Five patients underwent peripheral iridectomy during clear lens extraction as the angles were found to be occludable. The mean hyperopic spherical equivalent refraction was + 6.66 ± 2.17 D (range + 4.75 to + 13.0 D). The IOL power was calculated using the Holladay 2 formula. The patients were followed up for an average of 16.96 months (range from 6 to 35 months).

Preoperative mean uncorrected visual acuity (UCVA) was 0.10 ± 0.09 (range from 0.03 to 0.25). Mean UCVA after surgery was 0.45 ± 0.25 (range from 0.1 to 1.0). The UCVA improved by an average of 3 lines after surgery. Mean BCVA was 0.63 ± 0.3 and improved by an average of 1 line after surgery. Three patients gained 2 lines of BCVA and two patients 1 line of BCVA. One patient lost 1 line of BCVA. Seventy percent of the patients achieved refraction within + 0.5 D of intended refraction.

Discussion

The refractive surgical correction of hyperopia has lagged far behind the advances that have occurred in the treatment of myopia and astigmatism. Clear lens extraction for the correction of high myopia is a concept known since at least 1800. After the invention of sterilization, clear lens extraction for myopia was done by Fukala and Vacher.[14]

The hyperopic eye with a smaller axial length, small anterior chamber, and small corneal diameter is more vulnerable to intraoperative and postoperative complications. However, clear lens extraction with IOL implantation for hyperopia is considered to have the same safety and efficacy as modern small incision cataract techniques, except in extremely hyperopic eyes like nanophthalmos. For presbyopic hyperopes, clear lens extraction with IOL implantation has a great appeal.[15]

There have been various studies of clear lens extraction for hyperopia in the last decade. In the study of Siganos et al, using the SRK II formula for IOL power calculation, 100% of the eyes were within ± 1.0 D of emmetropia.[16] It was found to be a safe, effective procedure for the treatment of hyperopia from + 6.75 D to + 13.75 D. The SRK II formula proved superior to the SRK-T formula for IOL power calculation.[16] In the study of Lyle et al, 89% of the patients achieved 20/40 or better UCVA, all eyes had 20/25 or better BCVA. IOL power was calculated using Holladay formula as it reduced the chance of postoperative residual hyperopia.[17] They found that this method was less accurate for hyperopia less than + 3.0 D.[17] Isfahani and colleagues reported the safety of clear lens extraction for the correction of hyperopia. They have reported a close association between achieved spherical equivalence and predicted spherical equivalence using the Holladay Consultant formula for IOL power calculation. They have suggested that clear lensectomy is superior for the correction of moderate to high hyperopia in patients aged 35 or older. They reported

A

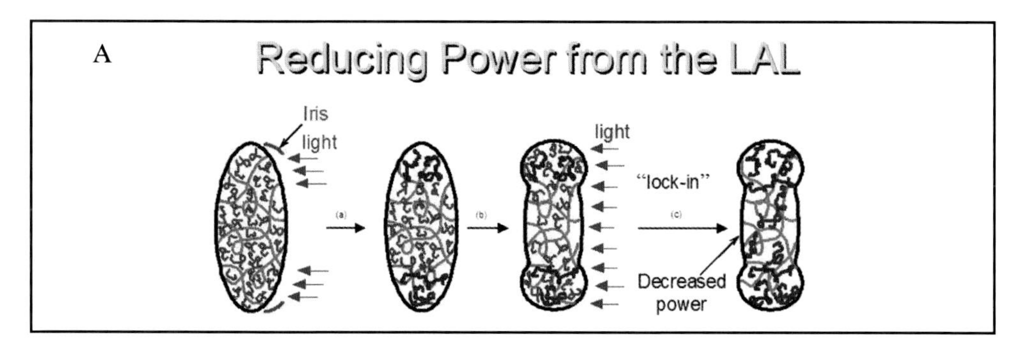

B

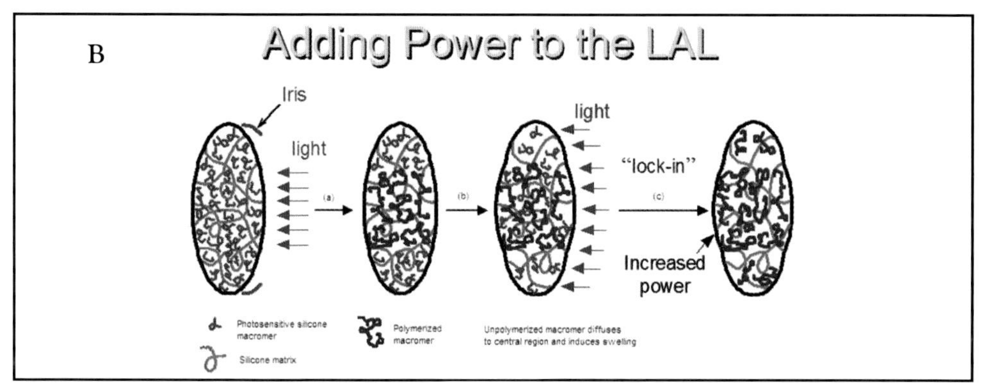

Figure 15-4. **A**. The Calhoun Vision Light Adjustable IOL (LAL)—Cross sectional schematic illustration of mechanism for treating myopic correction. a) Selective irradiation of peripheral portion of lens polymerizes macromer, creating a chemical gradient between irradiated and non-irradiated regions; b) macromer from the central zone diffuses peripherally leading to swelling of the peripheral lens; c) irradiation of the entire lens polymerizes the remaining macromer and "locks-in" the new lens shape with less power. (Photo courtesy of Calhoun Vision, Inc. Reprinted with permission from Agarwal A. *Bimanual Phaco: Mastering the Phakonit/MICS Technique*. Thorofare, NJ: SLACK Incorporated; 2005.) **B**. Cross sectional schematic illustration of mechanism for treating hyperopic correction. (a) Selective irradiation of central portion of lens polymerizes macromer, creating a chemical gradient between irradiated and non-irradiated regions; (b) in order to re-establish equilibrium, macromer from the peripheral lens diffuses into the central irradiated region leading to swelling of the central zone; (c) irradiation of the entire lens polymerizes the remaining macromer and "locks-in" the new lens shape. (Photo courtesy of Calhoun Vision. Reprinted with permission from Agarwal A. *Bimanual Phaco: Mastering the Phakonit/MICS Technique*. Thorofare, NJ: SLACK Incorporated; 2005.)

postoperative malignant glaucoma in one nanophthalmic eye and recommended peripheral surgical iridectomies in all eyes with axial length less than 20 mm.[18] In our study, 12 (60%) of the eyes achieved BCVA of more than 20/40. Clear lens extraction was done in amblyopic eyes also. Three patients achieved the intended refraction whereas 16 (80%) eyes were within + 1.0 D of the intended refraction. We use the Holladay 2 formula for the IOL power calculation. The Holladay, Hoffer Q, and SRK-T formulas are better than the older formulas for hyperopia (see Chapter 22). Hyperopic eyes with shallower anterior chambers are more prone to angle closure. All eyes in our series underwent gonioscopic evaluation preoperatively and surgical peripheral iridectomies were done in five eyes (25%) with occludable angles. We recommend preoperative gonioscopy in all patients who undergo clear lens extraction for hyperopia.

Nanophthalmos

Such eyes are more prone to intraoperative and postoperative complications such as uveal effusion, retinal detachment, intraocular hemorrhage, and malignant glaucoma. Foldable piggyback IOLs may be required in such nanophthalmic eyes (see Chapter 22). Piggyback IOLs in the bag have been associated with interlenticular pseudophakic opacification and a hyperopic shift.[19] Hence, one IOL must be placed in the bag and the other in the sulcus to avoid interlenticular pseudophakic opacification. In our study, the dioptric power of IOL ranged from + 27 to + 37 D. Eyes requiring more than + 30 D were implanted with PMMA IOLs. We did not implant piggyback IOLs in our series because higher power IOLs are now available. However, a PMMA IOL would require a larger incision, thereby negating the advantages of a watertight environment, which is particularly desirable in small eyes, especially nanophthalmic eyes.

Summary

LASIK has been suggested as an alternative modality for hyperopia correction. However, Ditzen and colleagues suggested preoperative corneal radius to be an important factor.[20] There was increased incidence of undercorrections and epithelial ingrowth with hyperopia (especially more than 6.0 D), due to problems with the suction ring and the microkeratome.[11] Regression and undercorrection have been reported as major concerns in LASIK for hyperopia. Goker and colleagues reported a regression and undercorrection of more than 2.00 D in 12.9% eyes that underwent LASIK for hyperopia.[21] Lack of a special nomogram to achieve results comparable to LASIK for myopia was pointed out in study by Tabbara and colleagues.[22] Postoperative glare is a common side effect.[23] Dry eye, particularly in females, was reported after LASIK for hyperopia, which was associated with refractive regression.[24] Thus, choice of LASIK for correction of hyperopia should be made with caution. Clear lens extraction with IOL implantation is a safe and effective procedure for the correction of hyperopia with minimal complications especially in patients in the presbyopic age group. However, care should be taken while doing surgery in nanophthalmic eyes. Further refinement is needed in the calculation of the IOL power in patients with hyperopia.

Key Points

1. The approach used is temporal clear corneal. If the axis is plus at 90°, a superior incision is made.
2. It is essential to use the air pump because gas-forced infusion helps deepen the anterior chamber. This will prevent endothelial damage.
3. Do an iridectomy by using a vitrectomy probe.
4. Hyperopic eyes with shallower anterior chambers are more prone to angle closure.
5. Nanophthalmic eyes are more prone to intraoperative and postoperative complications such as uveal effusion, retinal detachment, intraocular hemorrhage, and malignant glaucoma.

References

1. Abrams D. Hypermetropia. *Duke–Elder's Practice of Refraction*. 10th ed. London: Churchill Livingstone; 1997: 45.
2. Schallorn SC, Mcdonnell PJ. History and overview of refractive surgery. In: Krachmer JH, Mannis MJ, Holland EJ, eds. *Cornea*. St. Louis: CV Mosby; 1997.
3. Grandon SC, Sanders DR, Anello RD, Jacobs D, Biscaro M. Clinical evaluation of hexagonal keratotomy for treatment of primary hyperopia. *J Cataract Refract Surg* 1995;21(2):140–149.
4. Neumann AC, Sanders D, Raanan M, De Luca M. Hyperopic Thermokeratoplasty: clinical evaluation. *J Cataract Refract Surg*. 1991;17(6):830–838.
5. Thomson VM, Seiler T, Durrie DS, Cavanaugh TB. Holmium: YAG laser thermokeratoplasty for hyperopia and astigmatism: an overview. *Refract Corneal Surg*. 1993;9(3):236.
6. Nano HD, Muzzin S. Noncontact Holmium:YAG laser thermal keratoplasty for hyperopia. *J Cataract Refract Surg*. 1998;24(6):751–757.
7. Villasenor RA. Keratophakia Long term results. *Ophthalmology*. 1983;90(6):673–675.
8. Werblin TP, Blaydes JE. Epikeratophakia: existing limitations and future modifications. *Aust J Ophthalmol*. 1983;11(3):201–207.
9. Ehrlich MI, Nordan LT. Epikeratophakia for the treatment of hyperopia. *J Cataract Refract Surg*. 1989;15(6):661–666.
10. Dausch D, Smecka Z, Klein R, Schroder E, Kirchner S. Excimer laser photorefractive keratectomy for hyperopia. *J Catarac t Refract Surg*. 1997;23(2):169–176.
11. Sanders DR, Martin RG, Brown DC, Shepherd J, Deitz MR, De Luca M. Posterior chamber phakic intraocular lenses for hyperopia. *J Refract Surg*. 1999;15(3):309–315.
12. Fechner PU, Singh D, Wulff K. Iris-claw lens in phakic eyes to correct hyperopia: Preliminary study. *J Cataract Refract Surg*. 1998;24(1):48–56.
13. Boyd B. IOL power calculation in standard and complex cases—preparing for surgery. In: Boyd B, ed. *The Art and Science of Cataract Surgery*. Panama: Highlights of Ophthalmology: 47–48.
14. Seiler T. Clear lens extraction in the 19th century—an early demonstration of premature dissemination. *J Refract Surg*. 1999;15(1):70–73.
15. Kohnen T. Advances in the surgical correction of hyperopia. From the Editor. *J Cataract Refract Surg*. 1998;24(1):1.
16. Siganos DS, Pallikaris IG. Clear lensectomy and intraocular lens implantation for hyperopia from 17 to 114 diopters. *J Refract Surg*. 1998;14(2):105–113.
17. Lyle WA, Jin GJ. Clear lens extraction to correct hyperopia. *J Cataract Refracr Surg*. 1997;23(7): 1051–1056.

18. Isfahani AH, Rostamian K, Wallace D, Salz JJ. Clear lens extraction with intraocular lens implantation for hyperopia. *J Refract Surg*. 1999;15(5):316–323.
19. Shugar JK, Schwartz T. Interpsuedophakos Elschnig's pearls associated with late hyperopic shift: a complication of piggy-back posterior chamber intraocular lens implantation. *J Cataract and Refract Surg*. 1999;25:863–67.
20. Ditzen K, Huschka H, Pieger S. Laser in situ keratimileusis for hyperopia. *J Cataract Refract Surg*. 1998;24(1):42–47.
21. Goker, Hamdi ER, Cezmi Kahvecioglu. Laser in situ keratomiluesis to correct hyperopia from 14.25D to 18.00D. *J Refract Surg*. 1998;14(1).
22. Tabbara KF, El-Sheikh, Islam SM. Laser in situ keratomileusis for the correction of hyperopia from 10.50 to 111.50D with the Keracor 117C laser. *J Refract Surg*. 2001;17(2):123–8.
23. Prochazkova S, Kuchynka P, Novak P, Klecka D.Treatment of intermediate hypermetropia using laser in situ keratomilieusis—retrospective study (1995–1999). *Cesk Slov Oftalmol*. 2001;57(1):17–21.
24. Albeitz JM, Lenton LM, McLean SG. Effect of laser in situ keratomileusis for hyperopia on tear film and ocular surface. *J Refract Surg*. 2002;18(2):113–23.

Chapter 16

CATARACT SURGERY IN DRY EYE

Suresh K. Pandey, MD; Brighu Swamy, MBBS (Hons), M Med (Clin Epi);
Amar Agarwal, MS, FRCOphth, FRCS

INTRODUCTION

Patients with dry eyes who have cataract surgery are reported to have a relatively less favorable outcome (Figures 16-1 and 16-2). Patients with an age-related decrease in tear flow and deficient tear surfacing are also prone to complications. Complications such as superficial punctuate keratitis, recurrent filamentary keratitis, secondary infections including conjunctivitis and infectious keratitis, persistent or recurrent epithelial defects, stromal keratolysis, and corneal ulceration have been reported in patients after conventional extracapsular cataract extraction (ECCE). In conventional cataract surgery, a large incision is made at the limbus, denerving the superior half of the cornea. This leads to corneal desensitization with subsequent complications. Combined with the presence of sutures and prolonged use of topical steroids and antibiotics postoperatively, this often precipitates these complications, sometimes with a devastating outcome.[1]

ETIOLOGY AND PATHOGENESIS

There is a multifactorial etiology for the less favorable outcome post-cataract surgery in patients with dry eyes. It is reported that the loss of corneal sensitivity after cataract surgery often persists for more than 2 years and can be permanent. The sensory denervation interferes with the normal physiology of the corneal epithelium and decreases epithelial cell mitosis, delaying wound healing. The inability of the epithelium to reestablish the continuity of the corneal surface also triggers cell-biologic and biochemical mechanisms. The deficiency in the aqueous layer and an unstable tear film make the cornea susceptible to epithelial cell breakdown, leading to superficial punctuate keratopathy, erosions, or ulceration of the cornea.

There is an increased risk of infection in dry eyes, with *Staphylococcus* and *Streptococcus* the most common causes. Dry eyes have impaired ocular immunological defense mechanisms as a result of decreased quantities of various protective enzymes, lactoferrin, b-lysins, and immunoglobulins.

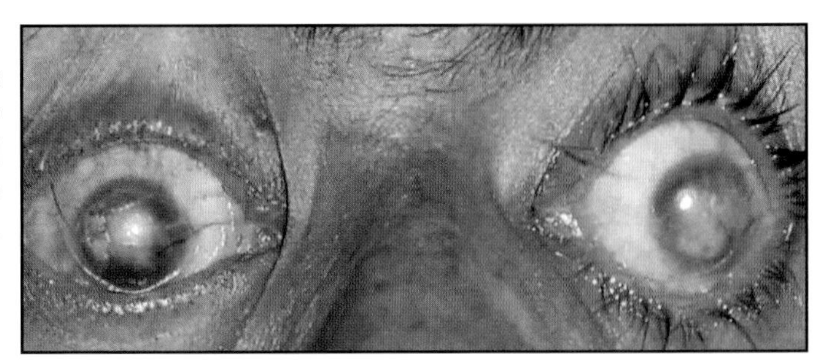

Figure 16-1. Patient with Stevens-Johnson syndrome presenting with severe dry eye, corneal opacity and age related cataract. (Photo courtesy of Abhay R. Vasavada, MD, FRCS, Ahmedabad, India.)

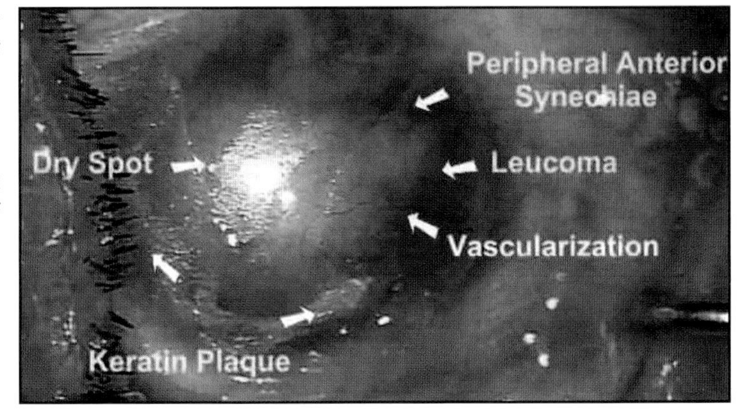

Figure 16-2. Ocular manifestations of Stevens-Johnson syndrome associated with total cataract in the only seeing right eye. (Photo courtesy of Abhay R. Vasavada, MD, FRCS, Ahmedabad, India.)

The use of topical steroids and poor compliance with dry-eye treatment have also been identified as risk factors for postoperative complications and a poor visual outcome.

Surgical Method of Choice in Patients With Dry Eyes

The tremendous advancement in cataract surgical techniques, implants, and other adjuncts (Table 16-1) during the past several years was helpful to enhance safety of cataract surgery in routine cases, and helpful to increase visual outcome in cataract associated with dry eye. Previously extracapsular extraction was the first choice for patients with cataracts and dry eye syndrome or other ocular comorbidities. However, with the currently preferred surgical technique, such as phacoemulsification and intraocular lens (IOL) implantation, and evolving techniques of ultra-small incision cataract surgery using phakonit and microphakonit, the situation has changed.[2,3] It is now believed that phacoemulsification and other techniques of microincision cataract surgery[4–25] may be associated with minimum complications in patients with dry eye. An air pump (gas-forced infusion) helps prevent shallowing of the anterior chamber. However, these patients must be counseled on the possible postoperative complications and the need to be compliant with their dry eye treatment to minimize such complications. Phacoemulsification and

Table 16-1.

Evolution of Techniques for Cataract Surgery

Technique	*Year*	*Author/Surgeon*
Couching	800 BC	Susutra
ECCE* (inferior incision)	1745	J. Daviel
ECCE (superior incision)	1860	von Graefe
ICCE** (tumbling)	1880	H. Smith
ECCE with PC-IOL***	1949	Sir H. Ridley
ECCE with AC-IOL****	1951	B. Strampelli
Phacoemulsification	1967	C.D. Kelman
Foldable IOLs	1984	T. Mazzocco
CCC	1988	H.V. Gimbel and T. Neuhann
Hydrodissection	1992	I.H. Fine
In-the-bag fixation	1992	D.J. Apple/E.I. Assia
Accommodating IOLs	1997	S. Cummings/Kamman
Phakonit (bimanual phaco)	1998	A. Agarwal
Air pump to prevent surge (gas-forced infusion)	1999	S. Agarwal
FAVIT technique	1999	A. Agarwal
MICS terminology	2000	J. Alio
Microphaco terminology and using a 0.8-mm phaco needle	2000	R. Olson
Dye enhanced cataract surgery	2000	S.K. Pandey/L. Werner/ D.J. Apple
Sealed Capsule Irrigation	2001	A.J. Maloof
Factors for PCO Prevention	2002 to 2004	D.J. Apple/L. Werner/ S.K. Pandey
Microincisional coaxial phaco 2.2 mm	2004/2005	T. Akahoshi
Microphakonit cataract surgery with a 0.7-mm tip	2005	A. Agarwal

*ECCE: extracapsular cataract extraction.
**ICCE: intracapsular cataract extraction.
***PC-IOL: posterior chamber intraocular lens.
****AC-IOL: anterior chamber intraocular lens.

other techniques of microincision cataract surgery offer advantages over conventional extracapsular cataract extraction (ECCE) in patients with dry eye. These include:

- A much smaller incision which causes less corneal desensitization.
- Minimal tear-film surfacing problems.
- Smaller risk of infection because there are no sutures.
- Faster visual rehabilitation of patients permit rapid tapering of topical drops.

Cataract surgery can worsen preexisting dry eye symptoms or surgically induce dry eyes. The management of cataract surgery in dry eyes involves preoperative, surgical, and postoperative methods.[2]

Preoperative Management

Diagnosis of dry eye syndrome is essential. If dry eyes are suspected, a series of investigations including tear-film breakup time (BUT) and fluorescein staining of the corneal epithelium should be done prior to surgery. If superficial punctuate keratitis exists, artificial drops or eye drops containing hyaluronic acid should be prescribed. Preservative containing eye drops should be avoided.

Surgical Procedure

Topical anesthetic application to the cornea should be minimized in patients with dry eyes. Anesthetic techniques for cataract surgery have advanced significantly. Table 16-2 presents the evolution of anesthetic techniques for cataract surgery. Currently, topical anesthesia is preferred in phacoemulsification using eye drops application, sponge anesthesia, eye drops plus intracameral injection, and most recently a combination of viscoelastic and anesthetic agent termed "viscoanesthesia". Recent reports indicate that phacoemulsification can be performed by a highly experienced, skilled surgeon without causing an unacceptable level of pain using no-anesthesia cataract surgery, as first shown by Dr. Amar Agarwal.

The exposure to the light source of the operating microscope should be kept to a minimum as well. Tear-film BUT can be increased for up to 1 month postsurgery. The nature of the surgical incision does not seem to be an important factor for phacoemulsification. Cataract surgery in patients with dry eye can be challenging, necessitating several tools and techniques. Most surgeons are familiar with conventional cataract surgical procedure using small incision cataract surgery. We believe it will be pertinent to provide brief details of ultra-small incision cataract surgery. Ultra-small incision cataract surgery techniques are currently evolving, and experience in cataract surgery in dry eye cases is limited at present. Nevertheless, as we gain more experience, it is clear that these minimally invasive surgical methods will be helpful to enhance visual outcome following cataract surgery in dry eye cases.

Ultra-small incision cataract surgery, also called phakonit, bimanual microphacoemulsification, or microincision cataract surgery (MICS), allows removal of cataract using sub 1.4 mm incision. The term "phakonit" represents bimanual phacoemulsification (**phako**) being done with a needle (**n**) opening via an incision (**i**) and with the phaco tip (**t**). In phakonit, the phaco needle is used without a sleeve and an irrigating chopper is used in the other hand. Once the nucleus is removed, bimanual cortical aspiration is done. The only limitation to realizing the goal of astigmatism neutral cataract surgery was the size of the foldable IOL, because the wound had to be extended for implantation of the currently available foldable IOLs. With the advent of the foldable IOLs, the advantage of the phakonit

Table 16-2.

Evolution of Anesthetic Techniques for Cataract Surgery

Technique	Year	Author
General anesthesia	1846	—
Topical cocaine	1881	Koller
Injectable cocaine	1884	Knapp
Orbicularis akinesia	1914	Van Lint, O'Briens, & Atkinson
Hyaluridinase	1948	Atkinson
Retrobulbar (4% cocaine)	1884	Knapp
Posterior peribulbar	1985	Davis & Mandel
Limbal	1990	Furata et al.
Anterior peribulbar	1991	Bloomberg
Pinpoint anesthesia	1992	Fukasawa
Topical	1992	Fichman
Topical plus intracameral	1995	Gills
No anesthesia	1998	Agarwal
Cryoanalgesia	1999	Gutierrez-Carmona
Xylocaine jelly	1999	Koch & Assia
Hypothesis, no anesthesia	2001	Pandey & Agarwal
Viscoanesthesia	2001	Werner, Pandey, Apple, et al.

incision could be realized because the ultra-small incision lenses could pass through a 1.5-mm incision.

On May 21, 2005, for the first time a 0.7-mm phaco needle tip with a 0.7-mm irrigating chopper was used by Dr. Agarwal to remove cataracts through the smallest incision presently possible. This is called "microphakonit". The instruments are made by Larry Laks from MicroSurgical Technology (Redmond, Washington). At the time of this writing, this is the smallest one that can be used for cataract surgery. With time, we will be able to go smaller with better instruments and devices. The problem at present is the IOL. We have to get good quality IOLs going through sub 1-mm cataract surgical incisions so that the real benefit of microphakonit can be given to the patient.

It is important to remember that cataract surgery in dry eye cases may be associated with suboptimal visibility intraoperatively, and therefore the surgeon should use the familiar surgical technique to help overcome intraoperative difficulties and to minimize complications. Trypan blue is an indispensable tool to enhance vision when white cataract is combined with corneal opacity. The staining combined with frequent regrasping allowed capsulorrhexis to be successfully performed. Work on dye-enhanced cataract surgery was done extensively by Suresh Pandey.[26] The blue-stained rim aided in confining phacoemulsification maneuvers to the posterior plane. Implementing the soft-shell technique partitioned the anterior chamber into a viscoelastic occupied space and a surgical zone protecting the delicate endothelial cells from fluid turbulence.

Key Points

1. Patients with dry eyes who have cataract surgery are reported to have a relatively less favorable outcome. Patients with an age-related decrease in tear flow and deficient tear surfacing are also prone to complications.
2. It is reported that the loss of corneal sensitivity after cataract surgery often persists for more than 2 years and can be permanent. The sensory denervation interferes with the normal physiology of the corneal epithelium and decreases epithelial cell mitosis, delaying wound healing.
3. If dry eyes are suspected, a series of investigations including tear-film breakup time (BUT) and fluorescein staining of the corneal epithelium should be done prior to surgery. If superficial punctuate keratitis exists, artificial drops or eye drops containing hyaluronic acid should be prescribed. Preservative-containing eye drops should be avoided.
4. Topic anesthetic application to the cornea should be minimized in patients with dry eyes.
5. Previously, ECCE was the first choice for patients with cataracts and dry eye syndrome or other ocular comorbidities. However, with the development of modern techniques, such as phacoemulsification, phakonit, and microphakonit, the situation has changed.

Postoperative Management

Eye drops containing preservatives tend to cause epithelial disturbances. Nonsteroidal anti-inflammatory drugs such as diclofenac sodium can cause corneal epithelial breaches. For patients already diagnosed with dry eyes only an antibiotic and steroid regimen are used. Additional use of artificial eye drops will increase the stability of the tear film. If SPK is severe, stopping all eye drops except the artificial eye drops will need to be considered. In treatment-resistant cases, serum eye drops may be prescribed. Finally, intracanalicular plugs can be used to prevent drainage of tears and provide a stable and moist corneal surface postoperatively. Rarely, severe cases of dry eye (associated with autoimmune disorders, eg, Stevens-Johnson syndrome) may require additional procedures such as amniotic membrane transplantation, stem cell transplantation, or penetrating keratoplasty.

References

1. Ram J, Gupta A, Brar G, Kaushik S. Outcomes of phacoemulsification in patients with dry eye. *J Cataract Refract Surg*. 2002;28:1386.
2. Bissen-Miyajima H. Cataract surgery in the presence of other ocular co-morbidities. In: Steinert R, ed. *Cataract Surgery: Technique, Complications, and Management.* Philadelphia: WB Saunders; 2004: 369–373.
3. Agarwal A, Agarwal S, Agarwal At. No anesthesia cataract surgery. In: Agarwal A, Agarwal A, Sachdev MS, Mehta KR, Fine IH, Agarwal A, eds. *Phacoemulsification, Laser Cataract Surgery, and Foldable IOLs*. 1st ed. Delhi, India: Jaypee Brothers; 1998: 144–154.
4. Pandey SK, Werner L, Agarwal A, Agarwal S, Agarwal At, Apple DJ. No anesthesia cataract surgery. *J Cataract Refract Surg*. 2001;28:1710.

5. Agarwal A, Agarwal S, Agarwal At. Phakonit: A new technique of removing cataracts through a 0.9 mm incision. In: Agarwal A, Agarwal A, Sachdev MS, Mehta KR, Fine IH, Agarwal A, eds. *Phacoemulsification, Laser Cataract Surgery, and Foldable IOLs*. 1st ed. Delhi, India: Jaypee Brothers; 1998:139–143.
6. Agarwal A, Agarwal S, Agarwal At. Phakonit and laser phakonit: lens surgery through a 0.9 mm incision. In: Agarwal A, Agarwal A, Sachdev MS, Mehta KR, Fine IH, Agarwal A, eds. *Phacoemulsification, Laser Cataract Surgery, and Foldable IOLs*. 2nd ed. Delhi, India: Jaypee Brothers; 2000:204–216.
7. Agarwal A, Agarwal S, Agarwal At. Phakonit. In: Agarwal A, Agarwal A, Sachdev MS, Mehta KR, Fine IH, Agarwal A, eds. *Phacoemulsification, Laser Cataract Surgery, and Foldable IOLs*. 3rd ed. Delhi, India: Jaypee Brothers; 2003: 317–329.
8. Agarwal A, Agarwal S, Agarwal At. Phakonit and laser phakonit. In: Boyd B, Agarwal A, eds. *LASIK and Beyond LASIK*. Panama: Highlights of Ophthalmology; 2000: 463-468.
9. Agarwal A, Agarwal S, Agarwal At. Phakonit and laser phakonit—cataract surgery through a 0.9 mm incision. In Boyd, Agarwal, eds. *Phako, Phakonit and Laser Phako*. Panama: Highlights of Ophthalmology; 2000: 327-334.
10. Agarwal A, Agarwal S, Agarwal At. The Phakonit Thinoptx IOL. In: Agarwal A, ed. *Presbyopia*. Thorofare, NJ: SLACK Incorporated; 2002: 187–194.
11. Agarwal A, Agarwal S, Agarwal At. Antichamber collapser. *J Cataract Refract Surg*. 2002;28:1085.
12. Pandey SK; Wener L, Agarwal A, Agarwal S, Agarwal At, Hoyos J. Phakonit: cataract removal through a sub 1.0 mm incision with implantation of the Thinoptx rollable IOL. *J Cataract Refract Surg*. 2002;28:1710.
13. Agarwal A, Agarwal S, Agarwal At. Phakonit: phacoemulsification through a 0.9 mm incision. *J Cataract Refract Surg*. 2001;27:1548–1552.
14. Agarwal A, Agarwal S, Agarwal At. Phakonit with an acritec IOL. *J Cataract Refract Surg*. 2003;29:854–855.
15. Agarwal S, Agarwal A, Agarwal At. *Phakonit with Acritec IOL*. Panama: Highlights of Ophthalmology; 2000.
16. Shearing S, Relyea R, Loaiza A, Shearing R. Routine phacoemulsification through a 1.0 mm non-sutured incision. *Cataract*. 1985;Jan; 6–8.
17. Hara T, Hara T. Clinical results of phacoemulsification and complete in the bag fixation. *J Cataract Refract Surg*. 1987;13;279–86.
18. Tseunoka H, Shiba T, Takahashi Y. Feasibility of ultrasound cataract surgery with a 1.4 mm incision. *J Cataract Refract Surg*. 2001;27;934–940.
19. Tseunoka H, Shiba T, Takahashi Y. Feasibility of ultrasound cataract surgery with a 1.4 mm incision- Clinical results. *J Cataract Refract Surg*. 2002;28;81–86.
20. Alio J. What does MICS require. In: Alios J, ed. *MICS*. Panama: Highlights of Ophthalmology; 2004: 1–4.
21. Soscia W, Howard JG, Olson RJ. Microphacoemulsification with Whitestar. A wound-temperature study. *J Cataract Refract Surg*. 2002;28;1044–1046.
22. Soscia W, Howard JG, Olson RJ. Bimanual phacoemulsification through two stab incisions. A wound-temperature study. *J Cataract Refract Surg*. 2002;28;1039–1043.
23. Olson R. Microphaco chop. In: Chang D, ed. *Phaco Chop: Mastering Techniques, Optimizing Technology, and Avoiding Complications*. Thorofare, NJ: SLACK Incorporated; 2004: 227–237.
24. Chang D. Bimanual phaco chop. In: Chang D, ed. *Phaco Chop: Mastering Techniques, Optimizing Technology, and Avoiding Complications*. Thorofare, NJ: SLACK Incorporated; 2004: 239–250.

25. Kanellopoulos AJ. New laser system points way to ultrasmall incision cataract surgery. *Eurotimes*. 5/2000.
26. Pandey SK, Werner L, Escobar-Gomez M, et al. Dye-enhanced cataract surgery. Part I. Anterior capsule staining for capsulorhexis in advanced/white cataracts. *J Cataract Refract Surg*. 2000;26:1052.

Supported in part by an unrestricted grant from Research to Prevent Blindness, Inc., New York, NY.

The authors have no financial or proprietary interest in any product mentioned in this chapter.

Chapter 17

Phacoemulsification in Patients With Uveitis

Jorge L. Alio, MD, PhD; Herminio Negri, MD

Introduction

Cataract formation is a common complication of chronic or recurrent uveitis and appears at an early age in the general population. In many forms of uveitis, the incidence of cataract occurs in up to 50%.[1] Intraocular inflammatory phenomena, as well as the drugs used to control them, are considered the main etiological agents. The most common type of cataract in uveitis patients is nuclear (66.1%).[2] Cataract surgery in uveitic eyes remains a challenge to ophthalmologists. The uncertainty of the postoperative process, the existence of an underlying systemic pathology, the poor tolerance of intraocular lenses (IOLs) observed in some cases, and the many technical difficulties make the handling of these patients very difficult before, during, and after the cataract operation. Establishing the diagnosis, thorough eye examination, careful patient selection, and meticulous control of perioperative inflammation are key elements to a successful visual outcome.

Specific Considerations Related to the Patient With Uveitis

The ophthalmologist should remember the following considerations when dealing with uveitic patients:

1. There are four indications for cataract surgery in patients with uveitis:
    a) Phacoantigenic uveitis (active inflammation as a result of leakage of lens proteins); this situation must be resolved immediately.
    b) Visually significant cataract if inflammation has been controlled.
    c) Cataract that impairs the evaluation of the fundus in a patient with suspected fundus pathology.
    d) Cataract that does not provided adequate visualization of the posterior segment in a patient undergoing posterior segment surgical procedure.
2. A systematic approach to establishing the diagnosis begins with a comprehensive ocular and systemic history, and an extensive review of medical systems that gives the possibility to create a differential diagnosis.

3. Good control of the underlying systemic disorder is required. In many cases, the presence of the base inflammatory pathology with long-standing and unpredictable evolution will condition the existence of recurrent inflammation. Its medical control may even require a multidisciplinary approach for this purpose.
4. Control of the ocular inflammation is needed prior to the surgical procedure. This preoperative control may require the use of topical and systemic steroids or immunosuppressive drugs. The treatment should be aimed at achieving a reduction in cellularity in the anterior chamber, as well as little or no vitreous activity. The inflammatory activity should be assessed only by the presence of cells and not by the amount of flare present. The definition of "controlled" inflammation is a patient with no cells and up to one (+) of flare in the anterior chamber; and cell (+), no active retinal inflammation, no macular edema. *It is very important that the surgery is performed in an "undisturbed" eye with an inflammatory reaction that has been controlled for at least 3 months prior to surgery.*
5. Cataract surgery is sometimes complicated by the presence of iris atrophy, sclerosis of the pupillary sphincter, cyclitic membranes, posterior synechiae, anterior capsular sclerosis, and poor visualization because of absence of red reflex or corneal PK and possible hemorrhage from the iris and angle neovascularization. The surgery is certainly more difficult because of the frequent presence of miosis refractory to pharmacological dilatation, anterior and posterior synechiae (festooned pupil) (Figure 17-1), harder white cataract, and glaucoma. A precise and delicate surgery is mandatory. Keep in mind that surgery can exacerbate the underlying inflammatory process by the release of lens material and by the surgical trauma itself. *The best anti-inflammatory is a good, atraumatic surgery.*
6. The IOL selection is another challenge. This is possibly the most controversial topic. IOL implantations trigger a number of reactions, including foreign body and inflammatory responses, complement and coagulation cascades. This leads to cellular adhesion to the anterior surface of the implant and the proliferation of lens epithelial cells (LEC), resulting in posterior capsular opacification and anterior capsular phimosis. In the last few years, many studies have focused on the biocompatibility of lenses and their interaction with uveitis patients,[2-5] reaching encouraging results and opening new perspectives.
7. The strict control of the postoperative inflammation is imperative. The necessary use of topical, and in most cases, periocular and systemic steroids can give rise to problems such as steroid-dependent ocular hypertension and even problems related to their progressive and full withdrawal. The postsurgical inflammatory reaction can produce a series of complications such as high intraocular pressure (IOP), corneal edema, endothelial damage, and cystoid macular edema, among others.
8. The mechanical stimulation of the iris has been known to induce the release of prostaglandins. Prostaglandins have been proven to play a role in ocular inflammatory reactions, particularly in those in which mechanical iris scraping was performed. Another factor that has been linked to postoperative destruction is the activation of complement by the classic or alternative route. The activation of the alternative course has been known to start by the presence of IOLs in contact with metabolically active tissues. Some polymers, especially prolene, cause activation of complement although some studies did not show a significant difference on activation of complement comparing prolene with polymethylmethacrylate (PMMA).[6] There are materials such as hydrogel that did not cause any significant activation of this factor. The introduction of phacoemulsification, viscoelastic materials, highly sophisticated instruments, new anti-inflammatory drugs, and new IOL materials has reduced the number of complications in these patients.

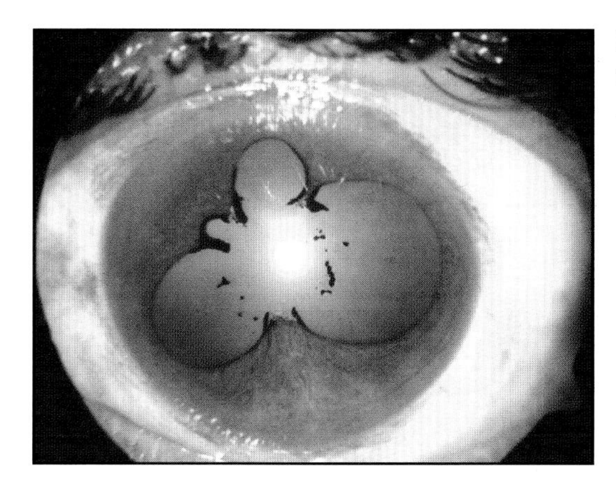

Figure 17-1. Festooned pupil. Note the posterior synechiae. (Photo courtesy of Dr. Agarwal's Eye Hospital.)

PATIENT PREPARATION

The goal of most cataract surgeries is successful visual rehabilitation. In uveitic cataract, this is more difficult than in ordinary age-related cataract, because successful visual outcome depends not only on the results of the surgery, but also on the degree of prior permanent structural damage that uveitis may have caused. After the decision to perform surgery, all patients have to be free of intraocular inflammations for a minimum period of 3 months. Good pupillary dilation must be achieved when possible to avoid manipulation of the iris during surgery. However, surgical dilation may be required. (Angle neovascularization may be treated by argon laser focal photocoagulation at the area of the surgical incision. It is performed by using a 100 micron spot size, 0.2 sec of exposure, and enough energy to blanch the vessels in three different places along its course.) Proper control of the IOP is recommended 2 to 3 weeks prior to surgery. The use of cholinergic drugs should be avoided in these patients because they alter the hematoaqueous barrier and tend to increase synechiae formation. Control is generally obtained by using beta-blockers and topical or occasionally systemic carbonic anhydrase inhibitors. Preoperative hypotony in patients with uveitis can also be found and is frequently due to the formation of cyclitic membrane, ciliary body dialysis, and severe inflammation causing severe decrease in aqueous production.

PREOPERATIVE CONTROL OF INFLAMMATION

The use of topical and/or periocular steroids can be sufficient for handling both pre- and postoperative inflammation in a large number of patients. Although administration of systemic steroids is controversial, it is mandatory to recommend it to patients who have required systemic or periocular administration of steroids in a previous inflammatory stage. The administration of 60 to 80 mg/day of prednisolone must be considered starting 2 weeks prior to the scheduled surgery. In general, the use of corticosteroids in children should not go beyond 3 months due to their possible side effects on growth. If steroids alone are insufficient, immunosuppressive agents should be added.[7] These drugs must be administered for at least 2 weeks prior to the surgery because of their latency period. Among these drugs, Methotrexate, Azathioprin, and Cyclosporin A are available.[8]

The following schedule is recommended:

1. Preparation should include full control of the underlying inflammatory process for at least 3 months prior to the surgery.
2. Prednisolone 1% should be added eight times a day starting 1 week before surgery.
3. One mg/kg/day of oral prednisone should be administered starting 1 week prior to the surgery, depending on the amount of inflammation.
4. Periocular steroid injection of Triamcinolone can help in handling severe inflammatory complications not controlled by topical or systemic medications.
5. Topical (Diclofenac 0.1%, flubiprofen 0.03%, Surprofen 1%) four times daily and systemic use of nonsteroidal anti-inflammatory drugs (NSAIDS), such as celecoxib 100 mg orally twice a day, is considered in cases of cystoid macular edema.[9]

In a recently published study, we demonstrated that a simplified criteria for patient preparation and follow up, independent from uveitis etiology and type of inflammation, is effective. Alio et al[2] classified uveitis into complicated and uncomplicated cases. Uncomplicated cases included patients whose ocular inflammation was controlled with topical treatment only within the past year. Complicated cases were patients who required systemic/periocular steroids within the year before surgery to control inflammation or those in whom the surgery was judged to be difficult by the surgeon based on a subjective impression of the eye. Uncomplicated cases received topical dexamethasone 0.1% four times daily 1 week before surgery. In complicated cases, 1 mg/kg/day of oral prednisolone was added to the usual prescription 1 week before surgery. With this new protocol, it is possible to obtain a standard preoperative medical preparation methodology with good results.

Surgical Technique

Good surgery is the most important "anti-inflammatory" element for the postoperative patient. If the uveitis has remained inactive, an anterior approach is undertaken, which is performed in the majority of cases. We prefer phacoemulsification for cataract removal in these patients. We think that microincision cataract surgery (MICS) is a promising technique to approach these difficult cases. Intracapsular surgery is reserved for the situation in which an important lens-induced component was present in prior contralateral surgery. If the inflammatory reaction persists or a chronic macular edema is present, a combined procedure should be performed (phacoemulsification and vitrectomy). Some authors have proposed performing this combined procedure through an anterior approach because of the frequent presence of total vitreous detachment in these patients.[10] Most surgeons opt for conventional pars plana vitrectomy techniques.[11-12]

Phacoemulsification

Phacoemulsification is our procedure of choice. It requires a small (corneal) incision, causes minimal trauma, and minimizes postoperative inflammation. Young patients and patients on high doses of steroids benefit from this technique. General anesthesia is not necessary, but is frequently requested by young patients. Local anesthesia by retrobulbar or peribulbar block is preferred. Topical anesthesia is not contraindicated, but we prefer not to use it in these cases. Clear corneal incision is our preferred approach (Figure 17-2) if no lens or a foldable lens is implanted, and if the implantation of a rigid PMMA lens is planned, a limbal approach with a short scleral tunnel is performed.

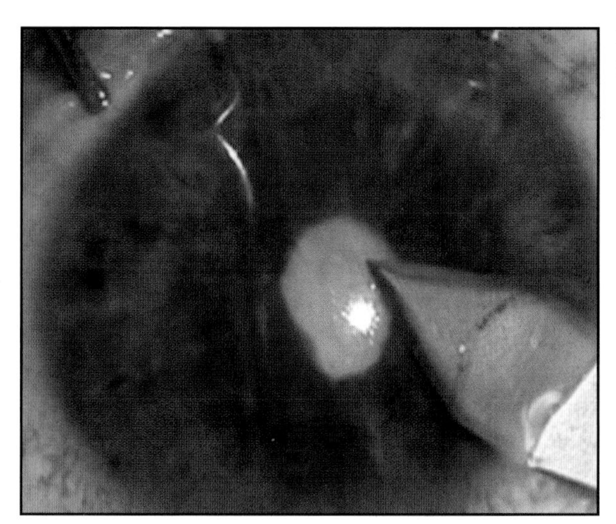

Figure 17-2. Clear corneal incision in a uveitic patient with cataract.

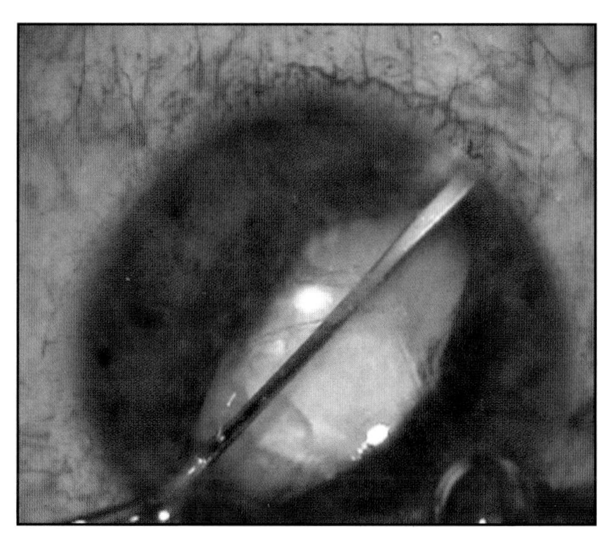

Figure 17-3. Distending and stretching the pupil.

Viscoelastic materials are routinely used to release adhesions. The combination of hyaluronic acid and chondritin sulphate (Viscoat) is preferred, but high viscosity materials (Healon GV Amvisc plus) can be used as well. Many patients with uveitis have sclerosis of the dilator muscle or severe posterior synechiae, and in these cases synechiolysis is performed with an iris spatula. If further mydriasis is desired, stretching technique is performed (Figure 17-3) and/or flexible iris retractors are used. Continuous curvilinear capsulotomy (CCC) is always attempted. Sometimes it is necessary to use capsular stain to visualize the anterior capsule. We use trypan blue and we generally use air to perform this maneuver. It is not unusual to find fibrotic anterior capsule and it may be necessary to use scissors or a sharper instrument to tear the capsule (Figures 17-4 and 17-5). If unsuccessful, a can-opener capsulotomy is done, but phacoemulsification is performed with caution.

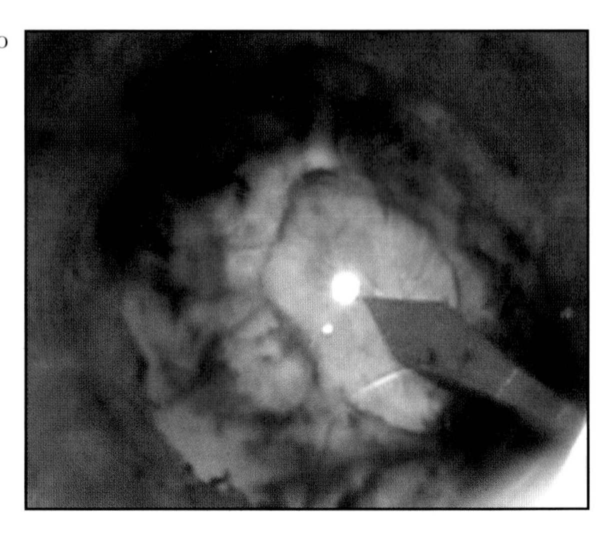

Figure 17-4. Sharp instrument used to enter the fibrotic capsule.

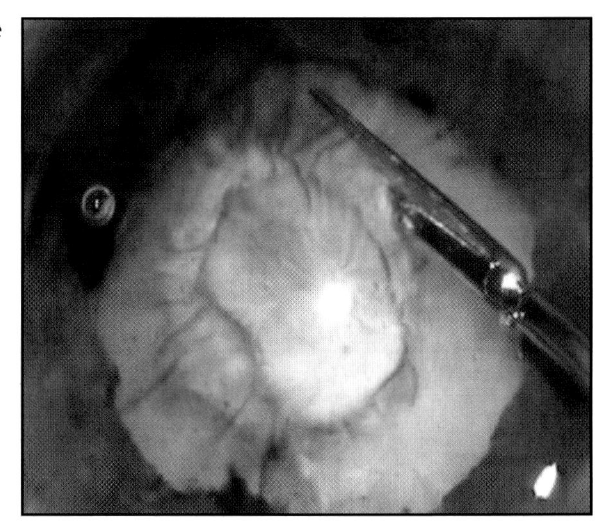

Figure 17-5. Scissor used to cut the anterior capsule.

Phaco chop techniques are used for removing a hard nucleus (Figure 17-6). In young patients with a soft nucleus, phacoaspiration may be all that is needed. Intensive cortical clean up is mandatory to eliminate one of the sources of postoperative inflammation reaction and the posterior surface of the anterior capsule must be vacuumed. Implantation of a foldable, three-piece hydrophobic acrylic lens into the capsular bag is our preferred procedure (Figure 17-7).

There are some situations in which a prophylactic peripheral iridectomy may be recommended, as in cases of uveitis with high tendency for synechia formation. Patients in whom a vitrectomy has been performed with removal of the posterior capsule do not require an iridectomy. In cases where there is an extensive membrane formation in the anterior vitreous, vitrectomy after posterior central capsulorrhexis must be considered. If the vitreous cavity shows extensive fibrosis and exudates formation, transcleral pars plana vitrectomy may be indicated.

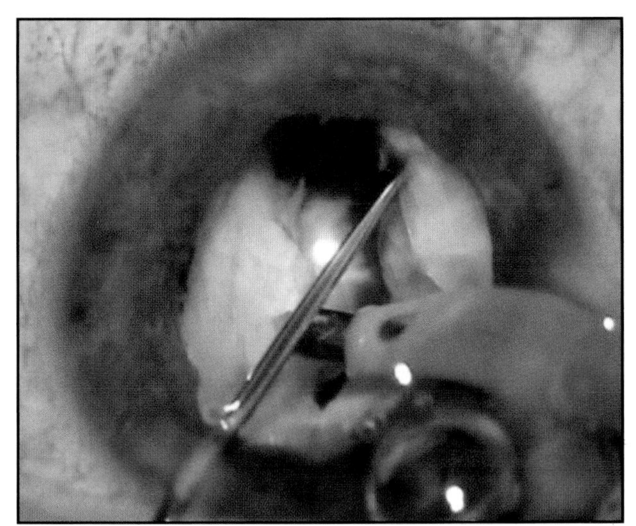

Figure 17-6. Phacoemulsification being performed.

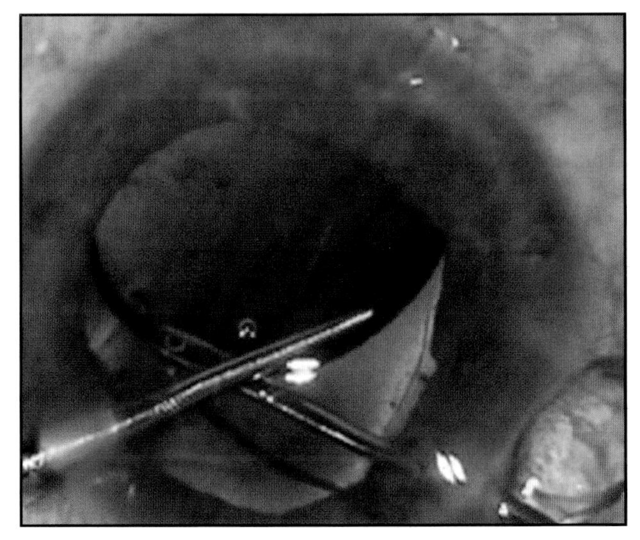

Figure 17-7. Foldable IOL implantation.

Microincision Cataract Surgery

Evolution of cataract surgery to a smaller incision has been the dream of many ophthalmologists since Kelman invented the phacoemulsification technique. A few years ago, a new technique was introduced in which you can perform cataract surgery through an incision of 1.4 mm or less. A small size incision correlates directly with a lower inflammatory rate postoperatively, which is why we consider MICS to be less invasive and it will be the best way to approach these patients. Although these are difficult cases, in the future, when IOL materials and biocompatibility are improved, this will be the preferred technique.

We perform two side-port incisions of 1.2 mm at 90°. There are special instruments designed to work through small incisions that make this surgery as safe and predictable as a standard phacoemulsification. One can use a special scissors (Katena) to break the posterior synechiae and to tear the fibrotic anterior capsule. We perform a CCC with a microutrata (Katena), a prechopper technique is used to divide the nucleus and with a chopper irrigation instrument (Katena) we perform a chop technique. Intensive cortical clean up is mandatory to eliminate one of the sources of postoperative inflammation reaction and the posterior surface of the anterior capsule must be vacuumed. Implantation of foldable, one-piece hydrophobic acrylic into the capsular bag is then performed. Suturing the incision is advocated.[13]

Combined Cataract-Vitrectomy Techniques

Pars plana vitrectomy combined with lensectomy can be the procedure of choice in cases of uveitis with vitritis refractory to medical treatment. This technique can be useful in patients with chronic juvenile arthritis or pars planitis. Technically speaking, if the lensectomy is performed through pars plana, corneal distortion is avoided. However, some disadvantages are associated with this technique, including the need for sulcus fixation of the posterior chamber IOL. In addition, removal of a dense nuclear sclerotic cataract may be difficult to perform.

In our hands, the combined phacoemulsification and pars plana vitrectomy technique has many advantages over other techniques.[14-15] IOL implantation after completion of the vitrectomy, if required, allows fast visual rehabilitation and functional unaided vision in patients who are considered poor candidates for aphakic contacts lens wear. If a limbal approach to the cataract posterior pars plana vitrectomy is intended, the scleral incisions for the vitrectomy should be made first. The fixed infusion method and upper sclerotomies occluded with scleral plugs are used. A capsulotomy or posterior capsulorrhexis must be performed upon completion of the vitrectomy because of the high opacification rate and because it allows a free connection between the anterior and posterior segment of the eye, facilitating the access of anti-inflammatory drugs in the postoperative period. Macular edema, retinal detachment, and glaucoma have been described as possible complications.[16-17]

Intraocular Lenses

Until recently, the existence of chronic uveitis has been regarded by most surgeons as a relative contraindication to IOL implantation.[18] For these reasons, sulcus or anterior chamber has always been contraindicated and capsular bag placement has been controversial. On the other hand, several researchers have suggested that inserting a posterior chamber lens into the capsular bag poses no additional threat to ocular mobility in selected uveitic eyes, provided proper perioperative treatment for inflammation is given.[2-5,19-21]

The use of anterior chamber IOLs should not be recommended in any type of uveitis. The first IOL used in uveitic eyes was rigid PMMA single-piece and they appear to have some advantages because they do not activate the complement cascade, a phenomenon associated with the presence of polypropylene haptics. Some authors advocated the use of single-piece PMMA lenses.[22] Also, there is a significantly lower prevalence of IOL cellular deposits as well as the number of anterior chamber cells, and a lower tendency of synechiae formation with the use of heparin surface modified IOL. The heparin surface modified IOL is created by inducing electrostatic absorption of heparin onto the surface of a PMMA IOL. Heparin coated IOLs are recommended for patients with uveitis, as they decrease the number and severity of deposits on the surface of the IOLs and although the IOL will not prevent or inhibit the development of fibrinous uveitis, the formation of adhesions to the IOL is likely to be retarded.[23-25] It has been suggested that heparin surface modified models provided an impressive cell-free IOL surface and greater protection from inflammatory complications than with unmodified lenses.[26] On the other hand, if cellular adhesion is reduced by implanting heparin surface modified lenses, the IOL will be clear and the visual acuity enhanced.[27] A recent report has shown that the mechanical irritation procedure destroys the heparin layer on PMMA IOLs in the grasp area. Clinical consequences are not yet known.[28]

Lately, very important information has been published studying the biocompatibility of different IOL materials in uveitic eyes. The use of phacoemulsification and the implantation of foldable IOLs in the bag in uveitic eyes have been recently studied.[2-5,29] The foldability of lenses allows their insertion through a small incision. Acrylic, but not silicone, foldable IOLs have also been shown to have better biocompatibility than PMMA IOLs. Acrylic hydrophobic lenses provided a lower incidence of postoperative complications in comparison with other lenses, especially silicone lenses. This might be based on the inert character and biocompatibility of acrylic hydrophobic material in uveitic eyes and the special design of the lens (sharp edge, adhesiveness to posterior chamber proteins) decreasing the incidence of LEC migration. Further research must be done to completely understand the uveal and capsular biocompatibility of the IOLs. However, we think that, at this moment, the first option is to perform a phacoemulsification and to implant a foldable three-piece hydrophobic acrylic IOL in the capsular bag (Acrysof).[2]

Postoperative Treatment

Postoperative care should include the maintenance of prior medications required for the control of the disorder with gradual reduction.

Suggested postoperative medications are:

1. The topical steroids treatment should be continued with prednisolone 1%, eight times a day for the first week, to be gradually decreased over a period of month.
2. Diclofenac four times a day for 2 weeks.
3. Tropicamide 1% three times a day for 4 weeks.
4. If the IOP is elevated, beta blockers, dorzolamide, or systemic acetozolamide are used.
5. Oral prednisone 1 mg/kg/day for 2 weeks, tapering it down for another 2 weeks for a total of 1 month.

The postoperative treatment of the uncomplicated cases is topical dexamethazone 0.1% every 8 hours for the first and second week, every 12 hours for the third week, and every 24 hours for the fourth week and the last week. In addition to the topical treatment used in the uncomplicated cases, complicated cases receive systemic steroids started preoperatively that continue for 2 weeks and are gradually tapered over 15 days.

Persistent uncontrolled glaucoma will require filtration surgery with the use of mytomicin C 0.02% applied for 2 minutes under the scleral flap. Pupillary membranes after cataract surgery can be removed by pars plana vitrectomy techniques. Cystoid macular edema is the most serious postoperative complication in patients with chronic uveitis who undergo cataract extraction. This complication occurs in 19 to 35% of the cases (angiographic diagnosis) and is present in 80% of eyes with less than 20/40 of postoperative visual acuity. Cystoid macular edema may be treated with oral acetozolamide, a topical NSAID, or topical, periocular, intravitreal injection and systemic steroids.

Other Therapeutic Alternatives for Patient Presentation and Follow-Up

Recently, the efficacy of two preoperative steroid regimens for cataract surgery in uveitic patients was compared. Group 1 received a single dose of IV methylprednisolone

(15mg/kg) 30 min before surgery, and group 2 received a 2-week course of oral prednisolone (0.5 mg/kg), which was tapered postoperatively. The conclusion was that the 2-week course of oral prednisolone produces a better recovery following cataract surgery in patients with uveitis.

Future Surgical Improvements: New Intraocular Medications

Routes of delivery of steroid compounds include systemic, periocular, and intraocular. Systemic administration is simple but carries the risk of systemic adverse effects associated with the high doses required for efficacy. Intraocular delivery, which has received the most recent interest, allows delivery of the medication directly to the site of action at a much smaller dosage, albeit at higher risk of ocular complications.

What is exciting about drug research is not only the new agents available, but also the possibility of new delivery options. Research has led to pellets, polymers, and even IOLs and contact lenses that can deliver drugs to the eye. One day, we may be able to treat chronic ocular disease or achieve postsurgical prophylaxis without the patient having to instill multiple drops. Drug delivery systems implanted during cataract surgery appear to offer continued prophylaxis against infection and quell inflammation. In one study, an implant containing fluocinolone acetonide effectively controlled inflammation for 3 years in cataract surgery patients who also had posterior uveitis and/or panuveitis.[30] The most significant risk was an IOP spike; average IOP among these patients went from 12 mmHg preop to 17 mmHg postop.

Elsewhere, surgeons implanted two drug delivery systems containing ciprofloxacin and dexamethasone in the anterior chambers of 64 cataract surgery patients.[31] No patient developed endophthalmitis, and average aqueous flare (measured in photon counts/ms) went from 9.2 at day 1 to 7.6 and 7.4 at days 4 and 30, respectively. One patient developed steroid-induced glaucoma.

IOLs themselves may become the drug delivery system. Hydrophilic acrylic IOLs can absorb and release liquids. Researchers placed one such IOL in 0.5% levofloxacin for 24 hours prior to surgery. The idea was that after implantation, the IOL would slowly release the fluoroquinolone directly into the anterior chamber. Using fluorescein, they observed this release in animal models over time, concluding that hydrophilic IOLs can serve as a drug delivery system for water soluble drugs such as fluoroquinolones.[32] There is an exciting future in the area of ophthalmic drug delivery systems. One day, this may eliminate the need for topical medications in complex, chronic ocular pathologies and following common surgical procedures.

Cataract Surgery in Children With Uveitis

In the pediatric age group, uveitis represents approximately 6% to 10% of all uveitis cases.[33,34] Moreover, 30% of patients develop one or more complications during the course of the uveitis. Juvenile rheumatoid arthritis is the most frequent underlying cause of uveitis in children (40% of all uveitis and 70% of the anterior uveitis group).[35] Patients are usually young females affected by monoarticular or pauci-articular juvenile rheumatoid arthritis with positive test for antinuclear antibodies and HLA DR5 and have the highest rate of complications, with an incidence of cataract up to 70%; band keratopathy, 65% glaucoma 30% and chronic hypotony or phthisis, 17%.[35-36] Most of these patients develop these complications in the first decade of life. The primary goal in the management of uveitis in children is early diagnosis and aggressive treatment to prevent ocular complications of the disease.

The average age at the time of the operation varies between series from 10 to 19 years,[37] but children as young as 4 years old may need surgery as well. Patients with juvenile rheumatoid arthritis have exacerbation of the uveitic process after cataract surgery. Surgery on these patients involves serious intraoperative complications, with vitreous loss and retains cortical material in good percentage of patients. Vision of 20/200 or worse is found in up to 60% of the cases.[38] Uveitis associated with juvenile rheumatoid arthritis is at present a contraindication for IOL implantation. Phacoemulsification without IOL implantation, whether associated or not with pars plana vitrectomy, is the preferred technique.[39]

Cataract Surgery in Specific Cases of Uveitis

Phacoemulsification in Fuchs' Heterochromic Cyclitis

The uveitis associated with Fuchs' Heterochromic Cyclitis (FHC) tends to be chronic and of low intensity. Posterior synechiae are rarely formed and the patients are usually unaware of the problem until the first complication arises cataracts or vitreous opacities.[40] The implantation of IOLs in patients with FHC is generally satisfactory with good visual outcome. Some authors have reported the use of heparin-surface modified lenses for all patients with FHC in whom implantation is indicated.[41] There are reports that suggest that the foldable hydrophobic acrylic IOL is the most suitable one for this type of uveitis.[42]

Fuchs' Heterochromic Cyclitis patients have few postoperative complications, although some isolated cases of vitreitis, hyphema, increase intraocular pressure and cyclitic membrane formation have been reported.[43] Posterior capsular opacification has been described in 8 to 20% of the patients. The problem with greatest visual significance is the development of glaucoma which appears in approximately 10% (3 to 35%) of the patients, and up to 70% of them may require filtration surgery.[40] Some risk factors have been identified in these patients. If glaucoma is present preoperatively, it may worsen postoperatively. In cases of severe iris atrophy, the risk of postoperative uveitis appears to be higher. When rubeosis iridis is present and hemorrhage occurs during surgery, the risk of both postoperative glaucoma and uveitis is higher.

Ocular Toxoplasmosis

Cataract surgery was regularly reported to induce exacerbations in different types of intraocular inflammations, therefor a group studied and reported an increase in the risk of reactivation of ocular toxoplasmosis following cataract extraction.[44] There was a reactivation rate of 36% for ocular toxoplasmosis within four month after cataract surgery and it may be taken into consideration a prophylactic treatment with antiparasitic drugs for patients with ocular toxoplasmosis at risk of visual loss.

Behcet's Disease, Vogt-Koyanagi-Harada, and Multifocal Chorioretinitis

There are few reports on cataract surgery or phacoemulsification in patients with Behcet's disease, Vogt-Koyanagi-Harada, and multifocal chorioretinitis. The incidence of phthisis bulbi and hypotony has been reported to decrease from 25% to 2% when limited vitrectomy was performed in combination with cataract extraction.[34] It is not clear, however, whether vitrectomy combined with cataract extraction can alter the course of inflammation. Visual prognosis is significantly worse in eyes with Behcet's disease than other types of uveitis because of the severe posterior segment complications, particularly optic atrophy.[45] Phacoemulsification or ECCE and vitrectomy in multifocal chorioretinitis with panuveitis have little therapeutic benefit. When an IOL is implanted, a visual improvement of one or two lines can be expected, but visual acuity returns to preoperative values within 6 months. Multifocal chorioretinitis remains poorly understood in terms of its etiology and suitable treatment.[46]

Tips and Pearls

1. Control of the preoperative inflammatory state is mandatory. A minimum of 3 months of quiescence is necessary before surgery is indicated. Topical, periocular, and systemic medications can be used for this purpose.
2. It will require a delicate surgery, maximum mydriasis, and the use of a dispersive viscoelastic.
3. Corneal 3.0 mm incision is recommended. Careful cortical material removal and posterior capsular polishing are important steps to prevent or delay posterior capsular opacification frequently found in these patients. It is also important to perform a CCC as regular as possible to overlap the IOL optics. This will decrease posterior capsular opacification as well. An anterior vitrectomy can be performed if vitreous opacities are present at the time of surgery.
4. IOLs can be implanted in the majority of uveitic patients. Until further studies are performed in this area, implantation of a foldable hydrophobic acrylic lens is the best approach.
5. The postoperative control of inflammation is extremely important in these patients, since the complications associated with it may be severe.
6. Chronic juvenile arthritis tends to exacerbate uveitis after cataract surgery. In these patients, a careful decision for IOL implantation must be made.
7. In children, the surgery will be of no value unless intensive treatment of amblyopia is performed immediately after the surgery.

Key Points

1. It is very important that the surgery is performed in an "undisturbed" eye with an inflammatory reaction that has been controlled for at least 3 months prior to surgery.
2. The mechanical stimulation of the iris has been known to induce the release of prostaglandins. Prostaglandins have been proven to play a role in ocular inflammatory reactions, particularly in those in which mechanical iris scraping had been performed.
3. Good surgery is the most important "anti-inflammatory" element for the post-operative patient.
4. Viscoelastic materials are routinely used to release adhesions.
5. Pars plana vitrectomy combined with lensectomy can be the procedure of choice in cases of uveitis with vitritis refractory to medical treatment.

REFERENCES

1. Okharavi N, Lightman SL, Towler HMA. Assessment of visual outcome after cataract surgery in patients with uveitis. *Ophthalmology*. 1999;106:710–722.
2. Alio JL, Chipont E, Benezra D, Fakhry M. Comparative performances of intraocular lenses in the eyes with cataract and uveitis. *J Cataract Refract Surg*. 2002;28:2096.
3. Abela-Formanek C, Amon M, Schild G, Schauersberger J, Nepp J, Kruger A. Results of hydrophilic acrylic, hydrophobic acrylic and silicon intraocular lenses in uveitic eyes with cataract. *J Cataract Refract Surg*. 2002:1141–1152.
4. Abela-Formanek C, Amon M, Schild G, et al. Inflammation after implantation of hydrophilic acrylic, hydrophobic acrylic, or silicon intraocular lenses in eyes with cataract and uveitis. *J Cataract Refract Surg*. 2002:1153–1159.
5. Abela-Formanek C, Amon M, Schild G, et al. Uveal and capsular biocompatibility of 2 foldable acrylic intraocular lenses in patient with uveitis or pseudoexfoliation syndrome. *J Cataract Refract Surg*. 2002:1160–1171.
6. Mondino BJ, Rao H. Effect of intraocular lenses on complacent levels in human serum. *Acta Ophthalmol*. 1983;61:76–94.
7. Kaplan HJ. Discussion of Foster CS, Fong LP, Singh G. Cataract surgery and intraocular lenses implantation in patients with uveitis. *Ophthalmology*. 1989;96:287–288.
8. Foster CS. Vitrectomy in the management of uveitis. *Ophthalmology*. 1988;95:1011–1012.
9. Foster CS, Barrett F. Cataract development and cataract surgery in patients with juvenile arthritis-associated iridociclitis. *Ophthalmology*. 1993;100:809–817.
10. Dangel ME, Stark WJ, Michels RG. Surgical management of cataract associated with chronic uveitis. *Ophthalmic Surg*. 1983;14:145–149.
11. Diamond JG, Kaplan HJ. Lensectomy and vitrectomy for complicated cataract secondary to uveitis. *Arch Ophthalmol*. 1978;75:1798–1804.
12. Girard IJ, Rodriguez, Mailman MI, Romano TJ. Cataract and uveitis management by pars plana lensectomy and vitrectomy by ultrasonic fragmentation. *Retina*. 1985;5:107–114.
13. Chipont E, Martinez JJ. Intrastromal corneal suture for small incision cataract surgery. *J Cataract Refract Surg*. 1996;22:671–675.
14. Koening SB, Han DP, Mieler WF, Abrams GW, Jaffe GJ, Burgon TC. Combined phacoemulsification and pars plana vitrectomy. *Arch Ophthalmol*. 1990;108:362–364.
15. MacKool RJ. Pars plana vitrectomy and posterior chamber intraocular lens implantation in diabetic patients. *Ophthalmology*. 1989;96:1679–1680.
16. Nove RJ, Kokoris D, Diddie KR. Lensectomy-vitrectomy in chronic uveitis. *Retina*. 1993;3:71–76.
17. Nolthenius PA, Deutman AF. Surgical treatment of the complications of chronic uveitis. *Ophthalmologica*. 1983;186:11–16.
18. Lichter PR. Intraocular lenses in uveitis patients. *Ophthalmology*. 1980;96:279–280.
19. Hooper PI, Rao NA, Smith RE. Cataract extraction in uveitis patient. *Surv Ophthalmology*. 1990;35:120–143.
20. Foster CB, Fong LP, Singh G. Cataract surgery and intraocular lens implantation in patients with uveitis. *Ophthalmology*. 1989;96:281–287.
21. Lowenstein A, Bracha R, Lazar M. Intraocular lens implantation in an eye with Behcet's uveitis. *J Cataract Refract Surg*. 1991;17:95–97.
22. Foster CB, Fong LP, Singh G. Cataract surgery and intraocular lens implantation in patients with uveitis. *Ophthalmology*. 1989;96:281–287.
23. Ygge J, Wenzel M, Philipson B. Cellular reactions on heparin surface-modified versus regular PMMA lenses during the first postoperative month. *Ophthalmology*. 1990;97:1216–1223.
24. Miyake K, Mackubo K. Comparison of heparin surface modified and ordinary PCLS: a Japanese study. *European J Implant Refract Surg*. 1991;3:95–97.

25. Borgioli M, Coster DJ, Fan RFT. Effect of heparin surface modification on polymethymethacrylate intraocular lenses on signs of postoperative inflammation after extracapsular cataract extraction. *Ophthalmology*. 1992;99:1248–1255.
26. Percival SPB, Pai V. Heparin-modified lenses for eyes at risk for breakdown of the blood-aqueous barrier during cataract surgery. *J Cataract Refract Surg*. 1993;19:760–765.
27. Jones NP. Extracapsular cataract surgery with and without intraocular lens implantation in Fuchs heterochromic uveitis. *Am J Ophthalmol*. 1989;108:310–314.
28. Dick B, Kohen T, Jacobi KW. Alteration of heparin coating on intraocular lenses caused by implantation instruments. *Klin Moatsbl Augenheilkd*. 1995;206:460–466.
29. Rauz S, Stavrou P, Murray P. Evaluation of foldable Intraocular lenses in patients with uveitis. *Ophthalmology*. 2000;107:909–919.
30. Denny JP, Carlson A, McCallum R, et al. Combined fluocinolone acetonide sustained drug delivery system implantation and phacoemulsification/intraocular lens implantation in patients with severe uveitis. ARVO, 2003.
31. Theng J, Chee SP, Ti SE, et al. Prospective clinical trial on the combined use of Suroquine Drug Delivery System (DDS) containing ciprofloxacin and Surodex DDS containing dexamethasone in phacoemulsification cataract surgery without need for eyedrops. ARVO, 2003.
32. Kobayakawa S, Tanaka K, Tsuji A, et al. Drug delivery intraocular lens. ARVO, 2003.
33. Kimura SJ, Hogan MJ, O Connor GR, Epstein WV. Uveitis and joint diseases. Clinical findings in 191 cases. *Arch Ophthalmol*. 1967;77:309–316.
34. Kanski JJ, Shun-Shin G. Systemic uveitis syndromes in childhood: an analysis of 340 cases. *Ophthalmology*. 1984;91:1247–1252.
35. Tugal-Tutkun I, Havrkikova K, Power WJ, Foster CS. Changing patterns in uveitis of childhood. *Ophthalmology*. 1996;103:375–383.
36. Dana MR, Merayo-Lloves J, Schaumberg DA, Foster CS. Visual outcomes prognosticators in juvenile rheumatoid arthritis–associated uveitis. *Ophthalmology*. 1997;104:236–244.
37. Pivetti-Pezzi P, Monacada A, Torce MC, Santillo C. Causes of reduced visual acuity on long term follow up after cataract extraction in patients with uveitis and juvenile rheumatoid arthritis. *Am J Ophthalmol*. 1993;115:926–827.
38. Key Sn III, Kimura SJ. Iridocyclitis associated with juvenile rheumatoid arthritis. *Am J Ophthalmol*. 1975;80:425.
39. Michelson JB, Nozik RA, Smith RA. Uveitis surgery. In: Tasman W, Jaeger EA, eds. *Duane's Clinical Ophthalmology*. 4th ed. Philadelphia: JB Lippincott Co; 1991.
40. Liesegang TJ. Clinical features and prognosis in Fuch's uveitis syndrome. *Am J Ophthalmol*. 1982;100:1622–1626.
41. Jones NP. Cataract Surgery using heparin surface modified intraocular lenses in Fuch's heterochromic uveitis. *Ophthalmic Surg*. 1995;26:49–52.
42. Foster C, Rashid S. Management of coincident cataract and uveitis. *Curr Opin Ophthalmol*. 2003;14:1–6.
43. Mills KB, Rosen ES. Intraocular lens implantation following cataract extraction in Fuch's heterochromic uveitis. *Ophthalmol Surg*. 1982;13:467.
44. Bosch-Driessen LH, Plaisier MB, Stilma JS, Van der Lelij A, Rothova A. Reactivations of ocular toxoplasmosis after cataract extraction. *Ophthalmology*. 2002;109:41–45.
45. Ciftci OU, Ozdemir, O. Cataract extraction comparative study of ocular Behcet's disease and idiopathic uveitis. *Ophthalmologica*. 1995;209:270–274.
46. Nolle B, Eckart C. Vitrectomy in multifocal chorioretinitis. *Ger J Ophthalmol*. 1993;2:14–19.

Chapter 18

Refractive Cataract Surgery

Pandelis A. Papadopoulos, MD, PhD, FEBO

Introduction

With the current advances in small incision cataract surgery and intraocular lens (IOL) technology, there is an increasing demand for the ophthalmic surgeon to perform "refractive" cataract surgery. The goal is to choose a surgical strategy that permits the correction of the patient's total refractive error in *one* operation. This may be accomplished by choosing the appropriate combination of wound construction, placement, and closure, as well as using techniques of incisional keratotomy. Precise axial length measurement is very important in refractive cataract surgery. Inaccurate ultrasound biometry or IOL miscalculation can lead to refractive errors that will destroy the final surgical outcome and to patient dissatisfaction. Multifocal, pseudoaccommodative and toric IOLs have enriched the surgeon's armamentarium lately, and will play a significant role towards less spectacle dependency. In some cases piggyback or negative-power IOLs will also help the surgeon in correcting high refractive errors in cataract patients.

Biometry

Measurement of axial length constitutes the largest source of error in IOL power calculation.[1] An error of 0.1 mm in axial length can cause an error of 0.3D in IOL power. Measurement accuracy is considered satisfactory if there is no more fluctuation than 0.15 mm in the same eye and 0.3 mm between the fellow eyes.

Ultrasound Biometry

Several methods were tested to improve the accuracy of axial length measurement. Among these, immersion A-scan technique (Figure 18-1) is reported to be the most accurate and reproducible.[2,3] There seems to be no statistically significant difference between

Figure 18-1. Immersion A-scan biometry in a high myopic eye with posterior staphyloma (C = cornea, La = anterior lens surface, Lp = Posterior lens surface, R = retina).

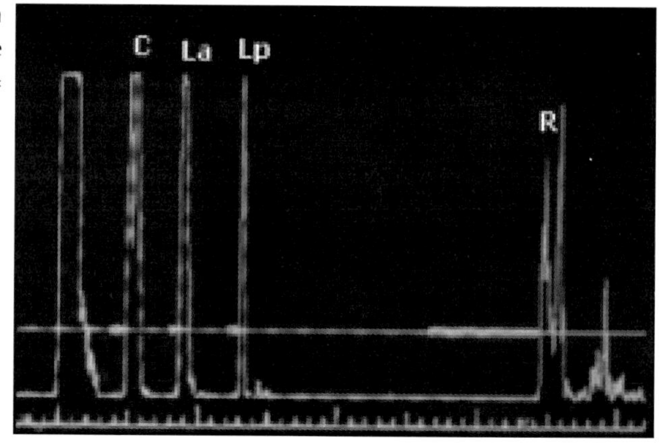

hand-held and slit-lamp attached A-probe measurements.[4] Manual rather than automated A-scan measurements are indicated in eyes with asteroid hyalosis.[5] Falsely short axial length measurements may be obtained using automated A-scan biometry, leading to significant errors.

Falsely longer axial length measurements may occur if:[6]

1. A drop of fluid or methylcellulose increases the distance between the probe and the corneal surface in applanation biometry.
2. The probe is not aligned with the optical axis.
3. Low gain is used, which can lead to confusion of retinal and scleral peaks.
4. Higher than indicated ultrasound velocity is used.
5. A posterior staphyloma exists. In these cases, B-mode-guided vector-A-mode biometry can help to determine the position of the fovea.[7]
6. The eye is filled with silicone oil.
7. The eye has a scleral buckle after retinal detachment surgery.

Falsely shorter axial length measurements may occur if:

1. Pressure is applied on the cornea in applanation biometry. This error does not occur in immersion biometry.
2. The probe is not aligned with the optical axis.
3. Membranes or opacities (asteroid hyalosis) in vitreous exist.
4. A retinal detachment is present.
5. An IOL is present.
6. The choroid is thickened.
7. Lower than indicated ultrasound velocity is used.

Frequent evaluation of the surgical outcomes and personalizing of A-constants can further reduce the postoperative refractive error. Flowers, McLeod, McDonnell, et al studied the use of personalized formula constants and concluded that they can significantly reduce the mean absolute predictive error for the SRK II, SRK/T, and Holladay formulas.[8]

Husain, Kohnen, Maturi, et al found that the computerized videokeratography (CVK)-derived corneal curvature values to be slightly less accurate than standard keratometry in predicting IOL power.[9] However, CVK provides important corneal curvature data for IOL calculations in patients with abnormal or surgically altered corneal surfaces.

The accuracy of IOL power calculation remains a major problem in very long and very short eyes. The accuracy of the newer generation theoretical IOL power calculation formulas and of the empirical SRK I and II formulas was evaluated in a series of 500 IOL implantations including a series of unusually long and short eyes.[10] The prediction error of the theoretical formulas was found to be largely unaffected by the variation in axial length and corneal power, while the prediction of the SRK I formula was less accurate in the short and long eyes. The prediction of the SRK II formula was more accurate than the SRK I in that no systematic offset error with axial length could be demonstrated. However, because of a relatively larger scatter in the long eyes and a significant bias with the corneal power, the absolute error of the SRK II formula was higher than that of the theoretical formulas in the long eyes. The higher accuracy of the newer generation theoretical formulas was attributed to their improved prediction of the pseudophakic anterior chamber depth (ACD).

The following guidelines can help the surgeon reduce errors of axial length measurements and IOL power calculations:

1. Usage of theoretical formulas (eg, SRK/T) if the axial length is shorter than 22 mm or longer than 25 mm.
2. Repetition of measurements if there is an AXL difference of more than 0,3 mm between the eyes.
3. Multiple measurements if axial length is shorter than 22 mm or longer than 25 mm.
4. Multiple measurements if the corneal curvature is less than 40 D or more than 47 D.
5. Repetition of measurements if the astigmatic cylinder power difference is more than 1 D between the fellow eyes.
6. Repetition of measurements if the refractive cylinder differs significantly from keratometric cylinder.
7. Repetition of measurements if the axial length is incompatible with the refraction of the eye (eg, long axial length in a hyperopic eye).
8. Repetition of measurements in patients with poor fixation or poor cooperation.
9. Usage of B-mode guided vector A-mode biometry in eyes with posterior staphyloma and age-related macular degeneration.
10. Calculation of personalized A-constant for each IOL type used.
11. Frequent analysis of refractive outcomes in order to localize the sources of error.

Optical Biometry

In recent years, noninvasive optical biometry methods based on the principle of partial coherence interferometry (PCI) have been developed.[11] The advantage of PCI is that this noncontact method neither requires local anesthesia nor represents a risk of infection.[12] In addition, the method precludes an additional source of error in axial length measurement caused by the indentation of the cornea. Moreover, pupil dilation is unnecessary in optical biometry using PCI, which has a high longitudinal and transversal resolution. In various publications, the accuracy is reported to be between 5 mm and 30 mm.[13,14] The main drawback of optical biometry is its limited usability in cases of fixation problems or advanced cataract.[11,14] In U/S biometry, the axial length is determined by measuring the reflection of the anterior surface of the cornea and the limiting membrane.

The IOLMaster (Carl Zeiss) is the first commercially available instrument using optical biometry (Figures 18-2 and 18-3). It was introduced in Germany in September 1999 and was approved by the US Food and Drug Administration in March 2000. It is able to measure the corneal curvature, the ACD, and the corneal diameter (white-to-white). The software includes various IOL calculation formulas (Haigis, SRK/T, SRK II, Hoffer, etc). The IOLMaster measures the distance from the anterior surface of the cornea to the pigmented epithelium. Due to this difference, the IOLMaster measurements are on average 0.23 mm longer for the same eye.[15] A different A-constant should be used when the axial length is measured by the IOLMaster. Several study groups have compared axial length and corneal radius measurements taken with the IOLMaster with those taken using traditional U/S systems and with keratometry measurements. The IOLMaster provides axial length measurements comparable to those by the immersion method.[16] The resulting correction factors were integrated in the software of the IOLMaster so that the IOL calculation formulas use

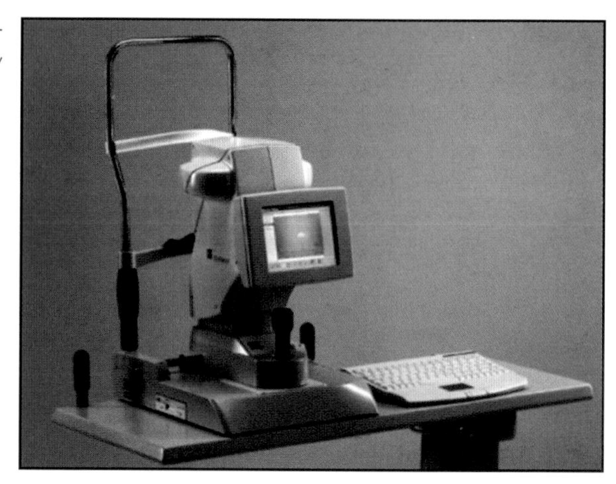

Figure 18-2. The Zeiss IOLMaster utilizes partial coherence interferometry to measure the axial length.

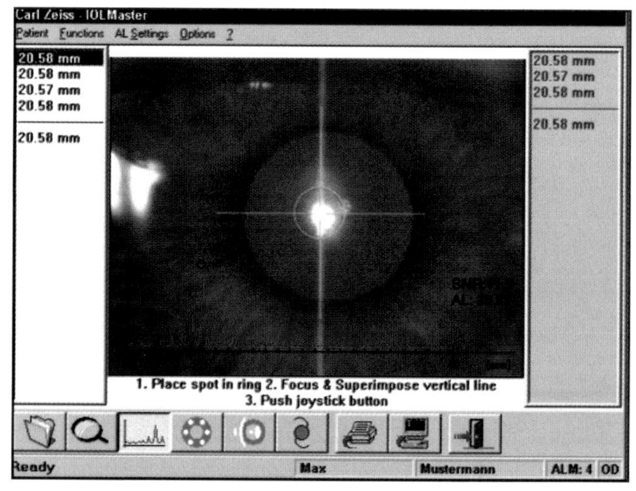

Figure 18-3. Measuring axial length with the IOLMaster.

customized constants. Updated optical A-constants of older and newer IOLs can be downloaded from the ULIB (User Group for Laser Interference Biometry) web site, found at URL: http://www.augenklinik.uni-wuerzburg.de/eulib/.

Intraocular Lenses for the Correction of Presbyopia

Monovision With Monofocal Intraocular Lenses

Monovision is a means of presbyopic correction in which one eye is corrected for distance vision and the other eye for near vision. In clinical practice, the dominant eye is commonly corrected for distance. This practice is based on the assumption that it is easier to suppress blur ín the nondominant eye than in the dominant eye. Monovision limitations in refractive cataract surgery have not been clearly defined in the current ophthalmic literature, although the monovision success rate with contact lens correction is high. Ideally, the patient with monovision should be able to see clearly at all distances. The binocular clear vision range should be continuous and equal to the sum of the monocular clear ranges without interference from blurred images in one eye. However, input from the dominant eye produces a greater response to a given stimulus. Success and patient satisfaction in monovision patients were significantly influenced by the magnitude of ocular dominance.[17] In monovision, the postoperative target refraction may range from –1.5 to –2.75 D, depending from the intended working distance. Any reduction in intermediate vision created by the choice of full distance and near correction was well tolerated and accepted by highly motivated patients.[18,19]

Multifocal Intraocular Lenses

Multifocal IOLs provide patients with an accommodative capacity, allowing multiple focal distances independent of ciliary body function and capsular mechanics. This pseudoaccommodation results in full distance visual acuity and increased depth of focus, including sufficient near visual acuity. Controversy exists over the quality of vision offered by these lenses. These IOLs have simultaneous multiple focal areas and therefore, multiple light distribution, which causes less light at every focal point.

The AMO Array is the most widely studied small-incision foldable multifocal IOL available at present time.[21-23] It has a five-zone refractive, progressive, aspheric configuration designed to provide true multifocality through a wide depth of focus and good visual acuity and contrast sensitivity for distance, which results from the lens preponderant distance correction (50% for distance, 37% for near, 13% for intermediate).

According to a study by Vaquero-Ruano, Encinas, et al, contrast sensitivity was found to be decreased at low contrasts with this IOL.[24] The most important subjectively reported optical side effects disappeared after the first 2 months. At 18 months, 6% of the cases reported ghosting and 4% reported glare. In the same study, 28% of the patients could read J1+ without spherical addition, however the other 72% required a mean near addition of only 1.03 D. This could be explained by the 35% light distribution of the near area in the far preponderance design of the lens and the low refractive power. In another study by Papadopoulos, Katsavavakis, Kotsiris, et al, 37.5% of the patients could read J1 without correction at 3 months.[25]

Bilateral multifocal IOL implantation is reported to give the best multifocal effect. Forty percent of the multifocal group were able to do without spectacles, compared to 11% of the monofocal group. Careful selection of appropriate candidates is important for a satisfactory outcome. Accurate biometry is essential. Glare and ghosting were reported during night driving. Postoperative automated refractometry can be misleading because of the variable refractive power in the central zone.[25] Absolute and relative contraindications for multifocal IOL implantation are summarized in Table 18-1.

A different concept of multifocality employs a diffractive design. Diffraction creates multifocality through constructive and destructive interference of incoming rays of light. An earlier multifocal IOL by 3M employed a diffractive design. It encountered difficulty in acceptance, not because of its optical design, but rather, due to poor production quality and the relatively large incision size required for its implantation. Alcon has recently completed clinical trials of a new diffractive multifocal IOL based on the 6-mm foldable three-piece AcrySof acrylic IOL, the Restor IOL. The diffractive region of this lens is confined to the center, so that the periphery of the lens is identical to a monofocal acrylic IOL. The inspiration behind this approach comes from the realization that during near work, the synkinetic reflex of accommodation, convergence, and miosis implies a relatively smaller pupil size. Putting multifocal optics beyond the 3-mm zone creates no advantage for the patient and diminishes optical quality. In fact, bench studies performed by Alcon show an advantage in modulation transfer function for this central diffractive design, especially with a small pupil at near and a large pupil at distance.[19]

Table 18-1.

Contraindications for Multifocal IOL Implantation

Ocular & Systemic Diseases (loss of contrast sensitivity)

- Foveal impairment (eg, maculopathy, diabetic retinopathy, retinal detachment surgery with macular involvement)
- Optic nerve anomalies (eg, glaucoma, optic neuropathy)
- Corneal disorders (eg, dystrophy, scar leukoma, tear film dysfunction)
- Vitreous opacities
- Amblyopia
- Multiple sclerosis, Parkinson's, diabetes (with and without retinopathy)

Other Conditions

- Astigmatism >1.00 D
- Miosis <2.0 mm
- Age >85 years

Factors Compromising Multifocal Function (preoperative or surgically induced)

- Biometric error
- Astigmatism >1.00 D
- Abnormal pupil
- IOL tilt and decentration
- Capsular opacity

The Acritec Acritwin IOLs are refractive/diffractive aspheric IOLs implanted bilaterally. One eye receives the 447 D IOL with 70% of the light intensity in the distance focus, while in the accompanying eye, the IOL type 443 D with 30% of the light intensity in the distance focus is implanted. The Acritec company has recently introduced the first multifocal MICS (microincision cataract surgery) IOL, the Acri.Smart 366D MICS, that can be implanted through a sub 2 mm incision.

Accommodative IOLs

Another approach to the correction of presbyopia has been introduced in the last few years with the accommodative IOLs. True pseudophakic accommodation could be achieved by an anterior shift of the IOL optic during ciliary muscle contraction. In an eye of usual dimensions, an anterior shift of 600 mm of the IOL corresponds to an accommodative effect of 1 D. Current IOLs are too rigid to change position significantly during ciliary body contraction, so recent attempts have been concentrated mainly on more flexible, accommodative IOL designs. A thin, flexible hinge at the haptic-optic junction is common to all current models. Two such IOLs (1CU, HumanOptics, and AT-45, Eyeonics Crystalens) are commercially available (Figure 18-4), whereas others are prototypes. Unfortunately, recent single or multicenter studies by independent researchers have shown that near-point accommodation did not induce significant movement of the so-called accommodating IOLs. In a study conducted by the author, 78% of the eyes implanted with the 1CU IOL had a visual acuity of 1.0 uncorrected for distance, but only 11% had J2 uncorrected for near. The overall satisfaction rate for near vision was very low. All patients required reading glasses.[41]

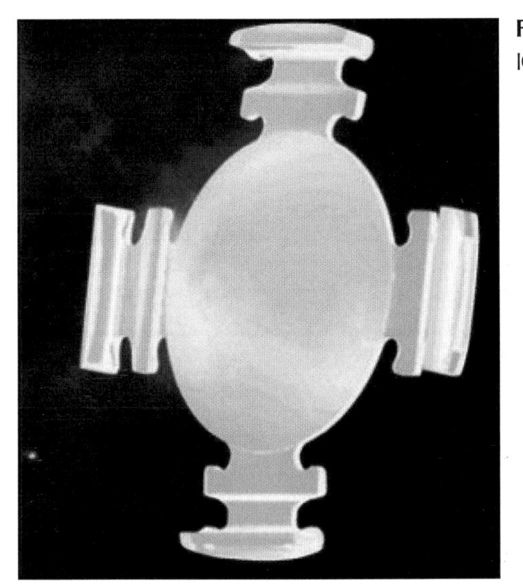

Figure 18-4. The Humanoptics 1CU Accommodative IOL.

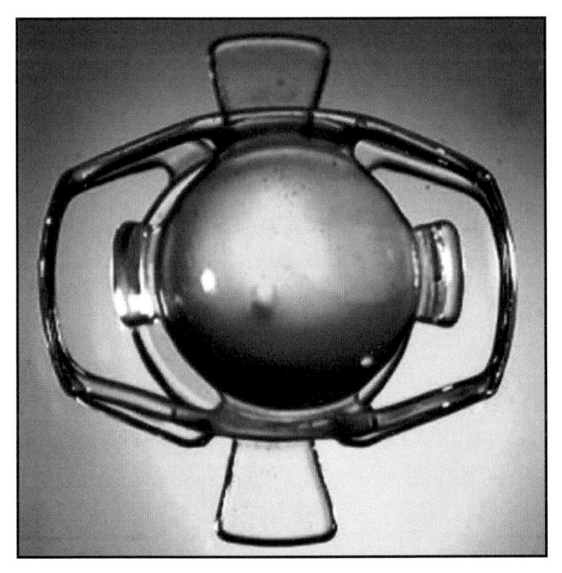

Figure 18-5. The dual-optics Visiogen Synchrony IOL.

Several dual-optic lenses are currently on the drawing board and in early clinical trials. The Visiogen Synchrony Dual Optic IOL, a one-piece, silicone lens consisting of a high plus-powered (front) optic attached by flexible bridges to a low minus-powered (back) optic, fits within the capsular bag (Figure 18-5). In a nonaccommodated state, the distance between the two optics is shorter than in an accommodative state, when the bag slackens and the compressible haptics push the plus-powered optic forward.

Lenstec has developed the Tetraflex accommodating IOL, an acrylic, square-edged, one-piece microincision lens with equiconvex optics. According to the manufacturing company, the specially designed haptics and a 5-degree anterior angulation allow the lens to move forward during the accommodating process. The optic acts like a sail in the wind, catching the wave of the vitreous.

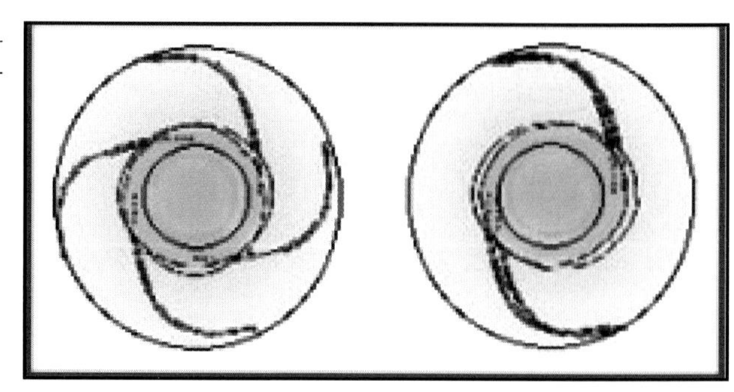

Figure 18-6. The piggyback IOL haptics can be inserted in a parallel or perpendicular fashion.

PIGGYBACK IOLS

Piggyback IOLs (Polypseudophakia) can provide appropriate pseudophakic optical correction for patients requiring very high IOL powers.[26,27] Since primary polypseudophakia is considered for highly hyperopic eyes with small anterior segments, using thin, high-index optics allows two lenses to fit well into the capsular bag and remain optically stable. Acrylic IOLs with high refractive index are currently preferred because they offer several advantages.[28,29] The material's high index of refraction (usually 1.54), allows the biconvex optics to have flatter surfaces than plate-haptic silicone lenses, which by their design, have more steeply curved surfaces in view of their lower index of refraction (usually 1.41). Alignment of the optical zones of the two plate lenses could be tenuous because the capsular bag contracts around silicone optics postoperatively. Therefore, optical stability is more likely to be achieved with piggyback acrylic IOLs than with silicone or other lens materials.

With the first IOL, placing the loops within the bag can be achieved by any commonly practiced method. However, when placing the second set of loops, additional viscoelastic must be added to the bag and the loops presented in longitudinal fashion rather than having them open posteriorly over the first IOL. This will avoid displacing the first IOL from the bag or entwining the loops of the two IOLs. The question of whether the loops of the two lenses should be left parallel or perpendicular to each other still remains unanswered (Figure 18-6). Negative-power IOLs are used in a piggyback fashion to correct high myopia. Fortunately, many IOL manufacturers have today a very large range of dioptric powers from –10 D up to +40D.

Recently, Humanoptics has introduced two foldable toric IOLs (MicroSil 614TPB and MS 714 TPB) to be implanted in a piggyback fashion in the ciliary sulcus to correct residual astigmatism in conjunction with a standard or multifocal IOL.

CONTROL OF ASTIGMATISM

An important goal in refractive cataract surgery is to control, and in some patients, to reduce, corneal astigmatism. Several options for modulating astigmatism are available, including modifying incision placement, length, and construction; astigmatic keratotomy; limbal and corneal relaxing incisions (LRIs and CRIs), and toric IOL implantation.

The surgeon's major goal in managing astigmatism intraoperatively should be to preserve preoperative corneal asphericity, reduce a small amount of preexisting astigmatism, or reduce high preoperative astigmatism without shifting the meridian. If the fellow eye is similar in astigmatic power and meridian, surgical astigmatic correction may not be indicated.

The temporal clear corneal, beveled single-plane or hinge incisions with a width of less than 3.3 mm retain the preoperative corneal cylinder within ±0,5D of astigmatism. The astigmatically neutral incision allows the surgeon to perform predictable incisional keratotomy for the correction of preoperative astigmatism.

Table 18-2.

Modified Gills Nomogram to Correct Astigmatism With Cataract Surgery

Astigmatism (D)	*Incision Type*	*Length (mm)*	*Optical Zone*
1	One LRI	6.0	At limbus
1–2	Two LRIs	6.0	At limbus
2–3	Two LRIs	8.0	At limbus
>3	Two LRIs+CRIs as indicated 3 months postoperatively	Lindstrom Surgical Nomogram for astigmatism	7–8 mm at cornea

Limbal Relaxing Incisions

The potential advantages of limbal relaxing incisions are preservation of the optical qualities of the cornea, less risk of inducing postoperative glare, less discomfort and more rapid recovery of vision.

They are placed at the limbus and can be made according to a modified Gills nomogram (Table 18-2), based on preoperative corneal astigmatism as determined with standard keratometry and computerized videokeratography. The location of the steep axis is determined on the corneal topographic map and then the location relative to any significant landmark on the conjunctiva or limbus is noted. If a clear landmark is not evident preoperatively, the 6 and 12 o'clock semimeridians are marked with a 25 gauge needle in the corneal epithelium with patient sitting upright. Alternatively, a marking pen can be used to mark these semimeridians. A guarded diamond knife is set to at a depth of 600 mm. The incisions can be made before or after cataract surgery. Some surgeons prefer to perform the incisions at the conclusion of the surgery in the event that a complication occurs, altering the astigmatic strategy.

According to a study by Budak, Friedman and Koch, patients achieved a mean reduction in astigmatism of 1.47 D at 1 month postoperatively.[30] The mean with the wound (WTW) change was –0.70+–0.44 D. Preoperative astigmatism was greater than 1.50 D in 83.3% of the eyes preoperatively, compared with 25% postoperatively. No overcorrections were observed. None of the patients reported postoperative distortion in vision, glare or discomfort. Based on their early results, the authors suggested a surgical nomogram for the correction of astigmatism during cataract surgery (Table 18-3).

In a similar approach, Nichamin and Dillman developed a nomogram for clear corneal phaco and arcuate keratotomies[31] (Table 18-4). As seen in the nomogram, patients who are relatively spherical receive only a single-plane, beveled temporal incision placed just inside the vascular arcade. For those patients with modest preexisting against-the-rule astigmatism, rather than enlarging the temporal incision, a peripheral nasal arcuate relaxing incision is placed according to the age-adjusted nomogram. If higher levels of astigmatism are present, a temporal limbal arcuate incision is placed so that it encompasses the posterior entry of clear corneal incision.

For preexisting with-the-rule astigmatism, the surgeon has two choices: utilize a superior clear corneal phaco incision, with or without arcuate limbal corneal incisions over the steep vertical axis, or retain the neutral temporal clear corneal phaco incision and place intralimbal arcs along the steep vertical axis. Although this latter approach may involve a greater number of incisions, it has the advantages of working temporally and the movement around the operating table is avoided.

Table 18-3.

Nomogram for Correction of Astigmatism During Cataract Surgery

Astigmatism (D)	*Incisions* (mm)
<0,5	3.5 mm clear corneal temporal
With-the-rule	
0.5–1.25	3.5 mm superior limbal
	or
	3.5 mm clear corneal temporal plus LRIs
<=1.50	3.5 mm clear corneal temporal plus LRIs (±CRIs at 3 months)
	or
	3.5 mm superior limbal plus LRIs
	or
	6.0 mm superior scleral
Against-the-rule	
0.5–1.25	3.5 mm clear corneal temporal
1.5–1.75	3.5 mm clear corneal temporal LRIs (±CRIs at 3 months)
.2.00	3.5 mm clear corneal temporal LRIs CRIs at 3 months
Oblique	
0.5–1.25	3.5 mm clear corneal on steeper meridian
1.5–1.75	3.5 mm clear corneal on steeper meridian plus LRIs (12CRIs at 3 months)
>2.00	3.5 mm clear corneal on steeper meridian plus LRIs plus CRIs at 3 months

Table 18-4.

Nomogram for Clear Corneal Phaco and AK Surgery

ASTIGMATIC STATUS = **SPHERICAL**: (+0–75 X 90's +0.50 X 180')

Incision Design = 'Neutral' temporal clear corneal incision (TCC) (3.2 mm or less single plane)

ASTIGMATIC STATUS = **AGAINST-THE-RULE**: Steep axis (0 to 30°/150 to 180°): Intraoperative keratoscopy determines exact incision location

Incision Design = Neutral TCC along with the following peripheral arcuate incisions

Preop cylinder	*Age:*	*30–50 years*	*51–70 years*	*71–85 years*	*>85 years*
		Degrees of arc to be incised			
+0.75 to +1.50	Nasal limbal arc	50°	45°	30°	–
+1.75 to +2.50	Paired arcuate Incisions	60°	50°	45°	30°
+2.75 to +3.50	Paired arcuate incisions	90°	75°	50°	45°
+3.75 to +4.50	Paired arcuate incisions	Reduce OZ (ie, 7.0 mm)	90°	75°	60°

TCC incision followed by nasal and temporal peripheral arcuate incisions.
The temporal arc approximates the posterior border of the TCC.

ASTIGMATIC STATUS = **WITH-THE-RULE**: (Steep axis 45° to 145°): Intraoperative keratoscopy determines exact incision location

Incision Design = Neutral TCC along with the following peripheral arcuate incisions

Preop cylinder	*Age:*	*30–50 years*	*51–70 years*	*71–85 years*	*>85 years*
		Degrees of arc to be incised			
+1.0 to +1.75	Paired limbal arcs On steep axis	40°	35°	30°	-
+2.00 to +2.75	Paired limbal arcs On steep axis	60°	50°	45°	30
+3.00 to +3.75	Paired limbal arcs On steep axis	75°	60°	50°	40

Or

Continued

Table 18-4, continued

Nomogram for Clear Corneal Phaco and AK Surgery

Incision Design = Superior clear cornea (SCC) with the following peripheral arcuate incisions:

	Age:	*30–50 years*	*51–70 years*	*71–85 years*	*>85 years*
Preop cylinder		Degrees of	arc to be incised		
+1.5 to +2.00		SCC alone	SCC alone	SCC alone	—
+2.00 to +2.75	Inferior limbal arc	45°	30°	SCC alone	SCC alone
+3.00 to +3.75	*paired arcuate incisions	60°	45°	30°	SCC alone

*SCC incision followed by superior and inferior peripheral arcuate incisions. The superior arc approximates the posterior border of the SCC.

After verifying the steep meridian with intraoperative keratoscopy or other method, the appropriate degree of arc is marked on the corneal surface. The incisions are placed just inside the limbus, taking care to keep the blade's footplates parallel to the corneal surface.

Arcuate keratotomy at a later date can be an alternative for the reduction of preexisting or induced astigmatism. The number of incisions, the size of the optical zone, and the arc length of the incision can be determined with reference to various nomograms.[32-34] The Thornton Nomogram for the correction of astigmatism is shown in Table 18-5. However, surgical outcomes in pseudophakic eyes with history of ocular surgery can be different from those with intact eyes.[35] The predictability of astigmatic keratotomy after cataract surgery has been addressed in very few published papers[36,37] and needs further evaluation with larger studies.

A more convenient way to perform more precise arcuate keratotomies is the Terry-Schanzlin Astigmatome (Oasis) (Figure 18-7). It consists of an alignment speculum attached to a syringe to create suction and preset-depth single or double blades. Blade depth and optical zone are preset to provide consistent depth and reproducibility. Preset depth options are 500, 550, 600, 650 and 700µ for arcuate cuts at 8mm. Pachymetry is required to determine corneal depth. Measurements should be taken centrally and at the location of the incisions. The double-blade design is commonly used for the treatment of regular astigmatism where two simultaneous arcs are desired exactly 180° apart. A single-blade variation is available for nonorthogonal and asymmetric corrections.

Toric IOLs

The advantages of toric IOLs versus AK are: 1) there is no additional intervention during surgery, 2) no interference with corneal curvature, and 3) high predictability.[38] A potential problem is obtaining and maintaining the correct axis.

The STAAR Toric IOL (Figure 18-8), was the first foldable single-piece, plate-haptic silicone injectable IOL available commercially. It incorporates a cylindrical correction on the anterior surface of a spherical optic, thereby producing a toric or sphero-cylindrical refract-

Table 18-5.

Thornton Nomogram for Astigmatic Keratotomy

Assumes cuts 98% deep (almost to Descemet's membrane) along the full length of the incision.

Age: For every year below age 30, add 1/2% to the astigmatic error. For every year above age 30, subtract 1/2%.

Sex: In premenopausal women (under age 40), subtract 3 years from actual age.

IOP: For every mm IOP below 12, add 2% to the astigmatic error. For every mm IOP above 15, subtract 2%.

Add or subtract the sum of the modifiers (%) from the actual amount of cylinder for the "Theoretical Cylinder."

Cylinder Corrected by Paired Arcuate Transverse Incisions

Chord Length of One Pair
Arcuate Transverse Incisions
Incision at 7.0mm

Theoretical Cylinder	*Degrees Arc*
0.50 D	20
0.75 D	23
1.00 D	25
1.25 D	28
1.50 D	32
1.75 D	35
2.00 D	38
2.25 D	42
2.50 D	45

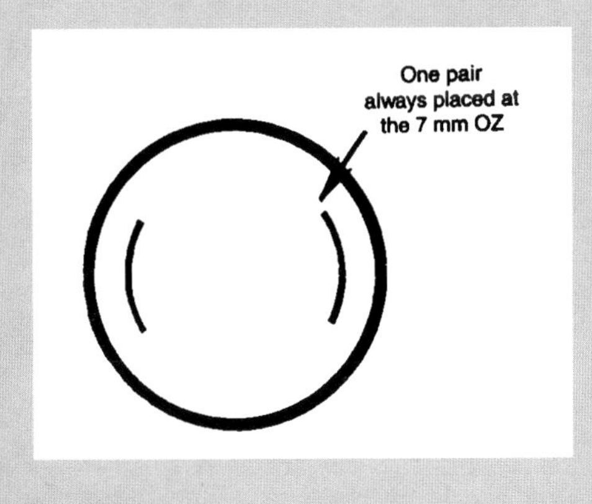

Chord Length of Two Pairs
Arcuate Transverse Incisions
Outer incision at 8.0mm – Inner incision at 6.0mm

Theoretical Cylinder	*Degrees Arc*
2.00 D	23
2.25 D	27
2.50 D	31
2.75 D	35
3.00 D	39
3.25 D	43
3.50 D	47
3.75 D	50

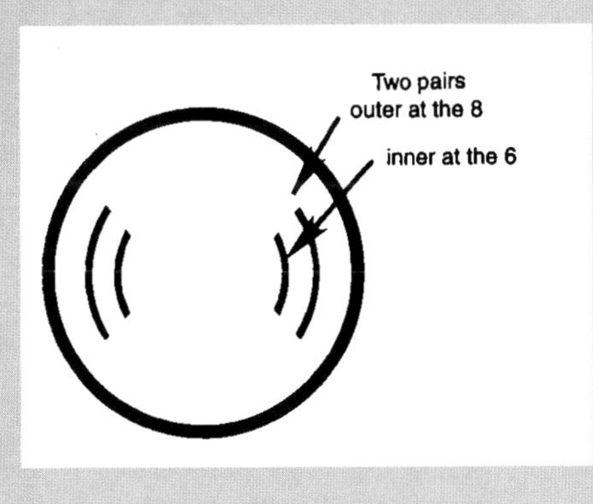

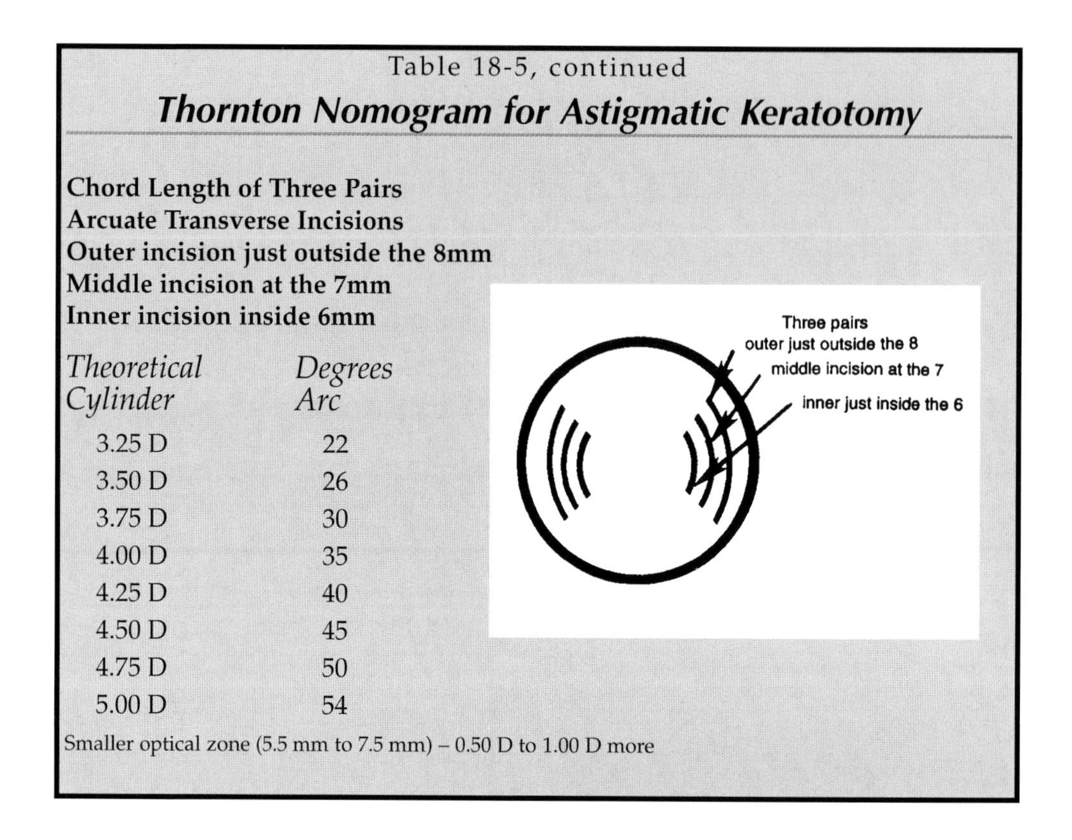

Table 18-5, continued

Thornton Nomogram for Astigmatic Keratotomy

Chord Length of Three Pairs
Arcuate Transverse Incisions
Outer incision just outside the 8mm
Middle incision at the 7mm
Inner incision inside 6mm

Theoretical Cylinder	*Degrees Arc*
3.25 D	22
3.50 D	26
3.75 D	30
4.00 D	35
4.25 D	40
4.50 D	45
4.75 D	50
5.00 D	54

Smaller optical zone (5.5 mm to 7.5 mm) – 0.50 D to 1.00 D more

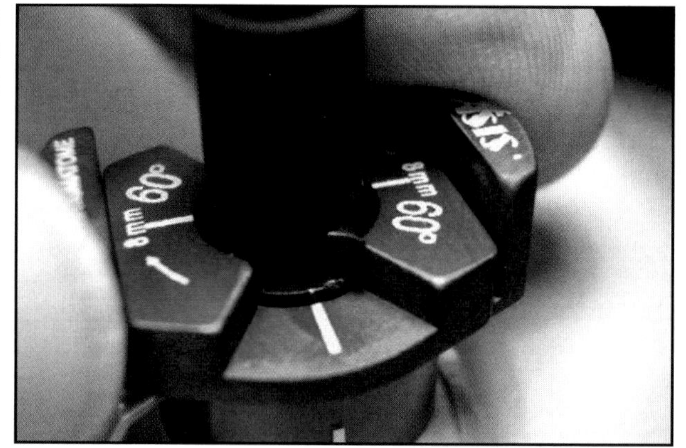

Figure 18-7. The Terry-Schanzlin Astigmatome to perform arcuate keratotomies during the cataract operation.

ing element. The lens is available in a complete range of spherical powers with cylindrical adds of 2.0 and 3.5 D. The 2.0 D Toric IOL is intended for use in cataract patients with 1.5 D to 2.25 D of preexisting corneal astigmatism. The 3.5 D Toric IOL is intended for use in cataract patients with 2.25 D to 3.5 D of preexisting astigmatism.[39]

The Toric IOL is indicated in cataract patients who will have a regular corneal astigmatism of 1.5 to 3.5D. On corneal topography these patients will exhibit symmetrical bow-tie or wedge-type patterns (Figures 18-9 and 18-10). On keratometry, they will have regular mires with the steep and flat corneal meridians at approximately 90° apart.

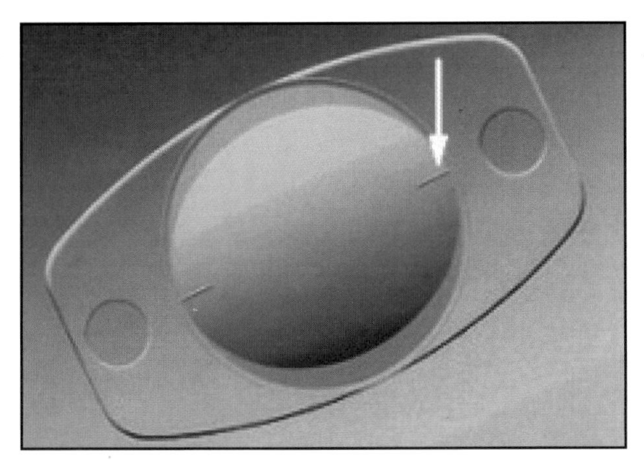

Figure 18-8. The STAAR Toric IOL. The axis is indicated by the markings at the haptic-optic junction (arrow).

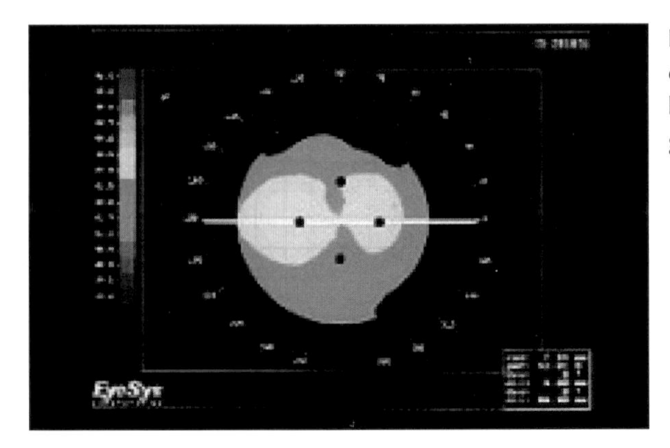

Figure 18-9. The Toric IOL is indicated in eyes with symmetrical bow-tie or wedge-shaped topographical patterns.

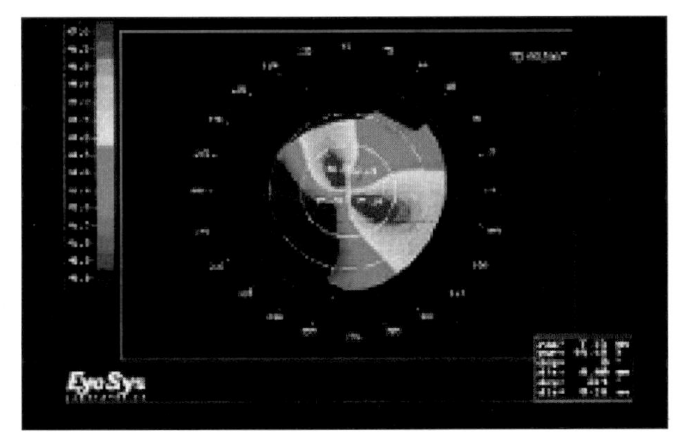

Figure 18-10. The Toric IOL is not indicated in eyes in which the steep and flat corneal meridians are not approximately 90° apart.

The steep meridian of the sphero-cylindrical optic is orientated along the short axis of the IOL, so that the axis of the cylindrical correction lies along the long axis of the IOL which is indicated by the two markings at the haptic-optic junction. When used in conjunction with astigmatically neutral cataract surgery, these markings are simply aligned with the steep corneal meridian in order to maximize the effect of the cylindrical correction afforded by the lens.

LIBRARY
POST GRADUATE CENTRE
KETTERING GENERAL HOSPITAL

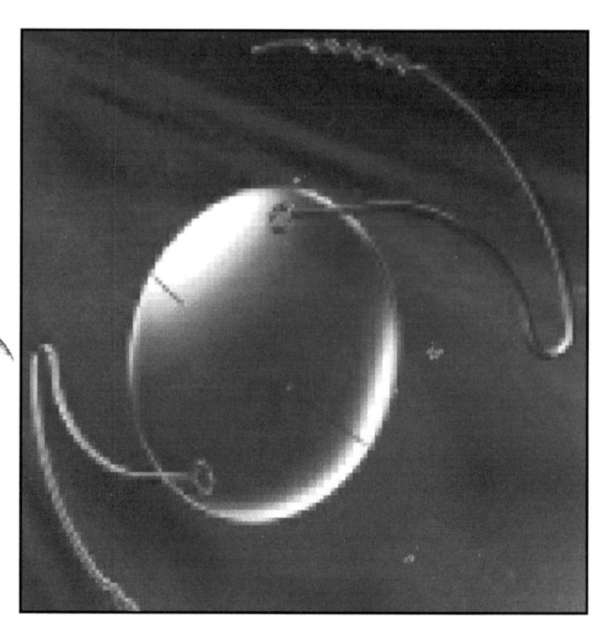

Figure 18-11. The Humanoptics MicroSil MS6116T has large serrated PMMA haptics that prevent IOL rotation.

The manufacturer of this IOL has developed software using the SRK/T formula to determine the IOL power and alignment axis. In addition, the probable postoperative astigmatism is displayed for misalignment up to 10°. If the axis of the lens is within 10° from the postoperative steep meridian it can be left uncorrected, but if it is greater than that postoperative realignment is indicated. At 30° misalignment, the toric correction is lost. Beyond that the cylindrical correction may be increased.

Of the eyes implanted with the 3.5D toric IOL, 42% had postoperative cylinder less than 0.5D, while 25% of the torics and 85% of the controls had greater than 1.5 D. Four of 175 IOLs in the FDA study had to be realigned within 1 week after the surgery.[40]

Another Toric IOL, the Humanoptics MicroSil MS6116T (Figure 18-11), is available in a wider dioptric range, from –3.0 D to +30.0 D and from 2.0 D to 12.0D for sphere and cylinder, respectively. This IOL has large serrated PMMA haptics that prevent IOL rotation.

The evolution and the refinement of all the current and future techniques will allow the cataract surgeon to correct the refractive error of any patient with high precision in a single operation. The true refractive cataract surgery has become a reality in the beginning of the 21st century.

Key Points

1. With the current advances in small incision cataract surgery and IOL technology, there is an increasing demand for the ophthalmic surgeon to perform "***refractive***" cataract surgery. The goal is to choose a surgical strategy that permits the correction of the patient's total refractive error in ***one*** operation.
2. Measurement of axial length constitutes the largest source of error in IOL power calculation. An error of 0.1 mm in axial length can cause an error of 0.3 D in IOL power.
3. In recent years, noninvasive optical biometry methods based on the principle of PCI have been developed. The advantage of PCI is that this noncontact method neither requires local anesthesia nor represents a risk of infection. The IOLMaster (Carl Zeiss) is the first commercially available instrument using optical biometry.

4. The AMO Array is the most widely studied small-incision foldable multifocal IOL available at present time. It has a five-zone refractive., progressive, aspheric configuration designed to provide true multifocality.
5. Diffraction creates multifocality through constructive and destructive interference of incoming rays of light. Alcon has a diffractive multifocal IOL based on the 6-mm foldable three-piece AcrySof acrylic IOL, the Restor IOL.
6. Another approach to the correction of presbyopia are the accommodative IOLs. True pseudophakic accommodation could be achieved by an anterior shift of the IOL optic during ciliary muscle contraction.
7. Piggyback IOLs (polypseudophakia) can provide appropriate pseudophakic optical correction for patients requiring very high IOL powers.
8. The potential advantages of limbal relaxing incisions are preservation of the optical qualities of the cornea, less risk of inducing postoperative glare, less discomfort, and more rapid recovery of vision.

References

1. Olsen T. Sources of error in intraocular lens power calculation. *J Cataract Refract Surg.* 1992;18(2):125-9.
2. Giers U, Epple C. Comparison of A-scan device accuracy. *J Cataract Refract Surg.* 1990;16(2):235-42.
3. Olsen T, Nielsen PJ. Immersion versus contact technique in the measurement of axial length by ultrasound. *Acta Ophthalmol.* 1989;67(1):101-2.
4. Whelehan IM, Heyworth P, Tabandeh H, McGuigan S, Foss AJ. A comparison of slit-lamp supported versus hand-held biometry. *Eye.* 1996;10(4):514-6.
5. Allison KL, Price J, Odin L. Asteroid hyalosis and axial length measurement using automated biometry. *J Cataract Refract Surg.* 1991;17(2):181-6.
6. Panidou I, Topouzidis H, Reptsis A, Alexandrou K, Zisiadis K. Biometric errors in IOL Power Calculation. Proceedings of the 31st Panhellenic Ophthalmological Congress, May, 1998.
7. Berges O, Puech M. B-mode-guided vector-A-mode versus A-mode biometry to determine axial length and IOL power. *J Cataract Refract Surg.* 1998;24:529-535.
8. Flowers CW, McLeod SD, McDonnell PJ, Irvine JA, Smith RE. Evaluation of intraocular lens power calculation formulas in the triple procedure. *J Cataract Refract Surg.* 1996;22(1):116-122.
9. Husain SE, Kohnen T, Maturi R, Er H, Koch DD. Computerized videokeratography and keratometry in determining intraocular lens calculations. *J Cataract Refract Surg.* 1996;22(3):362-6.
10. Olsen T, Thim K, Corydon L. Accuracy of the newer generation intraocular lens power calculation formulas in long and short eyes. *J Cataract Refract Surg.* 1991;17(2):187-93.
11. Hitzenberger CK. Optical measurement of the axial eye length by laser Doppler interferometry. *Invest Ophthalmol Vis Sci.* 1991;32:616-624.
12. Drexler W, Findl I, Menapace R, et al. Partial coherence interferometry: a novel approach to biometry in cataract surgery. *Am J Ophthalmol.* 1998;126:524-534.
13. Hitzenberger CK, Drexler W, Dolezal C, et al. Measurement of the axial length of cataract eyes by laser Doppler interferometry. *Invest Ophthalmol Vis Sci.* 1993;34:1886-1893.
14. Kuck H, Makabe R. Vergleichende axiale Biometrie des Auges. *Fortschr Ophthalmol.* 1985;82:91-93.
15. Papadopoulos PA, Tyligadi A. Accuracy of IOL calculations in Optical Biometry. Paper presented at 36th Panhellenic Congress of Ophthalmology, Crete, June, 2003.

16. Findl O, Drexler W, Menapace R, et al. Teilkoharenz- Laserinterferometrie: eine neue hochprazise Biometrie Methode zur Verbesserung der Refraktion nach Kataraktchirurgie. *Klin Monatsbl Augenheilkd*. 1998;212:29.
17. Handa T, Mukuno K, Uozato H, et al.Ocular dominance and patient satisfaction after monovision induced by intraocular lens implantation. *J Cataract Refract Surg*. 2004;30(4):769-74.
18. Greenbaum S. Monovision pseudophakia. *J Cataract Refract Surg*. 2002;28(8):1439-43.
19. Fine IH, Packer M, Hoffman RS. New lens technologies progress for correction of presbyopia. *Ophthalmology Times*. April 2003.
20. Kriechbaum K, Findl O, Koeppl C, Menapace R, Drexler W. Stimulus-driven versus pilocarpine-induced biometric changes in pseudophakic eyes. *Ophthalmology*. 2005;112(3):453-9.
21. Fine IH. Design and early clinical studies of the AMO array multifocal IOL. In: Maxwell A, Nordan LT, eds. *Current Concepts in Multifocal Intraocular Lenses*. Thorofare, NJ: SLACK Incorporated; 1991.
22. Percival SP, Setty SS. Prospectively randomized trial comparing the pseudoaccommodation of the AMO Array multifocal lens and a monofocal lens. *J Cataract Refract Surg*. 1993;19:26–31.
23. Jacobi PC, Konen W. Effect of age and astigmatism on the AMO Array multifocal intraocular lens. *J Cataract Refract Surg*. 1995;121:556–561.
24. Vaquero-Ruano M, Encinas JL. AMO Array multifocal versus monofocal intraocular lens: Long-term follow-up. *J Cataract Refract Surg*. 1998;24:118-123.
25. Papadopoulos PA, Katsavavakis D, Kotsiras I. Early Results with the Foldable Multifocal IOL AMO Array SA40. Paper presented at the 31st Panhellenic Ophthalmological Meeting, May, 1998.
26. Gayton JL. Implanting two posterior chamber intraocular lenses in nanophthalmos. *Ocular Surgery News*. 1994;64–65.
27. Holladay J, Gills J. Achieving emmetropia in extremely short eyes with two piggyback posterior chamber intraocular lenses. *Ophthalmology.* 1996;103:1118-1123.
28. Masket S. Piggyback intraocular lens implantation. *J Cataract Refract Surg*. 1998;24:569-570.
29. Shugar JK, Lewis C, Lee A. Implantation of multiple foldable acrylic posterior chamber lenses in the capsular bag for high hyperopia. *J Cataract Refract Surg*. 1996;22:1368-1372.
30. Budak K, Friedman N, Koch D. Limbal relaxing incisions with cataract surgery. *J Cataract Refract Surg*. 1998;24:503-508.
31. Nichamin L, Dillman D, Maloney WF. Peripheral arcuate astigmatic keratotomy partners with clear corneal phaco surgery. *Ocular Surgery News*. 1997;V17:N15.
32. Lindstrom RL. The surgical correction of astigmatism: a clinician's perspective. *Refr Corneal Surg*. 1990;6:441-454.
33. Thornton SP. Astigmatic keratotomy: a review of basic concepts with case reports. *J Cataract Refract Surg*. 1990;16:430-435.
34. Thornton SP. *Radial and Astigmatic Keratotomy*. Thorofare, NJ: SLACK Incorporated; 1994.
35. Georgaras S, Tsingos V, Papadopoulos PA. Correction of Postoperative Astigmatism. Proceedings of the 31st Panhellenic Ophthalmological Congress, May, 1998.
36. Guell JL, Manero F, Muller A. Transverse keratotomy to correct high corneal astigmatism after cataract surgery. *J Cataract Refract Surg*. 1996;22:331-6.
37. Oshika T, Shimazaki J, et al. Arcuate keratotomy to treat corneal astigmatism after cataract surgery. *Ophthalmology*. 1998;105:2012-2016.
38. Neuhann T. Ridley Medal Lecture, XVth ESCRS Congress, 1997 Prague.
39. STAAR TORIC IOL User's Guide, Staar Surgical, Monrovia, CA; 1996.
40. Sanders D. Preliminary Results of the FDA Trial for the STAAR TORIC IOL, XVth ESCRS Congress, 1997; Prague.
41. Papadopoulos PA, Georgaras SP. First Results with the Accommodative 1CU IOL. Presented at the 16th International Meeting of the HSIOIRS. Athens, February, 2002.

III

Anterior Segment—Worst Case Scenarios

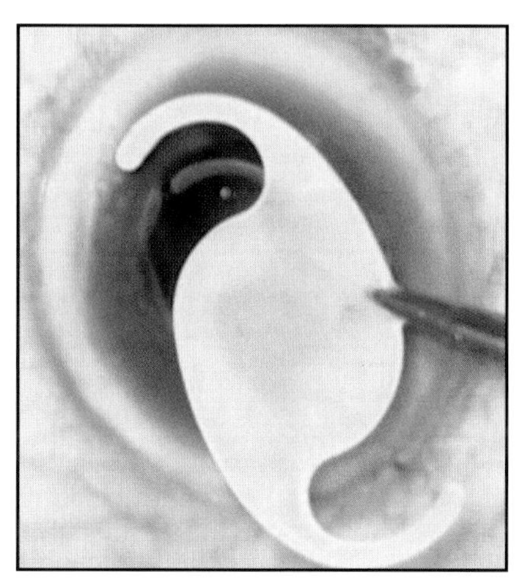

Opacified IOL.

Chapter 19

COMPLICATIONS IN PHACOEMULSIFICATION

L. Felipe Vejarano, MD; Alejandro Tello, MD

INTRODUCTION

Various complications can occur with phacoemulsification.[1–95] This can lead to phaco nightmares and so one should be careful when performing the surgery.

PROBLEMS CONSTRUCTING THE INCISION

Complications may arise from an incorrectly constructed incision (Figure 19-1). If the tunnel is too long (longer than 2.00 mm), passing the phaco tip through it and turning the tip downward to perform the procedure creates undue striae and makes visualization difficult. You can get oar locked as you try to manipulate the phaco needle. Moreover, the increased wound distortion will pose the risk of incisional burn. The tunnel can be too short (shorter than 1.4 mm) with a premature entry into the anterior chamber. The anterior chamber will tend to shallow, which can itself cause problems. Moreover, it is easier for iris prolapse to occur. To avoid this situation, angle the blade somewhat anteriorly when making the tunnel.

Using blunt blades (whether they are diamond or sapphire) may cause the incision roof to tear when you direct the tip of the blade downward to the anterior chamber. If you feel that you will need to apply too much pressure in order to make the blade enter into the anterior chamber, stop and change it. It is better to use a sharp metal blade than a blunt diamond blade. A Descemet's detachment can be created if a very blunt blade is used.

INCISIONAL BURNS

The technique of lens extraction by phacoemulsification has revolutionized cataract surgery. However, the production of ultrasound energy is associated with heat generation that can result in ocular tissue damage. Incisional burns are a risk whenever you use an

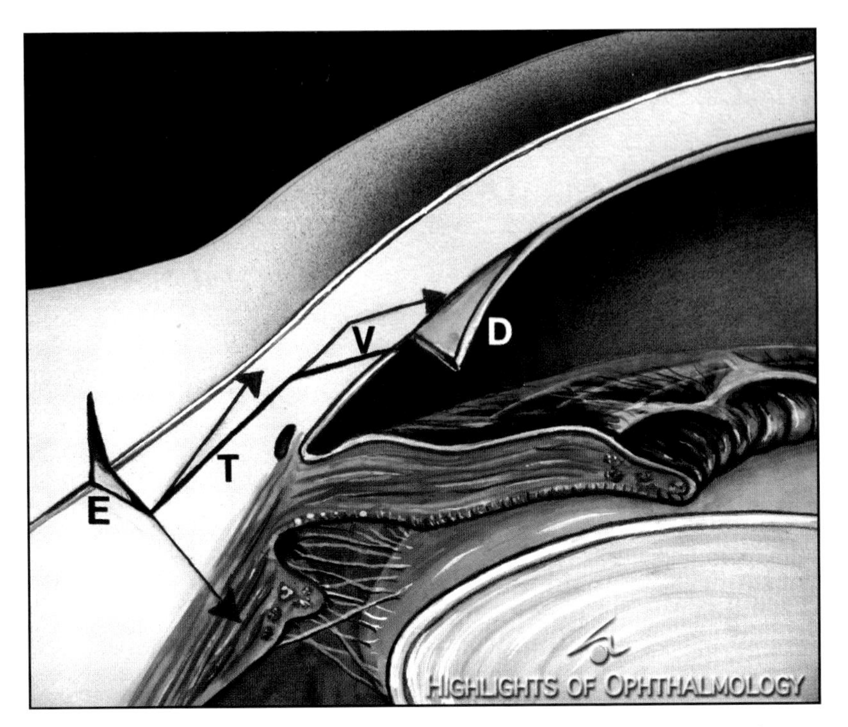

Figure 19-1. Problems from incorrect placement of tunnel incisions. The correct placement and performance of the sclero-corneal tunnel, limbal, or corneal incision is extremely important. In case of the sclero-corneal (E), it is made 1 to 2 mm from the limbus to a depth corresponding to 1/2 to 2/3 thickness of the sclera. A scleral tunnel (T) between 1.5 to 2 mm in length is made. With blade directed in a parallel path to the iris, the internal valve (V) opening is created. Common placement errors are shown by blue lines. Also shown is a detachment of Descemet's membrane (D), another uncommon complication. (Original illustration by Highlights of Ophthalmology, based on principles from Virgilio Centurion's book titled *"Complicações Durante a Facoemulsificação"*.) (Courtesy of Benjamin F. Boyd, Ed. *The Art and the Science of Cataract Surgery*. Highlights of Ophthalmology. English Edition, 2001.)

ultrasound tip.[2–3] The cause of an incisional burn is heat transfer from the needle to the tissue surrounding it; the degree of injury is directly related to the total amount of heat absorbed. Higher phaco power and a longer duration of phaco time (especially when using continuous mode) tend to increase the needle temperature. Therefore, the judicious use of phaco energy at lower power settings, the use of pulsed or burst modes, and the new options of turning off the energy during a period of time through the cycle of pulses, (WhiteStar's cool phaco [AMO Sovereign, Advanced Medical Optics, Santa Ana, California] or Infiniti's duty cycle and Legacy's Everest software (Alcon, Fort Worth, Texas)] or using hybrid phaco technology (NeoSoniX [Infiniti & Legacy, Alcon] and Staar Sonic Wave System, Staar Surgical, Monrovia, California] will also help reduce the risks for corneal burns.

Additional irrigation fluid will not enter the eye unless fluid or other materials, such as viscoelastic or the lens material, leave the eye. In an experimental study, both the cohesive and dispersive viscoelastic agents were associated with a delay from the onset of phaco power to the onset of irrigation flow, and this lack of irrigation and aspiration resulted in the greatest thermal rise and caused wound damage.[10] For these reasons, it is very important that just after inserting the phaco needle into the anterior chamber full of viscoelastic, you should aspirate for a while to ensure irrigation and aspiration flow, before the onset of phacoemulsification power.

It is important to watch for the production of a "milky" material while emulsifying the nucleus, which suggests poor irrigation and aspiration and, therefore, poor cooling. This is a warning sign indicating that a thermal injury may ensue if ultrasound is not stopped and the problem is not solved. Generally, the burn associated with phacoemulsification involves primarily the roof of the incision. It has a spectrum from a slight graying or whitening of the corneal tissue (which rarely have any lasting consequence) to collagen shrinking and extensive whitening of the anterior lip of the wound, resulting in gaping that may lead to difficulties with wound closure and different amounts of astigmatism. You can note this reflecting a ring on the corneal surface with the microscope light (the round reflex turns in oval toward the incision). The best approach to corneal burns is prevention. If it does occur, it needs suturing, as pouting of the lip will occur.

Shallow Anterior Chamber

Some eyes have a shallow anterior chamber. In these cases, it is very important to use viscoelastics to deepen the anterior chamber, but in eyes with extremely crowded anterior segments it could be difficult, and if too much viscoelastic is injected, the IOP will overly increase and may cause iris prolapse. In these eyes, performing capsulorrhexis is more risky due to the increased convexity of the anterior capsule, and endothelium is exposed to more trauma because of the decreased working space.[31] Although using Healon 5 (AMO) may be useful and effective in these cases,[22] some eyes with extremely shallow anterior chambers will still pose a challenge. Chang has described that an automated pars plana vitreous tap 3.5 mm behind the limbus with an automated vitrectomy cutter without infusion to remove a few tenths of millimeter of vitreous, is useful to expand the anterior segment when the anterior chambers do not deepen sufficiently with viscoelastic injection alone.[11,31] At the end of the case, the sclerotomy is closed with Vicryl (Ethicon).[31] Agarwal uses the air pump in all his cases and so does not have a shallow anterior chamber as more fluid enters the eye.

Shallowing during the procedure may be due to either extraocular or intraocular causes. To determine the origin, touch the eye gently and feel the intraocular pressure (IOP). If the eye is soft, the problem is external. It may be a tight lid speculum, tight drapes, or if you are using a recollecting bag it may be full of BSS.[15] If the IOP is high, it may be either a fluid misdirection syndrome or a suprachoroidal hemorrhage or effusion.[31] The cause of the misdirection is the presence of zonular dialysis that allows fluid to flow around the equator into the vitreous. Verify with the anesthesiologist if there are any cardiovascular contraindications, and use mannitol (0.75–1 gm/kg) intravenously to dehydrate the vitreous. It will take 10 to 15 minutes to lower the IOP. If it does not work, another option is to perform a sclerotomy to try to drain misdirected liquid from the vitreous cavity. Lower the bottle and decrease flow rates to achieve a lower flow-type emulsification to diminish the risk of fluid going back through the zonules and rehydrating the vitreous. If the IOP remains high after these measurements, it could be the result of a suprachoroidal effusion/hemorrhage, so surgery should be halted and the incision should be closed.[31] Use the indirect ophthalmoscope to confirm the diagnosis. Fortunately, with small incision cataract surgery, it is improbable that an effusion will turn into an expulsive hemorrhage. Never enlarge the incision to try to finish the case. The procedure must be finished in a second stage.

Lens-Iris Diaphragm Retropulsion Syndrome: Excessive Anterior Chamber Deepening

Lens-iris diaphragm retropulsion syndrome (LIDRS) is characterized by anterior chamber deepening, pupil dilation, and concave shape of the iris. The excessively deep chamber makes the surgery technically more challenging and painful for the patient under topical anesthesia. This can be caused by a reverse pupillary block, and so must be solved by equalizing the fluid pressure between the anterior chamber and the posterior chamber. It can be managed by simply separating the iris from the anterior capsule rim with the phaco needle, the irrigation/aspiration (I/A) tip, or any other second instrument. The iris immediately returns to a more physiologic position with correction of the chamber depth.[12]

Detached Descemet's Membrane

This uncommon complication may occur during a manipulation of the wound, including injection of viscoelastic, implantation of an IOL, passing of instruments into the eye, or enlargement of the incision (see Figure 19-1). When using dull blades, instead of sharply incising Descemet's membrane, the blades may catch it and push it ahead of them. When small, it is usually asymptomatic, but when it is severe enough it will cause serious corneal edema. A large Descemet's detachment may appear to be a retrocorneal membrane; however, this is contiguous with the normal Descemet's detachment and endothelium in the periphery. Agarwal has shown how one can diagnose this complication by injecting trypan blue inside the eye. The Descemet's detachment will stain blue (see Chapter 20). The differential diagnosis includes a residual fragment of anterior capsule.

The clue to avoiding this complication is careful placement of instruments inside the eye. Try to avoid pressing forcefully on the phaco tip or introduce it bevel down. A newly designed irrigation sleeve (Microsmooth, Alcon) with a more slippery material may diminish the friction when entering through the wound. Before injecting anything (viscoelastics, BSS, air), the surgeon must be sure that the tip of the cannula is entered into the anterior chamber, well beyond the incision, and not dissecting the Descemet's. If, upon placing an instrument within the eye, the surgeon feels unusual resistance, the instrument should be retracted and wound size or visualization should be improved before the instrument is again placed into the anterior chamber. If you've caught a piece of the membrane, the careful placement and removal of instruments becomes critical for the remainder of the procedure. For an intraoperatively diagnosed detachment, involving not more than one-fourth of the corneal area, the surgeon may make a stab incision in a location away from the wound, and inject air or a viscoelastic into the eye to force the membrane back to its original position. An injection of air at the end of the procedure may help to keep the Descemet's reattached, by compressing it to the cornea. However, for large detachments encompassing one-third or more of the corneal surface area, the best option is repositioning it surgically. A patient with this condition usually presents on the first postoperative day with a significant amount of corneal edema that does not resolve.

The Descemet's membrane can be reattached to the cornea using 10–0 monofilament sutures passed through the cornea, according with the classic technique described by Vastine.[13] The surgeon may make a new paracentesis site at the limbus to get a good approach to a site in the anterior chamber, where air or a viscoelastic can be injected to push the detached Descemet's membrane into its proper position. Then place the sutures starting posterior to the limbus, passing anteriorly into the anterior chamber, through Descemet's and into the cornea stroma.

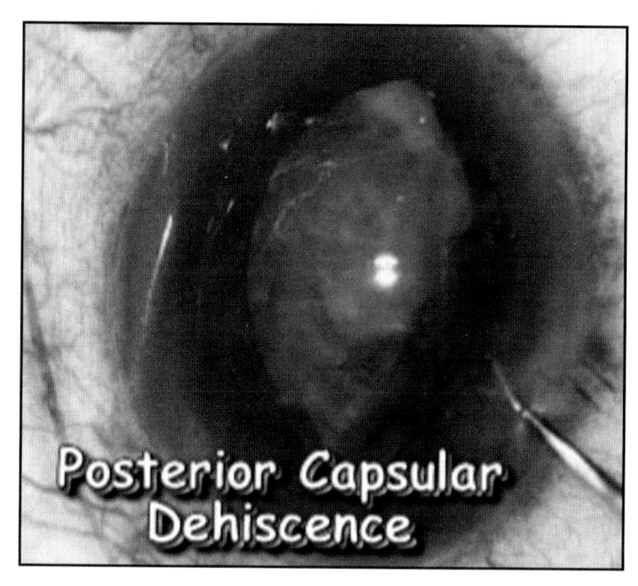

Figure 19-2. Posterior capsular dehiscence. Note the nucleus is subluxated and might fall into the vitreous cavity. (Photo courtesy of Dr. Agarwal's Eye Hospital.)

Another alternative is the injection of sulfur hexafluoride gas,[14] which may be used at the time of surgery or afterward if you notice a detachment postoperatively. The risk is the IOP increase, so it is mandatory to monitor it. A very good description of the procedure has been done by Dr. Fishkind.[15] A new technique for intracameral gas injection that can be performed by one person at the slit lamp microscope or in a minor operating room with minimal equipment has been described.[16]

Capsulorrhexis-Related Complications

The anterior continuous curvilinear capsulorrhexis (CCC) should be capable of preserving the integrity of the capsular bag against the asymmetric forces that occur during phacoemulsification (especially during modern endocapsular techniques) and IOL implantation.

In regard to the surgeon's control, a larger diameter capsulorrhexis is more challenging because the anterior capsular contour more rapidly slopes away from the instrument as it moves toward the periphery. Because of this, a smaller rhexis should be attempted if difficulty with visualization or control is encountered. If necessary, you may enlarge it, a maneuver that is safer to perform when the IOL is already in place. Always remember that when in the periphery, the capsulorrhexis tear can encounter a zonular attachment that can work as a straight edge, sending the tear out to the capsular fornix and possibly around and through the posterior capsule. Once an errant tear begins to extend radially, it becomes much harder to control.

If you are not careful, you can end up with a posterior capsular dehiscence (Figure 19-2). An IOL can get dislocated with nuclear fragments if there is a rupture (Figure 19-3). A retinal detachment might occur postoperatively in such cases as well (Figure 19-4).

Zonular Problems

Weakened zonules will dehisce more easily. Forceful maneuvers of the nucleus may shear zonules. Aspirating the anterior capsule or adherent lens material may break the

Figure 19-3. Posterior capsular rupture. Note the IOL sinking into the vitreous cavity. The white reflex indicates nuclear fragments also in the vitreous cavity. This patient was managed by vitrectomy, FAVIT (removal of the nuclear fragments) and the IOL repositioned in the sulcus. (Photo courtesy of Dr. Agarwal's Eye Hospital.)

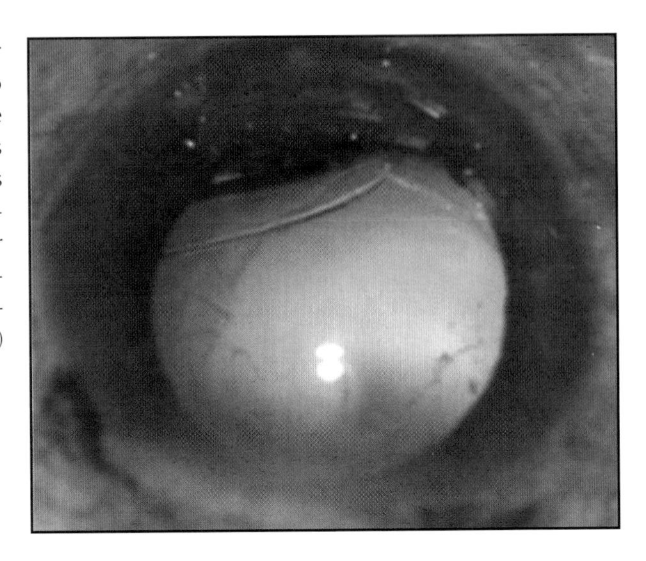

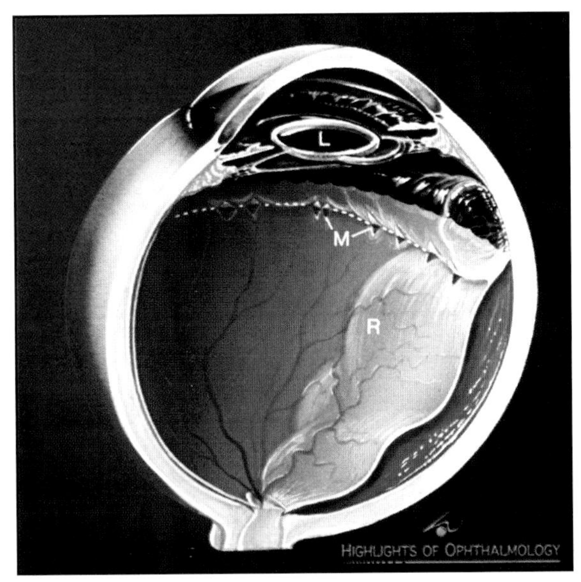

Figure 19-4. Difference between phakic and pseudophakic detachments. Classic pseudophakic retinal detachments differ from phakic retinal detachments in two major ways. Retinal detachments (R) with an intraocular lens (L) following cataract surgery are usually associated with more anteriorly located multiple breaks (M) along the posterior margin of the vitreous base (dotted line). Also with pseudophakos, these types of breaks tend to be in multiple quadrants. On the other hand, phakic detachments often tend to involve a single quadrant with one tear. The second major difference between phakic and pseudophakic detachments is in the reduced ability of the surgeon to see the peripheral retina in the case of pseudophakos (not shown). (Courtesy of Benjamin F. Boyd, Ed. *The Art and the Science of Cataract Surgery*. Highlights of Ophthalmology. English Edition, 2001.)

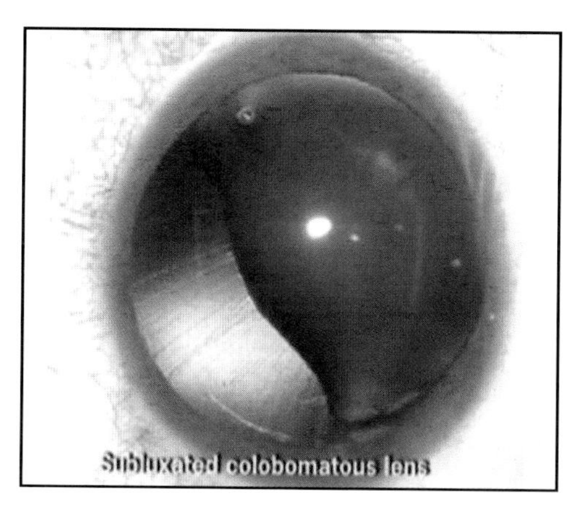

Figure 19-5. Subluxated colobomatous lens. The patient was managed with a Cionni endocapsular ring. (Photo courtesy of Dr. Lincoln L. Freitas.)

zonules in that location. Stripping the cortex tangentially rather than radially helps to distribute this force upon as large an area of zonules as possible. Moreover, inadequate zonular tension allows trampolining of the flaccid posterior capsule during epinuclear and cortical cleanup.

Hydrodissection is a crucial step in avoiding stress applied to zonules, and cortical cleaving as described by Fine,[32] loosens the adhesion of the cortex to the capsule. The more easily the cortex separates from the capsule, the less likely a floppy capsule will be pulled toward the aspirating instrument tip. Insertion of a capsular tension ring (CTR) is of tremendous help in the presence of zonular laxity. Figure 19-5 shows a case of subluxated colobomatous lens in whom a CTR was used.

Corneal Edema

When you note during the surgery that the cornea turns opaque or whitish, check the irrigation bottle, because sometimes it may happen due to a big mistake: changing of the BSS by NSS or worse by distilled water. The cornea may develop pseudophakic bullous keratopathy after cataract surgery, once the endothelial cell function and the endothelial cell population have been reduced to a significant level. A cell count of less than 600–800 per square millimeters, a pachymetry reading of more than 650 mm, morning edema, or epithelial microcyst may signal imminent decompensation of the cornea. In patients without IOLs, early signs of low corneal reserve may include thickening of the cornea, guttata, or mild Descemet folds.

Causes of a preoperatively compromised endothelium may include:[82]

- Advanced age
- Fuchs' dystrophy
- Previous intraocular surgery
- An attack of acute angle-closure glaucoma or trauma to the eye involving corneal injury or a flat anterior chamber
- A history of anterior uveitis

The already diminished preoperative endothelial cell population may be even more reduced by surgery, which may precipitate postoperative corneal edema. The average cell loss reported following cataract or implant surgery has varied widely, from 4% to 17% depending upon the expertise of the surgeon, the technique, and the type of viscoelastic used.[48–50]

If a patient exhibits corneal guttata or has a history of one of these problems, corneal pachymetry and specular microscopy should be performed preoperatively to evaluate the risk of surgery in relation to corneal decompensation. With this information, the physician can better explain to the patient the risks of postoperative corneal decompensation. The clinician should examine the eye closely for IOL endothelial touch or a detached Descemet's membrane, which demands surgical correction.

Agarwal suggests the preoperative use of a specular microscope in all cases. If the cell count is low, he suggests performing an ECCE.

Key Points

1. Measures that serve to cause the least wound distortion and so the least needle/sleeve/tissue compression, include: temporal approach, avoiding an excessively long corneal tunnel, and minimizing excess lifting or depression of the handpiece.
2. The best way to rescue a rhexis extending to the periphery is to refill the anterior chamber, fold the flap over the anterior capsule for better visualization, regrasp it close to the leading edge of the tear, and pull centripetally, rather firmly.
3. Beware of weak zonules, however, even the lower epinuclear vacuum setting may be too high if the zonules are lax. This is because the posterior capsule is able to "trampoline" toward the phaco tip if the weakened zonules do not keep it taut, and vacuum and flow must be lowered even further in this event.
4. Pseudoexfoliation syndrome, especially when significant zonular instability is present, poses a challenge in regard with long-term stability. Significant capsule phimosis despite ring placement in PXF cases can also occur.
5. In mature cataracts, damage to the corneal endothelium is still a concern and the surgeon must be very careful. Phaco in mature or hypermature cataracts is not for beginners. It is always better to do specular microscopy preoperatively.
6. Agarwal suggests the preoperative use of a specular microscope in all cases. If the cell count is low, he suggests performing an ECCE.

References

1. Lane S, Fine H. Perspectives in lens & IOL surgery. Getting to the bottom of clear cornea incisions—Part I. *Eye World*. October 2004.
2. Majid MA, Sharma MK, Harding SP. Corneoscleral burn during phacoemulsification surgery. *J Cataract Refract Surg*. 1998;24:1413.
3. Berger JW, Talamo JH, LaMarche KJ, et al. Temperature measurements during phacoemulsification and erbium:YAG laser phacoablation in model systems. *J Cataract Refract Surg*. 1996;22:372.
4. Bissen-Miyajima H, Shimmura S, Tsubota K. Thermal effect on corneal incisions with different phacoemulsification ultrasonic tips. *J Cataract Refract Surg*. 1999;25(1):60.
5. Tsuneoka H, Takuya S, Takahashi Y. Feasibility of ultrasound cataract surgery with a 1.4 mm incision. *J Cataract Refract Surg*. 2001;27:934.
6. Barrett, G.D. Improved fluid dynamics during phacoemulsification with a new (MicroFlow) needle design. ASCRS Symposium on Cataract, IOL and Refractive Surgery. Washington, USA, 1996.
7. Soscia W, Howard JG, Olson RJ. Bimanual phacoemulsification through 2 stab incisions. A wound-temperature study. *J Cataract Refract Surg*. 2002;28(6):1039.
8. Agarwal A, Agarwal S, Agarwal A. Phakonit: phacoemulsification through a 0.9 mm corneal incision. *J Cataract Refract Surg*. 2001;27:1548.
9. Tsuneoka H, Shiba T, Takahashi Y. Ultrasonic phacoemulsification using a 1.4 mm incision: clinical results. *J Cataract Refract Surg*. 2002;28:81.
10. Ernest P, Rhem M, McDermott M, Lavery K, Sensoli A. Phacoemulsification conditions resulting in thermal wound injury. *J Cataract Refract Surg*. 2001;27(11):1829.
11. Chang DF. Pars plana vitreous tap for phacoemulsification in the crowded eye. *J Cataract Refract Surg*. 2001;27:1911.
12. Cionni RJ, Barros M, Osher R. Management of lens-iris diaphragm retropulsion syndrome during phacoemulsification. *J Cataract Refract Surg*. 2004;30:953.
13. Vastine DW, Weinberg RS, Sugar J, Binder PS. Stripping of Descemet's membrane associated with intraocular lens implantation. *Arch Ophthalmol*. 1983;101(7):1042.
14. Ellis DR, Cohen KL. Sulfur hexafluoride gas in the repair of Descemet's membrane detachment. *Cornea*. 1995;14(4):436.
15. Fishkind WJ. Facing down the 5 most common cataract complications. *Review of Ophthalmology*. October 2001.
16. Kim T, Hasan SA. A new technique for repairing descemet membrane detachments using intracameral gas injection. *Arch Ophthalmol*. 2002;120:181.
17. Jeng BH, Hoyt CS, McLeod SD. Completion rate of continuous curvilinear capsulorhexis in pediatric cataract surgery using different viscoelastic materials. *J Cataract Refract Surg*. 2004;30(1):85.
18. Arshinoff SA. Dispersive-cohesive viscoelastic soft shell technique. *J Cataract Refract Surg*. 1999;25:167.
19. Horiguchi M, Miyake K, Ohta I, Ito Y. Staining of the lens capsule for circular continuous capsulorrhexis in eyes with white cataract. *Arch Ophthalmol*. 1998;116:535.
20. Melles G, de Waard P, Pameyer J, Beekhuis W. Trypan blue capsule staining to visualize the capsulorhexis in cataract surgery. *J Cataract Refract Surg*. 1999;25:7.
21. Dada V, Sharma N, Sudan R, Sethi H, Dada T, Pangtey MS. Anterior capsule staining for capsulorhexis in cases of white cataract: comparative clinical study. *J Cataract Refract Surg*. 2004;30:326.
22. Arshinoff SA. Using BSS with viscoadaptives in the ultimate soft-shell technique. *J Cataract Refract Surg*. 2002;28:1509.
23. Conner C. Rescuing an errant capsulorrhexis. Available at: www.ophthalmic.hyperguides.com.
24. Seibel BS. *Phacodynamics: Mastering the Tools and Techniques of Phacoemulsification Surgery*. 3rd ed. Thorofare, NJ: SLACK Incorporated; 1999.

25. Wilbrandt H. Comparative analysis of the fluidics of the AMO Prestige, Alcon, Legacy, and Storz Premiere phacoemulsification system. *J Cataract Refract Surg*. 1997;23:766.
26. Mackool R. Advancing phaco technology: an overview of the new Infiniti lens removal system. *Cataract and Refractive Surgery Today*, May 2003.
27. Chang DF. *Transition to Bimanual Microincisional Phaco*. Panama: Highlights of Ophthalmology; 2005.
28. Vejarano LF, Tello A, Vejarano A. The safest and most effective technique for cataract surgery. *Highlights of Ophthalmology*. 2004;32(2):13.
29. Vejarano LF, Tello A. Fluidics in Phakonit. In: Agarwal A, ed. *Bimanual Phaco: Mastering the Phakonit /MICS Technique*. Thorofare, NJ: SLACK Incorporated; 2004.
30. Chang DF. 400 mm Hg high vacuum bimanual phaco attainable with the Staar cruise control device. *J Cataract Refract Surg*. 2004;30:932.
31. Chang DF. *Phaco Chop: Mastering Techniques, Optimizing Technology, and Avoiding Complications*. Thorofare, NJ: SLACK Incorporated; 2004.
32. Fine IH. Cortical cleaving hydrodissection. *J Cataract Refract Surg*. 1992;18:508.
33. Witschel BM, Legler U. New approaches to zonular cases; the capsular ring. *Audiovisual J Cataract Implant Surg*. 1993;9(4).
34. Bayraktar S, Altan T, Kucuksumer Y, Yilmaz OF. Capsular tension ring implantation after capsulorhexis in phacoemulsification of cataracts associated with pseudoexfoliation syndrome. Intraoperative complications and early postoperative finding. *J Cataract Refract Surg*. 2001;27:1620.
35. D'Eliseo D, Pastena B, Longanesi L, et al. Prevention of posterior capsule opacification using capsular tension ring for zonular defects in cataract surgery. *Eur J Ophthalmol*. 2003;13:151.
36. Merriam JC, Zheng L. Iris hooks for phacoemulsification of the subluxated lens. *J Cataract Refract Surg*. 1997;23:1295.
37. Lee V, Bloom P. Microhook capsule stabilization for phacoemulsification in eyes with pseudoexfoliation-syndrome-induced lens instability. *J Cataract Refract Surg*. 1999;25:1567.
38. Mackool RJ. Capsule stabilization for phacoemulsification (letter). *J Cataract Refract Surg*. 2000;26:629.
39. Chang DF. Capsular tension rings versus capsule retractors. Stabilizing the weakened capsular bag during phacoemulsification. *Cataract and Refractive Surgery Today*. January 2004.
40. Cionni RJ, Osher RH. Management of profound zonular dialysis for weakness with a new endocapsular ring designed for scleral fixation. *J Cataract Refract Surg*. 1998;24:1299.
41. Cionni RJ. Suture fixation of the capsular bag. *Cataract and Refractive Surgery Today*. May 2004.
42. Maloney WF, Dillman DM, Nichamin LD. Supracapsular phacoemulsification: a capsule-free posterior chamber approach. *J Cataract Refract Surg*. 1997;23(3):323.
43. Koch PS, Katzen LE. Stop and chop phacoemulsification. *J Cataract Refract Surg*. 1994;20:566.
44. Chang DF. *Phaco Chop Techniques: Comparing Horizontal vs Vertical Chop*. Panama: Highlights of Ophthalmology; 2004.
45. Faschinger CW, Eckhardt M. Complete capsulorhexis opening occlusion despite capsular tension ring implantation. *J Cataract Refract Surg*. 1999;25:1013.
46. Masket S, Osher RH. Late complications with intraocular lens dislocation after capsulorhexis in pseudoexfoliation syndrome. *J Cataract Refract Surg*. 2002;28:1481.
47. Jehan FS, Mamalis N, Crandall AS. Spontaneous late dislocation of intraocular lens within the capsular bag in pseudoexfoliation patients. *Ophthalmology*. 2001;108:1727.
48. Zetterstrom C, Laurell CG. Comparison of endothelial cell loss and phacoemulsification energy during endocapsular phacoemulsification surgery. *J Cataract Refract Surg*. 1995;21(1):55.
49. Kreisler KR, Mortenson SW, Mamalis N. Endotelial cell loss following "modern" phacoemulsification by a senior resident. *Ophthalmic Surg*. 1992;23:158.
50. O'Brien PD, Fitzpatrick P, Kilmartin D J, Beatty S. Risk factors for endothelial cell loss after phacoemulsification surgery by a junior resident. *J Cataract Refract Surg*. 2004;30:839.

51. Sugar J, Mitchelson J, Kraff M. Endothelial cells trauma and intraocular lens insertion. *Arch Ophthalmol.* 1978;96:449.
52. Balyeat HD, Nordquist RE, Lerner MP, Gupta A. Comparison of endothelial damage produced by control and surface modified poly (methyl methacrylate) intraocular lenses. *J Cataract Refract Surg.* 1989;15(5):491.
53. Werner LP, Legeais JM, Durand J, Savoldelli M, Legeay G, Renard G. Endothelial damage caused by uncoated and fluorocarbon-coated poly(methyl methacrylate) intraocular lenses. *J Cataract Refract Surg.* 1997;23(7):1013.
54. Kraff MC, Sanders DR, Lieberman HL. Endothelial cell loss and trauma during intraocular lens implantation: A specular microscopic study. *Am Intraocular Implant Soc J.* 1978;4(3):107.
55. Balazs EA, Freeman MI, Klo¨ti R, et al. Hyaluronic acid and replacement of vitreous and aqueous humor. *Mod Prob Ophthalmol.* 1972;10:3.
56. Miller D, Stegmann R. Use of sodium hyaluronate in human IOL. Implantation. *Ann Ophthalmol.* 1981;13:7:811.
57. Stegmann R, Miller D. Extracapsular cataract extraction with hyaluronate sodium. *Ann Ophthalmol.* 1982;14(9):813.
58. Soll DB, Harrison SE. The use of chondroitin sulfate in protection of the corneal endothelium. *Ophthalmology.* 1981;88(Suppl):51.
59. Aron-Rosa D, Cohn HC, Aron JJ, Boquety C. Methylcellulose instead of Healon in extracapsular surgery with intraocular lens implantation. *Am Acad Ophthalmol.* 1983;90:1235.
60. Miller D, Stegmann R. Use of Na-hyaluronate in anterior segment eye surgery. *Am Intra-Ocular Implant J.* 1980;6:13.
61. Kerr Muir MG, Sherrard ES, Andrews V, Steele AD. Air, methylcellulose, sodium hyaluronate and the corneal endothelium. Endothelial protective agents. *Eye.* 1987;1(Pt 4):480.
62. Harfstrand A, Stenevi U, Schenholm M, et al. Sodium hyaluronate on the corneal endothelium. *Implant Ophthalmol.* 1990;4:83.
63. Rafuse PE, Nichols BD. Effects of Healon vs. Viscoat on endothelial cell count and morphology after phacoemulsification and posterior chamber lens implantation. *Can J Ophthalmol.* 1992;27(3):125.
64. Holzer MP, Tetz MR, Auffarth GU, et al. Effect of Healon 5 and 4 other viscoelastic substances on intraocular pressure and endothelium after cataract surgery. *J Cataract Refract Surg.* 2001;27:213.
65. Holmen J JB, Lundgren B. Scheimpflug photography study of ophthalmic viscosurgical devices during simulated cataract surgery. *J Cataract Refract Surg.* 2003;29(3):568.
66. Kiss B, Findl O, Menapace R, et al. Corneal endothelial cell protection with a dispersive viscoelastic material and an irrigating solution during phacoemulsification: low-cost versus expensive combination. *J Cataract Refract Surg.* 2003;29(4):733.
67. Miyata K, Namamoto T, Maruoka S, et al. Efficacy and safety of the soft-shell technique in cases with a hard lens nucleus. *J Cataract Refract Surg.* 2002;28:1546.
68. Behndig A, Lundberg B. Transient corneal edema after phacoemulsification: comparison of 3 viscoelastic regimens. *J Cataract Refract Surg.* 2002;28:1551.
69. Kim H, Joo CK. Efficacy of the soft-shell technique using Viscoat and Hyal–2000. *J Cataract Refract Surg.* 2004;30:2366.
70. Kim EK, Cristol SM, Geroski DH, et al. Corneal endothelial damage by air bubbles during phacoemulsification. *Arch Ophthalmol.* 1997;115:81.
71. Kim EK, Cristol S, Kang SJ, et al. Viscoelastic protection from endothelial damage by air bubbles. *J Cataract Refract Surg.* 2002;28:1047.
72. Kraff MC, Sanders DR, Lieberman HL. Specular microscopy in cataract and intraocular lens patients: a report of 564 cases. *Arch Ophthalmol.* 1980;98:1782.
73. Alió JL, Mulet ME, Shalaby AMM, Attia WH. Phacoemulsification in the anterior chamber. *J Cataract Refract Surg.* 2002;28:67.

74. Pirazzoli G, D'Eliseo D, Ziosi M, Acciarri R. Effects of phacoemulsification time on the corneal endothelium using phacofracture and phaco chop techniques. *J Cataract Refract Surg.* 1996;22(7):967.
75. Bourne RR, Minassian DC, Dart JK, Rosen P, Kaushal S, Wingate N. Effect of cataract surgery on the corneal endothelium: modern phacoemulsification compared with extracapsular cataract surgery. *Ophthalmology.* 2004;111(4):679.
76. Mannis MJ, Miller RB, Carlson EC, Hinds D, May DR. Effect of hypothermic perfusion on corneal endothelial morphology. *Br J Ophthalmol.* 1983;67:804.
77. McCarey BE, Edelhauser HF, Van Horn DL. Functional and structural changes in the corneal endothelium during in vitro perfusion. *Invest Ophthalmol.* 1973;12;6:410.
78. Edelhauser HF, Van Horn DL, Hydiuk RA, Schultz RO. Intraocular irrigating solutions: their effect on the corneal endothelium. *Arch Ophthalmol.* 1975;93:648.
79. Araie M. Barrier function of corneal endothelium and the intraocular irrigating solutions. *Arch Ophthalmol.* 1986;104(3):435.
80. Samuel MA, Desai UR, Strassman I, Abusamak M. Intraocular irrigating solutions. A clinical study of BSS Plus and dextrose bicarbonate fortified BSS as an infusate during pars plana vitrectomy. *Indian J Ophthalmol.* 2003;51(3):237.
81. Vejarano LF, Tello A. Outcomes with the ThinOptx IOL. Using the lens as part of microincisional cataract surgery. *Cataract & Refractive Surgery Today.* September 2004, 84.
82. Lindstrom RL, Smith SG. Corneal complications alter cataract surgery. Available on: www.ophthalmic.hyperguides.com.
83. Shepherd DM. The pupil stretch technique for miotic pupils in cataract surgery. *Ophthalmic Surg.* 1993;24:851–852.
84. Chang DF, Campbell JR. Intraoperative floppy iris syndrome associated with tamsulosin. *J Cataract Refract Surg.* 2005;31:664.
85. Oetting TA, Omphroy LC. Modified technique using flexible iris retractors in clear corneal surgery. *J Cataract Refract Surg.* 2002;28:596.
86. Smith GT, Liu CSC. Flexible iris hooks for phacoemulsification in patients with iridoschisis. *J Cataract Refract Surg.* 2000;26:1277.
87. Kershner RM. The Perfect Pupil Device and small pupil management. Available on: www.ophthalmic.hyperguides.com.
88. De Juan E Jr, Hickingbotham D. Flexible iris retractor [letter]. *Am J Ophthalmol.* 1991;111:776.
89. Nichamin LD. Enlarging the pupil for cataract extraction using flexible nylon iris retractors. *J Cataract Refract Surg.* 1993;19:793.
90. Graether JM. Graether pupil expander for managing the small pupil during surgery. *J Cataract Refract Surg.* 1996;22:530.
91. Kershner RM. Management of the small pupil for clear corneal cataract surgery. *J Cataract Refract Surg.* 2002;28:1826.
92. Nagahara K. Phaco-chop Technique Eliminates Central Sculping and Allows Faster Safer Phaco. *Ocular Surgery News International Edition.* 1993, pp. 12–13.
93. Vejarano LF, Tello A. Vejarano Safe Chop Makes Transition to Chopper Easier. *Ocular Surgery News.* March 2005.
94. Olson RJ. Micro phaco chop: rationales and technique. In: Chang DF, ed. *Phaco Chop: Mastering Techniques, Optimizing Technology and Avoiding Complications.* Thorofare, NJ: SLACK Incorporated; 2004.
95. Fry LL. Miscellaneous Surgical Procedures I Have Found Helpful. Presented at: Film Festival Symposium on Cataract, IOL, and Refractive Surgery; May, 1993; Seattle, Washington.

Chapter 20

Iatrogenic Descemetorhexis as a Complication of Phacoemulsification

Amar Agarwal, MS, FRCOphth, FRCS; Soosan Jacob, MS, DNB, FRCS, MNAMS, FERC; Ashok Kumar, MD, DO, FERC; Athiya Agarwal, MD, DO; Sunita Agarwal, MS, FSVH, DO

Introduction

The corneal endothelium is composed of a single layer of polygonal cells. Corneal transparency is maintained by the corneal endothelium. The corneal endothelium forms a physical barrier preventing aqueous from freely entering the cornea. It maintains the cornea in a dehydrated state by the active pumping action of the cells, mediated by the Na^+/K^+-ATPase,[1–5] and thus maintains the corneal transparency.

Endothelial Cell Count

Endothelial cell count in a normal human adult cornea is between 2000 and 2500 cells/mm^2. Corneal endothelial damage due to surgery, trauma, or underlying disease leads to corneal edema and loss of visual acuity. Loss of corneal transparency occurs when endothelial cell density is reduced below 500 cells/mm^2. This situation frequently results in the patient requiring a corneal transplant.

Iatrogenic Descemetorhexis

A 65-year-old woman presented to us with complaints of decreased vision in the left eye of 6 months duration. She gave a history of cataract surgery in the right eye 1 month back. Available records showed intraoperative posterior capsular rupture with secondary anterior chamber intraocular lens (ACIOL) implantation 1 week later. The patient had intermittent iritis in the eye. She also gave a history of glaucoma diagnosis and was on topical Betaxolol 0.5% twice daily. Examination of the patient revealed a best corrected visual acuity (BCVA) of finger counting at 1 meter in the right eye and 20/32 (6/9) in the left eye. Intraocular pressure (IOP) by applanation tonometry was 20 and 22 mmHg, respectively. Slit lamp examination showed a healed corneoscleral scar superiorly and pigmented keratic precipitates inferiorly. The pupil was distorted and an ACIOL was seen along with evidence of a posterior

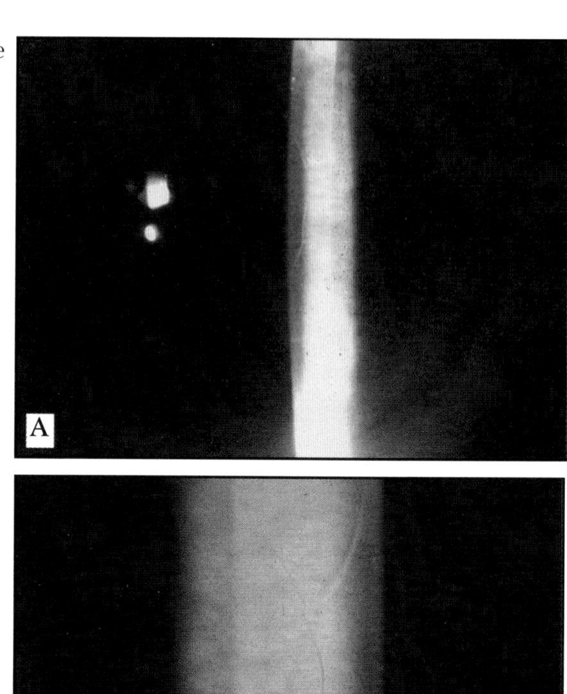

Figure 20-1 A,B. Margins of the descemetorhexis.

capsular rupture. The left eye showed peripheral cortical cataract with Grade II nuclear sclerosis. Fundus examination revealed a 0.8 cup to disc ratio through a hazy media in the right eye and 0.7 cup to disc ratio with a thin neuro-retinal rim and other evidence of glaucomatous changes in the left eye.

The patient was scheduled for superior trabeculectomy with temporal clear corneal phacoemulsification with foldable IOL implantation in the left eye. During surgery, after the superficial scleral flap for the trabeculectomy, the clear corneal temporal incision for phaco was made. The side-port incision was next made with a 26 gauge needle and viscoelastic was accidentally injected into the corneal stromal layers. As the surgeon (Am A) did not recognize this complication, a rhexis was performed in the space created by the viscoelastic substance. On attempting hydrodissection, the surgeon realized that the anterior lens capsule was intact and that he had inadvertently performed a "Descemetorhexis". Subsequently, a capsulorrhexis was performed and remainder of the phacoemulsification and the trabeculectomy were completed uneventfully. On the first postoperative day, the entire cornea was hazy with an IOP of 17 mmHg. Specular microscopy couldn't be done as it was not available at the time. The patient was kept on close follow-up and 1 month later, she had a BCVA of 20/20p (6/6p), N6 in the left eye and a pachymetry of 560 microns in the right eye and 556 microns in the left eye. The margins of the Descemetorhexis could be clearly seen at this time (Figure 20–1). The patient presented 6 months later with complaints of hazy vision in the left eye, which was determined to be due to a posterior capsular opacification. A YAG capsulotomy was done and this restored her vision to 20/20p

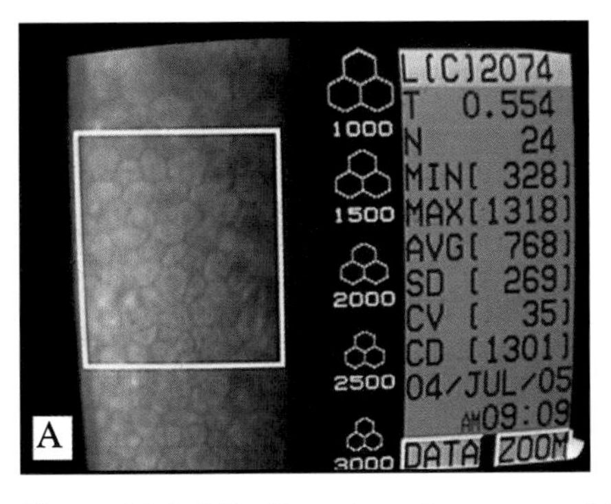

Figure 20-2 A,B. Specular microscopy of the corneal endothelium.

Table 20-1.

Specular Microscopy Evaluation of Corneal Endothelium

	Cell count	*Cell area*	*Range of cell area*	*Coefficient of variation*	*Pachymetry (Microns)*
Right eye	744	1344 1/2 542	484–2271	40	552
Left eye	1301	768 1/2 269	328–1318	35	554

(6/6p), N6. The patient's next visit was 1.5 years later, at which time her BCVA continued to remain 20/20p (6/6p) in the left eye with a clear cornea and the margins of the descemetorhexis being seen.

Polymegathism

The numerical density of endothelial cells in the central cornea (cells/mm^2) was estimated on photomicrographs taken with a noncontact specular microscope using the fixed frame technique (Figure 20–2). The cell count was 744 and 1301 in the right eye and left eye, respectively. There was evidence of pleomorphism and polymegathism (Table 20–1). Ultrasound pachymetry was 550 microns in the right eye and 560 microns in the left eye. IOP was under control without any medications. The patient remained satisfied with her vision in the left eye and had no specific complaints regarding the left eye.

Discussion

Descemet's membrane injury or stripping is a complication that has been known to occur in phacoemulsification surgery. It may occur due to the use of a blunt keratome or if the angle at which the anterior chamber is entered is too shallow. A blunt blade may catch the Descemet's membrane and pull it instead of sharply incising it. A small detachment while making the anterior chamber entry may later develop into a larger one if caught by the phaco or irrigation/aspiration (I/A) tip. Extension may also occur if irrigating solution or viscoelastic is forcibly pushed under a small detachment. Some patients have a weaker attachment of Descemet's membrane to the underlying stroma and such eyes may be more prone to develop a Descemet's detachment during surgery. Generally, injection of an air bubble at the end of surgery results in reattachment of Descemet's membrane. Accidental removal of Descemet's membrane and overlying endothelium will result in irreversible corneal decompensation. Descemet's detachment during surgery is a very commonly described complication and can be handled in most cases by injection of air into the anterior chamber at the end of surgery. In larger detachments, it may be necessary to suture it in place. In cases where it doesn't remain in place despite these measures, SF6 gas may be used intracamerally either intraoperatively or postoperatively. Once the membrane is up against the stroma, the endothelial pump sucks it in place. The expansile nature of SF6[6] helps to keep the Descemet's membrane in place. IOP must be monitored and some of the gas must be released to drop the IOP down to a normal level. Staining of the Descemet's membrane detachment can be done with trypan blue injected into the anterior chamber.

An iatrogenic descemetorhexis is an extremely rare complication.[7] Our case had a hazy cornea immediately postoperatively along with corneal edema, both of which had resolved by 1 month postoperatively and continued to remain clear at the 2-year postoperative follow-up. This is due to the reformed endothelial cell layer due to spreading and enlargement of the remaining endothelial cells.

The endothelial cell count averages[8] around 3000 cells/mm^2 at birth and then slowly declines with age.[9,10] The corneal thickness is also maximum at birth and then steadily decreases in thickness till the age of 3.[11,12] There is an insignificant decrease in corneal thickness after the age of 3.[13–18] A minimum endothelial count of 400–500 cells/mm^2 is required to maintain corneal clarity. As the endothelial cells have a limited capacity to regenerate,[8,19,20] any abnormality in the quantity or quality of corneal endothelial cells leads to corneal decompensation and loss of vision.

Damage to the corneal endothelium during surgery leads to transient edema and an increase in pachymetry. Studies have shown that this may remain so up to 6 months[21,22] or even 1 year postoperatively.[23] In our case, we see that the pachymetry was 556 microns 1 month postoperatively and at 2 years, the corneal endothelial count was 1301 and the corneal thickness was 554 microns. This proves that the ability of the cornea to repair large traumatic defects of Descemet's membrane and the endothelium is greater than we think. It was aided by the fact that the cornea was healthy preoperatively. However, this may not be possible for an already unhealthy cornea. Cornea with preexisting endothelial polymegathism show a slower return to preoperative pachymetry.[24] Previous studies have shown that in the case of a previously diseased endothelium, postoperative corneal edema is greater after 4 days and even at 6 months than in those with a healthy endothelium.[14]

In the previous report of iatrogenic descemetorhexis,[7] two patients were seen presenting 8 months and 5 years after surgery. In both these cases also, after initial corneal decompensation, transparency had improved markedly by the time of presentation. Confocal, slit-scanning videomicroscope of the corneae in these two cases revealed a relatively thick and highly reflective pseudo-Descemet's membrane, almost always covered by endothelial cells with ill-defined borders. Stromal alterations such as discrete edema and highly reflective spots representing detritus were seen.

To the best of our knowledge, this is the first report of the cornea regaining its clarity as early as 1 month after an iatrogenic descemetorhexis. This shows that the corneal endothelium is able to function with the remaining endothelial cells even after losing a large number of these cells. The left-over cells are able to maintain the thickness and clarity of the cornea. Thus we see that a healthy endothelium is able to maintain corneal deturgescence despite having a low endothelial cell count. Corneal thickness increases only when the number of endothelial cells has gone below a minimum physiological limit. Ventura et al[25] also corroborate this by stating that preoperative values of corneal thickness were restored by 3 and 12 months, even though significant endothelial cell losses had occurred. In their study, no correlation was seen between central corneal thickness and central corneal endothelial cell numerical density. Therefore, we see that as long as the endothelial cell count does not fall below the minimum physiological level, a moderate decrease in the count does not affect the endothelial function and does not lead to an increase in corneal thickness.

Key Points

1. The corneal endothelium forms a physical barrier preventing aqueous from freely entering the cornea. It maintains the cornea in a dehydrated state by the active pumping action of the cells, mediated by the Na^1/K^1-ATPase,[1–5] and thus maintains the corneal transparency.
2. Endothelial cell count in a normal human adult cornea is between 1,500 and 2,000 cells/mm^2. Loss of corneal transparency occurs when endothelial cell density is reduced below 500 cells/mm^2.
3. Descemet's detachment during surgery is a very commonly described complication and can be handled in most cases by injection of air into the anterior chamber at the end of surgery. In larger detachments, it may be necessary to suture it in place. In cases where it doesn't remain in place despite these measures, SF6 gas may be used intracamerally either intraoperatively or postoperatively.
4. Staining of the Descemet's membrane detachment can be done with trypan blue injected into the anterior chamber.
5. This is the first report of the cornea regaining its clarity as early as 1 month after an iatrogenic descemetorhexis. This shows that the corneal endothelium is able to function with the remaining endothelial cells even after losing a large number of these cells. The left-over cells are able to maintain the thickness and clarity of the cornea.

References

1. Hodson S. Evidence for a bicarbonate-dependent sodium pump in corneal endothelium. *Exp Eye Res*. 1971;11:20.
2. Maurice DM. The location of the fluid pump in the cornea. *J Physiol*. 1972;221:43.
3. Dikstein S, Maurice DM. The metabolic basis of the fluid pumps in the cornea. *J Physiol*. 221:29.
4. Fischbarg J, Lim JJ. Role of cations, anions and carbonic anhydrase in fluid transport across rabbit corneal endothelium. *J Physiol*. 1974;241:647.
5. Geroski HH, Matsuda M, Yee RW, et al. Pump function of the human corneal endothelium. Effects of age and cornea guttata. *Ophthalmology*. 1985;92:759.
6. Marcon AS, Rapuano CJ, Jones MR, Laibson PR, Cohen EJ. Descemet's membrane detachment after cataract surgery: management and outcome. *Ophthalmology*. 2002;109(12):2325.

7. Altmann G, Tympner J. Confocal corneal in-vivo microscopy in patients having a rhexis of Descemet's membrane. Kuckelkorn Dept. of Ophthalmology, RWTH Aachen, Pauwelsstr. 30, D-52074 Aachen.
8. Waring GO, Bourne WM, Edelhauser HF, et al. The corneal endothelium: normal and pathologic structure and function. *Ophthalmology*. 1982;89:531.
9. Bourne WM, Kaufman HE. Specular microscopy of human corneal endothelium in vivo. *Am J Ophthalmol.* 1976;81:319.
10. Bourne WM, O'Fallon WM. Endothelial cell loss during penetrating keratoplasty. *Am J Ophthalmol.* 1978;85:760.
11. Autzen T, Bjornstrom L. Central corneal thickness in premature babies. *Acta Ophthalmol.* 1991;69:251.
12. Ehlers N, Sorensen T, Bramsen T, et al. Central corneal thickness in newborns and children. *Acta Ophthalmol.* 1976;54:285.
13. Korey M, Gieser D, Kass MA, et al. Central corneal endothelial cell density and central corneal thickness in ocular hypertension and primary open-angle glaucoma. *Am J Ophthalmol.* 1982;94:610.
14. Olsen T. Light scattering from the human cornea. *Invest Ophthalmol Vis Sci*. 1982;23:81.
15. Rapuano CJ, Fishbaugh JA, Strike DJ. Nine point corneal thickness measurements and keratometry readings in normal corneas using ultrasound pachymetry. *Insight*. 1993;18:16.
16. Herse P, Yao W. Variation of corneal thickness with age in young New Zealanders. *Acta Ophthalmol.* 1993;71:360.
17. Li JH, Zhou F, Zhou SA. Research on corneal thickness at multi-points in normal and myopic eyes. *Chung Hua Yen Ko Tsa Chih*. 1994;30:445.
18. Lam AK, Douthwaite WA. The corneal-thickness profile in Hong Kong Chinese. *Cornea*. 1998;17:384.
19. Kaufman HE, Capella JA, Robbins JE. The human corneal endothelium. *Am J Ophthalmol.* 1966;61:835.
20. Capella JA. Regeneration of endothelium in diseased and injured corneas. *Am J Ophthalmol.* 1972;74:810.
21. Olsen T. Corneal thickness and endothelial damage after intracapsular cataract extraction. *Acta Ophthalmol.* 1980;58:424.
22. Olsen T, Eriksen JS. Corneal thickness and endothelial damage after intraocular lens implantation. *Acta Ophthalmol.* 1980;58:773.
23. Kohlhaas M, Stahlhut O, Tholuck J, et al. Changes in corneal thickness and endothelial cell density after cataract extraction using phacoemulsification. *Ophthalmologe*. 1997;94:515.
24. Rao GN, Shaw EL, Arthur EJ, et al. Endothelial cell morphology and corneal deturgescence. *Ann Ophthalmol.* 1979;11:885.
25. Sobottka Ventura AC, Wälti R, Böhnke M, et al. Corneal thickness and endothelial density before and after cataract surgery. *Br J Ophthalmol.* 2001;85:18.

Chapter 21

Posterior Capsule Rupture

L. Felipe Vejarano, MD; Alejandro Tello, MD

Introduction

One of the purposes of modern cataract surgery is to maintain the integrity of the posterior capsule, not only to support the intraocular lens (IOL), but to diminish the incidence of retinal complications like cystoid macular edema and retinal detachment.[1–74] Rupture of the posterior capsule and vitreous prolapse have been reported to occur in a wide range of incidence, from 0.45 to 8.22% of procedures performed by experienced surgeons.[1–6] The incidence of dislocation of lens fragments into the vitreous cavity has been reported between 0.06 % and 0.20%.[6,52]

Anterior Chamber Depth

Working space is an important issue in intraocular surgery. Variation in the amount of space in the anterior and posterior chambers may result from changes in the intraocular pressure (IOP) due to an alteration in the equilibrium between inflow and outflow of fluid. Diminished inflow may be secondary to insufficient bottle height, tube occlusion or compression, bottle emptying, too tight incisions compressing the irrigation sleeve, or the surgeon moving the phaco tip out of the incision, making the irrigation holes come out of the incision. It is a good habit to depress the foot pedal slightly to position 1 before entering the anterior chamber and to be in continuous irrigation (ie, in position 1) all the time. Excessive outflow may be caused by too high vacuum/flow parameters, or too large incisions with leakage. Another cause is the postocclusion surge. There are also intraocular factors influencing anterior chamber depth, such as fluid misdirection syndrome and suprachoroidal hemorrhage or effusion.[1,7] Dr. Agarwal suggests using the air pump or gas forced infusion to solve all these problems.

Posterior Capsule Rupture Pre-Phacoemulsification

Posterior polar cataracts (especially if calcified) are among high risk cases due to an increased incidence of posterior capsular rent (reported between 7.1 and 40%), attributable to adherence of the cataract to the posterior capsule.[9–16] In these cases, it is very important to look for preoperative signs of posterior capsule rupture, like small amounts of cortical material floating in the anterior vitreous, which may be seen at the slit lamp, moving like a "fish tail" in response to eye movements. Although most of the authors advise performing a very good hydrodelineation without hydrodissection, we have also found it useful, like Fine,[13] to perform gentle hydrodissection, with small amounts of balanced salt solution (BSS) to loosen the nucleus, checking that the posterior fluid wave advances only up to the middle peripheral zone of the lens and does not extend across the site of weakness or possible rupture. For this step, we employ a curved cannula (Katena Products, Inc, Denville, NJ) introduced up to the equator. It may cause the soft nucleus and epinucleus to hydrate and prolapse to the anterior chamber, where they are easily removed with aspiration assisted with slow-motion phacoemulsification. Another option may be to use viscodissection following the hydrodelineation to separate and lift the nucleus, leaving the epinucleus attached to the posterior capsule. Then it will be separated from the posterior plaque again using viscodissection. Avoid excessively increasing the IOP during the viscodissection, performing it slowly.[13] Vasavada described the inside-out hydrodelineation, which he finds useful in these cases.[15] He sculpts a central groove, introduces a specially-designed right-angled cannula through the main incision, and makes it penetrate the right wall of the groove, at a desired depth, causing a separation of epinucleus initiating from the inner portion of it. For epinucleus removal, low parameter aspiration is done.

If you find a hole in the posterior capsule when removing the epinucleus over the posterior plaque, never react by removing the handpiece. Maintain the handpiece irrigation while partially filling the anterior chamber with viscoelastic, and move to foot pedal position "0", but keep the handpiece inside until the anterior chamber is full of viscoelastic. Only at that time should you withdraw the handpiece, to avoid sudden prolapse of the vitreous. If vitreous is present, perform a careful two-port, limbal anterior vitrectomy, or a pars plana anterior vitrectomy.

Posterior Capsule Rupture During Phacoemulsification

Increased nuclear size and density increases the risk of posterior capsule rupture. Maneuvers such as sculpting, rotation (especially in these circumstances, where cortico-capsular adhesions may be present), and cracking all generate some lateral displacement of the nucleus, which applies stress to the capsule and the zonules.[7,8] The epinucleus helps to cushion the posterior capsule against these forces. However, as the endonucleus becomes larger, the epinucleus becomes proportionately thinner and may even be absent. The larger nucleus of a mature cataract is more difficult to bisect, and frequently has a leathery posterior plate, which requires the surgeon to perform maneuvers much closer to the posterior capsule.[7,8] Steinert has described the "viscoelastic vault": stopping phacoemulsification and injecting viscoelastic behind the hard nucleus. This substance functions as an artificial epinucleus to protect the posterior capsule.[7,66]

Another issue in damaging the capsule is the presence of a capsulorrhexis diameter less than 4.7 mm. A small capsulorrhexis poses a higher risk of catching the capsule edge with the phaco tip or the chopper, and moreover during hydrodissection, resistance to flow created by the small rhexis may lead to fluid accumulation behind the nucleus, increasing the pressure inside the bag and precipitating a posterior capsular tear. If the diameter of the rhexis is too small, it is preferable to enlarge it. During hydrodissection, inject fluid slowly, and then push the central nucleus gently to force the fluid behind it out. This maneuver will help in achieving a good hydrodissection, and will diminish the possibility of getting a posterior capsule rupture.

Once a posterior capsular tear occurs, subsequent surgical maneuvers and forces tend to expand its size, sometimes very quickly, so early diagnosis and management of posterior capsule rupture is critical, particularly while there is still nucleus present within the eye because of the risk of a dropped nucleus, the feared complication that was very rarely seen before the phacoemulsification era.

SIX SIGNS

David Chang outlined six signs of early posterior capsule rupture or zonular dehiscence:[7,8]

1. Sudden deepening of the chamber, with momentary expansion of the pupil.
2. Sudden, transitory appearance of a clear red reflex peripherally.
3. Apparent inability to rotate a previously mobile nucleus.
4. Excessive lateral mobility or displacement of the nucleus.
5. Excessive tipping of one pole of the nucleus.
6. Partial descent of the nucleus into the anterior vitreous space.

MANAGEMENT

Capsular Tear

If vitreous is present immediately after the capsular tear, it should not be removed until after the nucleus or nuclear fragments are emulsified, unless it is hindering the extraction of the material or there is vitreous loss through the incision, because it may provide support to keep the nucleus from falling to the posterior segment. If the nucleus is soft, only a small residual amount remains, and there is no vitreous prolapse, the procedure may be continued. If vitreous is already present, special care must be taken for preventing additional vitreous prolapse into the anterior chamber or to the wound. It is vital to avoid mingling vitreous and lens material. The vitreous will preferentially be attracted to the phaco tip, preventing aspiration of fragments, and causing traction, which will be transmitted to the retina, increasing the risk of causing a retinal tear. Unless vitreous can be isolated and compartmentalized away from lens remnants, the phaco handpiece should not be used to complete the removal of the nucleus.[62] In these cases, it is preferable to use the vitrector to remove vitreous and cortex in cutting-vacuum mode. Only if you are sure there is no vitreous should you switch to vacuum without cutting, to facilitate followability.[62] Manipulation of vitreous will increase not only the traction transmitted to the retina but also the inflammation in the posterior segment, and the risk of macular edema (Figure 21-1).

Reduce the Parameters

Lowering aspiration flow rate and decreasing the vacuum will control surge and will allow the bottle to be lowered, diminishing turbulence inside the eye. A slow motion phaco must be done (eg, bottle height 55 cm, flow 18 cc/min, and vacuum 100–150 mmHg). Use dispersive viscoelastics to tamponade the defect, and to move fragments away from it. Place cohesive viscoelastics below the lens nucleus to elevate it into the anterior chamber. It may be necessary to create a paracentesis opposite the incision, through which a hook can loosen and manipulate nuclear fragments into the proper position. Because the emulsification will take place in a viscoelastic filled environment, care must be taken to establish ade-

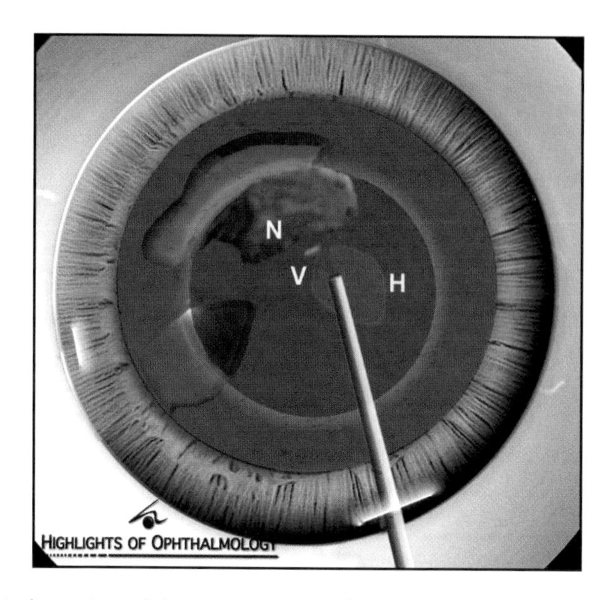

Figure 21-1. A disruption of the posterior capsule (H) is the most severe intraoperative complication. If no immediate action is taken, luxation of nucleus material (N) to the vitreous and retina may occur. If vitreous prolapse is present and it mixes with nucleus fragments, the vitreous should be addressed first. To solve this complication, the surgeon must stop the maneuvers of nucleus removal. Proceed immediately to inject viscoelastic (V) under the nucleus fragments to push the vitreous and lens fragments away from the posterior capsule tear. In this figure, only a "trickle" of viscoelastic (V) is seen between the tear and the nucleus fragments. The rest of the viscoelastic is underneath the nucleus attempting to push it away from the tear. At this time, it is indicated to perform a well-controlled anterior "dry vitrectomy" in which no infusion is used or one with a very low flow system. If abundant nuclear material still remains after these measures are taken, the surgeon may choose between converting to ECCE or very carefully continuing with phacoemulsification, decreasing significantly the phaco power. It depends on the surgeon's experience. (Courtesy of Benjamin F. Boyd, MD, FACS, Ed. *The Art and the Science of Cataract Surgery*. Highlights of Ophthalmology, English Edition, 2001.)

quate flow to avoid wound burn, aspirating for a while to ensure irrigation and aspiration flow, before the onset of phacoemulsification power[62,65] (Figure 21-2). If the rent is significant in size, a IOL Glide (Sheet) or a Phaco-Glide (Bobbit), (Visitec, Sarasota, Florida) can be placed beneath the fragments and the phaco tip.[28] IOL Glide (Sheet) is 5.0 mm wide x 35 mm long, and Phaco-Glide is 2.5 mm wide – tapered to 1.75 mm x 20 mm long. The nucleus should then be emulsified in the anterior chamber. If possible, the IOL can be placed prior to removal of the nuclear fragments.

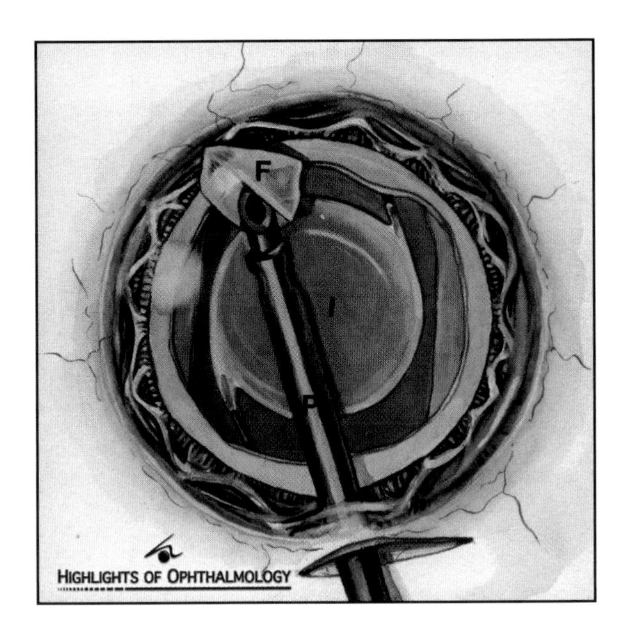

Figure 21-2. In the presence of a large posterior capsule rupture, an anterior vitrectomy is performed. Viscoelastic is infused in the anterior chamber. One alternative is for the lens fragments (F) to be moved or luxated by the surgeon to the anterior chamber with a bimanual maneuver. An IOL (I) is placed in the sulcus to shield the defect. Safe phacoemulsification (P) may continue with very low ultrasound energy. The surgeon may decide not to continue with the phaco technique and convert to ECCE. (Courtesy of Benjamin F. Boyd, ed. *The Art and the Science of Cataract Surgery*. Highlights of Ophthalmology, English Edition, 2001.)

Viscoexpression and Extracapsular Cataract Extraction

Another option to remove nuclear fragments is viscoexpression after enlarging the incision to 4.0 to 6.0 mm. Manual small incision extracapsular cataract extraction (ECCE) and the claw vectis technique using a dry technique, have also been advocated and may be an option to remove residual lens material.[29] If there is a sizeable amount of residual nucleus, and particularly if it is brunescent, it is advisable to convert to a large incision ECCE to minimize the possibility of a dropped nucleus. Viscoelastic should be injected underneath the nucleus to support it. Hydrate, or preferably suture, the temporal corneal or scleral incision and perform a superior scleral incision.

Bimanual Vitrectomy

Once nuclear emulsification or extraction is completed, a bimanual vitrectomy should be performed. This may be accomplished by establishing irrigation by means of a separate 23-gauge cannula through the paracentesis or using the bimanual irrigation port. Using a coaxial vitrector is not recommended because when positioning the tip inside the vitreous, the irrigation sleeve will forcefully inject fluid into the vitreous cavity, mobilizing and displacing the vitreous. The irrigation bottle is positioned at the appropriate height to just maintain the anterior chamber during vitrectomy. Vitrectomy should be performed with a high cutting rate (500 to 800 cuts per minute), an aspiration flow rate of 20 cc/min, and a vacuum of 150–200 mmHg.

Dry Cortical Aspiration

One good alternative is to use dry cortical aspiration with a 23-gauge cannula. If there is only a small amount of vitreous prolapse in the presence of a small capsular rent, a dry vitrectomy can be performed. In this case, a dispersive viscoelastic is first used to fill the anterior chamber. Without an irrigation sleeve, the vitrector is placed through the posterior capsule rent and into the vitreous. A limited vitrectomy is performed using the above parameters. The surgeon should have available the infusion tip or cannula and if the anterior chamber tends to collapse, may introduce any of those for a while and/or diminish the flow rate to 10 cc/min. Viscoelastic volume is augmented as is required, so usually no irrigation is necessary.

Pars Plana Vitrectomy

The other approach, which is gaining popularity and which we have found useful, is to perform a pars plana anterior vitrectomy. This placement may offer advantages such as permitting efficient removal of anterior chamber vitreous by drawing it down posteriorly, often limiting the total amount of vitreous that is removed. In the presence of zonular dehiscence, this approach may be safer because drawing vitreous back down lowers the risk of further unzipping the zonular apparatus.[62]

Viscoat Trap Method

Chang described the "Viscoat Trap" method, which combines the pars plana anterior vitrectomy with the use of a dispersive viscoelastic to keep the lens fragments anteriorly located and immobilized, as the vitrectomy is being carried out below. The viscoelastic filled anterior chamber is isolated from the vitrectomized posterior chamber.[7]

Triamcinolone Acetate

If residual vitreous strands are observed trapped in the phaco wound, use scissors to carefully perform a sponge vitrectomy, or if necessary insert a spatula via the side port, and pass it over the surface of the iris, to release them. Usually they will contract below the pupil; if not, additional dry vitrectomy may be performed. Check the entire anterior chamber for vitreous. Verify that the pupil is round and free of traction (indicating vitreous strands). The usage of the fiber of an endoilluminator, dimming the room lights and microscope lights, may be useful in cases of doubt, in order to identify vitreous strands. Another useful measure is the use of purified triamcinolone acetate suspension (Kenalog) to identify the vitreous described by Peyman[63] and adapted by Burke[64] for use in the anterior segment. Injectable triamcinolone (0.2 mL) (Kenalog) 40 mg/mL is captured in a 5 mm filter of a syringe filter (Sherwood Medical) and rinsed with 2 mL of BSS. It is then resuspended in 5 mL of BSS and recaptured to thoroughly remove the preservative. The Kenalog particles are ultimately resuspended in 2 mL of BSS and injected into the anterior chamber through a 27-gauge cannula. Kenalog particles remain trapped on and within the vitreous gel, making it clearly visible.[64] It is also a therapeutic measure, because although most of the drug is removed during the anterior vitrectomy, enough remains to exert some anti-inflammatory effect in the postoperative period.[62] Preservative-free triamcinolone is available. This vitreous staining method has also been advocated before beginning the vitrectomy to improve visibility.[7]

Dropped Nucleus

One of the most dreadful complications of posterior capsule rupture is a dropped nucleus. Facing this situation, surgeons must be prepared to act accordingly, to minimize the sequelae to the eye. The worst strategy for recovering a descending nucleus is to try to chase and spear the nucleus with the phaco tip.[32,33] The downward fluid infusion will flush more vitreous out, expanding the rent and propelling the nucleus away. Attempting to phacoemulsify or aspirate it may snag vitreous into the tip, potentially leading to retinal tears or detachment. In this situation (with a nucleus immersed in the vitreous cavity), it is better to perform a good anterior vitrectomy, leaving the anterior chamber free of vitreous; implant an IOL if it can be fixated securely in the anterior rhexis or in the sulcus; close the eye and refer the patient to a retina specialist, since a three-port pars plana posterior vitrectomy is required.

Undoubtedly the best strategy is avoiding nuclear material in the posterior segment, so when in front of an impending dropped nucleus it is necessary to take every measure to maintain it in the anterior segment. A good option is to levitate it into the pupillary plane or anterior chamber for extraction through a standard ECCE incision. However, depending upon its size and location, and due to the angle from which the instruments inserted through the phaco incision are approaching, it is often difficult to inject viscoelastic behind the nucleus. This is especially true if the capsulorrhexis is small and intact, if the pupil is small, if vitreous has already prolapsed around the nucleus, or if it has subluxated laterally or posteriorly.

PAL Technique

For this reason, Kelman described the "PAL" technique (posterior assisted levitation) utilizing a cyclodialysis spatula through a pars plana stab incision to push the nucleus up into the anterior chamber from below.[34,38] Packard modified the technique using a Viscoat cannula, inserting it through a pars plana stab incision located 3.5 mm behind the limbus. Viscoat is first slowly injected downward well behind the nuclear piece(s) to provide supplemental support. The nucleus is then elevated into the anterior chamber through a combination of additional Viscoat injection and manipulation of the cannula tip.

FAVIT

A technique described by Agarwal, "FAVIT" is an acronym for a technique to remove **FAll**en nucleus from the **VIT**reous. This can be done while performing phacoemulsification procedure (see Chapter 25).

Intraocular Lens Implantation

The other item that the surgeon must address in these cases is the IOL implantation. If the rupture in the posterior capsule is small and central, the surgeon can fashion a posterior capsulorrhexis and inject a three-piece or a single-piece acrylic posterior chamber IOL into the capsular bag.[62] The single-piece is easier to manipulate in a compromised capsular bag, without causing undue traction forces (Figure 21-3). Suturing of the IOL can also be done. Alternatively, one can use an Artisan IOL.

Summary

Rupture of the posterior capsule is a risk in any phacoemulsification procedure, and surgeons performing this procedure must be prepared to face it. The goal is to diminish the possibility of greater complications, like vitreous traction or dropped nuclear material,

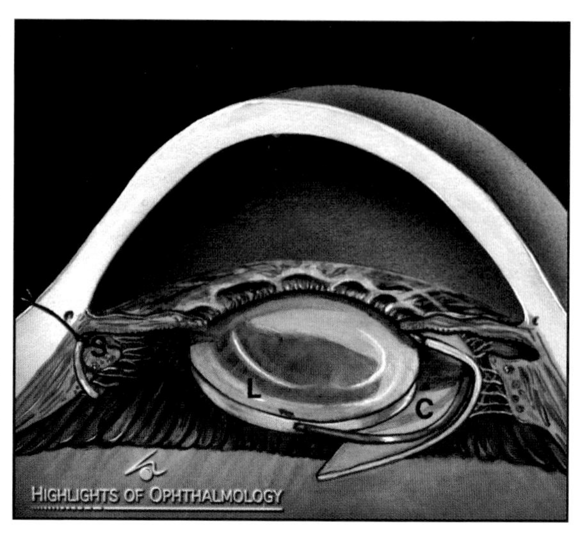

Figure 21-3. A large capsular disruption has occurred, resulting in partial absence of the upper half of the capsular bag. One alternative is for the surgeon to implant the IOL (L) with one haptic in the sulcus (S) above, and the other haptic within the remaining part of the capsular bag (C). The haptic in the sulcus above is secured by a single suture. (Courtesy of Benjamin F. Boyd, MD, FACS, Ed. *The Art and the Science of Cataract Surgery*. Highlights of Ophthalmology, English Edition, 2001.)

which may cause uveitis, macular edema, or retinal detachment, and if possible finish the case with a well-positioned IOL. The likelihood of posterior capsule related complications are higher in difficult cases (advanced cataracts, small pupils, shallow anterior chambers) and in procedures performed by surgeons beginning phacoemulsification, so additional caution is advised in these cases.

Key Points

1. The incidence of posterior capsule complications is related to the type of cataract and conditions of the eye, increases with the grade of difficulty of the case, and furthermore is influenced by the level of experience of the surgeon.
2. When suspecting or discovering a posterior capsule tear, first inject viscoelastic through the side port, avoiding abruptly removing the phaco or I/A tip or irrigating chopper in phakonit, because a sudden collapse of the anterior chamber will cause the posterior capsule to bulge forward and the anterior hyaloid face rupture, which will allow vitreous to prolapse through the defect toward the wound.
3. One approach gaining popularity in these cases is to perform a pars plana anterior vitrectomy, which may offer advantages such as permitting efficient removal of anterior chamber vitreous by drawing it down posteriorly, often limiting the total amount of vitreous that is removed; and in presence of zonular dehiscence lowers the risk of further unzipping the zonular apparatus.
4. In presence of a dropping nucleus, an immediate injection of viscoelastic may be performed by placing a short, disposable 25-gauge needle onto the Viscoat syringe and penetrating the conjunctiva and pars plana 3.5 mm behind the limbus.
5. In case of posterior capsule rent, the goal of all the maneuvers is to remove the remaining nucleus, epinucleus, and as much cortex as possible without causing vitreoretinal traction.
6. If the posterior capsule tear is too large or there is also significant zonular compromise with unreliable capsular support, a three-piece acrylic lens PC IOL may be sutured to the iris or sclera or an Artisan aphakic IOL (formerly known as Worst IOL) may be implanted over or underneath the iris.

References

1. Fishkind WJ. Facing down the 5 most common cataract complications. *Review of Ophthalmology*. October 2001.
2. Misra A, Burton RL. Incidence of intraoperative complications during phacoemulsification in vitrectomized and nonvitrectomized eyes: prospective study. *J Cataract Refract Surg*. 2005;31(5):1011.
3. Androudi S, Brazitikos PD, Papadopoulos NT, Dereklis D, Symeon L, Stangos N. Posterior capsule rupture and vitreous loss during phacoemulsification with or without the use of an anterior chamber maintainer. *J Cataract Refract Surg*. 2004;30(2):449.
4. Stefan C, Nenciu A, Asandi R. [Posterior capsule rupture in lens surgery]. *Oftalmologia*. 2002;55(4):92.
5. Gimbel HV, Sun R, Ferensowicz M, Anderson Penno E, Kamal A. Intraoperative management of posterior capsule tears in phacoemulsification and intraocular lens implantation. *Ophthalmology*. 2001;108(12):2186.
6. Pingree MF, Crandall AS, Olson RJ.Cataract surgery complications in 1 year at an academic institution. *J Cataract Refract Surg*. 1999;25(5):705.
7. Chang DF. *Phaco Chop: Mastering Techniques, Optimizing Technology, and Avoiding Complications*. Thorofare, NJ: SLACK Incorporated; 2004.

8. Chang DF, Conquering Capsule Complications: A Video Primer. Presented at: American Academy of Ophthalmology/PAAO Joint Meeting; 2002; Orlando, Fla.
9. Osher RH, Yu BC, Koch DD. Posterior polar cataracts: a predisposition to intraoperative posterior capsular rupture. *J Cataract Refract Surg*. 1990;16:157.
10. Vasavada AR, Singh R. Phacoemulsification with posterior polar cataract. *J Cataract Refract Surg*. 1999;25:238.
11. Allen D, Wood C. Minimizing risk to the capsule during surgery for posterior polar cataract. *J Cataract Refract Surg*. 2002;28(5):742.
12. Masket S. Posterior polar cataract: an "invitation" to posterior capsular rupture. Supplement to Cataract & Refractive Surgery Today. February 2003.
13. Fine IH, Packer M, Hoffman RS. Management of posterior polar cataract. *J Cataract Refract Surg*. 2003;29:16.
14. Gavris M, Popa D, Caraus C, et al. [Phacoemulsification in posterior polar cataract]. *Oftalmologia*. 2004;48(4):36.
15. Vasavada AR, Raj SM. Inside-out delineation. *J Cataract Refract Surg*. 2004;30(6):1167.
16. Vasavada AR, Raj SM. Approaches to a posterior polar cataract. *Cataract & Refractive Surgery Today*. April 2005.
17. Nichamin LD. Management of a Broken Posterior Capsule and Advanced Vitrectomy Technique. Available at: www.ophthalmic.hyperguides.com.
18. Nichamin LD. Posterior capsule rupture and vitreous loss: advanced approaches. In: Chang DF, ed. *Phaco Chop: Mastering Techniques, Optimizing Technology, and Avoiding Complications*. Thorofare, NJ: SLACK Incorporated; 2004.
19. Martin KR, Burton RL.The phacoemulsification learning curve: pre-operative complications in the first 3000 cases of an experienced surgeon. *Eye*. 2000;14(2):190.
20. Karp KO, Albanis CV, Pearlman JB, Goins KM. Outcomes of temporal clear cornea versus superior scleral tunnel phacoemulsification incisions in a university training program. *Ophthalmic Surg Lasers*. 2001;32(3):228.
21. Seward HC, Dalton R, Davis A. Phacoemulsification during the learning curve: risk/benefit analysis. *Eye*. 1993;7:164.
22. Prince RB, Tax RL, Miller DH. Conversion to small incision phacoemulsification: experience with the first 50 eyes. *J Cataract Refract Surg*. 1993;19:246.
23. Cruz OA, Wallace GW, Gay CA, Matoba AY, Koch DD. Visual results and complications of phacoemulsification with intraocular lens implantation performed by ophthalmology residents. *Ophthalmology*. 1992;99(3):448.
24. Allinson RW, Metrikin DC, Fante RG. Incidence of vitreous loss among third-year residents performing phacoemulsification. *Ophthalmology*. 1992;99:726.
25. Badoza DA, Jure T, Zunino LA, Argento CJ. State-of-the-art phacoemulsification performed by residents in Buenos Aires, Argentina. *J Cataract Refract Surg*. 1999;25:1651.
26. Colleaux KM, Hamilton WK. Effect of prophylactic antibiotics and incision type on the incidence of endophthalmitis after cataract surgery. *Can J Ophthalmol*. 2000;35(7):373.
27. Miller JJ, Scott IU, Flynn HW Jr, Smiddy WE, Newton J, Miller D. Acute-onset endophthalmitis after cataract surgery (2000–2004): incidence, clinical settings, and visual acuity outcomes after treatment. *Am J Ophthalmol*. 2005;139(6):983.
28. Michelson MA. Use of a Sheets' glide as a pseudo-posterior capsule in phacoemulsification complicated by posterior capsule rupture. *Eur J Implant Refract Surg*. 1993;5:70.
29. Akura J, Hatta S, Kaneda S, Ishihara M, Matsuura K, Tamai A. Management of posterior capsule rupture during phacoemulsification using the dry technique. *J Cataract and Refract Surg*. 2001;27:982.
30. Aasuri MK, Kompella VB, Majji AB. Risk factors for and management of dropped nucleus during phacoemulsification. *J Cataract and Refract Surg*. 2001;27:1428.

31. Stilma JS, van der Sluijs FA, van Meurs JC, Mertens DAE. Occurrence of retained lens fragments after phacoemulsification in The Netherlands. *J Cataract and Refract Surg*. 1997;23:1177.
32. Chang DF. Managing residual lens material after posterior capsular rupture. *Techniques in Ophthalmology. 2003;*1(4):201.
33. Lu H, Jiang YR, Grabow HB. Managing a dropped nucleus during the phacoemulsification learning curve. *J Cataract and Refract Surg*. 1999;25:447.
34. Kelman C. New PAL method may save difficult cataract cases. *Ophthalmology Times*. 1994;19:51.
35. Packard R. Technique prevents nucleus drop through capsular tear. *Ocular Surgery News*. 2001;19:14.
36. Chang DF, Packard R. Posterior assisted levitation for nucleus retrieval using Viscoat after posterior capsule rupture. *J Cataract and Refract Surg*. 2003;29:1860.
37. Lal H, Sethi A, Bageja S, Popli J. Chopstik technique for nucleus removal in an impending dropped nucleus. *J Cataract and Refract Surg*. 2004;30:1835.
38. Rao SK, Chan WM, Leung AT, et al. Impending dropped nucleus during phacoemulsification [Letter]. *J Cataract and Refract Surg*. 1999;25:1311.
39. Neuhann TT, Neuhann T. The Rhexis-Fixated Lens. Film methods of IOL optic capture through a capsulorhexis. Presented at the ASCRS Symposium on Cataract, IOL and Refractive Surgery; April 1991; Boston, Massachusetts.
40. Lifshitz T, Levy J. Posterior assisted levitation: long-term follow-up data. *J Cataract and Refract Surg*. 2005;31(3):499.
41. Worst JGF. L'implantation d'un cristallin artificiel (Iris Clip Lens de Binkhorst). *Bull. et Mém. Soc. Française d'Ophtalm*. 1971;84:547.
42. Menezo JL, Martinez MC, Cisneros AL. Iris-fixated Worst claw versus sulcus-fixated posterior chamber lenses in the absence of capsular support. *J Cataract and Refract Surg*. 1996;22(10):1476.
43. Hara T, Hara T. Ten-year results of anterior chamber fixation of the posterior chamber intraocular lens. *Arch Ophthalmol*. 2004;122(8):1112.
44. Oshima Y, Oida H, Emi K. Transscleral fixation of acrylic intraocular lenses in the absence of capsular support through 3.5 mm self-sealing incisions. *J Cataract and Refract Surg*. 1998;24(9):1223.
45. Galvis V, Galvis A, Ossma I. Long-Term Experience with the Artisan Phakic IOL: Safety and Efficacy. Paper presented at the ASCRS Symposium on Cataract, IOL and Refractive Surgery; 2005; Washington.
46. Galvis V, Ossma I, Tello A. Long term follow up of bioptics to correct high myopia. Paper presented at the ASCRS Symposium on Cataract, IOL and Refractive Surgery; 2002; USA.
47. Galvis V. Artisan: Our experience. Presented in the Meeting of the Colombian Ophthalmological Society; 2002; Cartagena, Colombia.
48. Blodi BA, Flynn HW Jr, Blodi CF, et al. Retained nuclei after cataract surgery. *Ophthalmology*. 1992;99:41.
49. Margherio RR, Margherio AR, Pendergast SD, et al. Vitrectomy for retained lens fragments after phacoemulsification. *Ophthalmology*. 1997;104:1426.
50. Kim JE, Flynn HW Jr, Smiddy WE, et al. Retained lens fragments after phacoemulsification. *Ophthalmology*. 1994;101:1827.
51. Borne MJ, Tasman W, Regillo C, et al. Outcomes of vitrectomy for retained lens fragments. *Ophthalmology*. 1996;103:971.
52. Kageyama T, Ayaki M, Ogasawara M, et al. Results of vitrectomy performed at the time of phacoemulsification complicated by intravitreal lens fragments. *Br J Ophthalmol*. 2001;85:1038.
53. Stefaniotou M, Aspiotis M, Pappa C, et al. Timing of dislocated nuclear fragment management after cataract surgery. *J Cataract Refract Surg*. 2003; 29:1985.

54. Scott IU, Flynn HW Jr, Smiddy WE, et al. Clinical features and outcomes of pars plana vitrectomy in patients with retained lens fragments. *Ophthalmology*. 2003;110(8):1567.
55. Kwok AK, Li KK, Lai TY, Lam DS. Pars plana vitrectomy in the management of retained intravitreal lens fragments after cataract surgery. *Clin Experiment Ophthalmol*. 2002;30(6):399.
56. Lai TY, Kwok AK, Yeung YS, et al. Immediate pars plana vitrectomy for dislocated intravitreal lens fragments during cataract surgery. *Eye*. 2004;24; [Epub ahead of print].
57. Teichmann KD. Posterior assisted levitation [letter]. *Surv Ophthalmol*. 2002;47:78.
58. Yan H, Chen J. Peripheral vitreo-retinal traction due to vitreous incarceration at sites of pars plana sclerotomies. Presented at the American Society of Retina Specialist 14th Annual Meeting; 1996; USA.
59. Sabti K, Kapusta M, Mansour M, Overbury O, Chow D. Ultrasound biomicroscopy of sclerotomy sites: the effect of vitreous shaving around sclerotomy sites during pars plana vitrectomy. *Retina*. 2001;21(5):464.
60. Liu W, Huang SY, Zhang P, et al. Bioptic significance of incarcerated contents at sclerotomy sites during vitrectomy. *Retina*. 2004;24(3):407.
61. Al-Harthi E, Abboud E, Al-Dhibi H, Dhindsa, H. Incidence of sclerotomy-related retinal breaks. *Retina*. 2005;25(3):281.
62. Arbisser LB. Comprehensive Strategy for Unplanned Vitrectomy Technique for the Anterior Segment Surgeon. Course presented at the ASCRS Annual Meeting; 2005; Washington.
63. Peyman GA, Cheema R, Conway MD, Fang T. Triamcinolone acetonide as an aid to visualization of the vitreous and the posterior hyaloid during pars plana vitrectomy. *Retina*. 2000;20:554.
64. Burk SE, Da Mata AP, Snyder ME, Schneider S, Osher RH, Cionni RJ. Visualizing vitreous using Kenalog suspension. *J Cataract Refract Surg*. 2003;29:645.
65. Ernest P, Rhem M, McDermott M, Lavery K, Sensoli A. Phacoemulsification conditions resulting in thermal wound injury. *J Cataract Refract Surg*. 2001;27(11):1829.
66. Chang DF. Strategies for handling the hard nucleus. In: Boyd S, ed. *New Outcomes in Cataract Surgery*. Panama: Highlights of Ophthalmology; 2005.
67. Osher RH. Managing posterior capsular problems with new technology. Presented at the ASCRS Annual Meeting; 2002.
68. Ahmed I. Approaching the patient with zonular weakness. *Techniques in Ophthalmology*. 2003;1(1):12.
69. Verma A, Singh D. Myopia, Phakic IOL. Available at: www.emedicine.com
70. Fechner PU, Singh D, Wulff K. Iris-claw lens in phakic eyes to correct hyperopia: preliminary study. *J Cataract Refract Surg*. 1998;24(1):48.
71. Cooper BA, Holekamp NM, Bohigian G, Thompson PA. Case-control study of endophthalmitis after cataract surgery comparing scleral tunnel and clear corneal wounds. *Am J Ophthalmol*. 2003;136:300.
72. Wallin T, Parker J, Jin Y, Kefalopoulos G, Olson RJ. Cohort study of 27 cases of endophthalmitis at a single institution. *J Cataract Refract Surg*. 2005;31(4):735.
73. Neuhann TH. Posterior chamber Artisan IOL implantation for eyes without capsule support. Paper presented at the Annual Meeting of ASCRS; 2004; San Diego, Calif.
74. Neuhann TH. Retropupillary IOL implantation in eyes with no capsule support. Paper presented at the Annual Meeting of ASCRS; 2005; Washington.

Chapter 22

Intraocular Lens Power Calculation in Complex Cases

Benjamin F. Boyd, MD, FACS; Samuel Boyd, MD; Luis W. Lu, MD, FACS

Introduction

Determination of intraocular lens (IOL) power through meaningful keratometer readings, a topographer, and axial length measurement through A-scan ultrasonography has become a standard of care. It is a challenging technique and crucial to the visual result and patient satisfaction. In small incision techniques, cataract surgery has attained the status of refractive surgery. Therefore, exact determination of the IOL power to end up with the specific planned postoperative refraction is essential.[1,2] The advent of multifocal foldable IOLs makes this an important though complex subject, as well as operating on eyes with different axial lengths: normal (Figure 22-1), short (as in hyperopia) (Figure 22-2), piggyback IOLs (Figure 22-3), and long (as in myopia) (Figure 22-4).

Specific Methods to Use in Complex Cases

Considering that there is no full agreement on specific methods for treating these patients, we recommend the use of third/fourth generation formulas, preferably more than one, and that the highest resulting IOL power should be used for the implant.[3] These formulas are preferably the Holladay 2, the SRK/T, or the Hoffer formulas. Do not use a regression formula (eg, SRK I or SRK II).[4] We also recommend that you use central topography's flattest curve as a keratometric method unless you are fortunate to have all the information needed in order to use the historical method. This reading is fed to the computer utilizing the selected formulas. The computer will then provide you with the power of the IOL to use. The modern formulas recommended are already available in most of the computers available today to calculate IOL power.

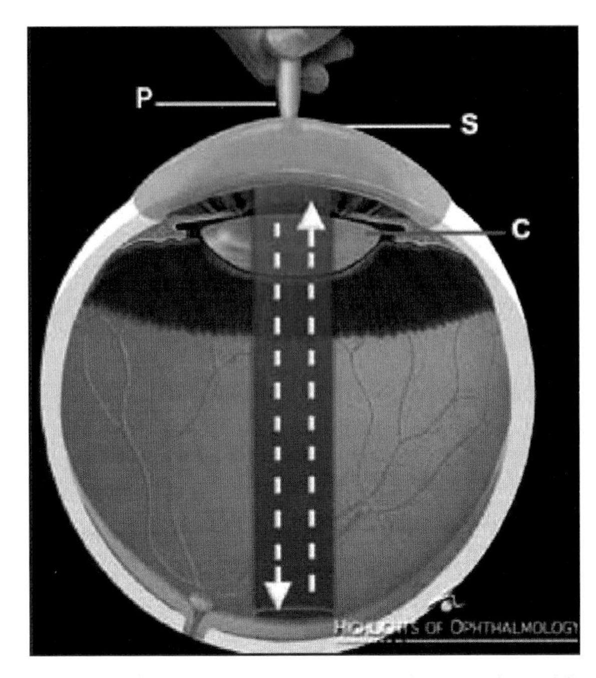

Figure 22-1. Determination of IOL power in patients with normal axial length (normal eyes)—mechanism of how ultrasound measures distances and determines axial length. The use of ultrasound to calculate the IOL power takes into account the variants that may occur in the axial diameter of the eye and the curvature of the cornea. The ultrasound probe (P) has a piezoelectric crystal that electrically emits and receives high frequency soundwaves. The soundwaves travel through the eye until they are reflected back by any structure that stands perpendicularly in their way (represented by arrows). These arrows show how the soundwaves travel through the ocular globe and return to contact the probe tip. Knowing the speed of the soundwaves, and based on the time it takes for the soundwaves to travel back to the probe (arrows), the distance can be calculated. The speed of the ultrasound waves (arrows) is higher through a dense lens (C) than through a clear one. Soft-tipped transductors (P) are recommended to avoid errors when touching the corneal surface (S). The ultrasound equipment computer can automatically multiply the time by the velocity of sound to obtain the axial length. Calculations of IOL power are based on programs such as SRK-II, SRK-T, Holladay, or Binkhorst (among others), which are installed in the computer. (Courtesy of Benjamin F. Boyd, MD, FACS, Ed. *The Art and the Science of Cataract Surgery*. Highlights of Ophthalmology, English Edition, 2001.)

Method for Choosing Formulas Based on the Axial Length

From a practical standpoint, if several formulas are available to the clinician, the first choice is as follows:

- Short eyes: AL, 22.00 mm: Holladay 2 or Hoffer Q, Haigis and Hoffer-Collenbrander. These constitute 8% of cases.
- AL (axial length) between 22.00 and 24.50 mm; 72% of the cases: mean of the three formulas: Hoffer, Holladay and SKR/T.
- AL higher than 24.00 mm; 20% of the cases: SRK/T formula.

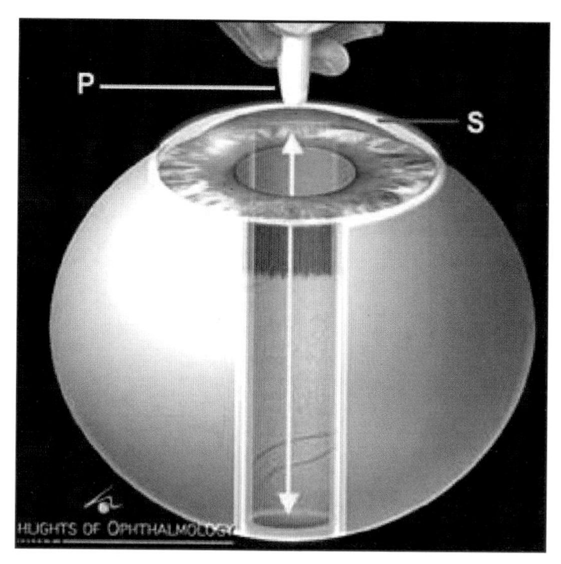

Figure 22-2. IOL power calculation in patients with very short axial length (hyperopia). In eyes with short or very short axial lengths, the third generation formulas such as Holladay 2 and Hoffer-Q seem to provide the best results. (P) represents probe, (S) represents corneal surface. (Courtesy of Benjamin F. Boyd, MD, FACS, Ed. *The Art and the Science of Cataract Surgery*. Highlights of Ophthalmology, English Edition, 2001.)

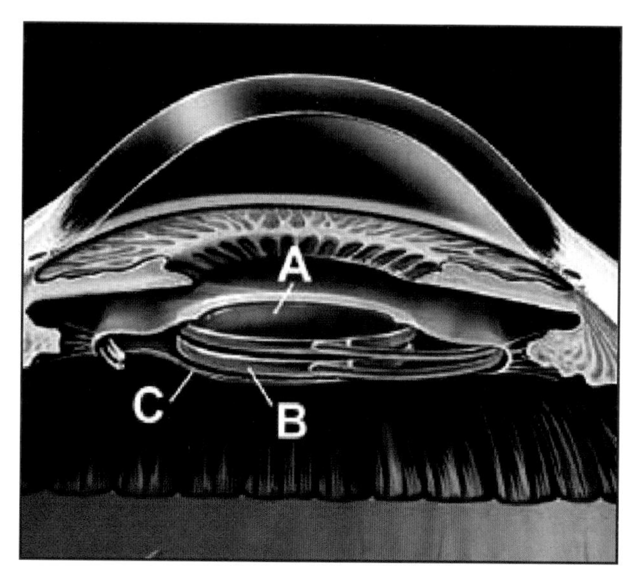

Figure 22-3. Concept of the piggyback high plus IOLs. In cases of very high hyperopia, a clear lens extraction may be done combined with the use of piggyback high-plus IOLs. One (A), two (B), or, some surgeons suggest, three or more IOLs can be implanted inside the capsular bag (C). This piggyback implantation technique may solve the problems of having to implant a lens of over +30 diopters with its consequent optical aberrations, but the procedure may give rise to postoperative complications (Courtesy of Benjamin F. Boyd, MD, FACS, Ed. *The Art and the Science of Cataract Surgery*. Highlights of Ophthalmology, English Edition, 2001.)

High Hyperopia

There are two main difficulties in measuring the axial length in these eyes: the utilization of the correct ultrasound velocity (Hoffer has recommended using 1560 m/sec) and dealing with the errors induced by the ultrasound contact techniques in these short eyes (perhaps it is more convenient to use immersion techniques).

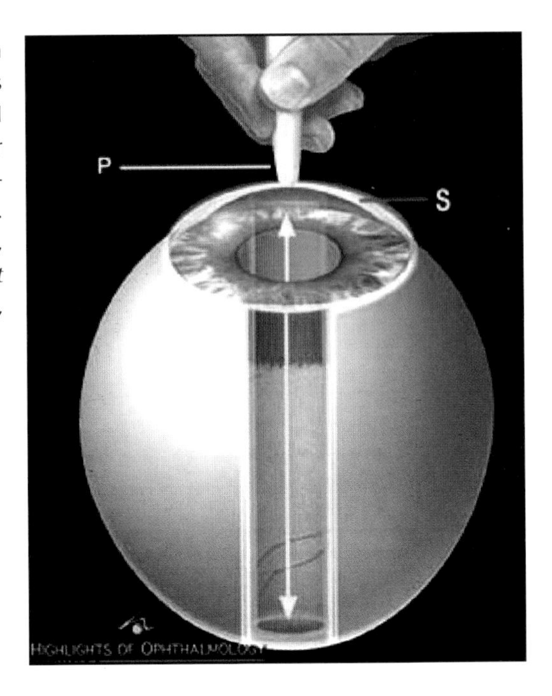

Figure 22-4. IOL power calculation in high myopia. In high myopia with axial lengths higher than 27.0 mm, the use of the SRK II formula with an individual surgeon's factor has shown good predictability of the refractive target. Probe (P), corneal surface (S). (Courtesy of Benjamin F. Boyd, MD, FACS, Ed. *The Art and the Science of Cataract Surgery*. Highlights of Ophthalmology, English Edition, 2001.)

In eyes with short or very short axial lengths (see Figure 22-2) the third generation formulas such as Holladay 2 and Hoffer-Q seem to provide the best results. Observing high refractive errors in extremely short eyes (<20.0 mm), Holladay[1] has discovered that the size of the anterior and posterior segments is not proportional, and has devised certain measurements to be used to calculate the parameters in these eyes. Assembling data from 35 international researchers, Holladay concluded that only 20% of short eyes present a small anterior segment; 80% present a normal anterior segment and it is the posterior segment that is abnormally short. This means that the formulas that predict a small anterior segment in a short eye provoke an 80% error margin, as they will predict an abnormally shallow anterior chamber which, in turn, can lead to hyperopic errors of up to 5 diopters. The Holladay 2 formula comprises the seven parameters previously described for IOL calculation: axial length, keratometry, anterior chamber depth (ACD), lens width, white-to-white corneal horizontal diameter, preoperative refraction, and age. This new formula has reduced 5 D errors to less than 1 D in eyes with high hyperopia.

The Use of Piggyback Lenses in Very High Hyperopia

For very short eyes (<22.00 mm in length), even though the Holladay 2 or the Hoffer Q formulas are a significant advance in calculating the IOL power needed, we do not have IOLs easily available with a power higher than +40 diopters because a higher diopter lens would have a marked, almost spherical curvature, which would cause major optical aberrations.[5] Such lenses can be customized but still may cause undesirable optical aberrations. In these cases, the piggyback method is employed, ie, the implantation of more than one IOL in a single eye, dividing the total power among the different lenses, placing 2/3 of the power in the posterior lens and 1/3 in the anterior lens (see Figure 22-3).

Gayton was the first to place two lenses in a single eye. He observed that placing multiple lenses in a single eye produces improved optical quality because there are fewer spherical aberrations than with very high diopter lenses.[6] Measuring the position of piggyback lenses, Holladay observed that contrary to what he supposed—the anterior lens would occupy a more anterior position—what effectively happens is that the anterior lens preserves its normal position while the posterior lens moves backwards because of the distensible nature of the capsular bag.[7] The latter may accommodate more than two IOLs and there are cases of patients with four piggyback lenses in the same eye.

The total power of the piggyback IOL implantation is calculated more precisely with the Hoffer-Collenbrander, or with a modification of the Holladay 2 formula.[9] Gayton and Apple described the presence of interlenticular opacification (ILO) in endocapsular piggyback implantation. The mentioned tissue consisted of retained/proliferative lens epithelial cells mixed with lens cortical material.[10] They recommended three surgical means that may help prevent this complication: meticulous cortical cleanup, especially in the equatorial region; creation of a relatively large continuous curvilinear capsulorrhexis (CCC) to sequester retained cells peripheral to the IOL optic within the equatorial fornix; insertion of the posterior IOL in the capsular bag and the anterior IOL in the ciliary sulcus to isolate retained cells from the interlenticular space.[11]

Echobiometry in highly hyperopic eyes, especially microphthalmic and nanophthalmic eyes, is still far from desirable.

High Myopia

According to Zacharias and Centurion's experience, results of cataract surgery in highly myopic eyes with axial lengths higher than 31.0 mm with implantation of low or negative power IOLs may be successful, without any more operative or postoperative complications than normal eyes.[5] The use of the SRK II formula with an individual surgeon's factor showed good predictability of the refractive target (see Figure 22-4). However, better formulas without the use of a personalized correction factor have yet to be developed.[8] There are technical difficulties in performing the echobiometry of patients with high myopia, especially when they have a posterior staphyloma. In those cases, one can obtain extremely irregular retinal echoes that cannot provide certainty in terms of really correct results of the IOL calculation. In addition, a posterior staphyloma may not always coincide with the macula, so the higher measurement is not necessarily the correct one, as is the case with normal eyes. In these patients it is useful to perform B type ultrasound to identify the existence of a staphyloma and its relation with the macula. Equally important is to have an ultrasound probe with a fixation light. The patient is asked to fixate at the light—which he will do with the macula— facilitating the measurement.

Determining Intraocular Lens Power in Patients With Previous Refractive Surgery

Patients who have undergone excimer laser procedures, radial keratotomy, or intracorneal segment rings, have had modifications to their corneal curvatures (Figures 22-5, 22-6, and 22-7). Accurate keratometric readings are fundamental in calculating IOL power.[12] IOL power calculation for cataract surgery in patients previously submitted to refractive surgery by modification of the corneal curvature is a new challenge for the cataract surgeon because of two features: 1) patients who previously decided to undergo refractive surgery are more psychologically resistant to using spectacles to correct residual ametropia. Consequently, their expectations for cataract surgery are unusually high; 2) so far there is no universally accepted formula to calculate these patients' IOL power accurately. Routine keratometry readings do not accurately reflect the true corneal curvature in these cases and may result in errors if used for IOL calculations. Therefore, standard keratometry readings should not be used for IOL calculations in these patients. If done, the standard IOL power-predictive formulas based on such readings commonly result in substantial undercorrection with postoperative hyperopic refraction or anisometropia, both of which are very undesirable.[13]

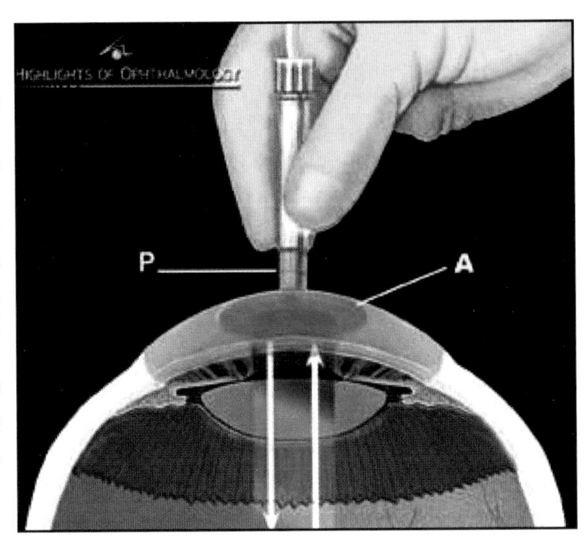

Figure 22-5. IOL power calculation in patients after excimer laser procedure. In this group of patients, even with the most advanced ultrasonic equipment, there is a degree of variation in the results of the IOL power calculation. This is the result of the varying modification in the curvature of the cornea after the excimer laser ablation (A). Ultrasound transducer (P), intracorneal rings (ICR). (Courtesy of Benjamin F. Boyd, MD, FACS, Ed. *The Art and the Science of Cataract Surgery*. Highlights of Ophthalmology, English Edition, 2001.)

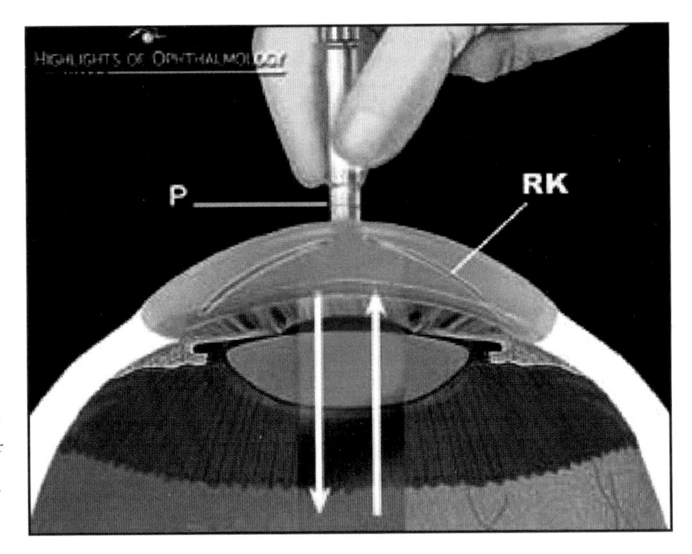

Figure 22-6. IOL Power Calculation in Patients After Radial Keratotomy. Patients who had RK with an optical zone smaller than 4.0 mm cannot have their central corneal curvature measured reliably with the standard keratometric methods. Ultrasound transducer (P), radial keratotomy incisions (RK). (Courtesy of Benjamin F. Boyd, MD, FACS, Ed. *The Art and the Science of Cataract Surgery*. Highlights of Ophthalmology, English Edition, 2001.)

Commonly Used Methods

There are three methods to determine the effective power of the cornea in these complex cases: 1) the "clinical history" method, also termed "the calculation method" by Holladay; 2) the contact lens method; and 3) the topography method. Holladay believes that the calculation or clinical history method and the hard contact lens trial are the two more reliable of the three, because the corneal topography instruments presently available do not provide accurate central corneal power following photorefractive keratectomy (PRK), LASIK, and RK with optical zones of 3 mm or less. In RK with larger optical zones, the topography instruments become more reliable. The great majority of cases, however, have had RK with an optimal zone larger than 3 mm, so they should also qualify for this method.

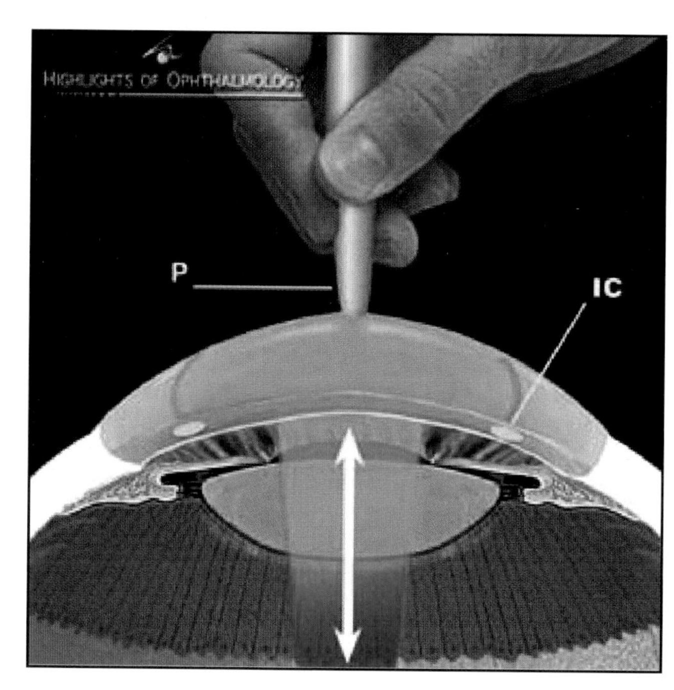

Figure 22-7. IOL power calculation after an intracorneal ring segment procedure. As with other refractive procedures on the cornea, this technique for correction of low myopia also modifies the central corneal curvature (arrows). Topography determines the present corneal curvatures. The surgeon uses the central flattest keratometric reading as a reference in cases where the pre-refractive procedure keratometry cannot be obtained. Ultrasound transducer (P), intracorneal rings (ICR). (Courtesy of Benjamin F. Boyd, MD, FACS, Ed. *The Art and the Science of Cataract Surgery*. Highlights of Ophthalmology, English Edition, 2001.)

The Clinical History Method

Holladay proposed this method based on the idea that refractive surgery has changed the corneal power and that this refractive change must be subtracted from the presurgical power of the cornea in order to estimate its present power.[14] You need to obtain:

1. A preoperative average K reading (Kp).
2. A preoperative spherical equivalent refractive error (Rp, before refractive corneal surgery).
3. A postoperative spherical equivalent refractive error (Ro, after the eye has healed following refractive surgery and visual acuity has stabilized but before cataract formation)

To calculate the eye's estimated corneal power (K), use the Hoffer formula:

K = Kp + (Rp) (Ro)

Remember to add algebraically and to change the sign when opening the second parenthesis.

Vertex-correcting the refractions is no longer recommended.

The Trial Hard Contact Lens Method

This method is based on the concept that, if a hard PMMA contact lens of known base curve (ie 36.00 D) and known power (ie, Plano) is placed on the cornea and the refraction does not change, the effective power of the cornea must be 36.00 D. If the power is different from plano and/or the difference in refraction is not zero, the formula will calculate the power. This method is limited to those cataractous eyes with a minimum best-corrected visual acuity (BCVA) of 20/80. The method will not work in eyes that are not able to be refracted.

You need to obtain:

1. A hard PMMA (not RGP) contact lens with a base curve (B) close to the estimated K reading and with a known power (P, easier if plano).
2. A bare manifest refraction without a contact lens (Rb).
3. A manifest overrefraction with a contact lens (Rc).

To calculate the eye's estimated corneal power (K), use the formula:
$K = B + P + Rc\ Rb$.
Remember to add algebraically and that vertex-correcting the refractions is no longer recommended.

The Corneal Topography Method

When information is not available for the clinical history method, it has been recommended that the keratometric reading be taken with the topography unit, using the flattest K found in the central 3 mm of the corneal mapping. Hoffer has suggested that after looking at the preceding methods, we should choose the lowest K reading from those calculated to use in the formula and then employ the Aramberri Double-K Method.

Aramberri Double-K Method

In 2001, Dr. Jaime Aramberri had the idea that the postsurgical flatter K reading should not be used in modern, theoretic formulas to calculate the estimated position of the IOL (estimated lens position [ELP], the visual axial distance from the apex of the cornea to the principal plane of the IOL, or ACD). This concept is based on the fact that the flattening and thinning of the cornea has not changed the biometric measurements of the anterior chamber structures; ie, the cornea has not changed its distance relationship with the crystalline lens and iris. Hoffer calls it the Aramberri Double-K Method.[15]

What you need to do is:

1. Use the preoperative K reading (Kp, eg, 43.50 D) in the part of the formula that predicts the ELP (ACD)
2. Use the postoperative (Ko, eg, 35.00 D) in the part of the formula that calculates the IOL power.

Presently this option is only available on the Hoffer Programs version 2.5. This method has not been tested for accuracy on a large reported series.

K-Method in Previous Radial Keratotomy

For patients with previous RK with optical zone of less than 4.0 mm, use the clinical history method if possible, otherwise use the flattest K of the central 3.0 mm in the topographic map, or both. Check the IOL power with the SRK/T formula of the Hoffer 2.5 software. If the optical zone is larger than 4.0 mm, use the measured K obtained with the keratometer because it will not be affected.[16–19]

In conclusion, in patients with previous Myopic LASIK/LASEK/PRK, use the clinical history method if possible, otherwise use the flattest K of the central 3.0 mm of the topographic map. In Hyperopic LASIK/PRK, conductive keratoplasty (CK), and intracorneal rings, the central corneal thickness is basically unaffected. In these cases, the K readings obtained can be used for the IOL power calculation. The clinical history method is utilized to double-check the corneal power.

The Importance of Detecting Irregular Astigmatism

Holladay has strongly recommended that biomicroscopy, retinoscopy, corneal topography, and endothelial cell counts be performed in all of these complex cases. The first three tests are primarily directed at evaluating the amount of irregular astigmatism. This determination is extremely important preoperatively because the irregular astigmatism may be contributing to the reduced vision as well as the cataract. The irregular astigmatism may also be the limiting factor in the patient's vision following cataract surgery. The endothelial cell count is necessary to recognize any patients with low cell counts from the previous surgery who may be at higher risk for corneal decompensation or prolonged visual recovery.

The potential acuity meter (PAM), super pinhole, and hard contact lens trial are often helpful as secondary tests in determining the respective contribution to reduced vision by the cataract and the corneal irregular astigmatism. The patient should be informed that only the glare from the cataract will be eliminated. Any glare from the keratorefractive procedure will essentially remain unchanged.

Intraocular Lens Power Calculation in Pediatric Cataracts

How to optically correct patients with bilateral congenital cataracts and monocular congenital cataract has been a major subject of controversy for many years. Some distinguished ophthalmic surgeons 20 years ago were strongly against performing surgery in monocular congenital cataract followed by treatment of amblyopia with a contact lens. Visual results were so bad that children with this problem must be amblyopic by nature, they thought, and the psychological damage to the children and the parents by forcing such treatment was to be condemned.

Surgery for bilateral congenital cataracts at a very early age followed by correction with spectacles and sometimes with contact lenses usually ended with no better than 20/60 vision bilaterally. This was again a source for belief that congenital cataracts (either unilateral or bilateral) were by nature associated with amblyopia, profound in cases of monocular cases and fairly strong in bilateral cataracts.

When posterior chamber IOL implantation in adults became established as the procedure of choice, strong influences within ophthalmology were adamantly opposed to their use in children for the following reasons: 1) the eye grows in length with consequent significant change in refraction. It was considered impossible to predict such change and consequently, the accurate IOL power adequate for each child; 2) there was opacification of posterior capsule in most cases. This required a second operation for posterior capsulotomy in the presence of an IOL.

The situation has now significantly changed. The previous failures with spectacles and contact lenses, the new developments in technology and surgical techniques and the fresh insight of surgeons of a new generation has led us to discard the previous thinking and very definitely implant posterior chamber IOLs in children. This has been made possible because of new medications that effectively prevent and/or control inflammation; the introduction of posterior capsule capsulorrhexis (Figure 22-8); high viscosity viscoelastics to facilitate intraocular surgery in smaller eyes; new, more appropriate IOLs and more refined technology that leads to a less difficult calculation of the IOL power.[20]

Different Alternatives

The limitations in calculating these lens powers (Figure 22-9) is due to the fact that the eye grows after cataract surgery and therefore refraction will change.[21] Two main methods of choosing an IOL power for pediatric patients are available:

1. Make the eye emmetropic at the time of surgery and thereby treat amblyopia immediately, taking advantage of a much better visual acuity. This is followed later by an IOL exchange or a secondary piggyback IOL implantation of a negative power or other means of treatment for the residual eventual myopia.

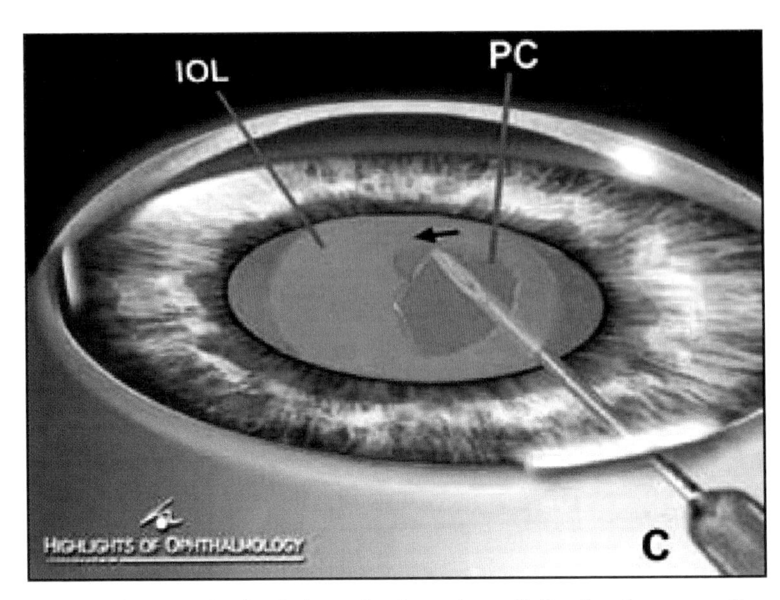

Figure 22-8. Posterior capsulorrhexis in pediatric patients. Following the conventional steps of phacoemulsification, an appropriate IOL for children is inserted with the required power in compliance with the criteria of the practitioner following the guidelines in the text. Once the IOL is located in the bag, and the tissues are properly protected with viscoelastics, a cystotome (C) is introduced through the limbal incision (I), and directed behind the IOL to perform a posterior capsule tear or posterior capsulorrhexis (PC). This opening in the posterior capsule at the time of the phaco procedure can provide permanent improved vision to the child. (Courtesy of Benjamin F. Boyd, MD, FACS, Ed. *The Art and the Science of Cataract Surgery*. Highlights of Ophthalmology, English Edition, 2001.)

2. Proceed with incomplete correction of the eye at the time of surgery (treated with glasses or contact lenses), taking advantage of the trend toward emmetropization that will occur as the eye grows. By "incomplete", we mean leaving the eyes hyperopic. As the eye grows in length with age (axial growth), the myopization that takes place in an eye artificially rendered hyperopic will lead to emmetropia or close to normal refraction. This measure avoids myopic anisometropia that may lead to an undesirable change of IOL surgically. In the meantime, the temporary hyperopia is managed with standard spectacles or contact lenses.

Alternatives of Choice

In the IOL power calculation in children younger than 1 year, keratometry is difficult and fortunately less important because the values change very rapidly during the first 6 months. Thus keratometry may be replaced by the mean adult average keratometry value of 44.00 D. Children less than 2 years old may be incompletely corrected +3.00 D to even +4.00 D; incompletely correct them +3.00 D in those closer to 3 and 12.50 D in those closer to 4 years. In children closer to 6 or 7, who have little chance of recovering from any amblyopia present but who are the ones that more frequently suffer from a unilateral traumatic cataract, overcorrect them by +1.00 D.[22–25]

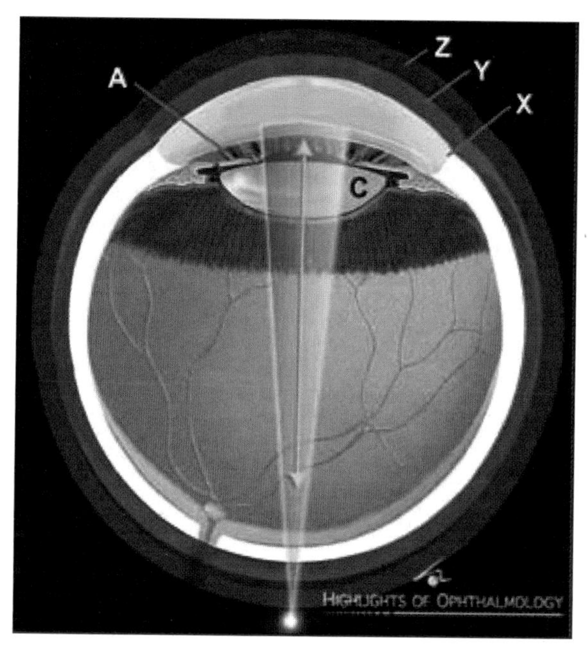

Figure 22-9. IOL power calculation in pediatric cataract. The growth of the ocular globe is ecographically registered until 18 years of age. However, the lens continues growing throughout the life of the individual. In normal conditions, anterior chamber (A) depth is reduced as the lens increases in size. In pathological conditions, such as the presence of cataracts, the opposite may happen: the ACD may increase due to reduction in the volume of the lens (C). In this illustration, we can see the changes in the size of the globe through the shaded images that outline the growth of the eye by stages. At birth, the axial diameter in the normal patient may measure approximately 17.5 mm; at 3 years of age it may measure 21.8 mm (X); at 10 years 22.5 mm identified in (Y), and in normal adulthood nearly 24 mm (Z). In selecting the lens power to be used, some surgeons choose to make the child hyperopic (arrows) with the intention that his growth will compensate hyperopia with the passage of time and will be eventually closer to achieving an emmetropic eye. Others prefer to calculate an IOL closer to emmetropia with the intention of keeping the child emmetropic during his growing years and prescribing eyeglasses in the future. (Courtesy of Benjamin F. Boyd, MD, FACS, Ed. *The Art and the Science of Cataract Surgery*. Highlights of Ophthalmology, English Edition, 2001.)

Intraocular Lens Power Calculation Following Vitrectomy

For the most part, IOL power calculation in eyes that develop a cataract following vitrectomy is very straightforward. The intravitreal gas is reabsorbed and slowly replaced by aqueous. If silicone oil was used, once it is removed aqueous fills the vitreous cavity. Since the refractive indices of aqueous and vitreous are identical (1.336), no corrections are needed in the IOL power calculation.

For patients who may undergo a silicone oil procedure at some point, it is wise to consider obtaining bilateral baseline axial length measurements by immersion A-scan biometry or by Optical Coherence Biometry (OCB) (IOL Master). This category would include

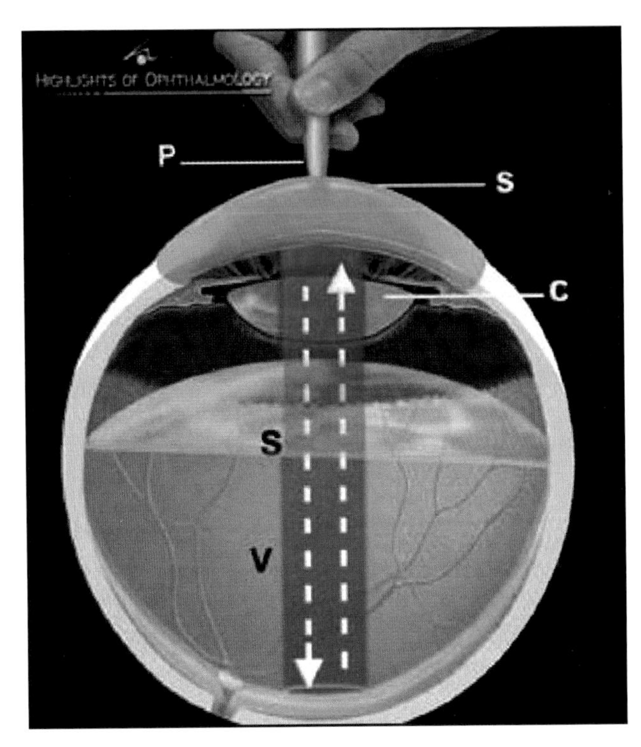

Figure 22-10. IOL power calculation in patients after vitrectomy procedure with silicone. If the patient is in the process of undergoing this procedure, it is recommended to calculate the IOL before using silicone in the vitreous cavity (V) and extracting the lens (C). PMMA lenses are recommended. Silicone foldable IOLs are not recommended because the silicone oil in the vitreous cavity sticks to the IOL and sometimes causes opacities. In the calculation of these lens powers, there may be differences in excess of 5 to 7 diopters. Errors can be frequent because if the vitreous cavity (V) is not filled completely with silicone (S), the movement of the bubble can induce errors in the calculation of the lens. In addition, in the eye filled with silicone, the ultrasound waves travel more slowly (arrows). This affects the axial diameter measurement during IOL power calculation. (Courtesy of Benjamin F. Boyd, MD, FACS, Ed. *The Art and the Science of Cataract Surgery*. Highlights of Ophthalmology, English Edition, 2001.)

any patient with a prior retinal detachment, moderate to high axial myopia, proliferative vitreoretinopathy, proliferative diabetic retinopathy, acquired immune deficiency syndrome, giant retinal tear, or history of a perforating ocular injury (Figure 22-10).[26]

Eyes that have undergone complicated retinal detachment repair with silicone oil placed in the vitreous cavity often require subsequent cataract surgery.[27] Accurate A-scan biometry can be very difficult in these eyes because silicone oil has a slower sound velocity than vitreous and often produces strong sound attenuation. These factors may prevent the display of a high-quality retinal spike and can contribute to significant measurement errors. Therefore, it is best to use OCB to measure theses eyes whenever possible.

Two densities of silicone oil are presently in use, each of which has a slower sound velocity than vitreous (1532 m/sec). The 1000 centistokes (cSt) silicone oil (eg, Silikon 1000, Alcon Laboratories, Fort Worth, Texas) has a sound velocity of 980 m/sec. The higher density 5000 cSt silicone oil (eg, Adato Sil-Ol 5000, Bausch & Lomb Surgical, Irvine, California) produces a velocity of 1040m/sec. It is important to know which density of silicone oil is present in the vitreous cavity before A-scan biometry so that the correct velocity setting can be used.

For eyes containing silicone oil, A-scan axial length measurements are best carried out with the patient seated as upright as possible. This is especially important if the vitreous cavity is only partly filled with silicone oil. In the upright position, silicone oil is more likely to remain in contact with the retina during the examination. Because of its lighter density with the patient fully recumbent, the entire mass of silicone oil often shifts away from the retina, toward the anterior segment, leading to confusion as to the true position of the retinal spike.[28]

If an incorrect sound velocity is used to measure the axial length of an eye containing silicone oil, the measurement displayed usually will be erroneously long. Measuring each component of the eye individually using the correct corresponding sound velocity avoids errors and gives good approximation of the true axial length. Examples of sound velocities include ACD at 1532 m/sec, crystalline lens thickness at 1641 m/sec, and vitreous cavity length at either 980 m/sec (for 1000 cSt silicone oil) or 1040 m/sec (for 5000 cSt silicone oil). Ideally, the biometer should have four electronic measuring gates and should allow the sound velocity to be modified when necessary. This allows for independent measurement of the individual components of the eye at the appropriate sound velocity. When the biometer provides only two gates and the sound velocities are not adjustable, a more complex approach is required.

The easiest way to measure the axial length of an eye containing silicone oil is to use OCB. Measurements can be made, without any special corrections, in phakic and aphakic eyes containing silicone oil. However, a large posterior subcapsular plaque or a dense nuclear cataract may make a reliable measurement impossible with this technique.

If the silicone oil is to be removed at some point, standard IOL power calculations can be performed after the true axial length has been determined. However, if the silicone oil is to remain in the eye indefinitely, a power adjustment must be made to prevent significant postoperative hyperopia.

When silicone oil is placed in the vitreous cavity, a higher-power IOL is required to achieve the same refractive result.[29,30] This is because the index of refraction for silicone is higher than that of normal vitreous. In addition, it is recommended that these patients receive a PMMA convex-plano lens; with the plano side oriented toward the vitreous cavity (and preferably over an intact posterior capsule). This approach prevents the silicone oil from altering the refractive power of the posterior surface of the IOL. The Holladay IOL Consultant software is very helpful for these cases because it has the ability to compensate for the different index of refraction of silicone oil compared to that of the vitreous.

For an average-length eye in which the vitreous cavity is filled with silicone oil, the additional power needed for a convex-plano PMMA IOL is typically between + 3.0 D to + 3.5 D. For example, the true axial length (TAL) of an eye with 1000 cSt silicone oil filling the vitreous cavity is 25.17 mm. The ACD is measured at 3.21 mm and the IOL power calculation calls for a plus 20.0 D convex-plano lens. In this circumstance, + 3.07 D of additional IOL power must be added at the level of the capsular bag to compensate for the differing refractive index of silicone oil. This will result in the implantation of a + 23.0 D lens.

If, however, removal of the silicone oil at a later date is anticipated, a possible alternative is to implant a + 20.0 D convex-plano PMMA IOL in the capsular bag and a + 3.0 D PMMA lens temporarily in the ciliary sulcus. The silicone oil and the ciliary sulcus lens could then be removed at the same time, thus avoiding a more complicated IOL exchange.

Meldrum, Aaberg, Patel, and Davis make the following recommendations:

- Measure the axial length using the velocity of sound in silicone oil.
- Calculate the IOL power to achieve emmetropia using the traditional formulas. To this IOL power, a correction factor must be added to obtain the IOL power to achieve emmetropia in silicone oil. The correction factors range from 2.79 D to 3.94 D, for axial lengths from 20 mm to 30 mm.

- Choose a convex-plano IOL if possible. If another type of lens is used, another correction factor must be added to obtain the total power of the IOL in the presence of silicone oil. For a convex-plano lens, no additional correction factor is required.

For instance, let us suppose that a patient requires indefinite intraocular tamponade with silicone oil and develops a cataract. Using the traditional formulas, assume that the IOL power is calculated to be 22 D based on a measured axial length of 23 mm. To this 22 D we must add a correction factor of 3.64 D[26] to correct for the axial length. Thus, for this patient a 25.5 D convex-plano lens should be implanted to achieve emmetropia in the presence of silicone oil. No additional correction factor for the IOL design is necessary.

Key Points

1. There are technical difficulties in performing the echobiometry of patients with high myopia, especially when they have a posterior staphyloma. In those cases, one can obtain extremely irregular retinal echoes that cannot provide certainty in terms of really correct results of the IOL calculation. In addition, a posterior staphyloma may not always coincide with the macula, so the higher measurement is not necessarily the correct one, as is the case with normal eyes.
2. The total power of the piggyback IOL implantation is calculated more precisely with the Hoffer-Collenbrander, or with a modification of the Holladay 2 formula.
3. For patients who may undergo a silicone oil procedure at some point, it is wise to consider obtaining bilateral baseline axial length measurements by immersion A-scan biometry or by OCB (IOL Master).
4. The potential acuity meter (PAM), super pinhole and hard contact lens trial are often helpful as secondary tests in determining the respective contribution to reduced vision by the cataract and the corneal irregular astigmatism.
5. Patients who have undergone excimer laser procedures, RK, or intracorneal segment rings have had modifications to their corneal curvatures. Accurate keratometric readings are fundamental in calculating IOL power.

References

1. Holladay JT. Intraocular lens power in difficult cases. In: Masket S, Crandal AS, eds. *Atlas of Cataract Surgery*. London: Martin Dunitz; 1999.
2. Lu LW, Fine IH. Phacoemulsification in Difficult and Challenging Cases. New York: Thieme; 1999.
3. Olsen T, Thim K, Corydon L. Theoretical versus SRK I and SRK II calculation of intraocular lens power. *J Cataract Refract Surg*. 1990;16:217.
4. Sanders DR, Retzlaff J, Kraff MC, Gimbel H, Raanan M. Comparison of the SRK/T formula and other theoretinal and regression formulas. *J Cataract Refract Surg*. 1990;16(3):341.
5. Zacharias W, Centurion V. Biometry and the IOL calculation for the cataract surgeon: its importance. *Faco Total*. 2000;66–88.
6. Gayton JL. Implanting two posterior chamber intraocular lenses in microphthalmos. *Ocular Surgery News*. 1994:64–5.
7. Holladay JT, Gills JP, Leidlein J, Cherchio M. Achieving emmetropia in extremely short eyes with two piggyback posterior chamber intraocular lenses. *Ophthalmology*. 1996;103:1118.
8. Zaldivar R, Schultz MC, Davidorf JM, et al. Intraocular lens power calculations in patients with extreme myopia. *J Cataract Refract Surg*. 2000;26:668.
9. Hoffer KJ. Ultrasound velocities for axial length measurement. *J Cataract Refract Surg*. 1994;20:554.

10. Gayton JL, Apple DJ, Peng Q, et al. Interlenticular opacification: clinicopathological correlation of a complication of posterior chamber piggyback intraocular lenses. *J Cataract Refract Surg.* 2000;26:300.
11. Buckley EG, Klombers LA, Seaber JH, et al. Management of the posterior capsule during intraocular lens implantation. *Am J Ophthalmol.* 1993;115:722.
12. Maeda N, Klyce SD, Smolek MK, McDonald MB. Disparity between keratometry-style reading and corneal power within the pupil after refractive surgery for myopia. *Cornea.* 1997;16:517.
13. Lacava AC Centurion V. Cataract surgery after refractive surgery. *Faco Total. Editora Cultura Medica.* 2000;269–276.
14. Hoffer KJ. The Hoffer Q formula: a comparison of theoretic and regression formulas. *J Cataract Refract Surg.*1993;19:700.
15. Aramberri J. Intraocular lens power calculation after corneal refractive surgery: Double K method. *J Cataract Refract Surg.* 2003;29:2063.
16. Hoffer KJ. Intraocular lens power calculation for eyes after refractive keratotomy. *J Cataract Refract Surg.* 1995;11:490.
17. Lyle WA, Jin GJC. Intraocular lens power prediction in patients who undergo cataract surgery following previous radial keratotomy. *Arch Ophthalmol.* 1997;115:457.
18. Celikkol L, Pavlopoulos G, Weinstein B, et al. Calculation of intraocular lens power after radial keratotomy with computerized videokeratography. *Am J Ophthalmol.* 1995;120:739.
19. Chen L, Mannis MJ, Salz JJ, et al. Analysis of intraocular lens power calculation in post-radial keratotomy eyes. *J Cataract Refract Surg.* 2003;29:65.
20. Brady KM, Atkinson CS, Kilty LA, Hiles DA. Cataract surgery and intraocular lens implantation in children. *Am J Ophthalmol.* 1995;120:1.
21. Kora Y, Shimizu K, Inatomi M, et al. Eye growth after cataract extraction and intraocular lens implantation in children. *Ophthalmic Surg.* 1993;24:467.
22. Ventura M, Ventura L, Endriss D. Updated management of pediatric cataracts. In: Boyd S, Dodick J, Freitas LL. *New Outcomes in Cataract Surgery.* Panama: Highlights of Ophthalmology; 2005:131-140.
23. Gimbel, HV. Posterior continuous curvilinear capsulorrhexis and optic capture of the intraocular lens to prevent secondary opacification in pediatric cataract surgery. *J Cataract Refract Surg.* 1997;23:652.
24. Gimbel HV, Basti S, Ferensowicz MA, DeBroff BM. Results of bilateral cataract extraction with posterior chamber intraocular lens implantation in children. *Ophthalmology.* 1997;104:1737.
25. Dahan E, Drusedan MUH. Choice of lens and dioptric power in pediatric pseudophakia. *J Cataract Refract Surg.* 1997;23:618.
26. Meldrum LM, Aaberg TM, Patel A, Davis JL. Cataract extraction after silicone oil repair of retinal detachments due to necrotizing retinitis. *Arch Ophthalmol.* 1996;114:885.
27. Grinbaum A, Treister G, Moisseiev J. Predicted and actual refraction after intraocular lens implantation in eyes with silicone oil. *J Cataract Refract Surg.* 1996;22:726.
28. McCartney DL, Miller KM, Stark WJ, et al. Intraocular lens style and refraction in eyes treated with silicone oil. *Arch Ophthalmol.* 1987;105:1385.
29. Grusha YO, Masket S, Miller KM. Phacoemulsification and lens implantation after pars plana vitrectomy. *Ophthalmology.* 1998;105:287.
30. Boyd B. Power calculation in standard and complex cases. In: Boyd B, ed. *The Art and Science of Cataract Surgery.* Panama: Highlights of Ophthalmology; 2001:37–58.

Chapter 23

POSTERIOR CAPSULE OPACIFICATION

Suresh K. Pandey, MD; David J. Apple, MD;
Liliana Werner, MD, PhD; John W. McAvoy, PhD; Anthony J. Maloof, MBBS, MBiomedE, FRANZCO, FRACS;
E. John Milverton, MBBS, DO, FRANZCO, FRCOphth

INTRODUCTION

Posterior capsule opacification (PCO, secondary cataract, after cataract) has been a nagging complication of cataract-intraocular lens (IOL) surgery since the beginning of extracapsular cataract surgery (ECCE) and IOL implantation. PCO needs to be eliminated because deleterious sequelae of this complication occur and Neodynium: Yttrium Aluminum Garnet (Nd: YAG) laser treatment now constitutes a major and unnecessary financial burden on the healthcare system. A successful expansion of ECCE-IOL surgery in the developing world depends on eradication of PCO, because patient follow-up is difficult and access to the Nd:YAG laser is not widely available. Advances in the surgical techniques, IOL designs/biomaterials have been instrumental in gradual, and unnoticed decrease in the incidence of the PCO. We strongly believe that the overall incidence of PCO and hence the incidence of Nd:YAG laser posterior capsulotomy is now rapidly decreasing from rates as high as 50% in the 1980s/early 1990s to less than 10% in the developed world. Our two decades of active research and information derived from other experimental and clinical studies from several other centers have revealed that the tools, surgical procedures, skills, and appropriate IOL designs are now available to significantly reduce this complication.

BACKGROUND

Opacification of the posterior capsule caused by postoperative proliferation of cells in the capsular bag remains the most frequent complication of cataract-IOL surgery.[1,2] In addition to classic PCO, postoperative lens epithelial cell (LEC) proliferation is also involved in the pathogenesis of anterior capsule opacification/fibrosis (ACO) and interlenticular opacification (ILO).[3–6] PCO has been recognized since the origin of ECCE and was noted by Sir Harold Ridley in his first IOL implantations.[7,8] It was particularly common and severe in the early days of IOL surgery (late 1970s/early 1980s) when the importance of cortical cleanup was less appreciated. Through the 1980s and early 1990s, the incidence of PCO ranged between 25% and 50%.[9] PCO is a major problem in pediatric cataract surgery, where the incidence approached 100%.[10–12]

One of the crowning achievements of modern cataract surgery has been a gradual, almost unnoticed decrease in the incidence of this complication. Our data at present show that with modern techniques and IOLs, the expected rate of PCO and the need for subsequent Neodynium: Yttrium Aluminum Garnet (Nd: YAG) laser posterior capsulotomy rate is decreasing to single digit (less than 10%).[13,14]

Reasons to Eradicate Posterior Capsule Opacification

Although cataract is the most common cause of blindness in the world, PCO is an extremely common cause as well. Jan G. F. Worst, MD has stated, "the most meaningful development in intraocular implant research in the next five years will be effective prevention of secondary cataract formation".[15] Eradication of PCO following ECCE has major medical and financial implications:

1. Nd: YAG laser secondary posterior capsulotomy, can be associated with significant complications. Potential problems include IOL optic damage/pitting, postoperative intraocular pressure (IOP) elevation, cystoid macular edema, retinal detachment, and IOL subluxation.[16–19]
2. Dense PCO and secondary membrane formation is particularly common following pediatric IOL implantation.[10–12] A delay in diagnosis can cause irreparable amblyopia.
3. PCO represents a significant cost to the US healthcare system. Nd:YAG laser treatments of almost 1 million patients per year have cost up to $250 million annually.[9]
4. A posterior capsulotomy can increase the risk of posterior segment complications in high myopes and patients with uveitis, glaucoma, and diabetic retinopathy.
5. PCO of even a mild degree can decrease near acuity through a multifocal IOL, and may interfere with the function of refractive/accommodating IOL designs.
6. A significant incidence of PCO means that cataract surgery, alone, may not restore lasting sight to the 25 million people worldwide who are blind from cataract.[20]
7. Finally, a successful expansion of ECCE-IOL surgery in the developing world depends on eradication, or at least diminishing of PCO, since patient follow-up is difficult and access to the Nd:YAG laser is not widely available.[20]

Etio-Pathogenesis

In the normal crystalline lens, the LECs are confined to the anterior surface at the equatorial region and the equatorial lens bow. This single row of cuboidal cells can be divided into two different biological zones (Figure 23-1):

1. The anterior-central zone (corresponding to the zone of the anterior lens capsule) consists of a monolayer of flat cuboidal, epithelial cells with minimal mitotic activity. In response to a variety of stimuli, the anterior epithelial cells ("A" cells) proliferate and undergo fibrous metaplasia. This has been called "pseudofibrous metaplasia" by Font and Brownstein.[21]
2. The second zone is important in the pathogenesis of "pearl" formation. This layer is a continuation of anterior lens cells around the equator, forming the equatorial lens bow ("E" cells). Unlike within the A-cell layer, cell mitoses, division, and multiplication are quite active in this region. New lens fibers are continuously produced in this zone throughout life.

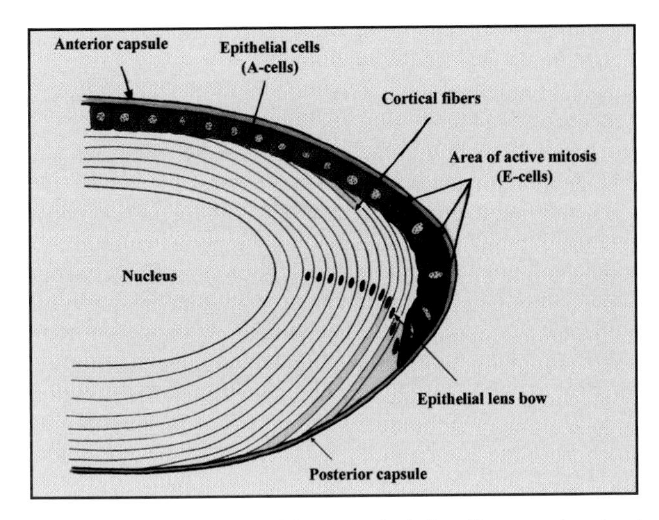

Figure 23-1. Postoperative proliferation of lens epithelial cells can also lead to postoperative opacification of capsular bag secondary to development of anterior capsule opacification/fibrosis (ACO) and interlenticular opacification (ILO). Schematic illustration of the microscopic anatomy of the lens and the capsular bag, showing the "A" cells of the anterior epithelium and the "E" cells, the important germinal epithelial cells of the equatorial lens bow. The primary cells of origin for posterior capsule opacification (PCO) are the mitotic germinal cells of the epithelial lens bow. These cells normally migrate centrally from the lens equator and contribute to formation of the nucleus or epinucleus throughout life. In pathologic states, they tend to migrate posteriorly to form such lesions as a posterior subcapsular cataract, as well as postoperative PCO following ECCE.

In addition to classic PCO, postoperative LEC proliferation is also involved in the pathogenesis of other entities, such as anterior capsule opacification/fibrosis (ACO)[3,4] and ILO; a more recently described complication related to piggyback IOLs.[5,6] Thus, there are three distinct anatomic locations within the capsular bag where clinically significant opacification may occur postoperatively (see Figure 23-1). Ophthalmic researchers are now developing surgical techniques/devices not only to eliminate PCO, but also to eliminate capsular bag opacification, secondary to proliferation of LECs.

Although both types of cells (from the anterior central zone and from the equatorial lens bow) have the potential to produce visually significant opacification, most cases of classic PCO are caused by proliferation of the equatorial cells. The term posterior capsule opacification implies that the capsule opacifies. Rather, an opaque membrane develops over the capsule as retained cells proliferate and migrate onto the posterior capsular surface.

The opacification usually takes one of two morphologic forms. One form consists of capsular *pearls*, which can consist of clusters of swollen, opacified epithelial "pearls" or clusters of posteriorly migrated equatorial epithelial (E) cells (bladder or Wedl cells). It is probable that both LEC types can also contribute to the *fibrous* form of opacification. Anterior epithelial (A) cells are probably important in the pathogenesis of fibrosis PCO, since the primary type of response of these cells is to undergo fibrous metaplasia. Although the preferred type of growth of the equatorial epithelial (E) cells is in the direction of bloated, swollen, bullous-like bladder (Wedl) cells, these also may contribute to formation of the fibrous form of PCO by undergoing a fibrous metaplasia. This is a particularly common occurrence in cataracts in developing world settings where cataract surgery has been delayed for many years, and where posterior subcapsular cataracts have turned into fibrous plaques.[22]

Capsulorrhexis contraction (capsular phimosis) is an important complication related to extreme fibrous proliferation of the anterior capsule.[2–4] Capsular phimosis can be avoided by not making the capsulorrhexis too small. In general, a diameter less than 5.0 mm is undesirable.

In contrast to the lesions of the anterior (A cells) capsule that cause phenomena related to fibrosis, the E cells of the equatorial lens bow tend to form cells that differentiate toward pearls (bladder cells) and cortex. Equatorial cells (E-cells) are also responsible for formation of a Soemmering's ring. The Soemmering's ring, a dumbbell or donut-shaped lesion that often forms following any type of rupture of the anterior capsule, was first described in connection with ocular trauma. The pathogenetic basis of a Soemmering's ring is rupture of the anterior lens capsule with extrusion of nuclear and some central lens material. The extruded cortical remnants then transform into Elschnig pearls. It is not widely appreciated that a Soemmering's ring forms virtually every time that any form of ECCE is done, whether manual, automated, or with phacoemulsification. This material is derived from proliferation of the epithelial cells (E-cells) of the equatorial lens bow. We have noted that these cells have the capability to proliferate and migrate posteriorly across the visual axis, thereby opacifying the posterior capsule. Because the Soemmering's ring is a direct precursor to PCO, surgeons should strive to prevent its formation.

Cells types other than lens epithelial cells may be involved in PCO. As ECCE is always associated with some breakdown of the blood-aqueous barrier, inflammatory cells, erythrocytes, and many other inflammatory mediators may be released into the aqueous humor. The severity of this inflammatory response may be exacerbated by the IOL. This foreign body elicits a three-stage immune response that involves many different cell types, including polymorphonuclear leukocytes, giant cells, and fibroblasts. Collagen deposition onto the IOL and onto the capsule may cause opacities and fine wrinkles to form in the posterior capsule. In most cases, however, this inflammatory response is clinically insignificant. Iris melanocytes also have been shown to adhere to and migrate over the anterior surface of the posterior capsule.

Lens Epithelial Cells Proliferation: Role of Growth Factors

Cataract surgery causes major changes in the ocular environment. Not only because of breakdown of the blood aqueous barrier, as mentioned above, but also through the release/activation of endogenous cytokines and growth factors from endogenous sources during wound healing. Aqueous and vitreous humors are rich in growth and regulatory factors and there is now abundant evidence that differences in the distribution of such factors between aqueous and vitreous compartments determine normal lens polarity and growth patterns; that is, factors in the vitreous environment promote the differentiation of fiber cells whereas the aqueous factors promote epithelial differentiation and growth.[23]

The lens itself expresses members of major growth factor families and a variety of growth factor receptors and molecules involved in a range of signaling pathways.[24] Studies over the last couple of decades have mostly concentrated on identifying the factor(s) that controls the differentiation of lens epithelial cells into fibers and there is now compelling evidence that members of the FGF growth factor family are required for induction of this process.[23] Recent studies have also indicated that the Wnt growth factor family plays a key role in promoting the differentiation of the epithelial sheet.[25] However, in relation to PCO, the most interesting studies have been on the transforming growth factor-beta (TGFβ) family.[26]

TGFβ is abundant in the lens, and the surrounding ocular media.[27] The effects of TGFβ on lens cells were initially studied in rats using epithelial explants and whole lens cultures.

TGFβ induces lens epithelial cells to commit to a differentiation pathway that is distinct from that seen in the normal lens. In cultured lenses, TGFβ induces the formation of subcapsular opacities.[27] These correspond to plaques of spindle-shaped cells that contain a-smooth muscle actin and desmin, and accumulations of extracellular matrix that include collagen types I and III, fibronectin and tenascin.[29] TGFβ also induces localized wrinkling of the capsule in epithelial explants and cultured lenses.[28,30] Similarly, overexpression of TGFβ in transgenic mice also results in the development of anterior subcapsular fibrotic plaques that grow progressively with age.[29,31] These studies clearly show that TGFβ disrupts the normal lens epithelial architecture and induces an epithelial-mesenchymal transition that is a central feature of the fibrotic growth that results in opacification and disturbed vision.

Similar patterns of aberrant growth and differentiation are found in subcapsular cataracts in humans. Following eye trauma, surgery, or associated with other disorders (eg, atopic dermatitis and retinitis pigmentosa), anterior subcapsular cataracts (ASC) can arise.[32] These exhibit similar fibrotic changes to that described for PCO. In this form of cataract in humans it also appears that members of the TGFβ family initiate the epithelial mesenchymal transition that is a central feature of this condition. In addition, it appears that an initial TGFb insult induces connective tissue growth factor, TGFβ-inducible gene-H3 and other autocrine signaling pathways, including endogenous TGFβ signaling, that promotes the progressive fibrosis that leads to cataract.[26,33,34]

As TGFβ is expressed by lens cells and the ocular media have abundant supplies, TGFβ bioavailability must be tightly regulated, otherwise all lenses would develop cataract. It appears that there may be multiple levels of TGFβ regulation. For example, it is well known that TGFβ is generally produced in a latent form that requires conversion to the mature (active) form. In addition, the ocular media, particularly vitreous, normally contain molecule(s) that inhibit active TGFβ and block its cataract-inducing effects.[33] The sensitivity of lens cells to TGFβ may also be modulated by many factors. For example, studies with rats have shown that estrogen can protect the lens from TGFβ-induced cataract.[35] This is consistent with epidemiological studies that report female hormones may help prevent or slow the development of some forms of cataract.[36]

In summary, during cataract surgery many growth factors are upregulated and/or activated in the lens and the ocular media. Not only does this disturb the normal distribution and activity of factors in the aqueous and vitreous compartments that are critical for determining normal growth patterns, but additional events such as activation of latent stores of TGFβ in the ocular media result in the induction of aberrant growth and differentiation in the lens. Clearly procedures that reduce the trauma of cataract surgery will be beneficial, as this will minimise disruption of the growth factor composition in and around the lens. A better understanding of lens cells biology also opens up possibilities of introducing molecules that will effectively kill residual lens cells. In addition, blockers of TGFβ could be included in irrigation solutions during surgery, and as coatings of IOLs, to ensure that any residual lens cells do not undergo epithelial mesenchymal transition, but rather maintain a normal epithelial phenotype.

Clinical Manifestations and Treatment

The interval between surgery and PCO varies widely, ranging anywhere from three months to four years after the surgery. Although the causes of PCO are multifactorial as reported in several studies[9,37,38] there is an inverse correlation with age. Young age is a significant risk factor for PCO, and its occurrence is a virtual certainty in pediatric patients.[10–12]

Visual symptoms do not always correlate to the observed amount of PCO. Some patients with significant PCO on slit lamp examination are relatively asymptomatic, while others have significant symptoms with mild apparent haze, which is reversed by capsulotomy.[39]

Visually significant PCO usually managed by creating an opening within the opaque capsule using the Nd: YAG laser. A surgical posterior capsulotomy may be indicated in children for dense PCO associated with secondary membrane formation. The technical details, parameters, preoperative and postoperative treatment, complications and recommendations for surgical and Nd: YAG laser posterior capsulotomy are discussed in literature.[16–19] In brief, indications for Nd: YAG laser capsulotomy include: presence of a thickened capsule leading to functional impairment of vision, and the need to evaluate and treat posterior segment pathology. However, caution should be exercised if there is any signs suggestive of intraocular inflammation, raised intra-ocular pressure, macular edema, and a predisposition to retinal detachment (eg, high myopia). As mentioned before Nd: YAG laser posterior capsulotomy may be rarely associated with complications such as transient rise in IOP, enhanced risk of retinal detachment, which is particularly marked in axial myopia, cystoid macular edema, IOL subluxation, lens optic damage/pitting, exacerbation of local endophthalmitis, and vitreous prolapse into the anterior chamber and anterior hyaloid disruption.

Surgical and Implant Related Factors for Prevention of Posterior Capsule Opacification

Based upon our 20 years of research experience on evaluation of ca. 17,500 IOL related specimens (7523 human eyes obtained postmortem; 6127 eyes implanted with rigid lenses and 1396 eyes implanted with foldable lenses) using Miyake-Apple technique, and published studies from our Center and other Centers,[1,9,13,14,20,40–45] we can review the principles of PCO prevention. These measures can be divided into two categories. One strategy is to minimize the number of retained/regenerated cells and cortex (including the Soemmering's ring) through thorough cortical cleanup. The second strategy is to prevent the remaining cells from migrating posteriorly. The edge of the IOL optic is critical in the formation of such a physical barrier.

We have identified three surgery-related factors and three IOL-related factors that are particularly important in the prevention of PCO (Table 23-1).[40–45]

Surgery-Related Factors to Reduce PCO

Hydrodissection-Enhanced Cortical Cleanup

A very important and underrated surgical step is hydrodissection. Dr. I. Howard Fine perfected and popularized this technique and coined the term cortical cleaving hydrodissection.[46] Until fairly recently, many surgeons had a rather fatalistic attitude regarding removal of lens cortex and cells during ECCE—either manual or automated—or with phacoemulsification. A common opinion was that removing all or even most equatorial cells from the bag is impossible. PCO was therefore considered an inevitable complication. This conclusion arose, in part, because PCO occurred in up to 50% of cases.

The necessary tenting up of the anterior capsule during subcapsular (or cortical cleaving) hydrodissection is best achieved by using a cannula with a bend at the tip allowing a flow of fluid toward the capsule to efficiently separate capsule from cortex (Figure 23-2). By freeing and rotating the lens nucleus, hydrodissection facilitates lens nucleus and cortex removal without zonular-capsular rupture.[47] We now know from autopsy and experimental studies that thorough cortical and cellular cleanup from the capsular bag can be accomplished

Table 23-1.

Factors That Significantly Influence the Formation of PCO

Six Factors to Reduce PCO

Surgery-Related Factors	IOL-Related Factors "Ideal" IOL
1. Hydrodissection-enhanced cortical clean-up	1. Biocompatible IOL to reduce stimulation of cellular proliferation
2. In-the-bag fixation	2. Maximal IOL optic- posterior capsule contact with angulated haptics, "adhesive" biomaterial to create a "shrink wrap" of the capsule
3. Small capsulorrhexis with anterior capsular edge on the IOL surface to sequester the capsular bag (shrink wrap the capsule around the IOL optic)	3. IOL optic geometry a square, truncated edge for 360°

in most cases.[42] Use of hydrodissection during cataract surgery allowed more efficient removal of cortex and LECs, (which in turn reduces PCO), when compared to control eyes where hydrodissection was not utilized.[42] A successfully performed cortical cleaving hydrodissection provides an easy way to remove the entire lens cortex as well as nucleus. Occasionally this can even occur without the need for cortical aspiration with a separate irrigation/aspiration instrument.

Surgeons use balanced salt solution (Alcon Inc., Fort Worth, TX., USA) while performing cortical cleaving hydrodissection. Recent experimental animal studies from our Center have shown that use of preservative-free lidocaine 1% during hydrodissection may diminish the amount of live LECs by facilitating cortical cleanup, by loosening the desmosomal area of cell-cell adhesion with decreased cellular adherence, or by a direct toxic effect.[48] Corneal endothelial toxicity continues to be a major concern of using hypo-osmolar agents (to loosen the cell-cell adhesion) during hydrodissection or any step of cataract surgery, in absence of a sealed capsular bag. However, it is now possible to irrigate the entire capsular bag using an injection-molded silicone disposable innovative device know as PerfectCapsule (Milvella Pty. Ltd., Sydney, Australia). Sealed capsule irrigation (SCI) isolates the internal lens capsule, and facilitates removal of residual cortical material as well as lens epithelial cells, and thus prevents/delays capsular bag opacification.[49,50] The SCI technique is pioneered by one of us (AJM), and discussed in details in later part of this chapter.

In-the-Bag (Capsular) IOL Fixation

The hallmark of modern cataract surgery is the achievement of consistent and secure in-the-bag (capsular) fixation (Table 23-1). The most obvious advantage of in-the-bag fixation is the accomplishment of good optic centration and sequestration of the IOL from adjacent uveal tissues. Numerous other advantages have been described elsewhere.[51,52] However, it is not often appreciated that this is also extremely important in reducing the amount of PCO.

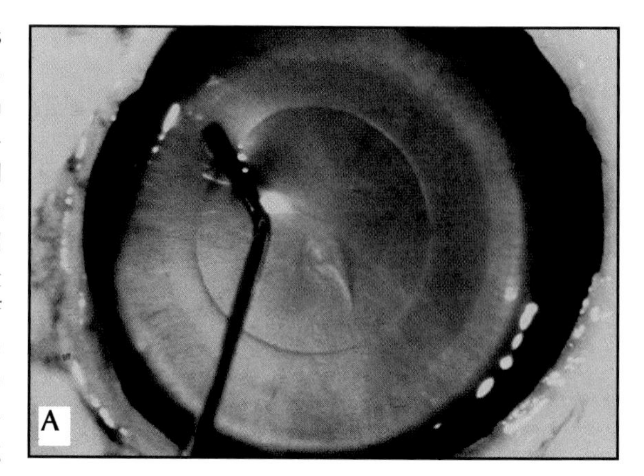

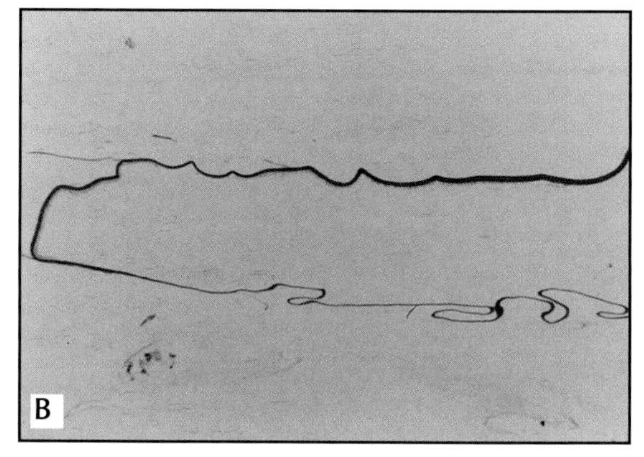

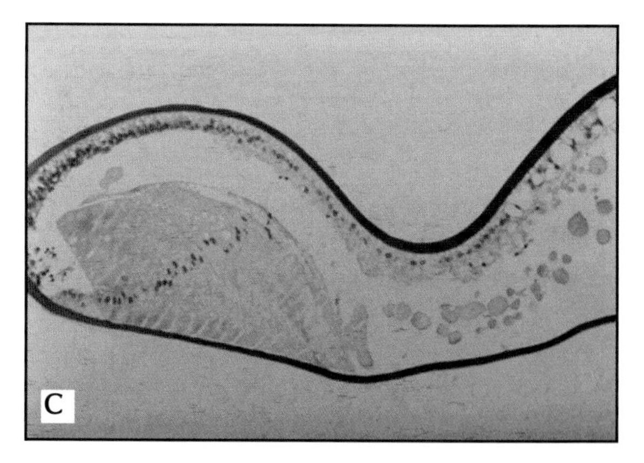

Figure 23-2. In our laboratory studies on human eyes obtained postmortem, we were pleasantly surprised that with copious hydrodissection and meticulous cortical cleanup, most cortex and most if not all lens epithelial cells from the equator (E cells) could be removed when compared to eyes without hydrodissection. **A**. Gross photograph of experimental surgery on a human cadaver eye from Anterior (surgeon's) view showing the technique of subcapsular hydrodissection (cortical cleaving hydrodissection). Note that the 27-gauge bent cannula is immediately under the edge of the capsulorrhexis. **B**. Photomicrograph of the lens capsular bag of one of the eye that underwent experimental cataract surgery associated with copious hydrodissection. Note excellent removal of lens material and E cells—a very clear capsular bag. (Periodic acid-Schiff stain, original magnification x750). **C**. Photomicrograph of a sagittal view of a crystalline lens without hydrodissection in human cadaver eyes. Note residual cortical material and equatorial lens epithelial cells. (Periodic acid-Schiff stain, original magnification 250x).

One desired goal of in-the-bag fixation is enhancing the IOL optic barrier effect, which is functional and maximal when the lens optic is fully in-the-bag with direct contact with the posterior capsule. In case one or both haptics are not placed in the bag, a potential space is created, allowing an avenue for cells to grow posteriorly toward the visual axis. The reader may recall the barrier ridge IOL design devised by Kenneth Hoffer in the 1980s, which did not function sufficiently at the time.[9] The reason was not a problem with the concept or the IOLs themselves, but rather that only about 30% of posterior chamber IOLs were implanted inside the bag at the time.

With non-phaco ECCE in-the-bag fixation of IOLs occurs about 60% of the time. One explanation is that many cases combined rigid design IOLs with can-opener anterior capsulotomies. Secure and permanent in-the-bag fixation only occurred in approximately 60% of cases.[40] However, when considering modern foldable lens implantation, the number rapidly rises to over 90%. It is not the foldable IOL itself, or even the small incision in and of itself that provides this positive result, but rather the fact that successful foldable IOL insertion generally requires meticulous surgery, with the necessity of performing a continuous curvilinear capsulorrhexis (CCC) and secures implantation of both IOL loops in the bag.[40]

Capsulorrhexis Edge on IOL Surface

A less obvious, but significant addition to precise in-the-bag fixation, is creating a CCC diameter slightly smaller than that of the IOL optic. For example, if the IOL optic were 6.0 mm, the capsulorrhexis diameter would ideally be slightly smaller, perhaps 5.0–5.5 mm. This places the cut anterior capsule edge on the anterior surface of the optic, providing a tight fit (analogous to a "shrink wrap") and helping to sequester the optic in the capsular bag from the surrounding aqueous humor (see Table 23-1). This mechanism may support protecting the milieu within the capsule from at least some potentially deleterious factors within the aqueous, especially some macromolecules, and some inflammatory mediators. The concept of capsular sequestration based on the CCC size and shape is subtle, but more and more surgeons appear to be applying this principle and seeing its advantages.

However, a recent study by Vasavada and Raj[53] suggested that with certain IOLs biomaterial such as 3-Piece AcrySof IOL, the relationship of the anterior capsule and the IOL does not seem to be a factor that relates to the development of central PCO. In a prospective, randomized, controlled trial, these authors evaluated the relationship of the anterior capsule and the AcrySof MA30BA IOL and its impact on the development of central PCO in 202 patients with senile cataracts. Patients were randomized prospectively to receive 1 of the three possibilities of anterior capsule and IOL optic relationship: group 1, total anterior capsule cover (360°) of the optic; group 2, no anterior capsule cover (360°) of the optic; group 3, partial anterior capsule cover (<360°) of the optic. After surgery, slit-lamp video photography was performed every 6 months for 3 years. The posterior capsule was divided into three zones: peripheral, central 3 mm, and midperipheral (the space between the peripheral and the central zones). At 3 years, the rate of central PCO was 6.4% in group 1, 7.1% in group 2, and 5.9% in group 3 ($P = 0.9$). Midperipheral PCO was present in 24.2% in group 1, 16% in group 2, and 20.6% in group 3 ($P = 0.9$). Peripheral PCO was seen in 100% of patients in all groups. The Nd:YAG posterior capsulotomy rate was 0% in all groups. The authors concluded that there was no significant difference in the incidence of development of central PCO among the three groups.

Implant-Related Factors to Reduce PCO

In addition to the three above-mentioned surgery-related factors, we will describe briefly the three IOL-related factors, which in our opinion play an important role in the eradication of PCO.

IOL Biocompatibility

Lens material biocompatibility (see Table 23-1) is an often-misunderstood term. It can be defined by many criteria, eg, the ability to inhibit stimulation of epithelial cellular proliferation. The less the cell proliferation the lower the chance for secondary cataract formation. In our large series of postmortem human eyes, the Alcon AcrySof IOLs presented with minimal to absent Soemmering's ring formation, PCO and ACO (Figure 23-3).[1–4,13,14,41,51] In

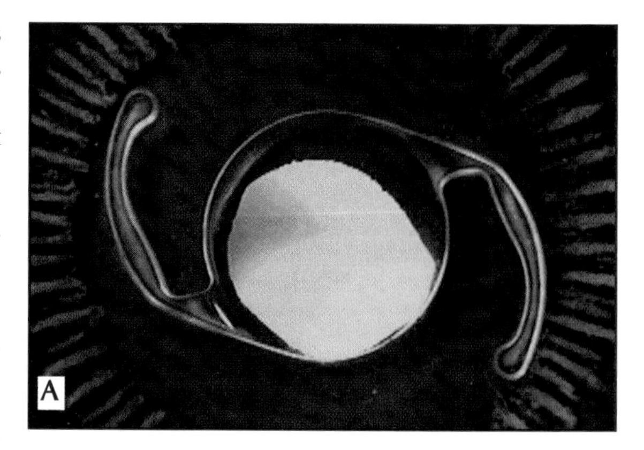

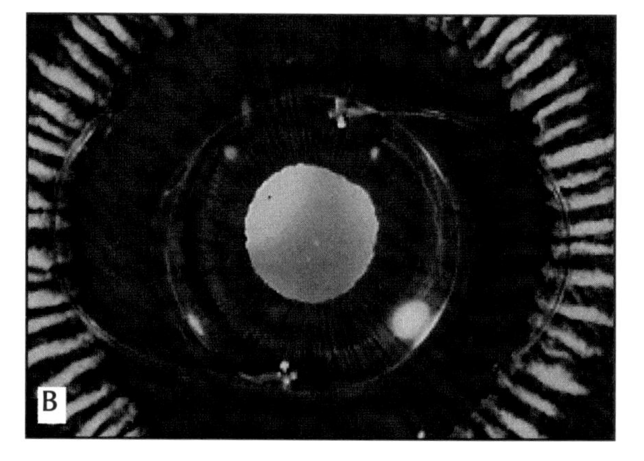

Figure 23-3. Among nine different types of rigid and foldable lens designs studies in pseudophakic human eyes, hydrophobic acrylic IOLs had the lowest PCO formation and therefore the Nd: YAG laser posterior capsulotomy rates. The lowest PCO score was confirmed by gross and histological evaluation. **A**. Human eye obtained postmortem, Miyake-Apple posterior photographic technique of a single-piece hydrophobic acrylic optic/haptics (Alcon AcrySof) PC-IOL showing a symmetric fixation and excellent centration. The surgical technique was excellent and there is virtually no retained/regenerative material (Soemmering's ring). This obviously represents good cortical clean-up, and also suggests good biocompatibility with minimal proliferation. **B**. 3-piece acrylic optic/PMMA haptics (Alcon AcrySof) showing a good example of excellent cortical clean-up, and also suggesting good biocompatibility, with minimal cellular proliferation.

addition, the amount of cell proliferation is greatly influenced by surgical factors, such as copious cortical clean up. Furthermore, the time factor also plays a role, such as the duration of the implant in the eye. Additional long-term studies are required to assess the overall role of "biocompatibility" in the pathogenesis of PCO.

Maximal IOL Optic-Posterior Capsule Contact

Other contributing factors in reducing PCO are posterior angulation of the IOL haptic and posterior convexity of the optic (Table 23-1). This is due to the creation of a "shrink wrap", a tight fit of the posterior capsule against the back of the IOL optic. The relative "stickiness" of the IOL optic biomaterial probably helps producing an adhesion between the capsule and IOL optic. There is preliminary evidence that the hydrophobic acrylic IOL biomaterial provides enhanced capsular adhesion, or "bioadhesion".[54–56]

RJ Linnola, MD, PhD proposed the sandwich theory for explanation of less PCO with hydrophobic IOL biomaterial.[54–56] According to this theory, if the IOL is made of a bioactive material it would allow a single lens epithelial cell layer to bond both to the IOL and the posterior capsule at the same time. This would produce a sandwich pattern including the IOL, the cell monolayer and the posterior capsule. The sealed sandwich structure would prevent further epithelial ingrowth. The degree of bioactivity of the IOL could explain the basic difference in the incidence of PCO and capsulotomy rates with different IOL materials.

The sandwich theory was tested in pseudophakic autopsy eyes implanted with PMMA, silicone, soft hydrophobic acrylate or hydrogel IOLs. Histological sections were prepared from the capsular bag and immunohistochemical analyses were performed for fibronectin, vitronectin, laminin and collagen type IV. Results of this study suggested that soft hydrophobic acrylate IOLs had significantly more adhesion of fibronectin to their surfaces than PMMA or silicone IOLs. Also, more vitronectin was attached to hydrophobic acrylate IOLs than to the other IOL materials. Silicone IOLs had more collagen type IV adhesion in comparison to the other IOL materials studied. In histologic sections a sandwich-like structure (anterior or posterior capsule-fibronectin-one cell layer-fibronectin-IOL surface) was seen significantly more often in eyes with hydrophobic acrylate IOLs than in PMMA, silicone or hydrogel IOL eyes. These studies support the sandwich theory for PCO after cataract surgery with IOLs. The results suggest that fibronectin may be the major extracellular protein responsible for the attachment of hydrophobic acrylate IOLs to the capsular bag. This may represent a true bioactive bond between the IOL and the LECs, and between the IOL and the capsular bag. This may explain the reason for clinical observations of less PCO and lower capsulotomy rates with the soft hydrophobic acrylate material of AcrySof IOLs compared to the other IOL materials studied.

Barrier Effect of the IOL Optic

The IOL optic barrier effect (see Table 23-1), plays an important role as a second line of defense against PCO, especially in cases where retained cortex and cells remain following ECCE. The concept of the barrier effect goes back to the original Ridley lens.[8] If accurately implanted in the capsular bag, it provided an excellent barrier effect, with almost complete filling of the capsular bag and contact of the posterior IOL optic to the posterior capsule ("no space, no cells"). A lens with one or both haptics "out-of-the-bag" has much less of a chance to produce a barrier effect. Indeed, the IOL optic's barrier function has been one of the main reasons that PC-IOLs implanted after ECCE throughout the decades did not produce an unacceptably high incidence of florid PCO.

A subtle difference between classic optics with a round tapered edge and optics with a square truncated edge became evident recently (Table 23-1). The effect of a square-edge optic design as a barrier was first discussed by Nishi et al[57,58] in articles related to PCO. In a clinicopathological study, our laboratory was the first to confirm this phenomenon in human eyes (Figure 23-4).[32,33] We reported our results of a large histopathological analysis covering the IOL barrier effect, with special reference to the efficacy of the truncated edge (see Figure 23-4). A truncated, square-edged optic rim appears to cause a complete blockade of cells at the optic edge, preventing epithelial ingrowth over the posterior capsule.[60–67] The enhanced barrier effect of this particular edge geometry provides another supplemental factor, in addition to the five above-mentioned factors, that has significantly diminished the overall incidence of clinical PCO.

Our past studies,[13,14] demonstrated that the original, three-piece MA60 AcrySof (Alcon, Fort Worth, Tex) IOL successfully combined these three IOL-related factors (see Table 23-1, Figures 23-3 and 23-4) in a way that produced a major PCO advantage. Other manufacturers have begun to incorporate these PCO preventing features, such as a sharp, or squared-posterior edge. The Cee-On 911 silicone IOL (Pfizer Inc., New York, NY) was the first silicone IOL to feature a squared edge. The Sensar hydrophobic acrylic (Advanced Medical Optics Inc., Santa Ana, Calif) and Clariflex silicone (Advanced Medical Optics Inc, Santa Ana, CA) IOLs now feature a sharp posterior edge, combined with a rounded anterior edge. Modification in the Centerflex one-piece hydrophilic IOL design (Rayner Inc., Hove East Sussex, UK) has been incorporated to prevent cellular ingrowth at the broad optic-haptic junction. The modified profile provides a square edge (barrier, ridge, wall) for 360° around the lens optic (enhanced square edge), eliminating the potential defect (Figure 23-5). This further minimizes the ingrowth of migrating LECs toward the visual axis.

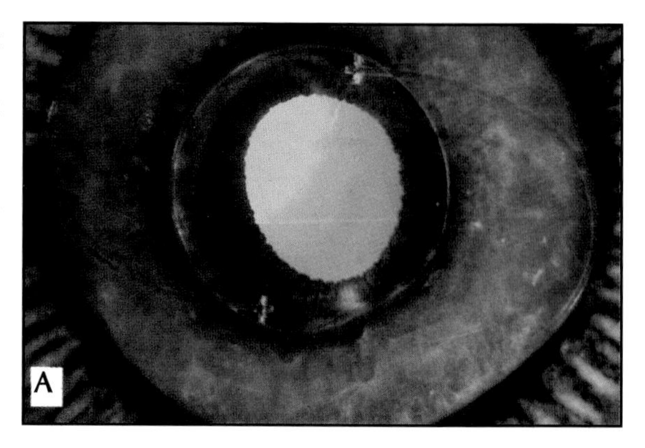

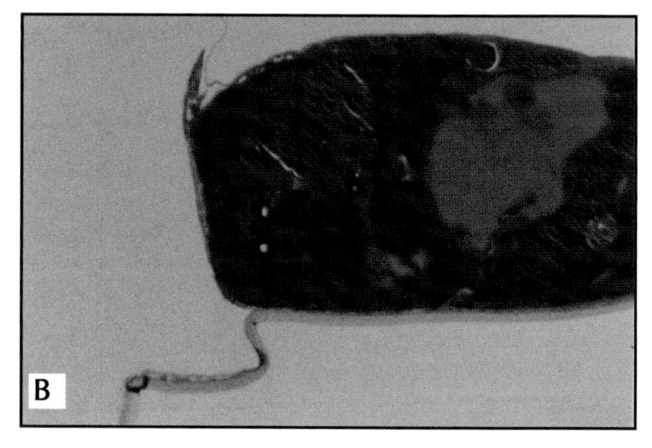

Figure 23-4. Even when a significant Soemmering's ring remains in the eye, a square truncated edge such as what exists on the AcrySof IOL provides a second line of defense against cortical ingrowth. Other IOLs with square or truncated optic edges include the Ciba Mentor MemoryLens, the Staar Surgical/Bausch and Lomb Surgical elastimide-polyimide silicone design, the Pfizer CeeOn Edge 911 silicone IOL, Advanced Medical Optics Sensar OptiEdge and plate haptic IOLs. **A**. Gross photograph from behind (Miyake-Apple posterior photographic technique) of a human eye obtained postmortem containing an AcrySof IOL. Some cortical remnants (a Soemmering's ring) remain peripherally but the optical zone remains totally cell free, with no encroachment of cells past the edge of the IOL optic. **B**. Photomicrograph of an eye in which an Alcon AcrySof IOL was implanted. Cleanup was not complete and a Soemmering's ring resulted. However, the Soemmering's ring remnants (red) were blocked by the square optic edge, leaving the posterior capsule cell-free. (Masson's trichrome stain, original magnification x 100.)

A major disadvantage of the truncated edge is the production of clinical visual aberrations, such as glare, halos and crescents.[68] Subtle changes in manufacturing are now helping alleviate glare and other optical complications.

Pharmacological Prevention of Posterior Capsule Opacification

Intraocular application of pharmacologic agents has also been investigated by several authors as a means to prevent PCO.[71–76] The idea was to selectively destroy the LECs and avoid toxic side effects on other intraocular tissues such as the sensitive corneal endothelium. Pharmacologic agents being investigated include cancer chemotherapeutic drugs (eg, antimetabolites such as methotrexate, mitomycin, daunomycin, 5-FU, colchicine, and daunorubicin), anti-inflammatory substances, hypo-osmolar drugs, and immunological agents.

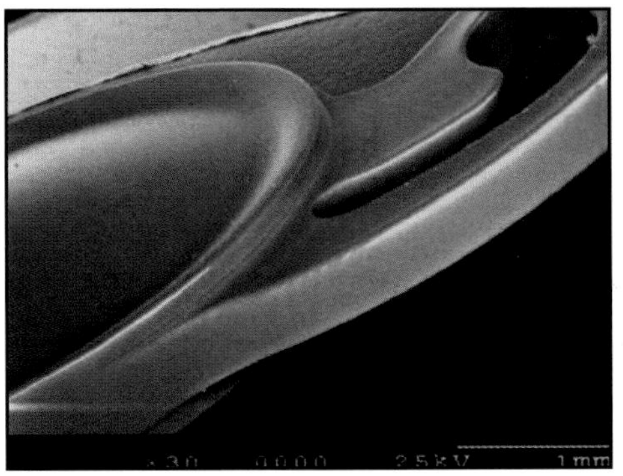

Figure 23-5. Scanning electron photograph obtained at the level of the optic-haptic junction of the Rayner Centerflex one-piece hydrophilic IOL. This profile provides a square edge (barrier, ridge, wall) for 360° around the lens optic, eliminating the potential defect. The round tapered edge of classic one-piece IOL design at the optic edge that subtends the optic-haptic junction represents a theoretical "Achilles' heel" in which when ingrowing cells may bypass the desired barrier.

We designed an intracapsular ring to prevent capsular bag contraction and also to inhibit LECs proliferation and metaplasia by sustained release of 5-FU.[77–79] The effects of the intracapsular ring on the prevention of PCO was prospectively studied by analyzing postmortem ocular specimens macroscopically using Miyake-Apple technique[81,82] and histologically. We also evaluated the toxic effects of 5-FU on the corneal endothelium, capsular bag and retina of rabbits.[77] Results of this study suggested that implantation of intracapsular ring may prevent central PCO after cataract surgery by mechanically blocking migration of lens epithelial cells towards the central visual axis. The potential pharmacological effect of 5-FU for PCO prevention was not demonstrated in this experimental study.[77]

Toxicity to corneal endothelium and other ocular structure remains one of the major concern for using cancer chemotherapeutic drugs, anti-inflammatory substances, hypo-osmolar drugs, and immunological agents, when intralenticular compartment is in direct contact with anterior chamber. However, with the development of a *SCI device*, it is now possible to precisely deliver the pharmacological/ hypo-osmolar agents to the lens epithelial cells within the capsular bag, while minimizing the potential for collateral ocular damage.[49,50]

Sealed Capsule Irrigation (SCI) device may allow the isolated safe delivery of pharmacologic agents into the capsular bag following cataract surgery (Figure 23–6).[49,50] Developed by one of the co-author (AJM), SCI is a form of Sealed Irrigation System applied to the internal eye, and may be applied elsewhere to the body. In the eye, the technique of capsular bag irrigation may be used with pharmacologic agents to target LECs, eliminate PCO and help maintain capsular bag transparency. We consider that SCI should meet the following requirements: it should be minimally invasive, be easy to use, fit through a small incision, be relatively inexpensive, provide a repeatable seal with the lens capsule, and be not add significantly to the duration of routine cataract surgery.

The intact human lens capsule is functionally a separate compartment within the eye. Once breached, the intralenticular compartment becomes continuous with the anterior chamber and the rest of the eye. However, since intact capsulorrhexis is now routinely performed, we devised a technique to reseal the capsular bag following lens removal. By resealing the capsular bag, we recompartmentalize the lens and allow for the selective irrigation of the internal contents of the capsular bag.

The SCI device called Perfect Capsule (Milvella Pty. Ltd., Sydney, Australia), which is made from biomedical grade soft silicone, allows the surgeon to reseal the capsular bag. The device consists of a rounded plate containing a suction ring, which abuts the anterior capsule, and an extension arm that passes through a phacoemulsification wound. This extension arm carries a vacuum channel which supplies vacuum to the suction ring, and a combined irrigation and aspiration channel. The irrigation and aspiration channels allow for communication between the sealed capsular bag and the external eye.

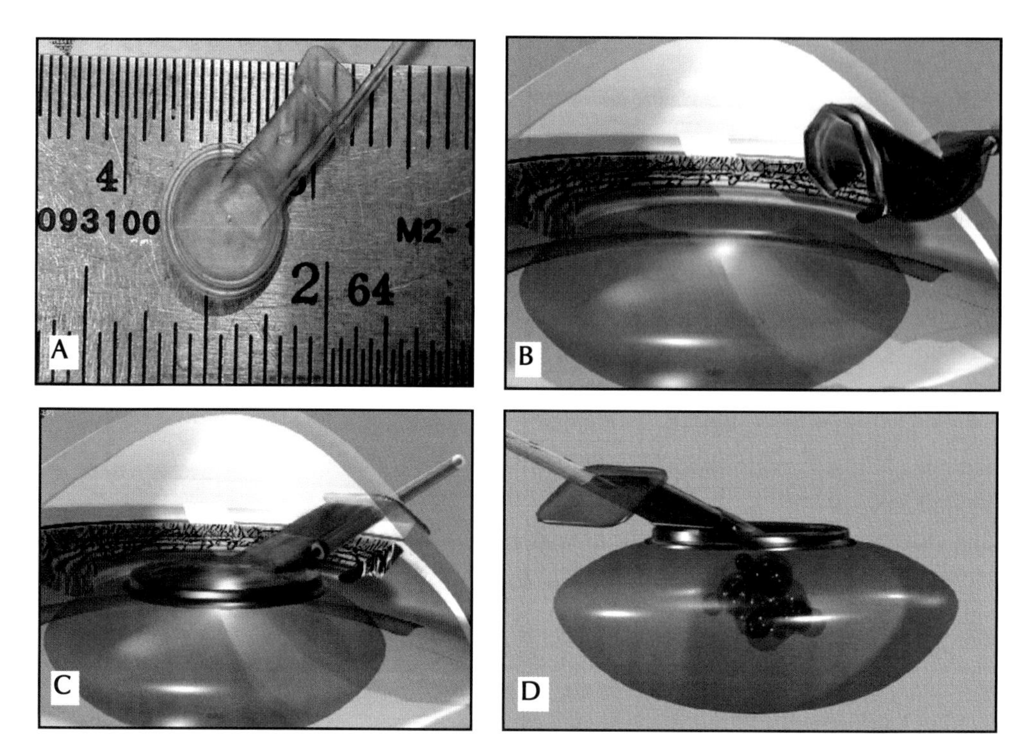

Figure 23-6. Schematic diagrams illustrating the concept of Sealed Capsule Irrigating device (PerfectCapsule, Milvella Pty. Ltd., Sydney, Australia). This device is designed to hold the capsular bag by means of a toroidal suction ring connected to a locking suction syringe. An irrigation/aspiration port allows fluids to be injected through the device into the empty capsule, significantly reducing the concentration of irrigation fluid able to contact other ocular structures and thus perform Sealed Capsule Irrigation. **A**. Sealed Capsule Irrigation device viewed from the top. It consists of a round plate that seals against the capsule and an extension arm that passes outside the wound to provide to the internal lens capsule. **B**. Sealed Capsule Irrigation device is folded and inserted through a 3-mm incision. The Sealed Capsule Irrigation device is placed onto the capsular bag and vacuum-activated by a syringe. Internal irrigation of the capsular bag using distilled water for 2 minutes is done. The Sealed Capsule Irrigation device prevents the endothelium from getting damaged by the distilled water. **C**. Illustration showing the Sealed Capsule Irrigation device fixed onto the anterior capsule once the cortex has been removed. **D**. The Sealed Capsule Irrigation device is then removed from the eye.

We have performed initial testing on postmortem porcine lens capsules and demonstrated the effectiveness of sealed capsule irrigation.[49] We have further refined the device to incorporate changes which would allow it to be used in small incision cataract surgery, and address the potential risk of pseudosuction, which would result in loss of sealing of the capsular bag. We considered the properties of the adult capsule to be less elastic than the pediatric capsule, and less prone to pseudosuction. To prevent pseudosuction, the device was modified to contain a vacuum manifold within the suction ring that ensures no focal occlusion of the suction ring is possible at any point, and that the vacuum is evenly distributed to the entire ring. This has been further developed using a cog-wheel design.

In performing product validation, 13 randomly chosen devices were subjected to testing on pig capsule. In all cases, the devices sealed the capsule using vacuum generated by a

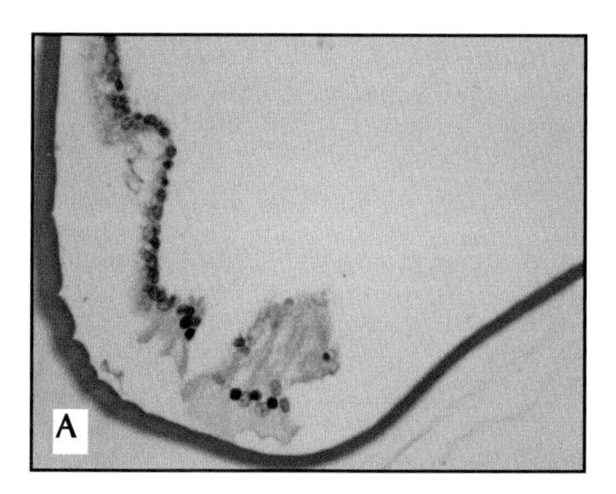

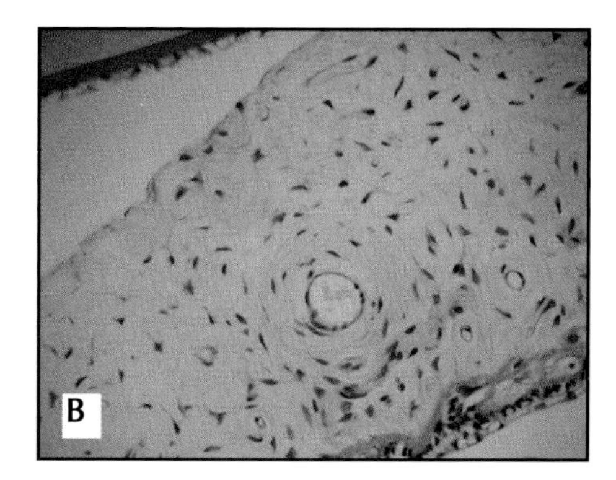

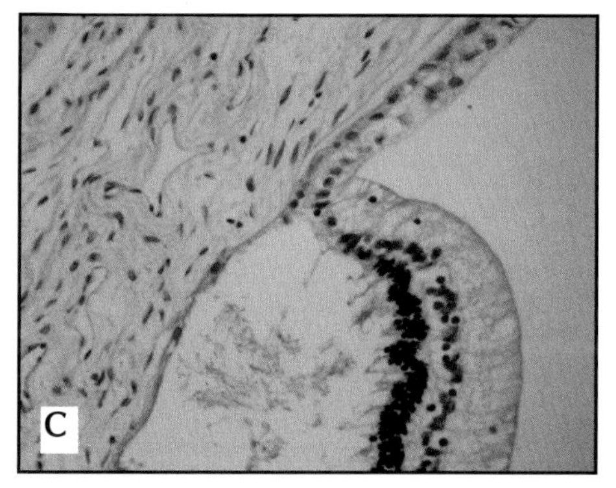

Figure 23-7. Histological findings of the rabbit eyes in Group 1 (phacoaspiration surgery without any treatment, Control Group). **A**. Photomicrograph showing the capsular bag. Note the presence of residual viable LECs with in the capsular bag. (Periodic acid-Schiff stain, original magnification x40). **B**. Photomicrograph showing healthy corneal endothelial cells and posterior iris epithelium. (Periodic acid-Schiff stain, original magnification x40). **C**. Photomicrograph showing undamaged retinal tissue and epithelium. There is postmortem artefactual detachment at the ora serata. (Periodic acid-Schiff stain, original magnification x40).

20mL lockable syringe resulting in a maximal vacuum pressure of greater than 700mmHg on application, with no evidence of pseudosuction with less than 2.5% reduction in vacuum pressure over a 1 minute period. One of these devices was then selected for repeat testing for a period of 10 minutes with less than 5% reduction in vacuum at 10 minutes.

We are continuing to demonstrate that selective capsular bag irrigation can be performed in animals and humans. In a rabbit study,[50] we assessed the ability to deliver a nonspecific extremely toxic agent directly to the LECs post crystalline lens removal, and assessed the eyes histologically for evidence of collateral damage (Figures 23-7 through 23-9). A total of six New Zealand White rabbit eyes were selected. The eyes were divided into three groups of four eyes. All eyes underwent phacoaspiration of the crystalline lens via a 3.2 mm corneal incision. Group 1 eyes were used as control. In Group 2 eyes, the capsular bag was irrigated with 1 % Triton X-100 and demineralised water for injection (DWI) for 5 minutes. In Group 3 eyes, the capsular bag was isolated from the anterior segment using the PerfectCapsule. Immediately after the surgery, all six rabbits were humanely euthanised. The enucleated eyes were immediately fixed in 10% neutral buffered formalin and histological analysis was performed to assess the corneal endothelium, iris, and retina. The capsular bag was also assessed and residual equatorial LECs were evaluated. There was no

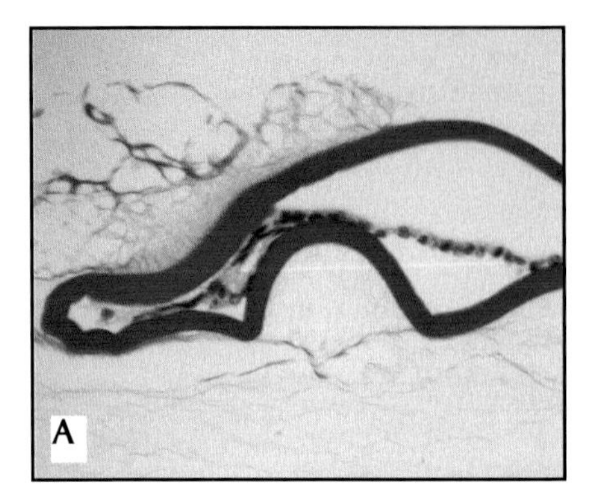

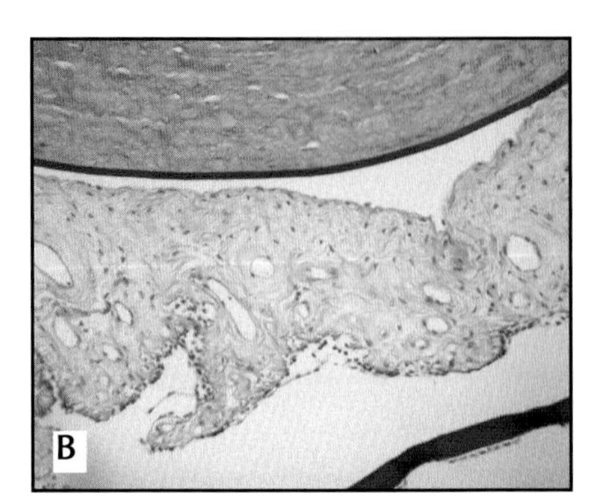

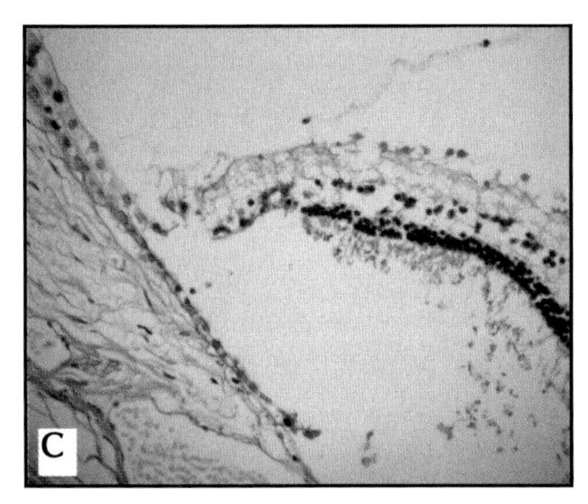

Figure 23-8. Histological findings of the rabbit eyes in Group 2 (phacoaspiration surgery and non-selective irrigation of the capsular bag with DWI & TTX-100 without SCI). **A**. Photomicrograph showing the collapsed fornices of the capsular bag. Note the presence of viable LECs at the anterior and equatorial region of the capsular bag. (Periodic acid-Schiff stain, original magnification x40). **B**. Photomicrograph showing almost total loss of corneal endothelial cells, with bare Descemet's membrane. There is a loss of integrity of posterior iris epithelium (Periodic acid-Schiff stain, original magnification x40). **C**. Photomicrograph of the peripheral retina showing significant disorganization of the retinal tissue and epithelium. (Periodic acid-Schiff stain, original magnification x40).

intraoperative complication in any eye. The capsular bag was sealed and inflated under SCI, PerfectCapsule in all treatment eyes in Group 3. Histological evaluation revealed no evidence of any collateral damage in Group 1 (control, group) and Group 3 (with SCI) (see Figures 23-7 and 23-9). Significant histological damage to the cornea, iris and peripheral retina was noted in Group 2 eyes, which underwent irrigation with DWI and Triton X-100 (without SCI). Histological evaluation of capsular bag suggests presence of LECs in Group 1 (control, group) and Group 2 (without SCI) (Figures 23–7 and 23–8). In the presence of SCI, Triton X-100 caused almost complete destruction of LECs in the capsular bag (Figure 23–9). Result of this pilot study suggest that SCI allows selective delivery of toxic agents directly into the capsular bag preventing collateral damage to surrounding intraocular structures in a rabbit eye. The SCI device kept the capsular bag well inflated intraoperatively and therefore it may allow the isolated safe delivery of pharmacological agents into the capsular bag during cataract surgery.

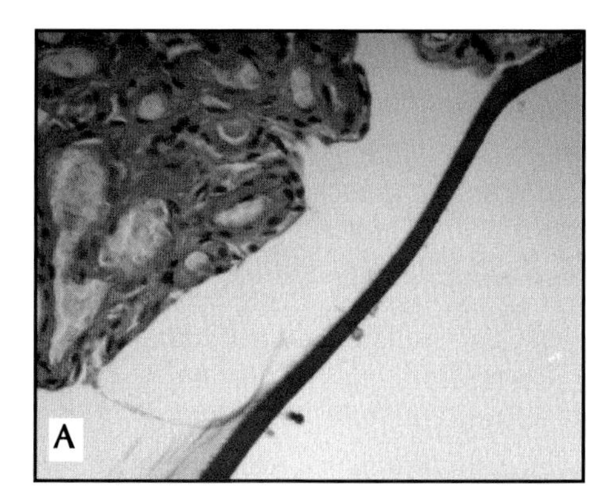

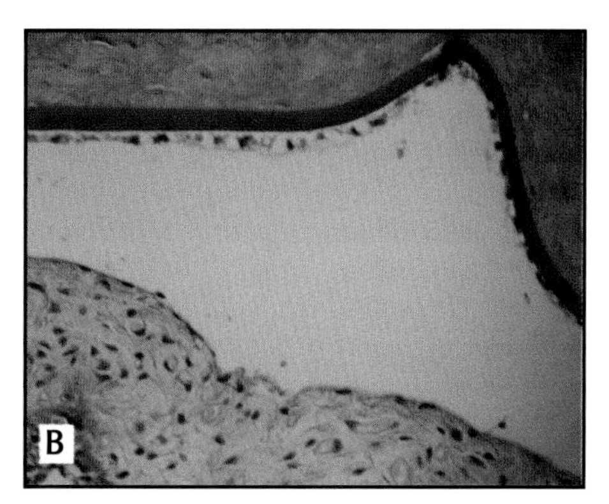

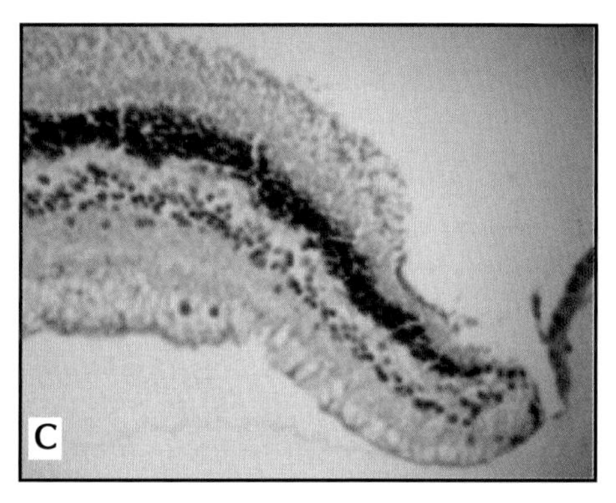

Figure 23-9. Histological findings of the rabbit eyes in Group 3 (phacoaspiration surgery and selective irrigation of the capsular bag with DWI & TTX-100 with SCI). **A**. Photomicrograph showing the capsular bag. Note the absence of viable LECs within the capsular fornices. Some nuclear remnants are visible lying on the capsule (Periodic acid-Schiff stain, original magnification x40). **B**. Photomicrograph showing healthy corneal endothelial cells and posterior iris epithelium. (Periodic acid-Schiff stain, original magnification x40). **C**. Photomicrograph showing undamaged peripheral retinal tissue and epithelium. (Periodic acid-Schiff stain, original magnification x40).

We have recently completed a 1-year follow up on a total of nine human eyes underwent cataract-IOL surgery using SCI with distilled water and silicone lenses (SI40NB, Clariflex, AMO, Santa Ana, Calif). A control group of nine eyes underwent cataract surgery with implantation of silicone lenses, without SCI. All eyes in the treatment Group, underwent internal irrigation of the capsular bag using 20cc of distilled water for 60 seconds to 90 seconds using the PerfectCapsule. Fluorescein sodium (0.01%) or trypan blue (0.01%) was used to identify any leakage into the anterior chamber during the SCI procedure. Slit lamp biomicroscopic examination was performed at 1 day, 1 week, 3, 6, and 12 months to evaluate anterior capsule opacification (ACO), capsular folds/wrinkling, capsular phimosis, and posterior capsule opacification (PCO) (area/severity). Intraoperatively, there was no visible leakage of fluorescein sodium/trypan blue dyes into the anterior chamber during SCI in all eyes in Group AA and AS, indicative of effective seal provided by the SCI device. Follow-up examination at 6 and 12 months demonstrated a significant reduction in ACO in all eyes, which had undergone SCI with distilled water treatment in comparison to control eyes. In addition, the degree of capsular phimosis was significantly reduced in treatment group, compared to control groups.

Using SCI technique, targeting of lens epithelial cells to prevent PCO can be safely conducted using precise delivery of known doses of pharmacologic agents, with much less fear of toxicity to surrounding intraocular structures. This method may be utilized to eliminate or modulate LEC activity after cataract surgery, which may lead to less postoperative inflammation and a theoretical reduction in the risk of postoperative cystoid macular edema, reduced anterior and posterior capsule opacification, and allow for definitive implantation of multifocal and accommodative lenses so that the treatment of presbyopia may finally become a reality. Clinical studies will be needed to test efficacy of SCI during pediatric cataract surgery. Theoretically, SCI may be helpful to elimination of LECs and therefore avoid the PCO/secondary membrane formation postoperatively. It may obviate the need for primary posterior capsulotomy with anterior vitrectomy intraoperatively.

Modulation of the Lens Epithelial Cells

The human lens capsular bag provides a unique environment within the body for selective specific targeting of tissue. Within this environment, an ideal approach would be to target LEC's for modulation of cell function, rather than cell death. Concern remains over the viability of a denuded lens capsule within the human eyes. It is not known how long the denuded lens capsule will support a lens and stay clear; to date, this has not been achieved. Conventional methods to destroy remaining LECs result in significant damage to surrounding structures.

The environment of the anterior chamber immediately following cataract surgery contains TGFB. There is breakdown of blood aqueous barrier and the presence of inflammatory mediators. Clinically, this corresponds with proliferation of LEC's, commonly seen at growing onto the surface of hydrophobic acrylic lenses 1 month, reaching a peak at 6 weeks, then stabilizing. In culture medium, LEC's are noted to very rapidly grow over capsule over 1 week under conditions of accelerated growth, and a similar effect may occur in the human eye. Modulation of the LECs can be another option to prevent visually significant capsular bag opacification. The effect of lithium chloride (LiCl) on the morphology and behavior of lens epithelial cells is profound. In low density, NaCl (20mM) treated cells display a loosely packed squamous profile with numerous pseudopodia. By contrast, LiCl (20mM) treated cells form aggregated islands and remain tightly packed with an apical-basal polarised profile and rounded cobblestone appearance. LiCl abrogates cell spreading over a concentration range of 10–40mM compared with NaCl controls.

LiCl has distinct and dichotomous roles in influencing the behavior of lens epithelial cells. LiCl is both a potent inhibitor of lens cell proliferation, migration and differentiation and, at similar concentrations, LiCl promotes cell adhesion and maintenance of epithelial characteristics i.e, apical-basal polarity. LiCl also blocks the TGFb-induced EMT. Evidence for the inhibition of GSK-3 by LiCl in lens cells was demonstrated by an increase in expression of active b-catenin (AbC). With LiCl, active b-catenin preferentially accumulates on membranes and does not move into the nucleus. However, under similar conditions, nuclear expression of AbC does occur with addition of a specific GSK-3 inhibitor. These results support the view that while LiCl promotes stabilization of AbC, this does necessarily result in nuclear transactivation. Our pilot study also implicate pathways other than Wnt/b-cateninin the LiCl response, these are: inhibition of proliferation and migration which coincides with abrogation of phospho-ERK expression, implying LiCl-induced modulation of the MAPK pathway; promotion of tight packing, polarised cells and increased expression of ZO-1 and MARCKS. MARCKS proteins bind and cross-link actin suggesting a role in stabilizing polarized cells. Therefore, LiCl promotes tight junction formation and membrane expression of AbC and ZO-1, through inhibition of GSK-3 and possibly activation of PKC. Inhibition of GSK3 promotes stabilization of b-catenin allowing canonical Wnt signaling. Formation of the Wnt/Frizzled/LRP complex activates b-catenin. In the nucleus, active b-catenin complexes with TCF and regulates gene expression. Active b-catenin also binds to E-cadherin and becomes localized at the cell membrane.

Removal of Lens Epithelial Cells Using AquaLase Liquefaction Device

AquaLase Liquefaction Device is a new advancement in lens removal technology which is a part of the newly introduced Infiniti Vision System (Alcon Inc., Fort Worth, Tex).[82] The AquaLase liquefaction hand piece proved to be effective to remove nuclear cataracts of up to grade 2 with reasonable efficiency, as of this writing, and this technology may have applications in polishing the capsule and removing lens equatorial cells thus minimizing the postoperative cellular proliferation of the LECs, thereby minimizing or eliminating the risk of capsular bag fibrosis (ACO/PCO).

The AquaLase tip is composed of a soft polymer and has soft, rounded edges. This design makes the instrument more capsule-friendly than metal ultrasound tips. The AquaLase hand piece propels small pulses of balanced saline solution (BSS) warmed to 57°C to liquefy lens material just inside the aspiration port of the tip. The BSS pulses are delivered at a maximum rate of 50 Hz, and the surgeon controls the magnitude of the pulses with the Infiniti™ foot pedal.

Summary

The tools, surgical procedures, skills, and appropriate IOLs are now available to eradicate PCO. Continued motivation to apply the 6 factors noted in this article, the efficacy of which have been further suggested in a recent study,[54] will help diminish this final major complication of cataract-IOL surgery exactly 50 years after Sir Ridley's first encounter with this complication. A major reduction of Nd: YAG laser capsulotomy rates towards single digits is now possible- because of application of aforementioned surgical factors and factors related to modern lens designs/biomaterials- at least in the industrialized world. This will obviously be of great benefit to patients in achieving improved long-term results and avoidance of Nd: YAG laser capsulotomy complications. Eradication of the Nd: YAG laser procedure will help control what has been the one of the most expensive costs to the health care System. To date one cannot precisely determine the relative proportion or contribution of IOL design vs. surgical techniques to the decrease of Nd: YAG laser rates observed here. However, this could be possible with continuing analysis including annual updates and increasing numbers of pseudophakic autopsy eyes.

In summary, we have ascertained various factors that help bring about the very positive conclusion that surgeons now have the sufficient tools and appropriate IOLs to help reduce the incidence of PCO. The recent advent of SCI is a significant step to eliminate PCO and to maintain long-term capsular bag clarity that is necessary for success of accommodative/refractive lenses. The SCI will also be helpful for maintaining the long-term clear visual axis in pediatric cataract-IOL surgery. However further experimental studies and multi-centric clinical trials are necessary to test its efficacy.

Key Points

1. In addition to classic posterior capsule opacification (PCO, secondary cataract, after cataract), postoperative lens epithelial cell (LEC) proliferation is also involved in the pathogenesis of anterior capsule opacification/fibrosis (ACO) and inter-lenticular opacification (ILO).
2. Nd: YAG laser secondary posterior capsulotomy, can be associated with significant complications. Potential problems include IOL optic damage/pitting, postoperative intraocular pressure elevation, cystoid macular edema, retinal detachment, and IOL subluxation.
3. Although both types of cells (from the anterior central zone and from the equatorial lens bow) have the potential to produce visually significant opacification, most cases of classic PCO are caused by proliferation of the equatorial cells. The term posterior capsule opacification implies that the capsule opacifies. Rather, an opaque membrane develops over the capsule as retained cells proliferate and migrate onto the posterior capsular surface.
4. One strategy to reduce posterior capsular opacification is to minimize the number of retained/regenerated cells and cortex (including the Soemmering's ring) through thorough cortical cleanup. The second strategy is to prevent the remaining cells from migrating posteriorly. The edge of the IOL optic is critical in the formation of such a physical barrier.
5. Sealed Capsule Irrigation (SCI) device may allow the isolated safe delivery of pharmacologic agents into the capsular bag following cataract surgery.

References

1. Apple DJ. Influence of intraocular lens material and design on postoperative intracapsular cellular reactivity. *Trans Am Ophthalmol Soc.* 2000;98:257–83.
2. Werner L, Apple DJ, Pandey SK. Postoperative proliferation of anterior and equatorial lens epithelial cells: A comparison between various foldable IOL designs. In: Buratto L, Osher R, Masket S, eds. *Cataract Surgery in Complicated Cases.* Thorofare, NJ: SLACK Incorporated; 2000.
3. Werner L, Pandey SK, Escobar-Gomez M, Visessook N, Peng Q, Apple DJ. Anterior capsule opacification: a histopathological study comparing different IOL styles. *Ophthalmology.* 2000;107:463–67.
4. Werner L, Pandey SK, Apple DJ, Escobar-Gomez M, McLendon L, Macky T. Anterior capsule opacification: correlation of pathological findings with clinical sequelae. *Ophthalmology.* 2001;108:1675–81.
5. Gayton JL, Apple DJ, Peng Q, et al. Interlenticular opacification: clinicopathological correlation of a complication of posterior chamber piggyback intraocular lenses. *J Cataract Refract Surg.* 2000;26:330–36.
6. Werner L, Apple DJ, Pandey SK, et al. Analysis of elements of interlenticular opacification. *Am J Ophthalmol.* 2002;133:320–26.
7. Ridley H. The origin and objectives of intraocular lenticular implants. *Trans Am Acad Ophthalmol Otolaryngol.* 1976;81:65–6.
8. Ridley H. Long-term results of acrylic lens surgery. *Proc R Soc Med.* 1970;63:309–10.
9. Apple DJ, Solomon KD, Tetz MR, et al. Posterior capsule opacification. *Surv Ophthalmol.* 1992;37:73–116.
10. Pandey SK, Wilson ME, Trivedi RH, et al. Pediatric cataract surgery and intraocular lens implantation: current techniques, complications and management. *Int Ophthalmol Clin.* 2001;41:175–96.

11. Pandey SK, Ram J, Werner L, Jain A, Barar GS, Gupta A. Visual results and postoperative complications of capsular bag versus sulcus fixation of posterior chamber intraocular lenses for traumatic cataract in children. *J Cataract Refract Surg*. 1999;25:1576–84.
12. Pandey SK, Wilson ME, Werner L, Ram J, Apple DJ. Childhood cataract surgical technique, complications and management. In: Garg A, Pandey SK. *Textbook of Ocular Therapeutics*. New Delhi, India: Jaypee Brothers; 2002:457–86.
13. Apple DJ, Peng Q, Visessook N, et al. Eradication of posterior capsule opacification. Documentation of a marked decrease in Nd:YAG laser posterior capsulotomy rates noted in an analysis of 5416 pseudophakic human eyes obtained postmortem. *Ophthalmology*. 2001;108:505–18.
14. Apple DJ, Peng Q, Visessook N, et al. Surgical prevention of posterior capsule opacification. Part I. Progress in eliminating this complication of cataract surgery. *J Cataract Refract Surg*. 2000;26:180–7.
15. Worst JGF. *International Intraocular Implant Club Report*. 1999;1:2.
16. Holweger RR, Marefat B. Intraocular pressure change after neodymium:YAG capsulotomy. *J Cataract Refract Surg*. 1997;23:115–21.
17. Hu CY, Woung LC, Wang MC. Change in the area of laser posterior capsulotomy: 3 months follow-up. *J Cataract Refract Surg*. 2001;27:537–42.
18. Richter CU, Steinert RF. Neodymium: Yttrium-Aluminium-Garnet laser posterior capsulotomy. In: Steinert RF, ed. *Cataract Surgery: Techniques, Complications and Management*. Philadelphia, PA: WB Saunders Co; 1995:378–388.
19. Koch D, Liu J, Gill P, Parke D. Axial myopia increases the risk of retinal complications after neodymium-YAG laser posterior capsulotomy. *Arch Ophthalmol*. 1989;107:986–90.
20. Apple DJ, Ram J, Foster A, Peng Q. Elimination of cataract blindness: a global perspective entering the new millennium. *Surv Ophthalmol*. 2000;45:S70–S99.
21. Font RL, Brownstein S. A light and electron microscopic study of anterior subcapsular cataracts. *Am J Ophthalmol*. 1974;78:972–84.
22. Peng Q, Hennig A, Vasavada AR, Apple DJ. Posterior capsular plaque: a common feature of cataract surgery in the developing world. *Am J Ophthalmol*. 1998;125:621–26.
23. McAvoy JW, Chamberlain CG. Growth factors in the eye. *Prog Growth Factor Res*. 1990;2:29–43.
24. Lang RA, McAvoy JW. Growth factors in lens development. In: Lovicu FJ, Robinson ML, eds. *Development of the Ocular Lens*. New York, NY: Cambridge University Press; 2004.
25. Stump RJ, Ang S, Chen Y, et al. A role for Wnt/beta-catenin signaling in lens epithelial differentiation. *Dev Biol*. 2003;259:48–61.
26. Wormstone IM. Posterior capsule opacification: a cell biological perspective. *Exp Eye Res*. 2002;74:337–47.
27. Gordon-Thomson C, de Iongh RU, Hales AM, Chamberlain CG, McAvoy JW. Differential cataractogenic potency of TGF-beta1, -beta2, and -beta3 and their expression in the postnatal rat eye. *Invest Ophthalmol Vis Sci*. 1998;39:1399–409.
28. Hales AM, Chamberlain CG, McAvoy JW. Cataract induction in lenses cultured with transforming growth factor-beta. *Invest Ophthalmol Vis Sci*. 1995;36:1709–1713.
29. Lovicu FJ, Schulz MW, Hales AM, et al. TGFbeta induces morphological and molecular changes similar to human anterior subcapsular cataract. *Br J Ophthalmol*. 2002;86:220–226.
30. Liu J, Hales AM, Chamberlain CG, McAvoy JW. Induction of cataract-like changes in rat lens epithelial explants by transforming growth factor beta. *Invest Ophthalmol Vis Sci*. 1994;35:388–401.
31. Srinivasan Y, Lovicu FJ, Overbeek PA. Lens-specific expression of transforming growth factor beta1 in transgenic mice causes anterior subcapsular cataracts. *J Clin Invest*. 1998;101:625–634.
32. Sasaki K, Kojima M, Nakaizumi H, Kitagawa K, Yamada Y, Ishizaki H. Early lens changes seen in patients with atopic dermatitis applying image analysis processing of Scheimpflug and specular microscopic images. *Ophthalmologica*. 1998;212:88–94.

33. Lee EH, Seomun Y, Hwang KH, et al. Overexpression of the transforming growth factor-beta-inducible gene betaig-h3 in anterior polar cataracts. *Invest Ophthalmol Vis Sci.* 2000;41:1840–5.
34. Saika S, Miyamoto T, Ishida I, et al. TGFb-Smad signalling in postoperative human lens epithelial cells. *Br J Ophthalmol.* 2002;86:1428–1433.
35. Hales AM, Chamberlain CG, Murphy CR, McAvoy JW. Estrogen protects lenses against cataract induced by TGFß. *J Exp Med.* 1997;185:273–280.
36. Younan C, Mitchell P, Cumming RG, Panchapakesan J, Rochtchina E, Hales AM. Hormone replacement therapy, reproductive factors, and the incidence of cataract and cataract surgery: the Blue Mountains Eye Study. *Am J Epidemiol.* 2002;155:997–1006.
37. Ram J, Kaushik S, Brar GS, Gupta A. Neodymium YAG capsulotomy rates following phacoemulsification with implantation of PMMA, silicone, and acrylic intraocular lenses. *Ophthalmic Surg Lasers.* 2001;32:375–82.
38. Schaumberg DA, Dana MR, Christen WG, Glynn RJ. A systematic overview of the incidence of posterior capsular opacification. *Ophthalmology.* 1998;105:1213–21.
39. Cheng CY, Yen MY, Chen SJ, Kao SC, Hsu WM, Liu JH. Visual acuity and contrast sensitivity in different types of posterior capsule opacification. *J Cataract Refract Surg.* 2001;27:1055–60.
40. Ram J, Apple DJ, Peng Q, et al. Update on fixation of rigid and foldable posterior chamber intraocular lenses. Part II. Choosing the correct haptic fixation and intraocular lens design to help eradicate posterior capsule opacification. *Ophthalmology.* 1999;106:891–900.
41. Apple DJ, Auffarth GU, Peng Q, Visessook N. *Foldable Intraocular Lenses: Evolution, Clinicopathologic Correlations, Complications.* Thorofare, NJ: SLACK Incorporated; 2000:157–215.
42. Peng Q, Apple DJ, Visessook N, et al. Surgical prevention of posterior capsule opacification. Part II. Enhancement of cortical clean up by focusing on hydrodissection. *J Cataract Refract Surg.* 2000;26:188–197.
43. Peng Q, Visessook N, Apple DJ, et al. Surgical prevention of posterior capsule opacification. Part III. Intraocular lens optic barrier effect as a second line of defense. *J Cataract Refract Surg.* 2000;26:198–213.
44. Vargas LG, Peng Q, Apple DJ, et al. Evaluation of 3 modern single-piece foldable intraocular lenses: clinicopathological study of posterior capsule opacification in a rabbit model. *J Cataract Refract Surg.* 2002;28:1241–50.
45. Vargas LG, Izak AM, Apple DJ, Werner L, Pandey SK, Trivedi RH. Single Piece AcrySof Implantation of a single-piece, hydrophilic, acrylic, minus-power foldable posterior chamber intraocular lens in a rabbit model: clinicopathologic study of posterior capsule opacification. *J Cataract Refract Surg.* 2003;29:1613–20.
46. Fine IH. Cortical cleaving hydrodissection. *J Cataract Refract Surg.* 1992;18:508–12.
47. Vasavada AR, Singh R, Apple DJ, Trivedi RH, Pandey SK, Werner L. Efficacy of hydrodissection step in the phacoemulsification for age related senile cataract. *J Cataract Refract Surg.* 2002;28:1623–28.
48. Vargas LG, Escobar-Gomez M, Apple DJ, Hoddinott DS, Schmidbauer JM. Pharmacologic prevention of posterior capsule opacification: in vitro effects of preservative-free lidocaine 1% on lens epithelial cells. *J Cataract Refract Surg.* 2003;29:1585–92.
49. Maloof AJ, Neilson G, Milverton EJ, Pandey SK. Selective and specific targeting of lens epithelial cells during cataract surgery using sealed- capsule irrigation. *J Cataract Refract Surg.* 2003;29:1566–68.
50. Maloof AJ, Pandey SK, Neilson G, Crouch R, Milverton EJ. Selective death of lens epithelial cells using demineralised water and Triton X-100 with PerfectCapsule™ sealed capsule irrigation: a histological study in rabbit eyes. *Arch Ophthalmol.* 2004.
51. Ram J, Apple DJ, Peng Q, et al. Update on fixation of rigid and foldable posterior chamber intraocular lenses. Part I: Elimination of fixation-induced decentration to achieve precise optical correction and visual rehabilitation. *Ophthalmology.* 1999;106:883–90.

52. Apple DJ, Reidy JJ, Googe JM, et al. A comparison of ciliary sulcus and capsular bag fixation of posterior chamber intraocular lenses. *J Am Intraocul Implant Soc.* 1985;11:44–63.
53. Vasavada AR, Raj SM. Anterior capsule relationship of the AcrySof intraocular lens optic and posterior capsule opacification: a prospective randomized clinical trial. *Ophthalmology.* 2004;111:886–94.
54. Linnola RJ. Sandwich theory: bioactivity-based explanation for posterior capsule opacification. *J Cataract Refract Surg.* 1997;23:1539–42.
55. Linnola RJ, Werner L, Pandey SK, Escobar-Gomez M, Znoiko SL, Apple DJ. Adhesion of fibronectin, vitronectin, laminin and collagen type IV to intraocular lens materials in human autopsy eyes. Part I: histological sections. *J Cataract Refract Surg.* 2000;26:1792–1806.
56. Linnola RJ, Werner L, Pandey SK, Escobar-Gomez M, Znoiko SL, Apple DJ. Adhesion of fibronectin, vitronectin, laminin and collagen type IV to intraocular lens materials in human autopsy eyes. Part II: explanted IOLs. *J Cataract Refract Surg.* 2000;26:1807–18.
57. Nishi O, Nishi K, Akura J, Nagata T. Effect of round-edged acrylic intraocular lenses on preventing posterior capsule opacification. *J Cataract Refract Surg.* 2001;27:608–13.
58. Nishi O, Nishi K, Menapace R, Akura J. Capsular bending ring to prevent posterior capsule opacification: 2 year follow-up. *J Cataract Refract Surg.* 2001;27:1359–65.
59. Kruger AJ, Schauersberger J, Abela C, Schild G, Amon M. Two year results: Sharp versus rounded optic edges on silicone lenses. *J Cataract Refract Surg.* 2000;26:566–70.
60. Kucuksumer Y, Bayraktar S, Sahin S, Yilmaz OF. Posterior capsule opacification 3 years after implantation of an AcrySof and a MemoryLens in fellow eyes. *J Cataract Refract Surg.* 2000;26:1176–82.
61. Meacock WR, Spalton DJ, Boyce JF, Jose RM. Effect of optic size on posterior capsule opacification: 5.5 mm versus 6.0 mm AcrySof intraocular lenses. *J Cataract Refract Surg.* 2001;27:1194–98.
62. Nishi O. Posterior capsule opacification. Part 1: Experimental investigations. *J Cataract Refract Surg.* 1999;25:106–17.
63. Nishi O, Nishi K. Effect of the optic size of a single-piece acrylic intraocular lens on posterior capsule opacification. *J Cataract Refract Surg.* 2003;29:348–53.
64. Hollick EJ, Spalton DJ, Ursell PG, Meacock WR, Barman SA, Boyce JF. Posterior capsular opacification with hydrogel, polymethylmethacrylate, and silicone intraocular lenses: two-year results of a randomized prospective trial. *Am J Ophthalmol.* 2000;129:577–84.
65. Buehl W, Findl O, Menapace R, et al. Effect of an acrylic intraocular lens with a sharp posterior optic edge on posterior capsule opacification. *J Cataract Refract Surg.* 2002;28:1105–1111.
66. Aasuri MK, Shah U, Veenashree MP, Deshpande P. Performance of a truncated-edged silicone foldable intraocular lens in Indian eyes. *J Cataract Refract Surg.* 2002;28:1135–40.
67. Auffarth GU, Golescu A, Becker KA, Volcker HE. Quantification of posterior capsule opacification with round and sharp edge intraocular lenses. *Ophthalmology.* 2003;110:772–80.
68. Masket S. Truncated edge design, dysphotopsia, and inhibition of posterior capsule opacification. *J Cataract Refract Surg.* 2000;26:145–47.
69. Ram J, Pandey SK, Apple DJ, et al. Effect of in-the-bag intraocular lens fixation on the prevention of posterior capsule opacification. *J Cataract Refract Surg.* 2001; 27:1039–46.
70. Ravalico G, Tognetto D, et al. Capsulorrhexis size and posterior capsule opacification. *J Cataract Refract Surg.* 1996;22:98–103.
71. Chung HS, Lim SJ, Kim HB. Efect of mitomycin-C on posterior capsule opacification in rabbit eyes. *J Cataract Refract Surg.* 2000;26:1537–42.
72. Power WJ, Neylan D, Collum LMT. Daunorubicin as an inhibitor of human lens epithelial cell proliferation in culture. *J Cataract Refract Surg.* 1994;20:287–90.
73. Rakic JM, Galand A, Vrensen GFJM. Lens epithelial cell proliferation in human posterior capsule opacification. *Exp Eye Research.* 2000;5:489–94.

74. Rootman J, Tisdall J, Gudauskas G, Ostray A. Intraocular penetration of subconjunctivally administered ^{14}C-fluorouracil in rabbits. *Arch Ophthalmol.* 1979;97:2375–78.
75. Legler UF, Apple DJ, Assia EI, Bluestein EC, Castaneda VE, Mowbray SL. Inhibition of posterior capsule opacification: the effect of colchicine in a sustained drug delivery system. *J Cataract Refract Surg.* 1993;19:462–70.
76. Tetz MR, Ries MW, Lucas C, Stricker H, Volcker HE. Inhibition of posterior capsule opacification by an intraocular–lens–bound sustained drug delivery system: an experimental animal study and literature review. *J Cataract Refract Surg.* 1996;22:1070–78.
77. Pandey SK, Cochener B, Apple DJ, Werner L, Bougran R, Colin J. Intracapsular ring sustained 5-fluorouracil delivery system for prevention of posterior capsule opacification in rabbits: a histological study. *J Cataract Refract Surg.* 2002;28:139–48.
78. Cochener B, Bougaran R, Pandey SK, Apple DJ, Colin J. Nonbiodegradable drug-sustained capsular ring for prevention of secondary cataract. Part I: In vitro evaluation. *J Fr Ophtalmol.* 2003;26:223–31.
79. Cochener B, Pandey SK, Apple DJ, Bougaran R, Colin J. Nonbiodegradable drug-sustained capsular ring for prevention of secondary cataract. Part II: In vivo evaluation. *J Fr Ophtalmol.* 2003;26:439–52.
80. Miyake K, Miyake C. Intraoperative posterior chamber lens haptic fixation in the human cadaver eye. *Ophthalmic Surg.* 1985;16:230–36.
81. Apple DJ, Lim ES, Morgan RC, et al. Preparation and study of human eyes obtained postmortem with the Miyake posterior photographic technique. *Ophthalmology.* 1990;97:810–16.
82. Mackool RJ, Brint SF. AquaLase: a new technology for cataract extraction. *Curr Opin Ophthalmol.* 2004;15:40–43.

Chapter 24

Intraocular Lens Opacification

Suresh K. Pandey, MD; Liliana Werner, MD, PhD; David J. Apple, MD

Introduction

It has been over 50 years since Harold Ridley's first implant and the cataract-intraocular lens (IOL) procedure has reached an extraordinarily high level of quality and performance. Still complications like IOL opacification do occur (Figure 24-1).

Delayed Opacification of PMMA IOL Optic Biomaterial: "Snowflake" or Crystalline Opacification

Over the past 50 years, PMMA has been rightly considered a safe, tried and true material for IOL manufacturing with high quality control. PMMA biomaterial was used as an optic biomaterial in Sir Harold Ridley's original IOL, manufactured by Rayner Intraocular Lenses Ltd, London, UK, and first implanted in 1949–1950.[1] Although surgeons in the industrialized world and in selected areas in the developing world have largely transitioned to foldable IOL biomaterials, PMMA does remain in widespread use in many regions. Biomaterial studies on PMMA IOL optics were rarely required. Until now, any untoward complications such as PMMA-optic material alteration/breakdown have not been seen with this material and its fabrication.

However, we have recently reported gradual but progressive late postoperative alteration/destruction of PMMA optic biomaterial causing significant decrease in visual acuity, sometimes to a severity that requires IOL explantation (Figure 24-2). The first clinical case of the type that we observed was a documentation of photographs sent to us by David Davis, MD, of Hayward, CA, in 1993. He noted "crystalline" formations in 7 IOPTEX Research (Azuza, CA) 3-piece PMMA IOLs. Over the past 4 years, 25 cases including 9 explanted IOLs were submitted to Center for Research on Ocular Therapeutics and Biodevices (Figure 24-2).[2,3]

All of the explanted IOLs were 3-piece posterior chamber (PC)-IOLs with rigid PMMA

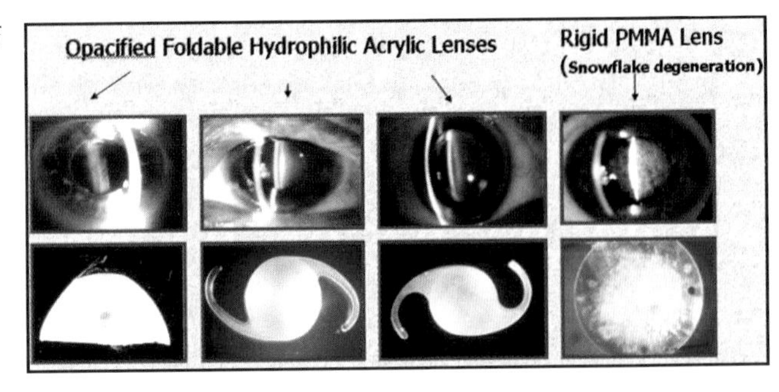

Figure 24-1. Opacification of rigid and foldable lenses.

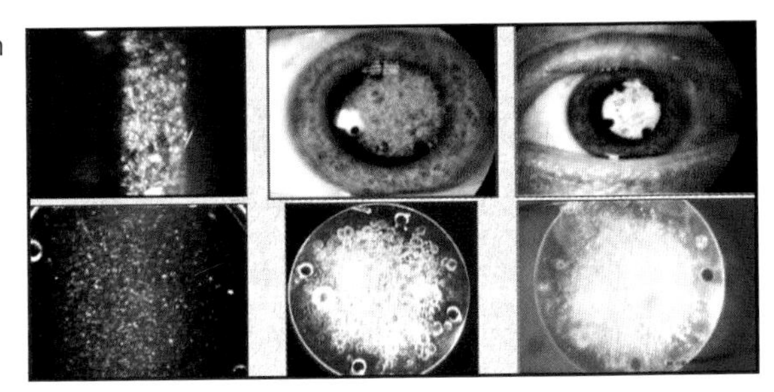

Figure 24-2. "Snowflake" opacification of PMMA IOLS.

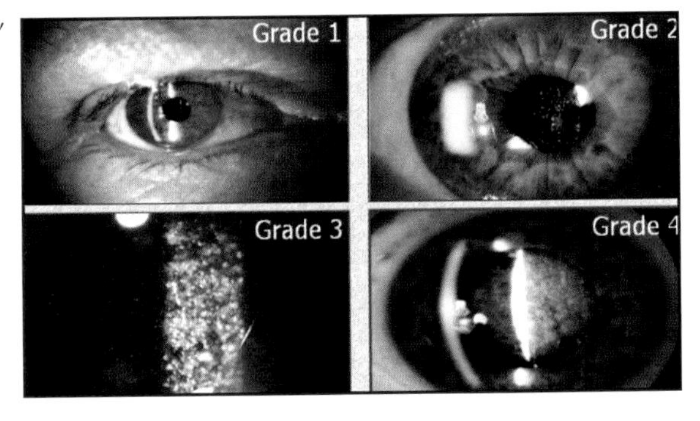

Figure 24-3. Classification of "Snowflake" lesion.

optical components and blue polypropylene or extruded PMMA haptics. These had been implanted in the early 1980s to early 1990s in most cases and the clinical symptoms appeared late postoperatively, 8 to 15 years after the implantation. The clinical, gross, light and electron microscopic profiles of all the cases showed almost identical findings, differing only in the degree of intensity of the "snowflake" lesions that in turn reflected the severity and probably the duration of the opacification. In the early stages of many of the cases, the lesions were first noted clinically by a routine slit lamp examination, in the absence of visual disturbances. Most examiners described the white-brown opacities within the IOL optics as "crystalline deposits" (Figure 24-3). They appeared to progress gradually in most cases. Clinically, the slowly progressive opacities of the IOL optics usually start as scattered white-brown spots within the substance of the IOL optic. These usually do not have an impact on the patients' VA. They gradually increase in intensity and number, eventually reaching a point where the VA loss necessitates removal or exchange of the IOL. In addition to visual loss the symptoms included decrease in contrast sensitivity and various visu-

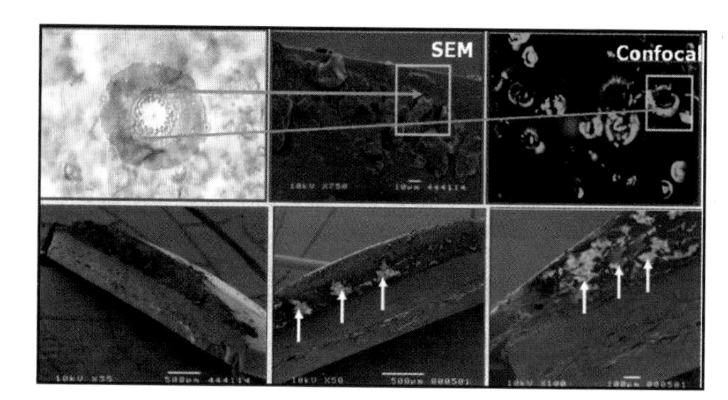

Figure 24-4. "Snowflake" lesions of PMMA IOL: microscopic, ultrastructural appearance.

al disturbances and aberrations, including glare. Figure 24-3 presents the classification of snowflake lesions as proposed by Apple and associates.[2,3]

Clinicopathological Study of Explanted Lenses

The opacities of the IOL optics may start as scattered white-brown spots within the substance of the IOL optic and remain stable or slowly progressive. Some may gradually increase in intensity and numbers, eventually reaching a point where a visual acuity loss may necessitate removal or exchange of the IOL. In addition to visual loss the reported symptoms included decrease in contrast sensitivity and various visual disturbances and aberrations, including glare. In early stages there was usually no effect on Snellen visual acuity but a gradual decrease of visual acuity was noted in the late stage of the process. Associated systemic disorders were not described. Metabolic imbalances have not been implicated as pathogenic factors. Because the lesions invariably appeared years later in a very late postoperative period there is almost certainly no direct connection between the opacities and substances used intraoperatively. In the examinations we performed to identify the nature of the deposits, including energy dispersive spectroscopy (EDS) we did not document any exogenous chemicals apart from elements present in PMMA itself (carbon, oxygen).

High power three-dimensional light microscopy (Figure 24-4, top left) and SEM (Figure 24-4, top middle) of the surfaces of bisected IOL optics were the most informative examinations with regard to determining the structure of the opacifications. The term "snowflake" applies best to the clinical and low power microscopic appearance of each lesion (Figure 24-4, top left). High power examination revealed that the lesions are spherical or stellate, the shape depending on the contour of the surrounding pseudocapsule (Figure 24-4). The interior of the sphere does not appear to contain fluid.

To date, there have not been any clinicopathologic reports on this complication nor any hypotheses regarding its pathogenesis. We suggest that manufacturing variations in some lenses fabricated in the 1980s/early 1990s may be responsible. It is possible that the late change in the PMMA material process is facilitated by long-term ultraviolet (UV, solar) exposure. This is supported by two pathologic observations. First, many opacities have been indeed clustered in the central zone of the optic, extending to mid-peripheral portion but often leaving the distal peripheral rim free of the opacities. This observations would support the hypothesis that the slow and sometimes progressive lesion formation noted here might relate to the fact that the IOL's central optic is exposed to ultraviolet radiation over an extended period, whereas the peripheral optic may be protected by the iris. Furthermore, the opacities are present most commonly and intensely within the anterior 1/3 of the optic's substance (Figure 24-4, bottom). Since the anterior strata of the optic are the first to encounter the ultraviolet light, this might explain why the opacities are seen more frequently in this zone.

Since it is plausible the lesions may be ultraviolet-induced, and it is highly unlikely that non-porous PMMA allows an entrance of aqueous into the optic substance, we postulate that the lesions are "dry" and that the PMMA disruption might be related to a specific manufacturing problem that leaves the optic susceptible to damage.

PMMA is manufactured by polymerization of the MMA monomer. This manufacturing process utilizes many different polymerization techniques, and various components such as UV absorbers and initiators. Therefore various impurity profiles are possible. An initiator substance starts such process. A frequently used initiator is azo-bis-isobutyryl nitrile (AIBN).[4–6] It is possible that UV radiation is a contributing factor, however, the exact pathogenesis can as of now only be hypothesized. Potential causes of a snowflake lesion include 1) insufficient post-annealing of the cured PMMA polymer; 2) excessive thermal energy during the curing process leaving voids in the polymer matrix; 3) non-homogeneous dispersement of the UV chromophore and/or thermal initiator into the polymer chain; 4) poor filtration of the pre-cured monomeric components (MMA, UV blocker, thermal initiator). Another possible pathogenic factor could be an inadvertent use of excessive initiator substance during the polymerization process that may facilitate the formation of the snowflake lesions. The N = N bond of the AIBN initiator may be disrupted by gradual UV exposure with a release of nitrogen gas (N_2). Such gas formation can be caused by either heat or UV light exposure. Indeed the normal polymerization process for PMMA synthesis consists in part of a heat-induced N_2 formation as a byproduct. During normal polymerization the N_2 escapes from the mixture. However, with a poor manufacturing process, for example using excessive initiator—more than the fractional amount required—unwanted initiator may be entrapped in the PMMA substance. Slow release of gaseous N_2within the PMMA substance trigged by long-term UV exposure would explain the formation of the cavitations within the snowflake lesions. The outer "pseudocapsule" might consist of PMMA, whereas the central space contains the N_2 gas admixed with convoluted material also possibly consisting of degenerated PMMA. There is nothing in the molecular structure of the PMMA that in and of itself could be compressed to form such an expansile material that might create the round circular cavitations of the snowflake lesions.

These hypothetical mechanisms have the potential to form micro-heterogeneity within the PMMA polymer that, over time and potentially with exposure to UV radiation, could result in a lesion within the polymer. Additional experimentation is necessary to determine if any of these proposed mechanisms for the formation of a snowflake lesion are realized.

Awareness of this delayed complication may be warranted in developing countries, where PMMA IOLs are still used in the majority of cases. Virtually all IOLs manufactured today appear to be satisfactory. However, one should always be aware that some early IOLs from American manufacturers, including some described in this report, have been delivered to the developing world over the years, sometimes implanted without regard to expiration dates on the packaging. It would be very unfortunate to see this complication showing up in underprivileged areas where patients have almost no recourse to treat visual loss/blindness of this type.

The emergence of this complication could have represented a true disaster, except for the fact that many of the patients implanted with these IOLs are now deceased. However, there are probably still sufficient number of patients living with varying stages of this complication. This necessitates that today's ophthalmologists to be aware of, to diagnose, and to know when not to explant and/or exchange these lenses. It is important to know the nature of this syndrome in order to spare by now elderly patients and their doctors unwarranted anxiety about the cause of his or her visual problems/loss and also to obviate request for unwarranted diagnostic testing.

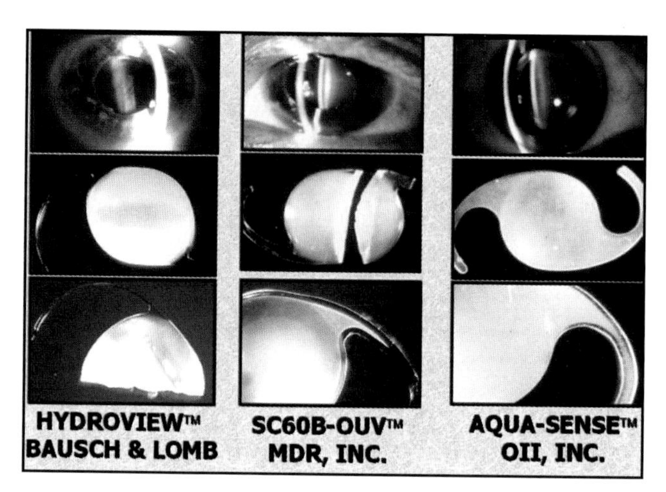

Figure 24-5. Hydrophilic acrylic lens designs presented with delayed postoperative opacification.

Opacification of Foldable Hydrophilic Acrylic Lenses

Introduction

Small incision cataract surgery with implantation of foldable lenses has evolved significantly over the past two decades. Presently available foldable intraocular lens (IOL) biomaterials include silicone, hydrophobic acrylic, and recently introduced hydrophilic acrylic or hydrogel materials. Foldable hydrophilic acrylic intraocular lenses (IOLs), also known as hydrogel lenses are not yet available in the United States but have been marketed by several firms for several years in international markets. Most of the currently available hydrophilic acrylic lenses are manufactured from different copolymers acrylic with water contents raging from 18% to 28%, and an incorporated UV absorber.[6,7] They are packaged in a vial containing distilled water or balanced salt solutions, thus being already implanted in the hydrated state and in their final dimensions. Hydration renders these lenses flexible, enabling the surgeons to fold and insert/inject them through small incisions. Many surgeons have adopted the use of hydrophilic acrylic IOLs because of their easier-handling properties and biocompatibility.[8,9] Although hydrophilic surfaces have been shown to lower the inflammatory cytological response to the IOL,[9] some currently available hydrophilic acrylic IOL designs have been associated to reports on late postoperative opacification caused by calcium precipitation.[10–35] Postoperative opacification of the foldable hydrophilic acrylic lens designs is a major concern among surgeons, and manufacturers. The majority of cases are reported from Asia, Australia, Canada, Europe, Latin America, and South Africa.

In the later section of the chapter on IOL opacification, we describe the analyses performed in our laboratory on hydrophilic acrylic lenses of 3 major designs during past 3 years (Figure 24-5). They were all explanted because of whitish discoloration of the optic component, or of the whole lens, related to different forms and degrees of dystrophic calcification.[36,37]

Figure 24-6 illustrates the first group of explanted hydrophilic acrylic lenses analyzed because of whitish discoloration, represented by the Bausch and Lomb Surgical (Rochester, NY) Hydroview IOL. Figure 24-7 represents the second group of the SC60B-OUV lens, which is another hydrophilic IOL to be recently associated with clinically significant post-

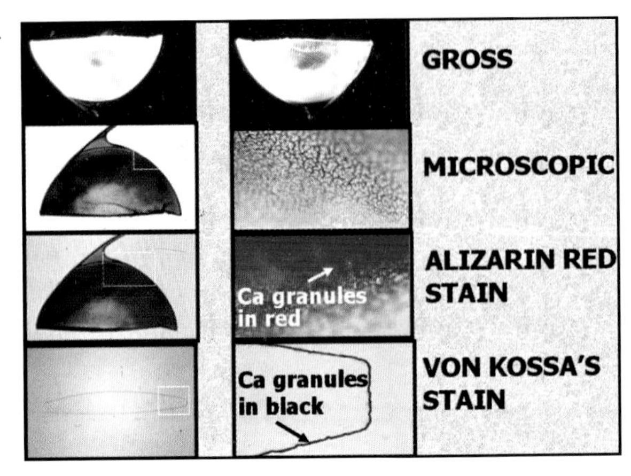

Figure 24-6. Hydroview IOL: microscopic and histochemical evaluation.

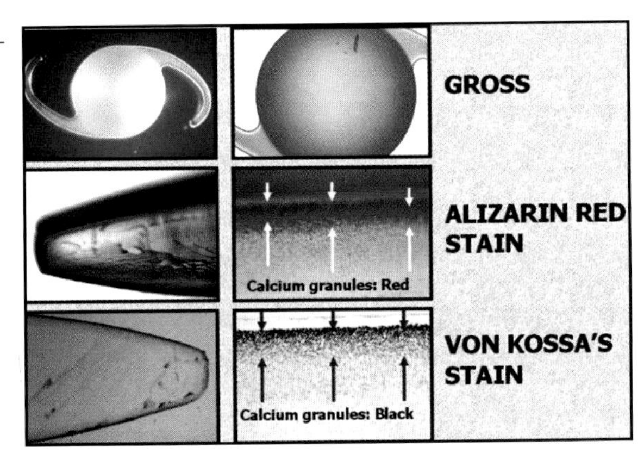

Figure 24-7. SC60B-OUV IOL: microscopic and histochemical evaluation.

operative optic opacification. The manufacturer and distributor of this design is Medical Developmental Research (MDR Inc., Clearwater, Fla). The clinical characteristics of these lenses were different from the previously described "granularity" covering the optical surfaces of the Hydroview design. The clinical appearance of the SC60B-OUV lenses was that of a clouding similar to a "nuclear cataract".

Figure 24-8 represents the explanted Aqua-Sense lenses, manufactured by Ophthalmic Innovations International, Inc. (OII), Ontario, Canada.[34,35] The clinical appearance of the Aqua-Sense lenses was also that of a clouding similar to a "nuclear cataract". As with the two above-mentioned designs, Nd: YAG laser was performed in some cases in an attempt to "clean" the optical surfaces, without success.

Clinicopathological Analyses

The explanted hydrogel IOLs were submitted by several ophthalmic surgeons from various countries (Australia, China, Sweden, Egypt, Germany, South Africa, Turkey, UK, and others) for pathological analysis. Gross (macroscopic) analysis of the explanted IOLs was performed and gross pictures were taken using a camera (Nikon N905 AF, Nikon Corporation, Tokyo, Japan) fitted to an operating microscope (Leica/Wild MZ-8 Zoom Stereomicroscope, Vashaw Scientific, Inc., Norcross, GA). The unstained lenses were then

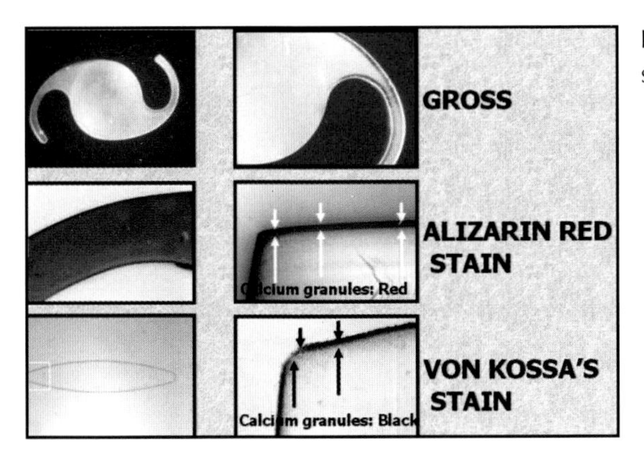

Figure 24-8. Aqua-Sense IOL: microscopic and histochemical evaluation.

microscopically evaluated and photographed under a light microscope (Olympus, Optical Co. Ltd., Japan). They were rinsed in distilled water, immersed in a 1% alizarin red solution (a special stain for calcium) for 2 minutes, rinsed again in distilled water and reexamined under the light microscope.[35, 38-40]

We then performed full thickness sections through the optic of the explanted lenses. Some of the resultant cylindrical blocks were directly stained with 1% alizarin red. Calcium salts stain in dark brown with this technique.[35, 38-40] Some lenses in each group were air-dried at room temperature for 7 days, sputter-coated with aluminum and examined under a JEOL JSM 5410LV scanning electron microscope (SEM) equipped with a Kevex X-ray detector with light element capabilities for energy dispersive X-ray analyses (EDS). Incisional biopsies of conjunctiva and iris were also obtained from one patient during removal and exchange of a Hydroview IOL.[18] This was done in order to rule out the presence of dystrophic calcification in those tissues.

Figures 24-6 through 24-8 summarize the gross, microscopic, and histochemical findings in three different types of opacified explanted foldable hydrophilic lenses manufactured by Bausch and Lomb, MDR, and OII Inc., respectively. Figure 24-6 illustrates the deposits on the surfaces of the Hydroview IOLs stained positive with alizarin red in all cases. Sagittal histological sections through the optic of this lens design, stained using von Kossa's method showed a continuous layer of dark brown, irregular granules on the anterior and posterior optical surfaces, and the edges of the lenses (see Figure 24-6). Histochemical evaluations of the conjunctiva and iris biopsies obtained from one of the patients were negative.

Alizarin red staining of the surfaces of the SC60B-OUV lenses was in general negative. Analysis of the cut sections (sagittal view) of the lens optics revealed multiple granules of variable sizes in a region beneath the external anterior and posterior surfaces of the IOLs. The granules were distributed in a line parallel to the anterior and posterior curvatures of the optics. They stained positive with alizarin red (see Figure 24-7). Sagittal histological sections stained with the von Kossa method also confirmed the presence of multiple dark brown/black granules mostly concentrated in a region immediately beneath the anterior and posterior optical surfaces (see Figure 24-7).

Staining with alizarin red revealed spots of granular deposits on the external surfaces of the Aqua-Sense lenses (see Figure 24-8). In some cases, a fine granularity was covering the lenses' external surfaces. Analysis of cut sections (sagittal view) of the lens optic revealed multiple granules of variable sizes in a region beneath the external anterior and posterior

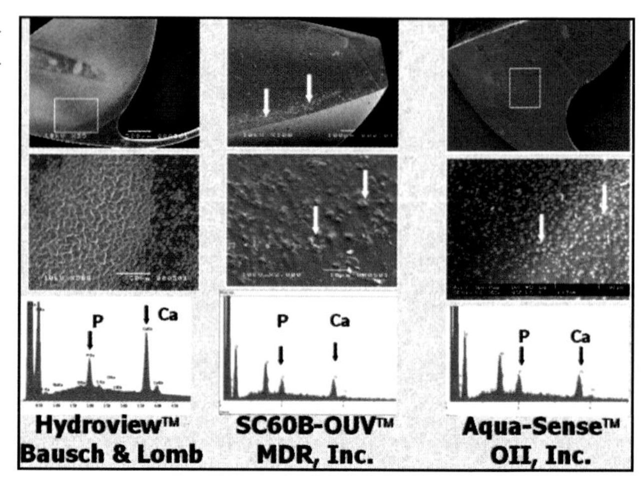

Figure 24-9. Opacified hydrogel lenses: ultrastructural evaluation.

surfaces of the IOLs. As with the previous lens design, the granules were distributed in a line parallel to the anterior and posterior curvatures of the optics and they stained positive with alizarin red and the von Kossa method (see Figure 24-8).

Scanning Electron Microscopy

Figure 24-9 summarizes the ultrastructural findings in three different types of opacified explanted foldable hydrophilic lenses manufactured by the Bausch and Lomb, MDR, and OII Inc., respectively. The aspect of the three lens designs observed under light microscopy was confirmed by SEM. Analyses of the anterior optical surfaces of some Hydroview lenses revealed granular deposits composed of multiple spherical-ovoid globules, scattered in some areas, and confluent in others. SEM analysis of cut sections (sagittal view) of the optic of some SC60B-OUV lenses confirmed that the region immediately subjacent to the IOLs outer surfaces as well as the central area of the optical cut sections were free of deposits. This also revealed the presence of the granules in the intermediate region beneath the anterior and posterior surfaces. With the Aqua-Sense lenses, SEM of the anterior surface revealed the presence of small granular deposits. Analyses of cut sections of this lens design demonstrated features similar to those described with the SC60B-OUV lens (see Figure 24-9).

Energy Dispersive X-Ray Spectroscopy

With the three lens designs, EDS performed precisely on the deposits revealed the presence of calcium and phosphate peaks (see Figure 24-9). EDS was also performed on areas free of deposits to serve as controls, showing only peaks of carbon and oxygen (see Figure 24-9).

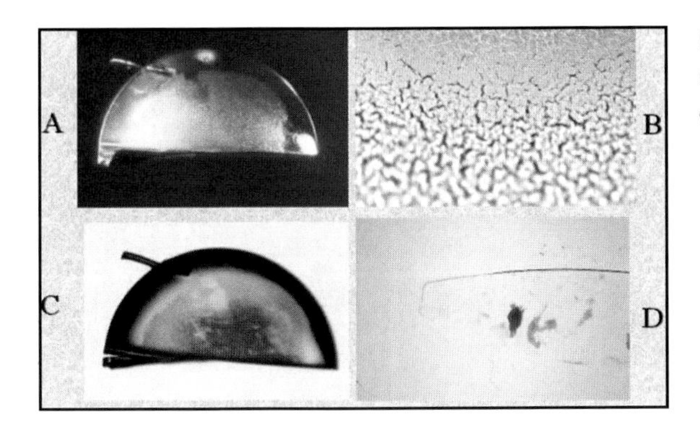

Figure 24-10. Opacification of memory IOL: gross and histochemical evaluation.

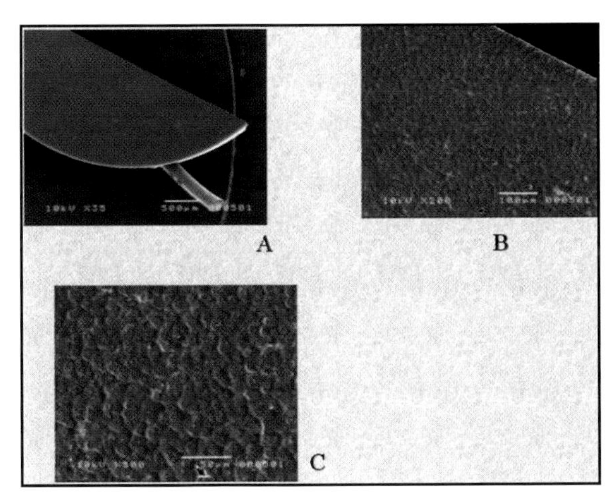

Figure 24-11. Opacification of memory IOL: ultrastructural evaluation.

Late Postoperative Opacification of Cibavision Memory Lens

We recently reported clinical, pathologic, histochemical, ultrastructural, and spectroscopic analyses of MemoryLens IOLs explanted from patients who had visual disturbances caused by postoperative opacification of the lens optic.[41] A total of 106 hydrophilic acrylic IOLs of the same design explanted from 106 different patients (Figures 24-10 and 24-11). All patients had decreased visual acuity at presentation approximately 2 years after cataract surgery, associated with a whitish fine granularity on the optical surfaces of the IOLs. The explanted IOLs were submitted to the John A. Moran Eye Center and were examined under light microscopy, histochemically, and with scanning electron microscopy (SEM) equipped with an energy dispersive x-ray spectroscopy detector with light element capabilities (EDS) (see Figures 24-10 and 24-11). The IOLs were examined for distribution, structure, and composition of the deposits causing opacification of their optic components. The average interval between lens implantation and opacification was 25.81/–11.9 months. The most frequently associated medical and ophthalmic conditions were diabetes and glaucoma. However, some patients did not have any preexisting medical or ophthalmic conditions. Most of the IOLs had been implanted in 1999 and 2000. Microscopic analyses revealed the presence of multiple fine, granular deposits of variable

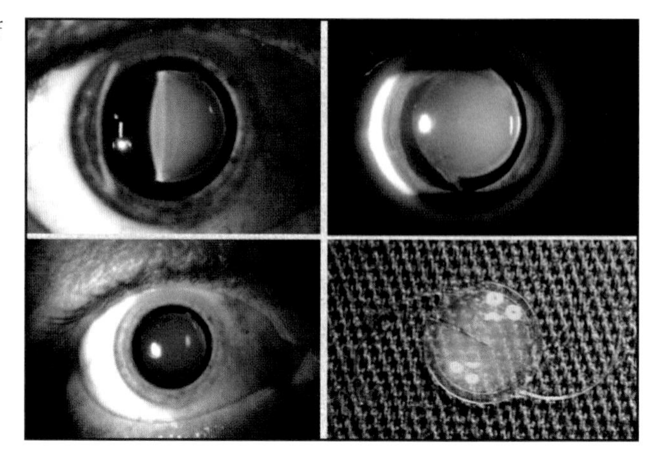

Figure 24-12. Opacification of silicone (AMO SI40) IOL.

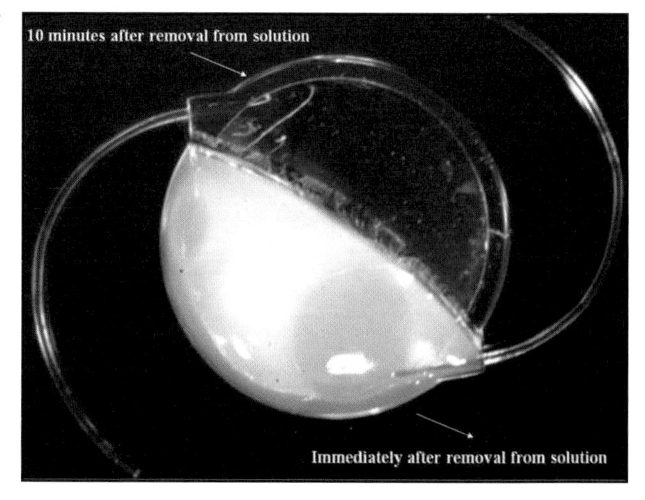

Figure 24-13. Opacification of AMO SI40 IOLs: gross evaluation.

sizes on the anterior and posterior optic surfaces, especially on the anterior surface (see Figures 24-10 and 24-11). The deposits stained positive for calcium. The EDS confirmed the presence of calcium and phosphate within the deposits. In conclusion, late postoperative opacification due to surface deposit formation in a series of 106 MemoryLens IOLs. The deposits were probably caused by an altered surface energy, which, under certain circumstances, allowed adsorption of proteins with the deposition of calcium on top of the protein film. Further studies should be undertaken to evaluate the possible interactions of biomaterials with their surroundings, as well as their stability in biological systems over time, as theoretically no material might be spared from the complication of calcification.

Opacification of the Silicone Lenses

Recently some cases of silicone IOL opacification (SI-40NB, AMO Inc.) was reported (Figures 24-12 and 24-13). The opacification was observed on the first postoperative day in all cases, who had phacoemulsification between April and June 2003. The appearance of the silicone IOLs ranged from milky gray to a yellow hue and affected the entire optical component homogeneously (see Figure 24-12). The patients did not complain about their vision, and visual acuity was only slightly affected; three of the four patients had a best corrected visual acuity of 20/30, and no anterior chamber reaction was observed. Contrast sensitivity was reduced in all cases.

We recently became aware of cases in which IOLs, analyzed elsewhere became cloudy in vivo, apparently after exposure to aerosol fumigants prior to implantation (see Figure 24-13). One explanted lens was sent for chemical analysis by gas chromatography/ mass spectrometry. The key finding was the presence of a chemical in the cloudy lens that was not present in a control lens. The chemical was not used in the IOL manufacturing process but was, however, the primary nonaqueous component in a disinfectant solution used in the operating theater at the site that submitted the lens for evaluation. Laboratory studies were subsequently conducted on clear IOLs by exposing them to gaseous diffusion from a disinfectant solution. These lenses became cloudy upon immersion in water. This supports the hypothesis that environmental conditions are capable of producing unexpected changes in IOLs during storage and that this may impact how the lenses behave when exposed to the aqueous environment of the eye. Most IOLs are enclosed in semipermeable packages to allow sterilization by ethylene oxide gas. This may also unexpectedly allow other aerosolized chemicals to seep into the unopened package and come into contact with the lens inside. Storage facilities and operating theaters that are sprayed with aerosolized disinfectants, insecticides, cleaning solutions or other volatile chemicals may be inadvertently introducing chemicals through the package and onto the lenses. As a general precautionary measure, all IOLs should be stored in a clean, dry environment, at room temperature, and be protected from potentially harmful fumigant sprays.

Prevention and Treatment

The opacification described in our reports have an entirely different appearance than classic posterior capsule opacification or anterior lens epithelial cell proliferation.

Excessive Nd: YAG laser treatment, in an attempt to clean the optical surfaces of the lenses may jeopardize implantation of a new lens in the capsular bag after explantation of the opacified lens. The adherence of the deposits to the optical surfaces of the lenses seems to be extremely strong and Nd: YAG laser treatment was proven to be ineffective in the cleaning of the lenses' surfaces. The cause of this condition seems to be multifactorial, and until the pathogenic mechanism is not fully clarified, explantation and exchange of the IOL is the only available treatment.

Surgeons usually face two important challenges during explantation of these opacified lenses. Firstly, fibrosis along the capsulorrhexis edge and secondly the capsular adhesions around the lens haptics. A few radial incisions may be helpful to increase the rhexis diameter and to remove the capsular flap. It is very important to well viscodissect the lens from the capsular bag, in order to liberate any adherence to this structure. The lens is removed after being folded inside the eye, bisected, or intact through a larger incision. The status of the capsular bag should then be carefully inspected, which will influence the decision about the site for fixation of the new lens. Methods for the prevention of this condition are also not completely defined to date. Long-term clinical studies will determine the efficacy of modifications performed on IOL polymers and packaging for prevention of lens calcification.

Summary

Each hydrophilic acrylic IOL design available in the market is manufactured from a different copolymer acrylic. To the best of our knowledge, the calcification problem described in this text cannot be generalized to all of the lenses in this category. The incidence of IOL explantation because of calcification remains low, much less than 1% in each of the 3 groups described here. The mechanism is not fully understood, but it does not seem to be directed related to substances used during the surgery as it occurred in the late postoperative period. Also, the substances used during the surgery were not the same in all cases. The majority of the patients involved had an associated systemic disease; therefore, the possibility of a patient-related factor, such as a metabolic imbalance cannot be ruled out.

Lot history, component history, process changes, surgical setting and techniques, environmental factors, preexisting patients conditions, and packaging have been examined. It is now important to carefully follow clinical outcomes of these lens designs in order to assure if this phenomenon will disappear following the changes in polymer source or packaging.

Acknowledgment

The authors would like to thank all the ophthalmic surgeons around the world for submitting the explanted rigid PMMA and hydrogel intraocular lenses for pathological analysis at the David J. Apple, MD Laboratory for Ophthalmic Devices Research, Moran Eye Center, Salt Lake City, Utah, USA.

Key Points

1. The opacities of the IOL optics may start as scattered white-brown spots within the substance of the IOL optic and remain stable or slowly progressive. Some may gradually increase in intensity and numbers, eventually reaching a point where a visual acuity loss may necessitate removal or exchange of the IOL.
2. In addition to visual loss the reported symptoms included decrease in contrast sensitivity and various visual disturbances and aberrations, including glare.
3. Surgeons usually face two important challenges during explantation of these opacified lenses. Firstly, fibrosis along the capsulorrhexis edge and secondly the capsular adhesions around the lens haptics.
4. The IOL can be removed after being folded inside the eye, bisected, or intact through a larger incision.
5. Methods for the prevention of this condition are also not completely defined to date.

References

1. Ridley NHL. Artificial intraocular lenses after cataract extraction. St. Thomas Hospital Reports 1951;7:12–4.
2. Apple DJ, Peng Q, Arthur SN, et al. Snowflake degeneration of poly(methyl methacrylate) (PMMA) posterior chamber intraocular lens optic material: A newly described clinical condition caused by an unexpected late opacification of PMMA. *Ophthalmology.* Sept. 2002.
3. Peng Q, Apple DJ, Arthur SA, et al. "Snowflake" opacification of poly(methyl methacrylate) intraocular lens optic biomaterial: a newly described syndrome. *Int Ophthalmol Clin.* 2001;41:91–108.
4. Park JB. *Biomaterials—An Introduction.* New York: Plenum Press; 1979:88–91.
5. Sugaya H, Sakai Y. Polymethylmethacrylate: from polymer to dialyzer. *Contributions to Nephrology.* 1999;125:1–8.
6. Christ FR, Buchen SY, Deacon J, et al. Biomaterials used for intraocular lenses. In: Wise DL, ed. *Encyclopedic Handbook of Biomaterials and Bioengineering.* New York: Marcel Dekker Inc.; 1995:1277.
7. Chehade M, Elder MJ. Intraocular lens materials and styles: A review. *Aust NZ J Ophthalmol.* 1997;25:255–63.
8. Schauersberger J, Kruger A, Abela C, et al. Course of postoperative inflammation after implantation of 4 types of foldable intraocular lenses. *J Cataract Refract Surg.* 1999;25:1116–20.
9. Hollick EJ, Spalton DJ, Ursell PG. Surface cytologic features on intraocular lenses: can increased biocompatibility have disadvantages? *Arch Ophthalmol.* 1999;117:872–8.
10. Chang BYP, Davey KG, Gupta M, Hutchinson C. Late clouding of an acrylic intraocular lens following routine phacoemulsification. *Eye.* 1999;13:807–8.
11. Murray RI. Two cases of late opacification of the hydroview hydrogel intraocular lens. *J Catract Refract Surg.* 2000;26:1272–3.
12. Fernando GT, Crayford BB. Visually significant calcification of hydrogel intraocular lenses necessitating explantation. *Clin Experiment Ophthalmol.* 2000;28:280–6.
13. Apple DJ, Werner L, Escobar-Gomez M, Pandey SK. Deposits on the optical surfaces of Hydroview intraocular lenses (letter). *J Cataract Refract Surg.* 2000;26:796–7.
14. Werner L, Apple DJ, Escobar-Gomez M, et al. Postoperative deposition of calcium on the surfaces of a hydrogel intraocular lens. *Ophthalmology.* 2000;107:2179–85.
15. Izak A, Werner L, Pandey SK, et al. Calcification on the surface of the Bausch & Lomb Hydroview intraocular lens. *Int Ophthalmol Clin.* 2001;41:62–78.
16. Apple DJ, Werner L, Pandey SK. Newly recognized complications of posterior chamber intraocular lenses (Editorial). *Arch Ophthalmol.* 2001;119:581–2.
17. Pandey SK, Werner L, Apple DJ, Kaskaloglu M. Hydrophilic acrylic intraocular lens optic and haptics opacification in a diabetic patient: Bilateral case report and clinicopathological correlation. *Ophthalmology.* 2002;109:2042–2051.
18. Pandey SK, Werner L, Apple DJ, Gravel JP. Calcium precipitation on the optical surfaces of a foldable intraocular lens: a clinicopathological correlation. *Arch Ophthalmol.* 2002;120:391–393.
19. Yu AFK, Shek TWH. Hydroxyapatite formation on implanted hydrogel intraocular lenses. *Arch Ophthalmol.* 2001;107:2179–85.
20. Yu AKF, Kwan KYW, Chan DHY, Fong DYT. Clinical features of 46 eyes with calcified hydrogel intraocular lenses. *J Cataract Refract Surg.* 2001;27:1596–1606.
21. Groh JMM, Schlotzer-Schrehardt U, Rummelt C, et al. Postoperative Kunstlinsen-Eintrubungen bei 12 Hydrogel-Intraokularlinsen (Hydroview). *Klin Monatsbl Augenheilkd.* 2001;218:645–8.
22. Shek TW, Wong A, Yau B, Yu Ak. Opacification of artificial intraocular lens: an electron microscopic study. *Ultrastruct Pathol.* 2001;25:281–3.
23. Buchen SY, Cunanan CM, Gwon A, et al. Assessing intraocular lens calcification in an animal model. *J Cataract Refract Surg.* 2001;27:1473–84.

24. Frohn A, Dick B, Augustin AJ, Grus FH. Late opacification of the foldable hydrophilic acrylic lens SC60B-OUV. *Ophthalmology*. 2001;108:1999–2004.
25. Mamalis N. Hydrophilic acrylic intraocular lenses (Editorial). *J Cataract Refract Surg*. 2001;27:1339–40.
26. Werner L, Apple DJ, Kaskaloglu M, Pandey SK. Dense opacification of the optical component of a hydrophilic intraocular lens: a clinicopathological analysis of 9 explanted lenses. *J Cataract Refract Surg*. 2001;27:1485–92.
27. Macky TA, Trivedi RH, Werner L, et al. Degeneration of UV absorber material and calcium deposits within the optic of a hydrophilic IOL lens (manufactured by Medical Developmental Research). *Int Ophthalmol Clin*. 2001;41:79–90.
28. Apple DJ, Werner L, Pandey SK. Opalescence of hydrophilic acrylic lenses (letter). *Eye*. 2001;15:97–98.
29. Izak AM, Werner L, Pandey SK, Apple DJ. Opacification of modern foldable hydrogel intraocular lens designs. *Eye*. 2003;17(3):393-406.
30. Sharma TK, Chawdhary S. The opalescence of hydrogel intraocular lens. *Eye*. 2001;15:97–98.
31. Sharma A, Ram J, Gupta A. Late clouding of an acrylic intraocular lens following routine phacoemulsification (letter). *Eye*. 2001;15:361.
32. Woodruff SA, Khan J, Dhingra N, et al. Late clouding of an acrylic intraocular lens following routine phacoemulsification (letter). *Eye*. 2001;15:362.
33. Pavlovic S, Magdowski G, Brueckel B, Pavlovic S. Ultrastructural analysis of opacities seen in a hydrophilic acrylic intracular lens. *Eye*. 2001;15:657–9.
34. Werner L, Apple DJ, Izak AM. Discoloration/opacification of modern foldable hydrogel intraocular lens designs. In: Buratto L, Zanini R, Apple DJ, Werner L, eds. *Phacoemulsification: Principles and Techniques*. Thorofare NJ: SLACK Incorporated; 2002:659–670.
35. Werner L, Izak AM, Apple DJ, Pandey SK, et al. Complete calcification of a hydrogel lens design: case reports and clinicopathological correlation. *Am J Ophthalmol*. (submitted).
36. Werner L, Apple DJ, Pandey SK. Late postoperative opacification of hydrophilic intraocular lens designs. Presented at the ASCRS Symposium on Cataract, IOL and Refractive Surgery, Best Paper of the Session; San Diego, CA; April 28, 2001.
37. Pandey SK, Werner L, Apple D, Kaskaloglu MM, Izak AM, Cionni RJ. Intraocular Lens Opacification. Second prize in the category Intraocular Lenses at the ASCRS/Alcon Annual Video Festival, Congress of the American Society of Cataract and Refractive Surgeons; Philadelphia, PA.
38. McGee-Russell SM. Histochemical methods for calcium. *J Histochem Cytochem*. 1958;6:22–42.
39. Carr LB, Rambo ON, Feichtmeir TV. A method of demonstrating calcium in tissue sections using chloranilic acid. *J Histochem Cytochem*. 1961;9:415–7.
40. Pizzolato P. Histochemical recognition of calcium oxalate. *J Histochem Cytochem*. 1964;12:333–6.
41. Neuhann I, Werner L, Pandey SK, et al. Opacification of the Memory Lens. Presented at the ASCRS Symposium on Cataract, IOL, and Refractive Surgery, San Diego, CA, May 2004.

The authors have no financial or proprietary interest in any product mentioned in this chapter.

IV

Posterior Segment—Worst Case Scenarios

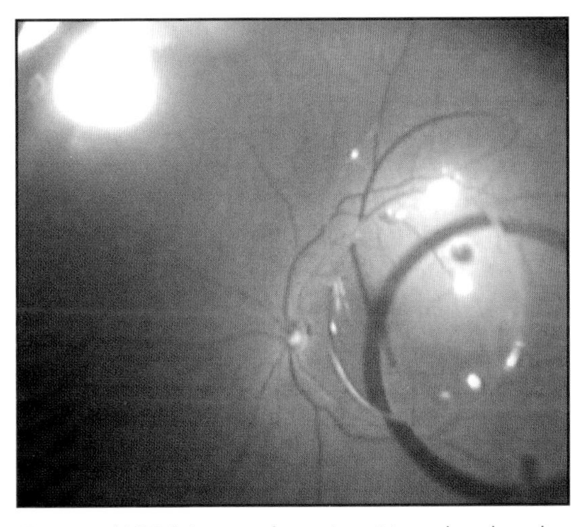

Dropped IOL lying on the retina. Note the chandelier illumination on the upper left hand corner.

Chapter 25

Managing Dislocated Lens Fragments

Clement K. Chan, MD, FACS

Introduction

Dislocation of lens fragments into the vitreous cavity occurs in a small percentage of cases of cataract extraction with phacoemulsification or phakonit but continues to be encountered on an intermittent basis with potentially serious consequences in the modern setting.[1] Small lens fragments consisting of mostly cortical material may gradually resolve with conservative medical management alone. However, large lens fragments with a sizeable nuclear component do not resolve easily, and may elicit a phacoantigenic response from the host.[2–5] The released lens proteins may not only induce persistent intraocular inflammation, but also block the trabecular meshwork, resulting in phacolytic (or lens particle) glaucoma.[6,7] In time, other serious anatomical complications with poor visual consequences may develop in the absence of appropriate management of the lens fragments, i.e. peripheral anterior synechiae of the iris, pupillary or vitreous membranes, cystoid macular edema, retinal breaks or detachment, and phacoanaphylaxis, etc.[1,2–5] Therefore, most retained and dislocated lens fragments with a substantial nuclear component require surgical removal.[1,5,8–10] Earlier clinical studies advocated the immediate removal of dislocated lens fragments.[11,12] In Blodi's report, those eyes undergoing surgery within 7 days had a lower incidence of long-term glaucoma.[11] However, subsequent reports by Gilliland et al and Kim et al demonstrated no difference in visual outcome and glaucoma development between those eyes undergoing lens fragment removal within 7 days and those after 30 days following the dislocation.[13,14] Despite such conclusions, expeditious surgical management of retained lens fragments within a limited time frame is the current standard of care that allows rapid visual rehabilitation and prevention of serious complications mentioned above.[1,11,12,14]

The Responsibility of the Cataract Surgeon

In the event of a rupture of the posterior lens capsule or zonular dehiscence leading to posterior migration of lens fragments, the cataract surgeon must avoid any uncontrolled and forceful surgical maneuvers in the vitreous cavity in an attempt to retrieve the sinking lens fragments. Any retrieval technique that does not provide for the appropriate management of the vitreous first creates the potential of immediate or subsequent retinal complications. Thus, the cataract surgeon must refrain from the temptation of passing a sharp instrument or lens loop into the mid or posterior vitreous cavity to engage the sinking lens fragments, or passing forceful irrigation fluid into the vitreous cavity to float the lens fragments.[1,15,16] Such maneuvers usually generate vitreoretinal traction resulting in retinal breaks and detachment. Instead, he should finish the clean up of the remaining cortical debris within the capsular bag and its vicinity, and then also perform a limited anterior vitrectomy in the event of vitreous prolapse into the anterior chamber and at the cataract wound.[1,5,11–14,16,17] An intraocular lens (IOL) may also be implanted in the absence of significant anterior segment complications, i.e. corneal decompensation, iridodialysis, hyphema, anterior chamber angle injury, etc.[1,13,14,16,17] An anterior chamber lens (ACIOL) can usually be safely implanted, but it may induce postoperative corneal pathology, chronic cystoid macular edema, and even glaucoma under certain circumstances.[18] Frequently, a posterior chamber implant (PCIOL) can be safely inserted at the ciliary sulcus or even into the capsular bag with the aid of a capsular tension ring for cases with limited capsular or zonular damages.[18–20] The surgeon should avoid the implantation of an IOL made of silicone material due to its potential of interfering with subsequent vitreoretinal surgery, particularly in the event of fluid-gas exchange or long term silicone oil tamponade.[21] The moisture condensation on the posterior surface of a silicone IOL due to its hydrophobic properties leads to a loss of visibility during fluid-gas exchange,[21] and silicone oil may erode into the silicone IOL with long term silicone oil tamponade subsequently. In addition, the surgeon should avoid the implantation of an IOL altogether in the presence of a rock-hard dislocated lens fragment, which may need to be removed intact through a limbal incision subsequently (see sections on cryoextraction and perfluorocarbon liquid).[1,17] Finally, a watertight wound closure is important in anticipation of postoperative intraocular pressure fluctuation and subsequent posterior surgical maneuvers for the lens fragments.[1,17] With the completion of the anterior segment maneuvers described above, the cataract surgeon is now ready to consider various options for managing the posteriorly dislocated lens fragments. In case of familiarity with vitreoretinal techniques, he may convert over to a posterior segment setup and utilize one of the methods described in the following sections for removing the lens fragments. Otherwise, a prompt referral of the patient to a vitreoretinal surgeon is recommended. At the same time, medical management with topical anti-inflammatory, antibiotic, as well as cycloplegic medications should be instituted. If necessary, hypotensive agents are also utilized.

Techniques for Removing Posteriorly Dislocated Lens Fragments

FAVIT

This innovative method was introduced by Agarwal et al.[22] FAVIT stands for (FA- Fallen and VIT- Vitreous) meaning a technique to remove fragments fallen into the vitreous. Its major advantage is that it allows the cataract surgeon familiar with vitreoretinal techniques to quickly convert over to posterior segment surgery with a limited amount of additional setup of instrumentation for removing the lens fragments (Figures 25-1 and 25-2). One can perform a two-port FAVIT. First, a vitrectomy probe with an infusion sleeve is passed

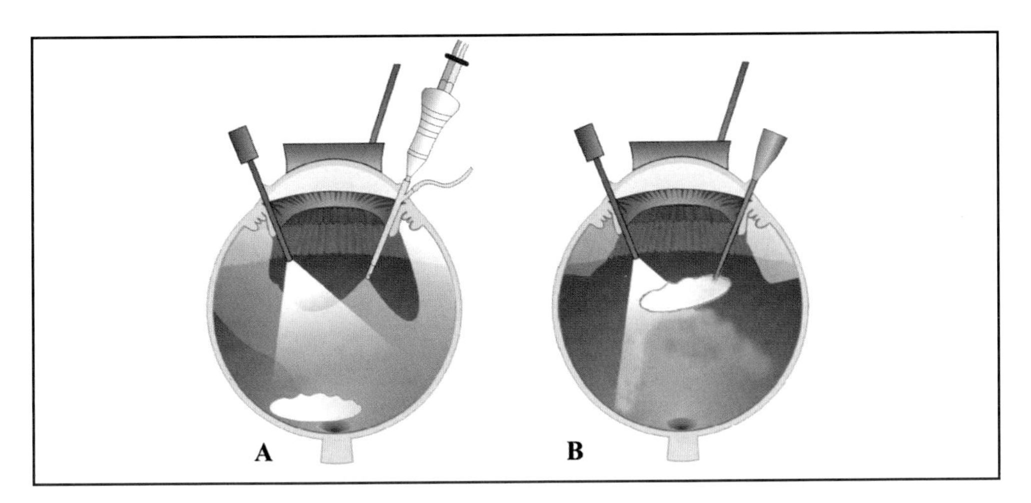

Figure 25-1. FAVIT technique. **A**. After completing the anterior lenticular cortical clean up and anterior vitrectomy, a two-port posterior vitrectomy is performed. The vitrectomy probe and endoilluminator are inserted through separate clear corneal or scleral tunnel incisions created at the start of cataract surgery, and a vitrectomy contact lens is applied firmly on the cornea by surgical assistant to allow adequate viewing of the posterior fundus for the surgeon. **B**. The vitrectomy probe is replaced with a phacoemulsification probe after completion of a posterior vitrectomy to engage the posteriorly dislocated nuclear lens fragment. Suction-only mode is activated to elevate the lens fragment, and the phaco tip is then embedded into the elevated lens fragment with a small burst of ultrasonic energy.

through the same clear corneal or scleral-tunnel cataract incision into the anterior chamber and the anterior vitreous cavity for removal of anterior lenticular cortical material and an anterior vitrectomy respectively. The peristaltic pump of the same phacoemulsification machine is used to drive the vitrectomy probe, and the microscope light may be used for illumination for this part of the procedure. A bimanual (two-port) technique is then required for the rest of the procedure. A fiberoptic endoilluminator is passed through a separate limbal incision and a vitrectomy contact lens is applied on the cornea to provide for appropriate visualization of the posterior vitreous cavity. The surgical assistant should apply the right amount of tension with the vitrectomy contact lens on the cornea to allow an adequate view for the surgeon, on account of the temporary disturbance of the normal corneal curvature induced by the two instruments passing simultaneously through the separate clear corneal incisions. Next, the surgeon performs a thorough posterior vitrectomy including the elimination of the vitreous fibers surrounding the retained lens fragments, in order to prevent subsequent vitreoretinal traction (Figure 25-1A). After the completion of the posterior vitrectomy, the surgeon replaces the vitrectomy probe with a phacoemulsification probe through the same incision (Figure 25-1B). With the ultrasonic power at 50 percent and the aspiration intensity at moderate setting, the surgeon activates the suction-only mode to elevate the lens fragment from the retinal surface. He quickly applies a small burst of ultrasonic energy to embed the probe tip into the elevated lens fragment, and then lifts the entire fragment anteriorly. The endoilluminator is also used at the same time to guide the lens fragment above the iris plane and into the anterior chamber (Figure 25-2A). Finally, the lens fragment is gradually removed with continuous phacoemulsification in the anterior chamber without pulsing or chopping to avoid dropping small fragments back into the vitreous cavity (Figure 25-2B). The endoilluminator can be exchanged with a cannula for infusion into the anterior chamber and prevention of chamber collapse. An excessively

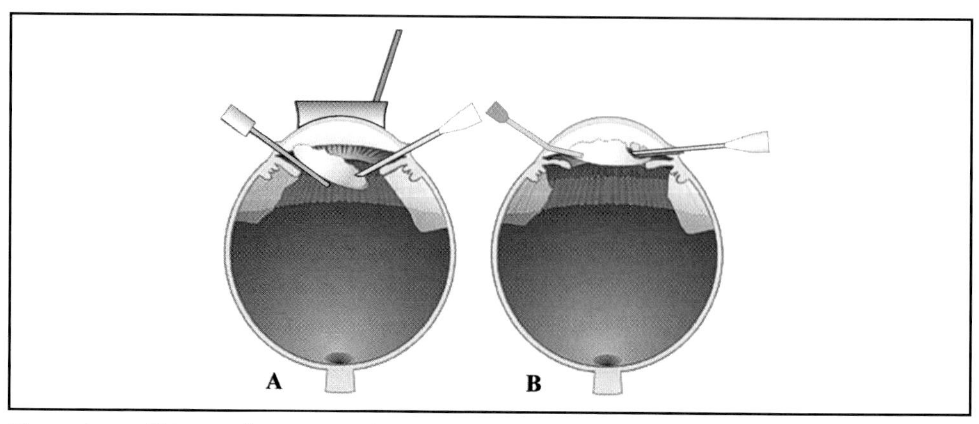

Figure 25-2. FAVIT technique. **A.** The lens fragment is lifted anteriorly with the phaco probe while the endoilluminator is used at the same time to guide the lens fragment above the iris and into the anterior chamber. **B.** Emulsification is performed on the lens fragment in the anterior chamber, while chopping and pulsing are avoided to prevent dropping smaller lens fragments back into the vitreous cavity. At present, Dr. Agarwal prefers to use the chandelier illumination and wide field contact lens while performing FAVIT.

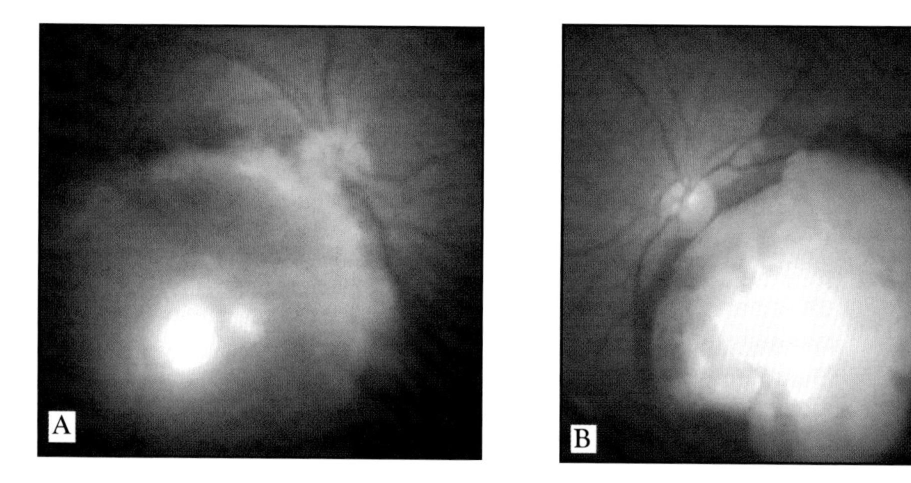

Figure 25-3. **A**. Hard nucleus lying on the retina. **B**. Nucleus lying on the retina. (Photos courtesy of Dr. Agarwal's Eye Hospital.)

large or hard nuclear fragment (Figure 25-3) may be removed through an enlarged limbal incision.[22]

Alternatively, one can do a 3-port FAVIT (Figures 25-4 through 25-6), which is better. First, an infusion cannula is fixated through the first port. An endoilluminator is then inserted through the second port, and a vitrectomy probe without an infusion sleeve is inserted through the third port. A phacofragmentation tip is exchanged for the vitrectomy probe subsequently. One may use an air pump to drive the irrigation through the infusion cannula so that no collapse of the eye occurs while removing the nucleus, and a precise intraocular pressure level is maintained at all time. The better method now is to use the microphakonit needle (phaco needle of 0.7 mm) to embed the nucleus and then remove it.

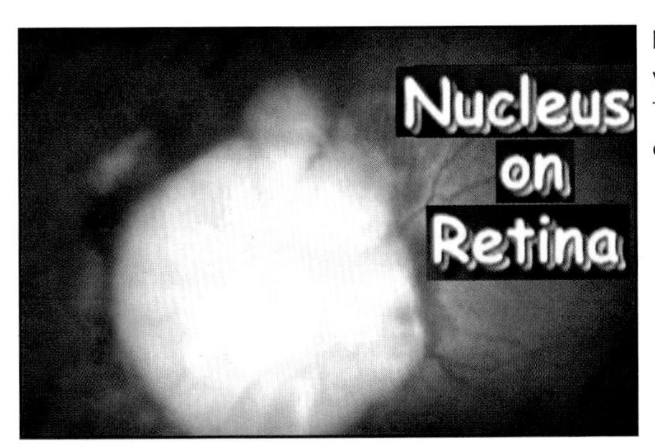

Figure 25-4A. Three-port FAVIT. The whole nucleus is lying on the retina. Three-port vitrectomy is done. (Photo courtesy of Dr. Agarwal's Eye Hospital.)

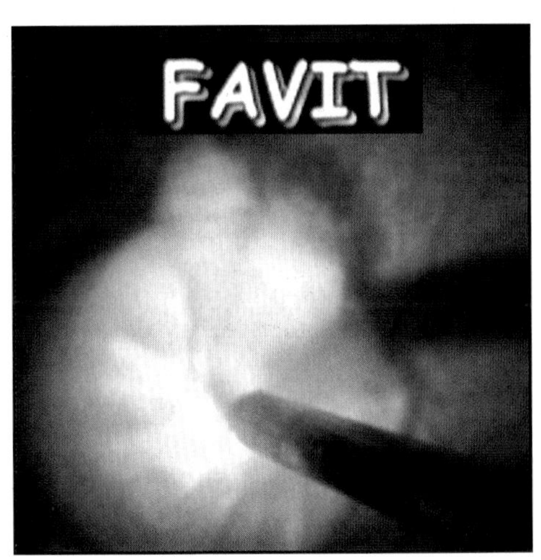

Figure 25-4B. Three port FAVIT. The phaco needle is taken and the nucleus aspirated. Once it is stuck on the needle, a little bit of ultrasound is applied to embed the nucleus. It is better to use a phaco needle of 0.7 mm (microphakonit needle). (Photo courtesy of Dr. Agarwal's Eye Hospital.)

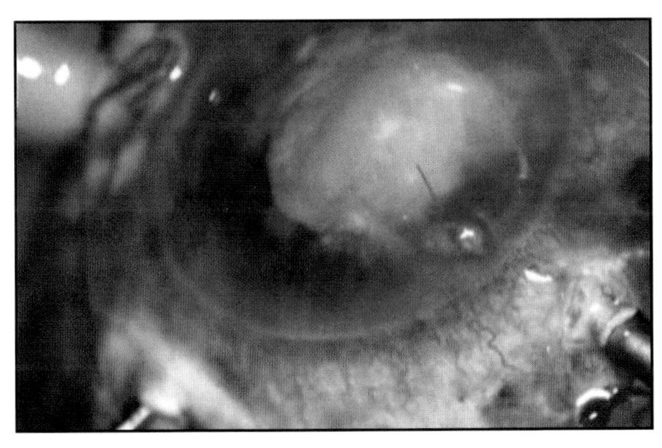

Figure 25-5. Three-port FAVIT. The nucleus is then brought anteriorly. Note the infusion cannula in the upper left hand corner. (Photo courtesy of Dr. Agarwal's Eye Hospital.)

If one uses a chandelier illumination system in which the light source is connected to the infusion cannula, one can do FAVIT as a proper bimanual vitrectomy. Preservative-free triamcinolone is first injected and vitrectomy done, which will help one know that the whole vitreous has been removed. One can do proper bimanual vitrectomy as one hand can hold the vitrectomy probe and the other the phaco needle probe (Figure 25-6A-D). Any adhesions of the vitreous can be cut with the vitrectomy probe while removing the nucleus. The phaco needle embeds the nucleus and it is then brought anteriorly.

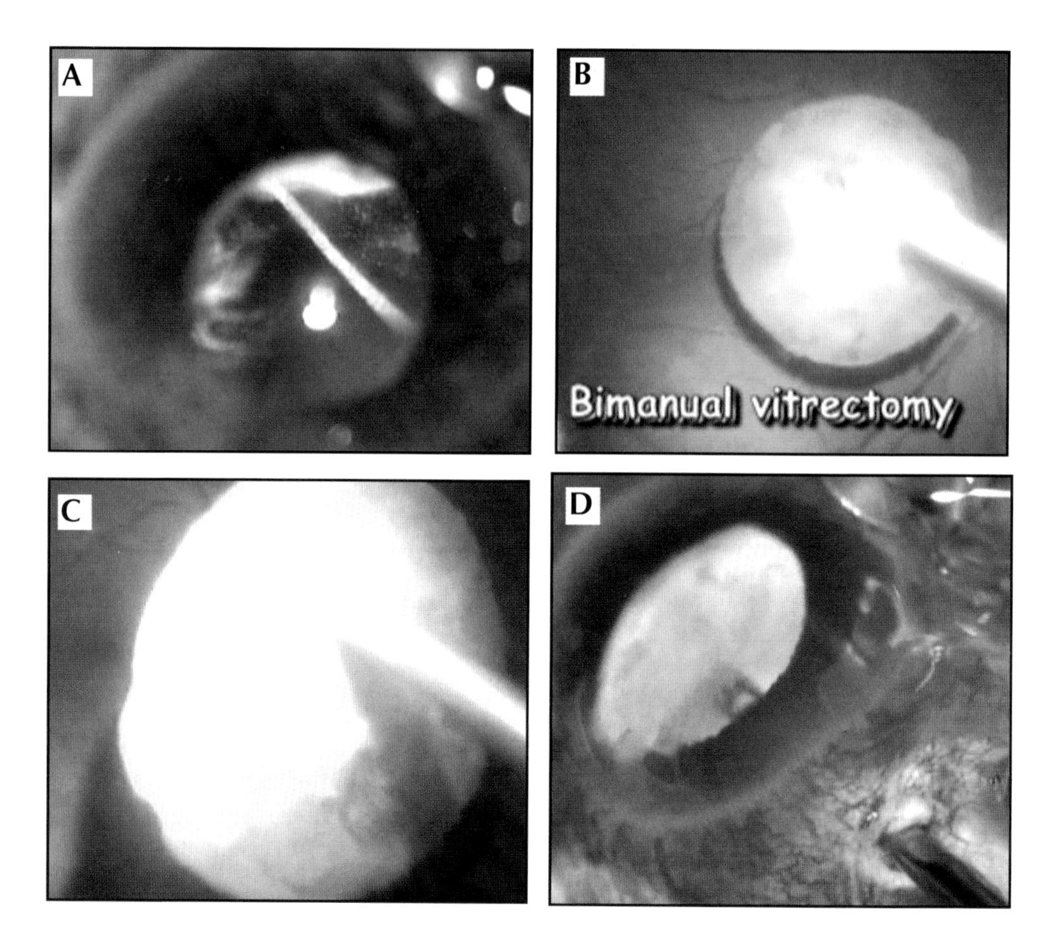

Figure 25-6A-D. Dropped nucleus removed by FAVIT and chandelier illumination. (Photos courtesy of Dr. Agarwal's Eye Hospital.) **A**. Triamcinolone injection. **B**. Nucleus lying on the retina. Illumination is through the chandelier illumination system. Bimanual vitrectomy being done. In the right hand is the microphakonit 0.7 mm phaco needle. In the left hand is the vitrectomy probe. Note there is no illuminator in the hand. A wide field contact lens is used for visualization so that the entire retina is seen. **C**. Nucleus embedded by the microphakonit needle. **D**. Nucleus brought anteriorly and then removed.

Vitrectomy and Phacofragmentation Techniques

The standard three-port pars plana vitrectomy approach is the most frequently employed method for the removal of posteriorly dislocated lens fragments in a safe and effective manner.[1,5,8–14,16,17] The first step involves the insertion of a posterior infusion cannula at the inferior temporal pars plana. In the event of a localized concomitant choroidal detachment in the inferior temporal quadrant, an alternative quadrant (eg, inferior nasal) may be chosen for the infusion cannula. Frequently, cloudy media resulting from dense lens fragments or in some cases hyphema and fibrin deposits surrounding the implant, may prevent an adequate view of the tip of the pars plana infusion cannula. In that situation, the surgeon may ascertain the proper intravitreal location of the infusion cannula tip by inserting a microvitreoretinal blade through one of the superior pars plana sclerotomies to rub against the cannula tip, before turning on the infusion fluid. Utilizing a longer infusion cannula (eg, 4- or 6-mm) is also advantageous in avoiding inadvertent subretinal or choroidal infusion.

Managing the Anterior Chamber Opacities and Herniated Vitreous

Cloudy lens material, hemorrhagic infiltrates, and fibrin deposits in the anterior chamber must be first eliminated before the performance of a posterior vitrectomy and phacofragmentation.[1,5,16,17] For the anterior chamber washout, a separate infusion cannula (eg, a 20- or 22-gauge angled rigid or flexible soft cannula) may be inserted at the limbus for anterior chamber infusion and prevention of chamber collapse. Microsurgical picks, hooks, bent needle tips, or forceps may be used to remove opaque membranes from the anterior and posterior surfaces of the implant.[1] Vitreous herniated into the anterior chamber and vitreous strands attached to the iris or the limbal surgical wound must be excised with a vitrectomy probe in order to reduce the chance of postoperative cystoid macular edema and other types of vitreoretinal complications. To further enhance anterior media clarity, intracameral viscoelastic substances can be injected to coat the corneal endothelium for reducing striate keratopathy, displace blood from the visual axis, or to achieve hemostasis associated with a persistent hyphema.[1,5] Unwanted residual lenticular capsular remnants may also be eliminated with the vitrectomy probe. Pupillary dilation may be maintained throughout surgery with the administration of topical and subconjunctival mydriatics, or intracameral epinephrine.[1,5] If necessary, temporary iris retractors can be inserted via multiple limbal incisions to maintain pupillary dilation during surgery.

Posterior Vitrectomy and Phacofragmentation

After completing the core vitrectomy, it is important for the surgeon to carefully remove all of the vitreous fibers surrounding the posterior lens fragments before proceeding with phacofragmentation, in order to prevent the occlusion of the phaco tip by formed vitreous elements during the phacofragmentation process and also prevent traction on the retina.[1,5,8–14,16,17] In fact, the surgeon should remove as much of the vitreous as he can safely achieve before performing phacoemulsification, in order to avoid unwanted vitreoretinal traction.[16] Perfluorocarbon liquid may be infused into the eye to serve as a cushion for protecting the underlying retina from the bouncing lens fragments during the process of lens emulsification (Figure 25-7). Only a limited amount of perfluorocarbon liquid should be injected, since excessive perfluorocarbon liquid with a convex meniscus tends to displace the lens fragments away from the central visual axis and toward the peripheral fundus and the vitreous base.[1] In case of peripheral displacement of the lens fragments, a layer of viscoelastic may be applied on top of the perfluorocarbon liquid to neutralize its convex meniscus, resulting in recentering of the lens fragments toward the visual axis, a simple maneuver described by Elizalde (Figure 25-8).[23]

At the start of the pars plana phacoemulsification process, each lens fragment is first engaged at the phaco tip with the machine set at the aspiration mode and then brought to the mid vitreous cavity for emulsification.[16,17,24] During the emulsification of the lens fragments, the ultrasonic power is kept at a low or moderate setting in order to decrease the tendency of blowing the fragments from the phaco tip and repeatedly dropping them on the retina.[16,17] The more advanced phacofragmentation units with sophisticated linear (proportional) ultrasonic and aspiration controls tend to reduce the erratic movements of the lens fragments at the phaco tip during the fragmentation process. The surgeon may also stabilize a large lens fragment in the mid vitreous cavity by using his other hand to spear

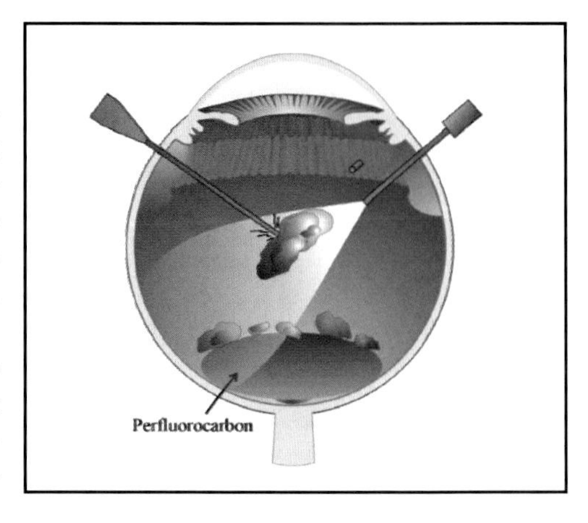

Figure 25-7. Insulating the retina with perfluorocarbon. A small amount of perfluorocarbon liquid may be infused on the retinal surface to protect it from dropped lens fragments during the process of lens emulsification. Excessive perfluorocarbon is avoided to decrease the propensity of peripheral displacement of the floating lens fragments toward the vitreous base due to the convex meniscus of the perfluorocarbon. During phacoemulsification, the ultrasonic power of the phaco probe is kept at a low to medium setting to reduce the tendency of blowing the lens fragments from the phaco tip toward the retina.

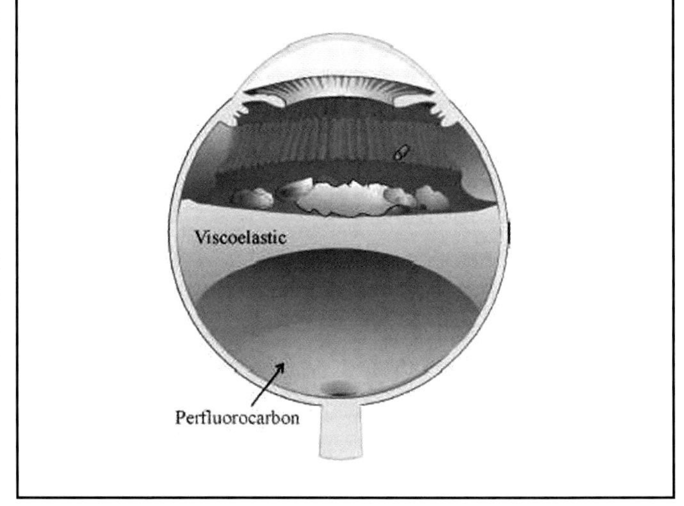

Figure 25-8. Recentering lens fragments on top of perfluorocarbon with viscoelastic. A layer of viscoelastic is applied on top of the perfluorocarbon liquid to neutralize its convex surface meniscus for recentering a peripherally displaced lens fragment toward the visual axis. (Based on an idea from Dr. J. Elizalde and adapted with permission.)

the fragment with an endoilluminator with a hook or pick at its tip for emulsification (Figure 25-9).[1,12] As an alternative, he may utilize the bimanual "crush" or "chopstick" technique, which involves the use of his other hand to methodically crush each lens fragment with the tip of an endoilluminator against the phaco tip before aspirating it from the eye through the phaco tip (Figure 25-10).[1,16] After emulsifying and removing the bulk of the lens fragments, the surgeon eliminates any remaining vitreous with the vitrectomy probe. He also carefully searches for and removes residual small lens fragments embedded at the vitreous base, as well as inspects the peripheral fundus with indirect ophthalmoscopy.[1] One can use a combination of perfluorocarbon liquids and FAVIT also (Figures 25-11 through 25-14). In this once vitrectomy is done PFCL is injected to raise the nuclear fragments from the retinal level. Then using the phaco needle they are removed. Retinal breaks and periph-

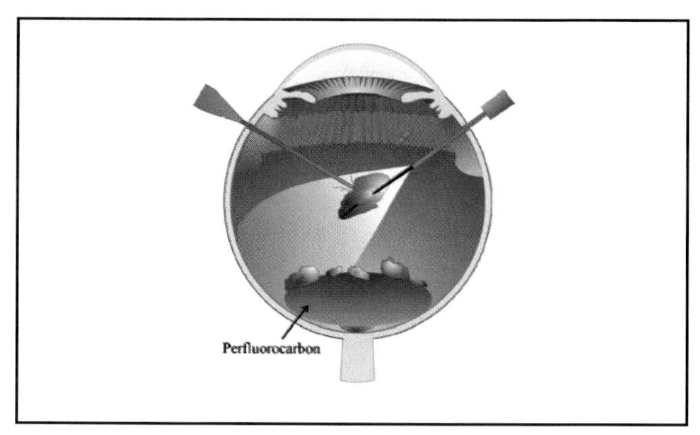

Figure 25-9. Stabilizing the lens fragment with a sharp instrument for emulsification. The surgeon may stabilize a lens fragment in the mid vitreous cavity by using his other hand to spear the fragment with an endoilluminator probe with a hook or pick at its tip for emulsification.

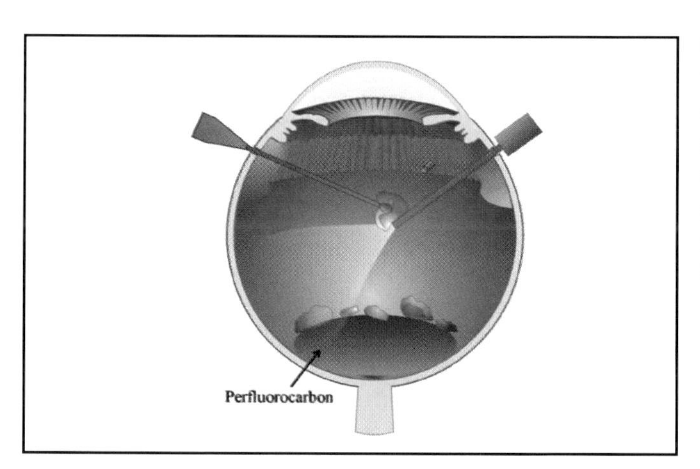

Figure 25-10. Crush method. The surgeon may also use his other hand to methodically crush each lens fragment with the endoilluminator tip against the phaco tip, before aspirating it from the eye through the phaco tip.

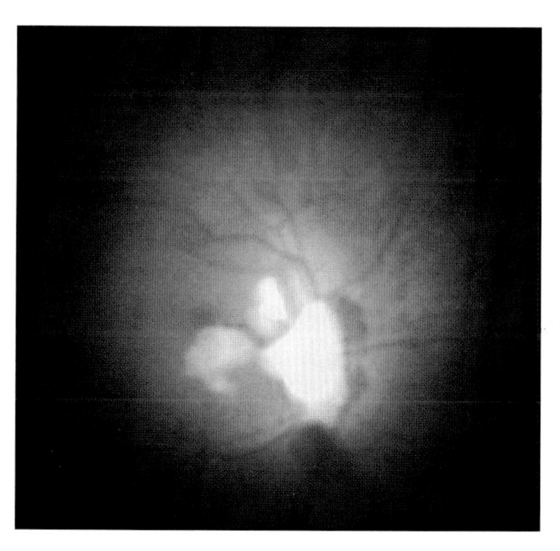

Figure 25-11. Combination of perfluorocarbon liquid (PFCL) and FAVIT. Small nuclear fragments are lying on the retina. (Photo courtesy of Dr. Agarwal's Eye Hospital.)

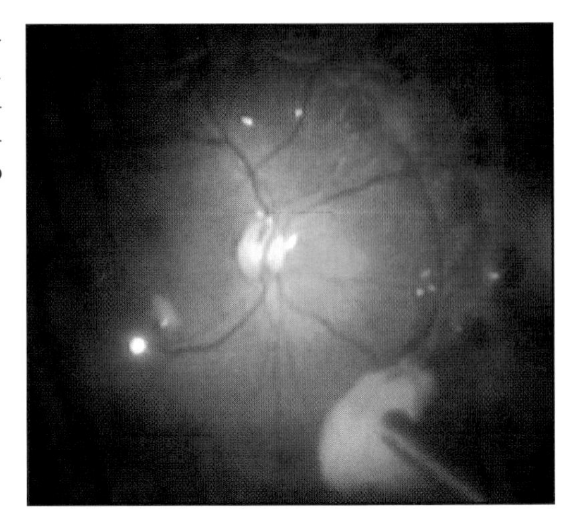

Figure 25-12. Combination of perfluorocarbon liquid (PFCL) and FAVIT. Perfluorocarbon liquid is injected once vitrectomy is done. Then using the phaco needle the nuclear pieces are removed. (Photo courtesy of Dr. Agarwal's Eye Hospital.)

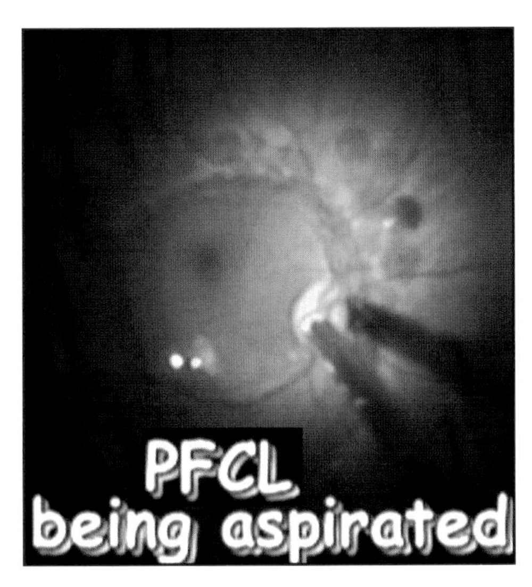

Figure 25-13. Combination of perfluorocarbon liquid (PFCL) and FAVIT. The perfluorocarbon liquid is then aspirated. (Photo courtesy of Dr. Agarwal's Eye Hospital.)

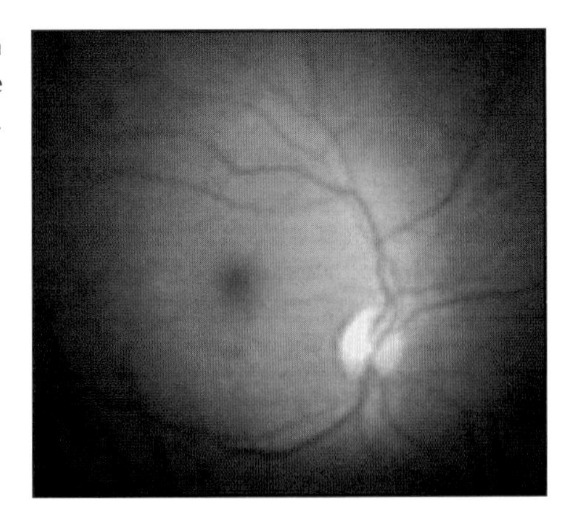

Figure 25-14. Combination of perfluorocarbon liquid (PFCL) and FAVIT. The retina as seen once the case is completed. (Photo courtesy of Dr. Agarwal's Eye Hospital.)

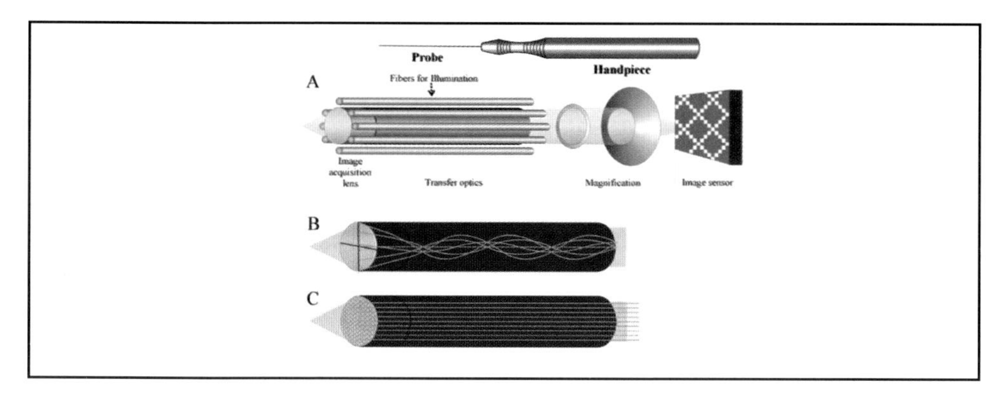

Figure 25-15. Principle of an ophthalmic endoscopic system. A. The image acquired at the tip of an endoscopic handpiece is transmitted through an optical pathway (GRIN solid-lens or a fiberoptic bundle). The image magnification and coupling to the CCD camera system take place at the proximal portion of the handpiece and the CCD camera unit. B. GRIN endoscope: The image acquired at the probe is transmitted along the length of a cylindrical pathway of the solid lens with a gradient index (index of refraction varies with the distance from the central axis) in a sinusoidal mode to a CCD camera unit. C. Fiberoptic endoscope: The image acquired with a GRIN lens at the distal end of a handpiece is transferred through a bundle of microfibers (via total internal reflection within each fiber) to a CCD camera unit.

eral retinal detachment discovered during the inspection are then promptly treated with the appropriate modality (eg, laser, cryotherapy, scleral buckling, fluid-air or gas exchange, etc.) Residual perfluorocarbon liquid is removed before closure. The postoperative therapy includes the application of topical steroidal or nonsteroidal anti-inflammatory medications, antibiotics, and cycloplegics.

Previous studies utilizing the phacoemulsification methods similar to the above description reported favorable visual outcome (ie, a final visual acuity of 20/40 or better with 52% to 87% of treated eyes.)[12,13,14,25]

Endoscopic Technique

The endoscopic approach is best suited for removing dislocated lens fragments from eyes with an opacified cornea, a miotic or occluded pupil, persistent hyphema, or a cloudy IOL, etc.[26–33] It also provides a clear and unimpeded view of lens fragments trapped at the vitreous base. It allows the surgeon to scrutinize peripheral fundus details and appreciate the precise anatomical relationship of various retro-irideal structures (eg, irido-capsular interface, haptic-ciliary junction, vitreous base, etc.) The magnified and undistorted images of the peripheral intraocular structures provided by the endoscope cannot be obtained through other methods. The endoscopic system includes an endoscopic hand piece with a probe, connected to a fiberoptic light source, a charged coupled device (CCD) video camera system and recorder, coupled with a high- resolution color video monitor.[26–33] For optimal viewing, a bright light source such as Xenon is preferred, although halogen lights can be used.[26–33] The two types of ophthalmic endoscopic systems that are commercially available include the gradient Index (GRIN) solid-rod endoscopes first developed by Eguchi,[26,27] and the fiberoptic endoscopes subsequently developed by Uram and Fisher.[27–31] Both types of devices share the principle of image acquisition and optics transfer through the distal probe , and then image magnification and coupling in the handpiece or the remote CCD camera unit (Figure 25-15A).[27] The GRIN solid rod endoscope employs a single long, slender, glass lens for optics transfer. The image acquired at the probe is transmitted along the length of a cylindrical pathway of the solid lens with a gradient index in a sinusoidal mode to a CCD camera unit (Figure 25-15B).[26,27] The index of refraction of the lens varies with the distance from the central axis. In the case of a fiberoptic endoscope, the image acquired with a GRIN lens at the distal end of a handpiece is transferred through a bundle of microfibers (via total internal reflection within each fiber) to a CCD camera unit (Figure 25-15C).[27–32] The fiberoptic endoscope allows for a lighter handpiece. However, its image resolution is limited by the pixel density of the CCD camera as well as the density of the microfibers, and its depth of field is less than the GRIN single-rod endoscope.[27] Besides vitrectomy and phacoemulsification, other surgical maneuvers including laser photocoagulation can be performed in conjunction with the endoscopic system.[27–29] Laser componentry can be built into the endoscopic system.[27–29] For instance, the endoscopic hand piece may contain an optical path for viewing, besides separate fibers for endoillumination and photocoagulation. Thus a single endoscopic handpiece can be constructed with the capability of performing multiple tasks simultaneously: viewing, endoillumination, and photocoagulation.[27–29] Even a channel for infusion can also be incorporated into the endoscope.[27] However, the multiple functions increase the bulk and weight of the handpiece. One commercially available fiberoptic endoscopic system offers a 20-gauge endoscopic handpiece with a 3000-pixel fiberoptic bundle allowing a 70-degree field of view and a depth of focus from 0.5 to 7.0 mm, or an18-gauge hand piece with a 10,000-pixel fiberoptic bundle allowing a 110-degree field of view and a depth of focus from 1 to 20 mm.[28,29] Drawbacks of the endoscopic method include the lack of a stereoscopic or three-dimensional view, and an initially steep learning curve for the surgeon.[1,33] Excellent surgical results can be achieved with this technique. In their study published in 1998, Boscher and associates reported consistently successful outcome in the use of the endoscopic method for managing a consecutive series of 30 eyes with dislocated lens fragments or IOLs.[33]

Further development in ophthalmic endoscopic systems holds the promise of providing unparalleled microscopic images of intraocular structures (even on a cellular level) that are not possible through conventional surgical instrumentation (eg, viewing of sensory retinal, retinal pigment epithelial, and choroidal components in the subretinal space during vitreoretinal surgery).[27] The construction of stereoscopic endoscopes is also technically feasible.

Removal by Cryoextraction

This method is reserved for removing an entire dislocated lens or a large and particularly hard lens nucleus that would otherwise require application of excessive intraocular ultrasonic energy and time-consuming manipulation with the conventional phacoemulsification approach.[24,34,35] When properly performed, it allows rapid delivery of a hard lens nucleus from the retinal surface to the anterior chamber and then out of the eye through a limbal incision, in the absence of an intraocular implant obstructing the passage of the lens nucleus. It is critical that the surgeon first performs a meticulous vitrectomy to eliminate all vitreolenticular and vitreoretinal traction. A fluid-air exchange is also required immediately before the insertion of the endocryoprobe to engage the dislocated lens nucleus.[1,24] The surgeon's failure to eliminate sufficient vitreous fluid from the eye before activation of the endocryoprobe may result in spreading of the freezing ice-ball throughout the residual vitreous fluid and the adjacent retina. Thus this seemingly simple surgical approach is associated with multiple potential hazardous complications. While delivering the hard lens nucleus anteriorly, the surgeon must apply a continuous freeze of sufficient intensity on the lens fragment to prevent its fall from the probe, but at the same time, avoid an excessive freeze that may damage the surrounding vital intraocular structures, including the retina, iris, and cornea, etc. This delicate balance and the intrinsically unpredictable behavior of the expanding ice-ball present a difficult challenge to the surgeon, particularly in the presence of poor visibility through a hazy cornea frequently encountered in such cases made even worse by the intraocular air.[1,35] Due to its potential of inducing retinal necrosis, vitreous hemorrhage, and even severe choroidal and expulsive hemorrhage, it is the authors' opinion that posterior cryoextraction should be limited to select cases of large dislocated hard lens nuclei and performed with extreme caution by an experienced surgeon.

Manipulation With Perfluorocarbon Liquid

High density, inert behavior, and low viscosity are unique properties of perfluorocarbon liquid that allow its use as an elegant surgical tool for removing dislocated lens fragments with minimal instrumentation in a safe and consistent manner.[35–38] As described in the previous section, perfluorocarbon liquid is frequently used to insulate the retina from injury by dropped lens fragments during phacoemulsification.[1] Perfluorocarbon is particularly effective when the surgeon is faced with the adverse condition of poor visibility through a hazy cornea and a dislocated nucleus with a rock-hard consistency.[1,35] In that situation, he may use perfluorocarbon alone without phacoemulsification to deliver the lens fragment anteriorly for its extraction through a limbal wound. Employing conventional phacoemulsification techniques to retrieve a hard lens nucleus may be time consuming and hazardous, particularly in the presence of marked ocular inflammation and a cloudy media with poor visibility.[35] Historically, several methods of removing a dislocated hard nucleus were utilized in the past.[35,39,40] With the exception of cryoextraction, these methods have been largely abandoned due to their technical difficulties and associated potential complications. They include trapping the lens nucleus with two needles passed across the globe with the patient in a prone position and buoying the lens nucleus anteriorly with sodium hyaluronate.[35,39,40] The needle-trapping technique is inherently difficult to apply and is associated with many potential hazards.[35,39] Although sodium hyaluronate is well tolerated by the eye, its relatively low density in comparison to perfluorocarbon does not allow the buoying of the lens nucleus on a consistent basis.[35] In contrast to perfluorocarbon liquid, clear visibility is required for the precise placement of the sodium hyaluronate with a cannula under the dislocated nucleus in order for it to float the nucleus. To avoid the premature dilution and extrusion of the sodium hyaluronate from the globe, the infusion fluid must also be turned off temporarily during the placement of the sodium hyaluronate. Such a maneuver may lead to hypotony and miosis with potentially serious consequences during surgery.[35,40] For the above reasons, perfluorocarbon liquid is superior to sodium hyaluronate and is currently the agent of choice for floating a posteriorly dislocated lens fragment for removal.[35–38]

Shapiro and associates reported the removal of dislocated hard lens nuclei with perfluoro-n-octane in 1991 (Figure 25-16).[35] Their technique includes an initial vitrectomy to eliminate vitreoretinal traction after a thorough clean up of the anterior lenticular cortical and capsular remnants. The subsequent intraocular infusion of perfluoro-n-octane floats the hard lens nucleus anteriorly toward the vitreous base. The nuclear fragment is displaced peripherally due to the convex meniscus of the perfluorocarbon, and temporarily wedged at the vitreous base between the surface of the perfluorocarbon and the iris and ciliary processes. No attempt is made to directly expulse the dislocated lens fragment into the anterior chamber and out of the limbal wound with the perfluorocarbon liquid, due to potential mechanical injury of the corneal endothelium and the iris by the hard lens nucleus with such a maneuver. Instead, a soft-tipped cannula is inserted through a sclerotomy to recenter the lens nucleus behind the pupil (Figure 25-16A). The lens nucleus is then gently floated further anteriorly with slow infusion of balanced salt solution on top of the perfluorocarbon, and carefully brought into the anterior chamber for delivery out of the eye with a lens loop through a limbal incision (Figure 25-16B). In the absence of poor integrity of

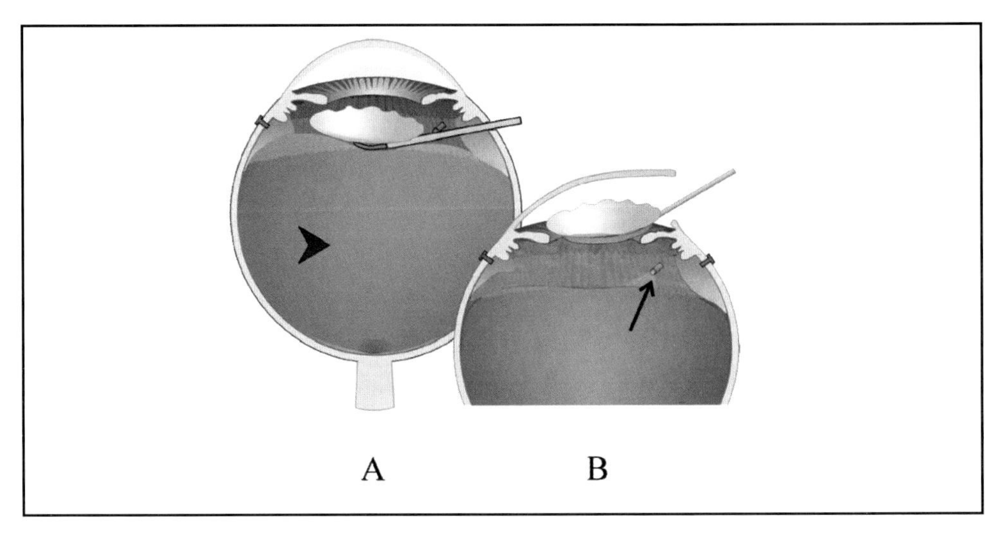

Figure 25-16. Removal of entire hard lens fragment with perfluorocarbon. **A**. After a thorough clean up of the anterior lenticular remnants and a posterior vitrectomy to eliminate vitreoretinal traction, perfluorocarbon liquid (arrow head) is infused via a pars plana sclerotomy into the vitreous cavity to float the hard lens fragment, until it is lodged at the vitreous base between the surface of the perfluorocarbon and the iris as well as the ciliary processes. A soft-tipped cannula is inserted through a sclerotomy to recenter the lens fragment behind the pupil. **B**. Slow infusion of balanced salt solution (arrow) on top of the perfluorocarbon allows the gentle floating of the lens fragment further anteriorly.

the cornea and the iris, a secondary IOL can be conveniently implanted through the same limbal incision before closure. Due to its low viscosity and tendency for posterior pooling, the surgeon can easily remove the perfluorocarbon liquid with a small aspiration cannula after the closure of the limbal wound at the end of surgery. Besides Shapiro's report, there have been a series of reports by multiple surgeons in the effective use of a variety of perfluorocarbon liquids to remove dislocated intraocular lens fragments. Similar to cryoextraction, this method of removing lens fragments is not appropriate for an eye with an IOL, unless the IOL is explanted first or at the time of the lens fragment removal.

The special properties of perfluorocarbon liquid make it especially suitable as an intraocular tool for atraumatic tissue manipulation when the surgeon encounters the situation of posteriorly dislocated lens fragments in conjunction with retinal breaks and a retinal detachment.[1,41] In the presence of a giant retinal tear or a large retinal dialysis, perfluorocarbon frequently becomes indispensable for a successful surgical outcome.[36] The retinal complications may be related to pre-existing retinal pathology, elicited by vitreoretinal traction associated with attempts to remove the lens fragments during the primary cataract surgery, or retinal injury from the dropped lens fragments subsequently.[1,5] The retinal breaks may also enlarge and a retinal detachment may progress during the process of lens fragment removal. In such a situation, perfluorocarbon liquid serves the dual purpose of stabilizing the retinal complications and preventing more retinal injury, while the lens fragments are floated anteriorly for phacoemulsification or removal through a limbal incision.[1,35,41] Any posterior hemorrhage from the retinal breaks may also be displaced anteriorly by the perfluorocarbon liquid for removal. With the retina held down by the perfluorocarbon liquid, standard vitreoretinal techniques are employed to repair the retinal breaks and detachment following the vitrectomy and elimination of the lens fragments. After the application of laser or cryotherapy and possible placement of a scleral buckle, fluid-air or gas exchange is performed to replace the perfluorocarbon liquid and to achieve appropriate retinal tamponade. In case of proliferative vitreoretinopathy, silicone oil may be required as the agent for prolonged retinal tamponade. Utilizing perfluorocarbon liquid in a manner similar to the above description, Lewis and others reported favorable outcome in managing dislocated lens fragments and IOLs.[41] Improved care and methods in the management of dislocated lens fragments during the primary cataract extraction and the subsequent surgery may be responsible for the much lower prevalence of associated retinal breaks and detachment in recent reports in contrast to earlier studies (3% to 5% versus 7% to 50%.)[42] In a recent study, Moore and colleagues reported a combined incidence of 13.4% for retinal detachment associated with retained lens fragments and their subsequent surgical management (6.4% before pars plana vitrectomy and 7.0% after pars plana vitrectomy).[43]

Conclusion

Modern vitreoretinal surgery offers a variety of effective techniques in the safe removal of posteriorly dislocated lens fragments. Besides the standard 3-port pars plana vitrectomy with phacoemulsification, FAVIT is an expedient alternative for the cataract surgeon familiar with vitreoretinal techniques to promptly remove the lens fragments with minimal additional setup during the primary surgery. Perfluorocarbon liquid is a highly valuable intraoperative tool in managing the dislocated lens fragments and underlying associated retinal complications at the same time. Although cryoextraction provides a simple and direct means of removing a large and hard lens nucleus from the posterior segment, severe ocular complications may be associated with this technique. Its use should be limited to select cases by an experienced surgeon familiar with its potential hazards. Under the adverse condition of markedly poor visibility due to various causes, endoscopy can provide unparalleled viewing of the retro-irideal structures to allow safe removal of dislocated lens fragments irrespective of the degree of transparency of the anterior segment of the eye. Employing one or more of the techniques described in this chapter, favorable visual outcome can be achieved for the majority of eyes with dislocated lens fragments.

Key Points

1. Small lens fragments consisting of mostly cortical material may gradually resolve with conservative medical management alone. However, large lens fragments with a sizeable nuclear component do not resolve and may elicit a phacoantigenic response from the host and so have to be removed.
2. In the event of a rupture of the posterior lens capsule or zonular dehiscence leading to posterior migration of lens fragments, the cataract surgeon must avoid any uncontrolled and forceful surgical maneuvers in the vitreous cavity in an attempt to retrieve the sinking lens fragments.
3. Any retrieval technique that does not provide for the appropriate management of the vitreous first has the potential of causing immediate or subsequent retinal complications.
4. The cataract surgeon must refrain from the temptation of passing a sharp instrument or lens loop into the mid or posterior vitreous cavity to engage the sinking lens fragments, or passing forceful irrigation fluid into the vitreous cavity to float the lens fragments. Such maneuvers usually generate vitreoretinal traction resulting in retinal breaks and detachment.
5. In case of familiarity with vitreoretinal techniques, one may convert over to a posterior segment setup and utilize one of the methods described in the following sections for removing the lens fragments. Otherwise, a prompt referral of the patient to a vitreoretinal surgeon is recommended.
6. Medical management with topical anti-inflammatory, antibiotic, as well as cycloplegic medications should be instituted. If necessary, hypotensive agents can also be utilized.
7. Modern vitreoretinal surgery offers a variety of effective techniques in the safe removal of posteriorly dislocated lens fragments. Besides the standard 3-port pars plana vitrectomy with phacoemulsification, FAVIT is an expedient alternative for the cataract surgeon familiar with vitreoretinal techniques to promptly remove the lens fragments with minimal additional setup during the primary surgery.
8. Perfluorocarbon liquid is a highly valuable intraoperative tool in managing the dislocated lens fragments and underlying associated retinal complications at the same time.
9. The chandelier illumination system helps give better visualization and results when doing vitrectomy for a dropped nucleus.

References

1. Chan CK, Lin SG. Management of dislocated lens and lens fragments by the vitreoretinal approach. In: Agarwal S, Agarwal A, Sachdev MS, et al, eds. *Phacoemulsification, Laser Cataract Surgery, and Foldable IOLs*. 2nd ed. New Delhi: Jaypee Brothers Medical Publishers, Ltd; 2000.
2. Verhoeff FH, Lemoine AN. Endophthalmitis phacoanaphalactica. *Am J Ophthalmol.* 1922;5:737.
3. Apple DJ, Mamalis N, Steinmetz RI, et al. Phacoanaphylactic endophthalmitis associated with extracapsular cataract extraction and posterior chamber intraocular lens. *Arch Ophthalmol.* 1984;102:1528.
4. Smith RE, Weiner P. Unusual presentation of phacoanaphylaxis following phacoemulsification. *Ophthalmic Surg.* 1976;7:65.

5. Fastenberg DM, Schwartz PL, Shakin JL, et al. Management of dislocated nuclear fragments after phacoemulsification. *Am J Ophthalmol.* 1991;112:535.
6. Epstein DL. In: *Chandler and Grant's Glaucoma.* 3rd ed. Philadelphia: Lea and Febiger; 1986:320.
7. Epstein DL. Diagnosis and management of lens-induced glaucoma. *Ophthalmology.* 1982;89:227.
8. Hutton WL, Snyder WB, Vaiser A. Management of surgically dislocated intravitreal lens fragments by pars plana vitrectomy. *Ophthalmology.* 1978;85:176.
9. Michels RG, Shacklett DE. Vitrectomy techniques for removal of retained lens material. *Arch Ophthalmol.* 1977;95:1767.
10. Ross WH. Management of dislocated lens fragments following phacoemulsification surgery. *Can J Ophthalmol.* 1993;28:163.
11. Blodi BA, Flynn HW Jr, Blodi CF, et al. Retained nuclei after cataract surgery. *Ophthalmology.* 1992;99:41.
12. Lambrou FH, Stewart MW. Management of dislocated lens fragments during phacoemulsification. *Ophthalmology.* 1992;99:1260.
13. Gilliland GD, Hutton WL, Fuller DG. Retained intravitreal lens fragments after cataract surgery. *Ophthalmology.* 1992;99:1263.
14. Kim JE, Flynn HW Jr, Smiddy WE, et al. Retained lens fragments after phacoemulsification. *Ophthalmology.* 1994;101:1827.
15. Verhoeff FH. A simple and safe method for removing a cataract dislocated into fluid vitreous. *Am J Ophthalmol.* 1942;25:725.
16. Charles S. Posterior dislocation of lens material during cataract surgery. In: Agarwal S, Agarwal A, Sachdev MS, et al, eds. *Phacoemulsification, Laser Cataract Surgery, and Foldable IOLs.* 2nd ed. New Delhi: Jaypee Brothers Medical Publishers, Ltd; 2000: 517.
17. Topping TM. Management of dislocated lens fragments during phacoemulsification, and, Retained intravitreal lens fragments after cataract surgery [Discussion]. *Ophthalmology.* 1992;99:1268.
18. Gimbel HV, Penno EA. Divide and conquer nucleofractis techniques. In: Agarwal S, Agarwal A. Sachdev MS, et al. (eds), *Phacoemulsification, Laser Cataract Surgery, and Foldable IOLs.* 2nd ed. New Delhi: Jaypee Brothers Medical Publishers, Ltd; 2000: 133.
19. Hara T. Endocapsular phacoemulsification and aspiration (ECPEA)—recent surgical technique and clinical results. *Ophthalmic Surg.* 1989;20:469.
20. Cionni RJ, Osher RH. Endocapsular ring approach to the subluxated cataractous lens. *Cataract Refract Surg.* 1995;21:245.
21. Eaton AM, Jaffe GJ, McCuen BW, et al. Condensation on the posterior surface of silicone intraocular lenses during fluid-air exchange. *Ophthalmology.* 1995;102:733.
22. Agarwal A, Siraj AA. FAVIT—a new method to remove dropped nuclei. In: Agarwal S, Agarwal A, Sachdev MS, et al, eds. *Phacoemulsification, Laser Cataract Surgery, and Foldable IOLs.* 2nd ed. New Delhi: Jaypee Brothers Medical Publishers, Ltd; 2000: 538.
23. Elizalde J. Combined use of perfluorocarbon liquids and viscoelastics for safer surgical approach to posterior lens luxation. [Poster]. The Vitreous Society 17th Annual Meeting; Rome, Italy; September 21–25, 1999.
24. Charles S. *Vitreous Microsurgery.* 2nd ed. Baltimore: Williams and Wilkins; 1987:48.
25. Ross WH. Management of dislocated lens fragments after phacoemulsification surgery. *Can J Ophthalmol.* 1996;31:234.
26. Eguchi S, Araie M. A new ophthalmic electronic videoendoscope system for intraocular surgery. *Arch Ophthalmol.* 1990;108:1778.
27. Grizzard WS. GRIN endoscopy. In syllabus: Subspecialty Day – Vitreoretinal Update 1998, pp 109–112, New Orleans

28. Uram M. Ophthalmic laser microendoscope endophotocoagulation. *Ophthalmology.* 1992;99:1829.
29. Uram M. Laser endoscope in the management of proliferative vitreoretinopathy. *Ophthalmology.* 1994;101:1404.
30. Fisher YL, Slakter JS. A disposable ophthalmic endoscopic system. *Arch Ophthalmol.* 1994;112:984.
31. Ciardella AP, Fisher YL, Carvalho C, et al. Endoscopic vitreoretinal surgery for complicated proliferative diabetic retinopathy. *Retina.* 2001;21:20.
32. Yaguchi S, Kora Y, Takahashi H, et al. A new endoscope for ophthalmic microsurgery. *Ophthalmic Surg.* 1992;23:838.
33. Boscher C, Lebuisson DA, Lean JS, et al. Vitrectomy with endoscopy for management of retained lens fragments and/or posteriorly dislocated intraocular lens. *Graefes Arch Clin Exp Ophthalmol.* 1998;236:115.
34. Barraquer J. Surgery of the dislocated lens. *Trans Am Acad Ophthalmol Otolaryngol.* 1975;76:44.
35. Shapiro MJ, Resnick KI, Kim SH, et al. Management of the dislocated crystalline lens with a perfluorocarbon liquid. *Am J Ophthalmol.* 1991;112:401.
36. Chang S. Perfluorocarbon liquids in vitreoretinal surgery. New approaches to vitreoretinal surgery. *Int Ophthalmol Clin.* 1992;32:153.
37. Rowson NJ, Bacon AS, Rosen PH. Perfluorocarbon heavy liquids in the management of posterior dislocation of the lens nucleus during phacoemulsification. *Br J Ophthalmol.* 1992;76:169.
38. Greve MD, Peyman GA, Mehta NJ, et al. Use of perfluoroperhydrophenanthrene in the management of posteriorly dislocated crystalline and intraocular lenses. *Ophthalmic Surg.* 1993;24:593.
39. Calhoun FP, Hagler WS. Experience with Jose Barraquer method of extracting a dislocated lens. *Am J Ophthalmol.* 1960;50:701.
40. Haymet BT. Removal of dislocated hypermature lens from the posterior vitreous. *Aust NZJ Ophthalmol.* 1990;18:103.
41. Lewis H, Blumenkranz MS, Chang S. Treatment of dislocated crystalline lens and retinal detachment with perfluorocarbon liquids. *Retina.* 1992;12:299.
42. Smiddy WE, Flynn HW Jr, Kim JE. Retinal detachment in patients with retained lens fragments or dislocated posterior chamber intraocular lenses. *Ophthalmic Surg Lasers.* 1996;27:856.
43. Moore JK, Scott IU, Flynn HW Jr, et al. Retinal detachment associated with retained lens fragments removed by pars plana vitrectomy [paper]. American Academy of Ophthalmology Annual Meeting; New Orleans, La; November 12, 2001.

The author has no commercial or proprietary interest in any products or techniques mentioned in the manuscript.

Please see Incredible Disasters video on enclosed CD-ROM.

Chapter 26

Surgical Management of the Malpositioned Intraocular Implant

Clement K. Chan, MD, FACS; Amar Agarwal, MS, FRCS, FRCOphth; Athiya Agarwal, MD, FRSH, DO; Sunita Agarwal, MS, FSVH, DO

Introduction

With ever more sophisticated and increasingly innovative technological advances in cataract surgery, more surgical complications are expected.[1-3] For instance, higher demands in surgical skills associated with microincisional phacoemulsification techniques requiring complex surgical maneuvers through an ever smaller surgical incision (eg, as in 0.7 mm tips used for microphakonit) may result in greater tendency for complications such as subluxation and dislocation of the intraocular lens (IOL) under certain circumstances. Thus, the ophthalmic surgeon engaged in modern microincisional surgery must be versatile in or familiar with the management of surgical complications associated with the malpositioned IOL.[3-56]

Management of a Malpositioned Intraocular Lens

Disturbing visual symptoms such as diplopia, metamorphopsia, and hazy images are associated with a dislocated IOL (Figure 26-1). Contemporaneous with advances in phakonit microsurgical techniques for treating cataracts, a number of highly effective surgical methods have been developed for managing a dislocated IOL (Figure 26-2). They include IOL manipulation with perfluorocarbon liquids, scleral loop fixation, use of a snare, employing 25-gauge IOL forceps, temporary haptic externalization, as well as managing the single plate implant and two simultaneous intraocular implants.[3–13] One excellent method is the use of diamond-tipped forceps to grasp the malpositioned IOL during a vitrectomy for its explantation or repositioning (Figure 26-3). The primary aim of such methods is to reposition the dislocated IOL close to the original site of the crystalline lens in an expeditious manner whenever possible, and with minimal morbidity, in order to optimize the outcome.

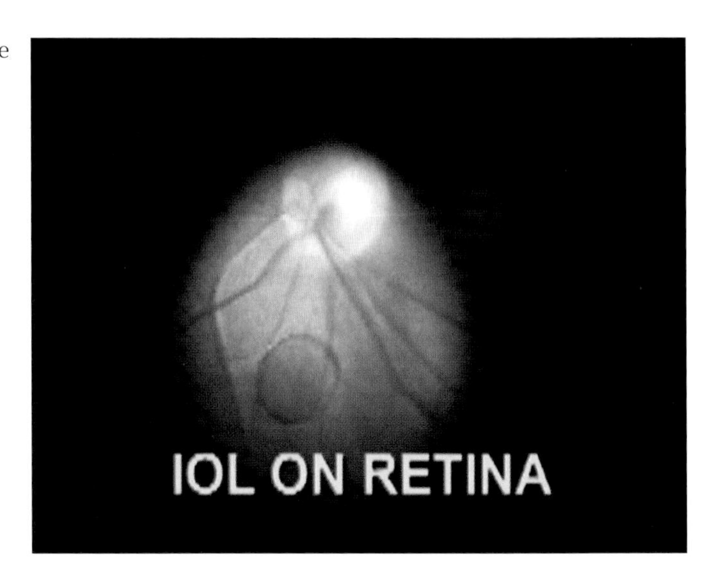

Figure 26-1. Dislocated plate haptic IOL on the retina.

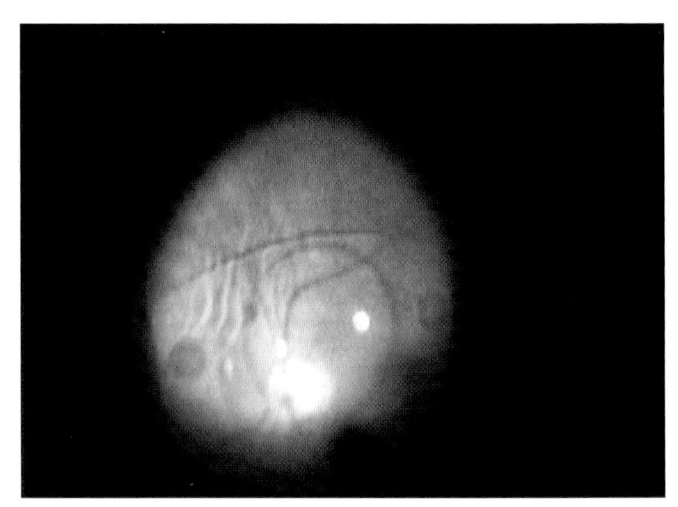

Figure 26-2. IOL lying over the disc.

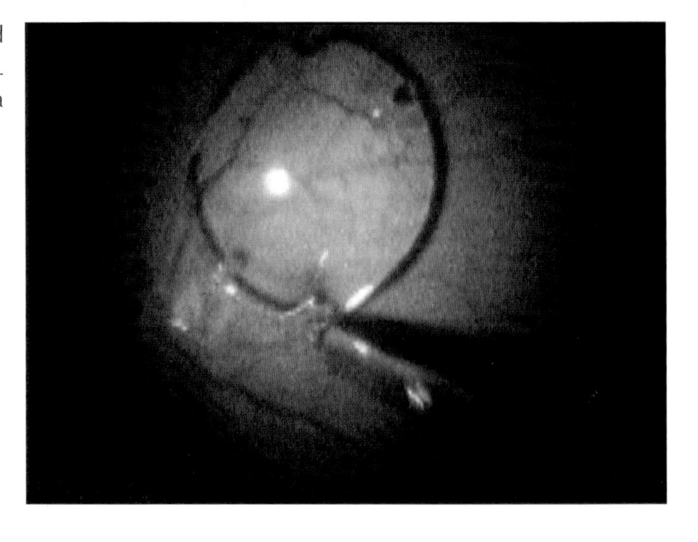

Figure 26-3. Diamond-tipped forceps lifting a looped IOL lying on the retina after a vitrectomy.

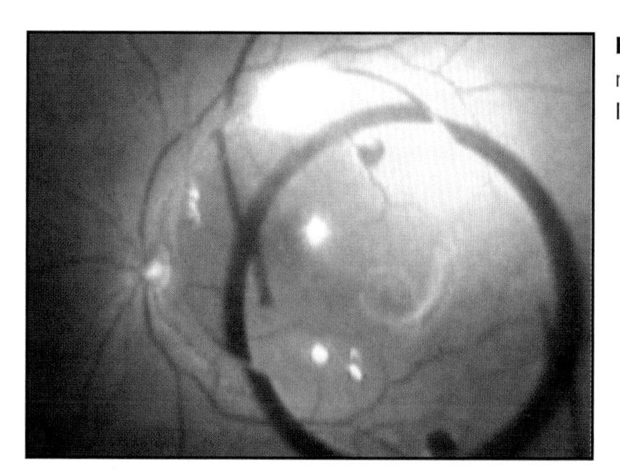

Figure 26-4A. View of chandelier illumination for removal of a dislocated IOL on the retinal surface.

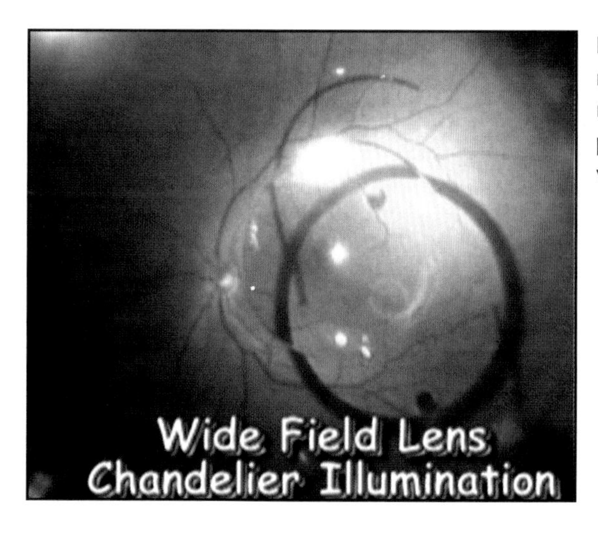

Figure 26-4B. View of an IOL on the macular surface. Notice the wide-field retinal image provided by a special panoramic contact lens with lighting via chandelier illumination.

Chandelier Illumination

The introduction of chandelier illumination supplemented with xenon lighting markedly enhances the surgical versatility of the ophthalmic surgeon for performing complex surgical maneuvers. This lighting system provides high-quality and diffuse illumination over a wide surgical field without the need of an endoilluminating fiberoptic probe. With this system, both hands are available for performing surgical tasks (Figure 26-4A-G). For instance, the surgeon may use one hand to excise vitreous adhesions with a vitrectomy probe and the other hand to grasp the dislocated IOL with diamond-tipped forceps (see Figure 26-4D). He may also perform bimanual manipulation of the dislocated IOL with separate forceps (hand-shake technique) for its removal or repositioning (see Figures 26-4 F and 26-4 G). For optimal viewing quality, special fiberoptic light sources providing high intensity and diffuse lighting are required for chandelier illumination, eg, PHOTON Light Source (Synergetics Inc., O'Fallon, Missouri, USA), and Alcon Xenon Light Source (Alcon Laboratories Inc., Fort Worth, Texas, USA).

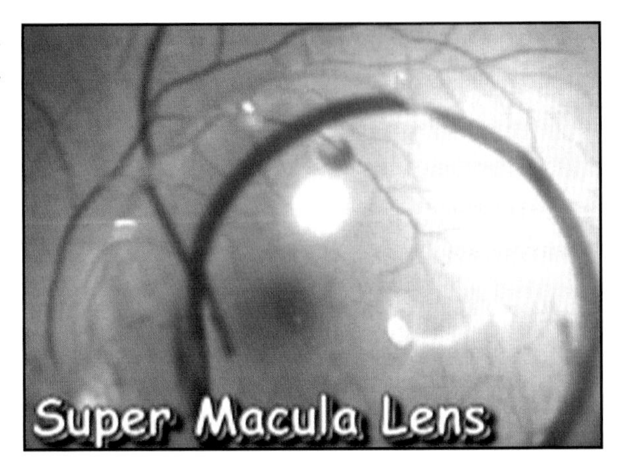

Figure 26-4C. View with the Supermacula Volk lens that provides stereoscopic macular images.

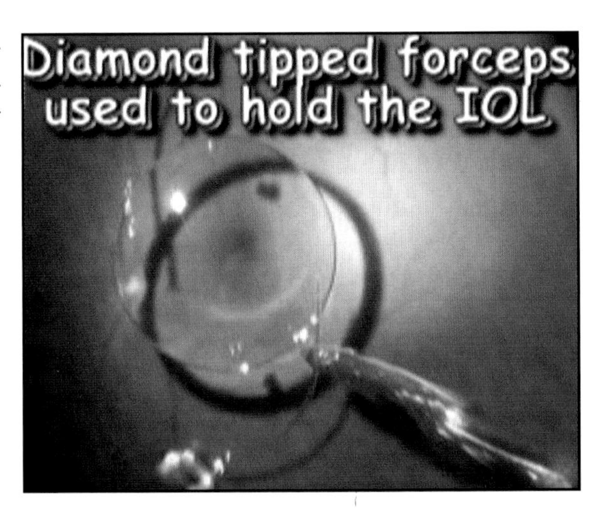

Figure 26-4D. View of diamond-tipped forceps lifting a looped IOL from the retinal surface after performance of a vitrectomy.

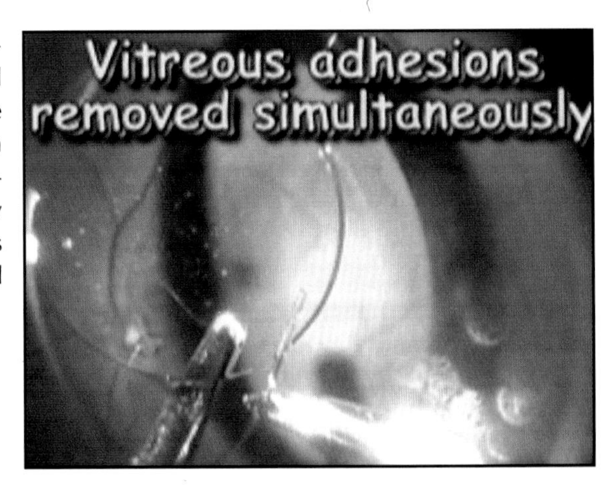

Figure 26-4E. View of bimanual technique in manipulating a dislocated IOL, whereby the surgeon uses one hand to grasp the dislocated IOL with forceps and his other hand to cut vitreous adhesion with a vitrectomy probe. Appropriate lighting for this bimanual technique is achieved through chandelier illumination.

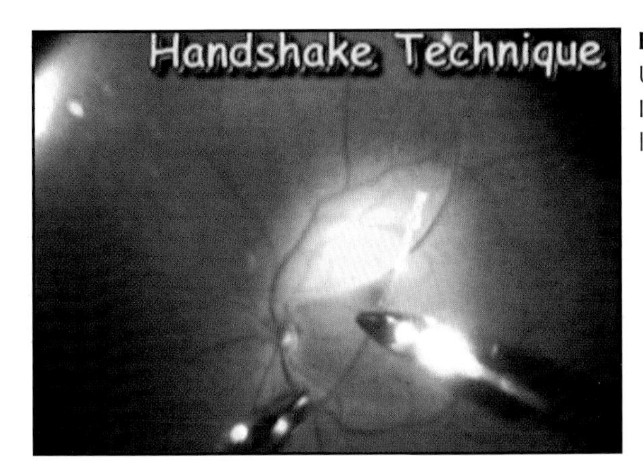

Figure 26-4F. Handshake technique. Using two forceps, one can hold the IOL comfortably and bring it anteriorly.

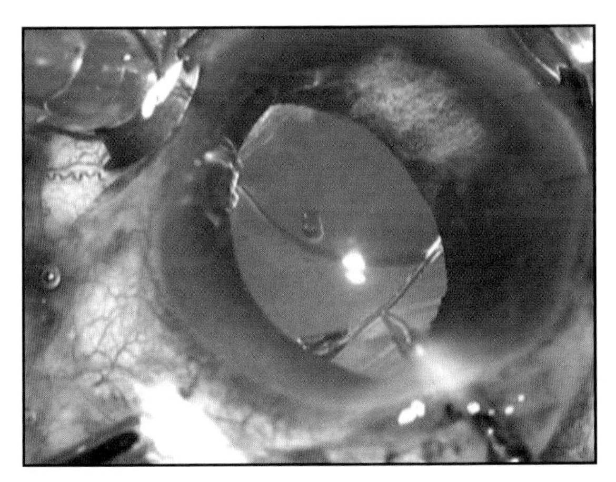

Figure 26-4G. View of explantation of a dislocated IOL through a limbal incision. Notice the presence of separate infusion cannulas at both the upper right and upper left corners of the surgical field. One cannula is for fluid infusion, whereas the other is for chandelier illumination. Fluid infusion and chandelier illumination can also be achieved through the same specially manufactured dual-function cannula.

Wide-Angle Viewing System

Modern panoramic viewing systems provide superior wide-angle viewing during a vitrectomy, previously not obtainable with conventional contact lenses. There are two different types of commercially available wide-angle viewing system, namely the noncontact and contact viewing systems. Both types of viewing systems have distinct advantages and disadvantages, and both have their proponents and detractors.

Noncontact Wide-Angle Viewing System

The SDI/BIOM noncontact wide-field viewing system manufactured by OCULUS Optikgeraete GmBH (Wetzlar, Germany) is the most common example of the first type of viewing system. With this system, a reduction lens and high-powered wide-angle front lenses (60°, 90°, or 120°) mounted on a metallic extension are attached to the bottom of the operating microscope and then positioned over the surgical eye during a vitrectomy. Since wide-field indirect (inverted) images are provided by this viewing system, a reinverting box (Stereoscopic Diagnostic Inverter) inserted within the optical path of the microscope is required for converting the inverted images to direct (upright) images for the surgeon during a vitrectomy. The surgeon can activate the reinverting mechanism either via a foot switch or a button mounted on the microscope. Autoclavable or disposable lenses are available.

In recent years, Möller-Wedel (Möller-Wedel GmbH, Wedel, Germany) introduced a noncontact wide-angle viewing system that provides erect images for the surgeon without the need of a reinverting box. Similar to the SDI/BIOM system, this system, known as the Erect Indirect Binocular Ophthalmic System (EIBOS), is also mounted on the bottom of the microscope.

The most important advantage of the noncontact viewing system is it does not require expensive contact lenses and the aid of highly skillful surgical assistants to stabilize those lenses on the cornea during a vitrectomy. However, there is a relatively steep learning curve in achieving optimal viewing of both the posterior and the peripheral fundus with the noncontact system.

Contact Wide-Angle Viewing System

The second type is the contact panoramic viewing system. Wide-angle viewing contact lenses constructed with special material are positioned on the cornea of the surgical eye to provide panoramic viewing during a vitrectomy. These lenses are attached with handles for the surgical assistants to stabilize and manipulate them on the surgical eye. One of the first contact wide-angle viewing systems (A.V.I. Panoramic Viewing System [Advanced Visual Instruments Inc., New York, USA]) was developed by Avi Grinblat under the guidance of Stanley Chang, MD in 1989. It consists of a stereoscopic image inverter, wide-field indirect aspheric contact lenses, lens handles, lens retaining ring, and fiberoptic chandelier illumination that fits through a single 20-gauge sclerotomy. The Volk Reinverting Operating Lens System (ROLS or ROLS plus) (Volk Optical Inc., Mentor, Ohio, USA), with single-element prism design is another example of a high-quality stereoscopic wide-angle viewing system. A series of wide-angle contact lenses are used with this system, eg, Super Macula lens for macular viewing (see Figure 26-4C), the Mini Quad and Mini Quad XL lenses for the peripheral fundus (up to 127° and 134° respectively), Dyna View 156° (full field fundus viewing). Wide-angle contact lenses with special high-index material manufactured by OCULUS and Ocular Instruments (Bellevue, Washington, USA) are also available for panoramic viewing during a vitrectomy, eg, OWIV-HM (100°), OLIV-EQ-2 (131°), and OLIV-WF (146°). All such systems provide panoramic viewing via special wide-angle contact lenses for the posterior fundus including the macula, the equator, and beyond, as well as the far peripheral fundus. Depending on the lenticular and refractive status of the surgical eye, viewing of the peripheral fundus may reach as far as the ora serrata with specific wide-angle lenses for certain eyes. Similar to the SDI/BIOM noncontact viewing system, the contact viewing systems also require the incorporation of a reinverting box along the optical pathway of the microscope to convert inverted images to erect images for the surgeon. Sterilization of these lenses may require ethylene oxide, steam sterilization, Steris or Sterad system, depending on the product specification.

The most valuable aspect of various contact panoramic viewing systems is the availability of both posterior and peripheral panoramic fundus images with unparalleled resolution via specially designed contact lenses. However, careful maintenance of expensive contact lenses and skillful stabilization of the contact lenses on the cornea are required.

Perfluorocarbon Liquids

Chang popularized the use of perfluorocarbon liquids for the surgical treatment of various vitreoretinal disorders.[3] Due to their heavier-than-water properties, and their ease of

Table 26-1.

Properties of Perfluorocarbon Liquids

Characteristic	*Perfluoron Octane*	*Perfluoro-tributylamine*	*Perfluoro-decaline*	*Perfluoro-phenanthrene*
Chemical formula	C_3F_{18}	$C_{12}F_{27}N$	$C_{10}F_{18}$	$C_{14}F_{24}$
Molecular weight	438	671	462	624
Specific gravity	1.76	1.89	1.94	2.03
Refractive index	1.27	1.29	1.31	1.33
Surface tension (Dyne/cm at 25°C)	14	16	16	16
Viscosity (Centistokes— 25°C)	0.8	2.6	2.7	8.03
Vapor Pressure (mm Hg at 37°C)	50	1.14	13.5	<1

intraocular injection and removal,[14–17] perfluorocarbon liquids are highly effective for flattening detached retina, tamponading retinal tears, limiting intraocular hemorrhage, as well as floating dropped crystalline lens fragments and a dislocated IOL.[18–27]

Types of Perfluorocarbon Liquids

Four types of perfluorocarbon liquids are frequently employed for intraocular surgery. They include:

1. Perfluoro-N-Octane
2. Perfluoro-Tributylamine
3. Perfluoro-Decaline
4. Perfluoro-Phenanthrene

Their physical properties are outlined in Table 26-1.

Intraocular Lens Manipulation With Perfluorocarbon Liquids

Due to their unique physical properties, perfluorocarbon liquids are well suited for floating dropped lens fragments and dislocated IOL, in order to insulate the underlying retina from damage. At the same time, the anterior displacement of the dislocated IOL by the perfluorocarbon liquids facilitates its removal or repositioning.[18–27]

Anterior Chamber Intraocular Lens

An anterior chamber intraocular lens (AC IOL) usually does not dislocate into the vitreous cavity because the iris serves as a natural physical barrier. However, decentration or subluxation of the AC IOL is not uncommon (eg, due to trauma), and requires surgical correction with special techniques.[28,29]

In case of subluxation of the ACIOL in the anterior chamber or anterior vitreous cavity, bimanual techniques for correcting the malpositioning with hooks and forceps can usually be accomplished without the need for a fiberoptic endoilluminating probe or a chandelier lighting system. It is important for the surgeon to excise any prolapsed vitreous surrounding the subluxated ACIOL first before its manipulation, in order to avoid harmful vitreoretinal traction. The bimanual maneuvers may be carried out simultaneously via two separate limbal incisions, two pars plana incisions, or one limbal and one pars plana incision.

External Approach

The external approach requires a large surgical incision for explanting the dislocated IOL first before IOL manipulation (eg, suture attachment) outside of the eye. Due to potentially excessive tissue trauma and astigmatic changes induced by a large surgical incision, this approach is only appropriate for special situations, such as in conjunction with penetrating keratoplasty and IOL exchange.

Internal Approach—Pars Plana Techniques

For this approach, surgical corrections of the malpositioned IOL are accomplished via small pars plana or limbal incisions that avoid excessive tissue trauma and allow maintenance of the integrity of the globe.[4-11,25,26,51,52]

Scleral Loop Fixation

This technique was first described by Maguire and Blumenkranz.[5] For this technique, microforceps are used to make simple knots or series of twists with a 9-0 or 10-0 polypropylene suture. The same microforceps are used to grasp the suture adjacent to the suture loop for insertion through an anterior sclerotomy corresponding to the location of the ciliary sulcus, following the excision of vitreous traction via a pars plana vitrectomy. The inserted suture loop is then used to capture one of the dislocated haptics for anchoring at the anterior sclerotomy. The opposite haptic is likewise anchored in the ciliary sulcus in the same manner.

The Grieshaber Snare

This technique requires the use of a snare to secure the dislocated IOL (Figure 26-5). The engaged IOL is moved anteriorly for suture fixation in the ciliary sulcus. The successful deployment of this technique for IOL repositioning was reported by Little et al.[3,6,9]

The 25-Gauge Intraocular Lens Forceps

The employment of the 25-gauge IOL forceps for managing a dislocated IOL was presented by Chang et al in 1994 (Figure 26-6).[6]

The proximal groove of the Chang forceps are designed for holding the haptic, and the smooth distal platforms are for grasping sutures or tissues. These forceps fit well into the scheme of bimanual surgical maneuvers via separate limbal, pars plicata, or pars plana incisions for IOL fixation in the ciliary sulcus (see Figure 26-6).

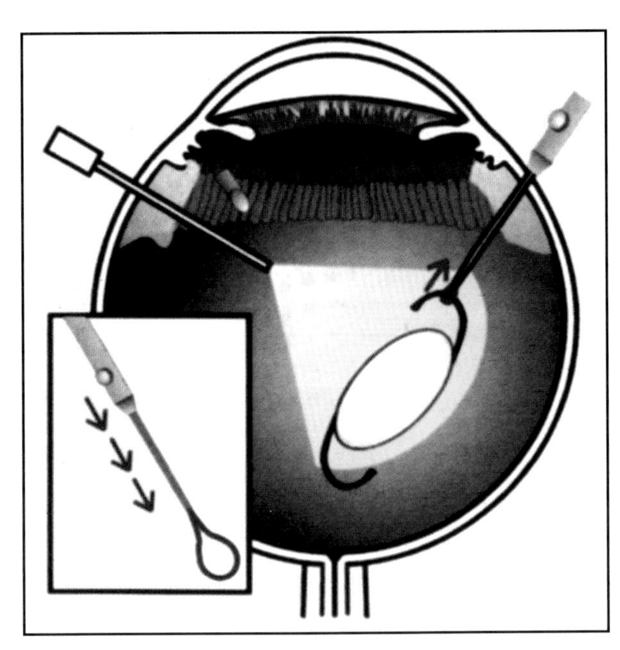

Figure 26-5. The Grieshaber snare consists of a 20-gauge tube and handle with a movable spring-loaded finger slide for adjusting the size of a protruding polypropylene suture loop. The suture loop is inserted posteriorly to engage a dislocated haptic. The external portion of the suture loop is then cut free and guided through a 30-gauge needle for anchoring at the sclera, after the engaged haptic is pulled up against the anterior sclerotomy.

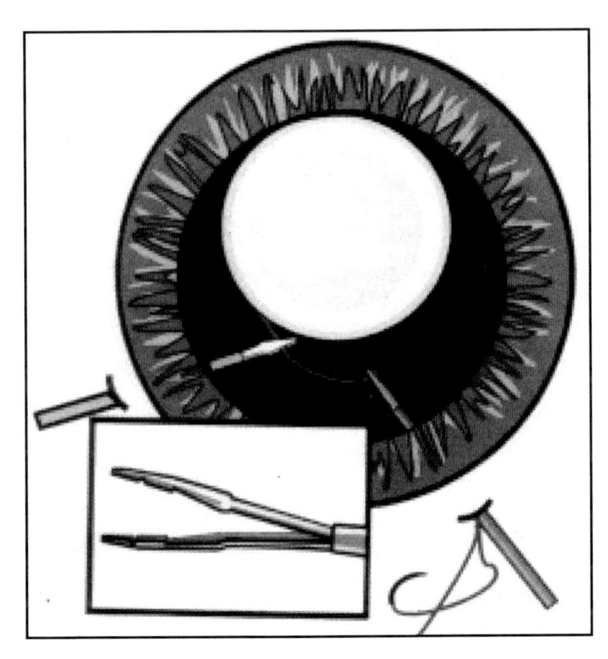

Figure 26-6. These 25-gauge Chang passive-action IOL forceps have smooth distal platforms for grasping tissues or sutures, and a proximal groove for gripping a haptic. A slip knot is inserted through a paralimbal scleral groove incision to engage the haptic of the IOL. The forceps are then used to regrasp the distal end of the haptic to prevent the slippage of the suture loop. After tightening the slip knot, the needle of the 10-0 polypropylene suture is anchored within the scleral groove for the implant fixation in the ciliary sulcus. (From Chan CK, Agarwal A, Agarwal S, Agarwal A. Management of dislocated intraocular implants. In: Nagpal PN, Fine IH, eds. *Ophthalmology Clinics of North America, Posterior Segment Complications of Cataract Surgery*. Philadelphia: W. B. Saunders; 2001:681. Reprinted with permission.)

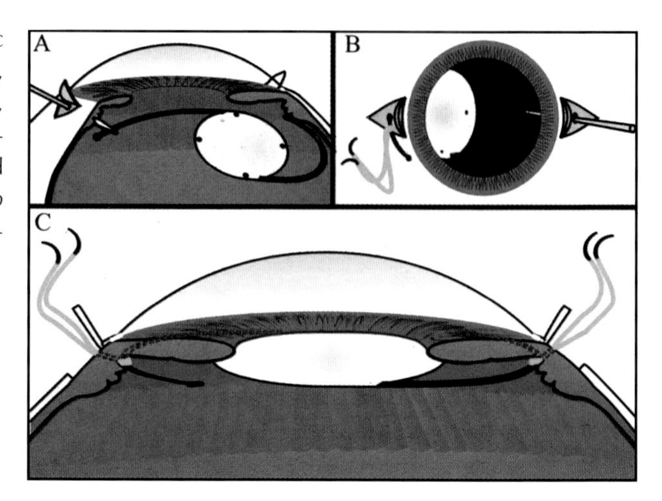

Figure 26-7. Temporary haptic externalization. (From Chan CK, Agarwal Am, Agarwal At, Agarwal S. Surgical management of the malpositioned intraocular implant. *Comp Ophthalmol Update*. 2004;5:103-15. Reprinted with permission.)

Temporary Haptic Externalization

Chan first described this method in 1992.[7] Its main features involve temporary haptic externalization for suture placement after a pars plana vitrectomy, followed by reinternalization of the haptics tied with 9–0 or 10–0 polypropylene sutures for secured anchoring by the anterior sclerotomies.[7] The details of this technique include the following:[7,8]

1. A 3-port pars plana vitrectomy is performed for the removal of the anterior and central vitreous adjacent to the dislocated IOL, in order to prevent any vitreoretinal traction during the process of manipulating the IOL.
2. Two diametrically opposed limbal-based partial thickness triangular scleral flaps are prepared along the horizontal meridians at 3 and 9 o'clock. Anterior sclerotomies within the beds under the scleral flaps are made at 1 to 1.5 mm from the limbus (Figure 26-7A). As an alternative to the scleral flaps, the anterior sclerotomies may be made within scleral grooves at 1 to 1.5 mm from the horizontal limbus.
3. A fiberoptic light pipe is inserted through one of the posterior sclerotomies, while a pair of fine nonangled positive action forceps (eg, Grieshaber 612.8) is inserted through the anterior sclerotomy of the opposing quadrant to engage one haptic of the dislocated IOL for temporary externalization (Figure 26-7B). A double-armed 9–0 (Ethicon TG 160–8 plus, Somerville NJ) or 10–0 polypropylene suture (Ethicon CS 160–6, Somerville, NJ) is tied around the externalized haptic to make a secured knot. The same process is repeated for the other haptic after the surgeon switches the instruments to his opposite hands.
4. The externalized haptics with the tied sutures are reinternalized through the corresponding anterior sclerotomies with the same forceps (Figure 26-7C). The surgeon anchors the internalized haptics securely in the ciliary sulcus by taking scleral bites with the external suture needles on the lips of the anterior sclerotomies. By adjusting the tension of the opposing sutures while tying the polypropylene suture knots by the anterior sclerotomies, the optic is centered behind the pupil, and the haptics are anchored in the ciliary sulcus.

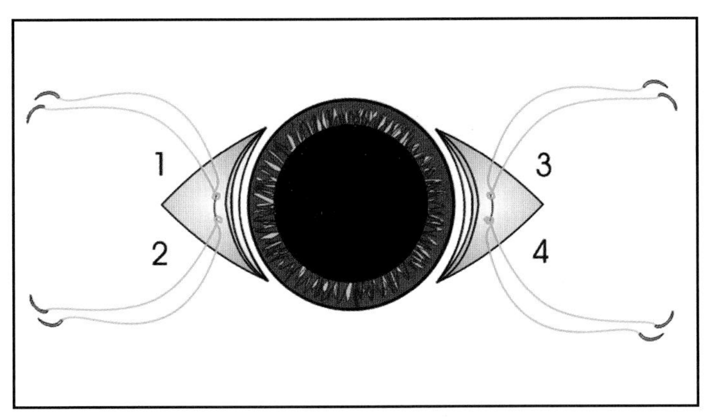

Figure 26-8. Four-point fixation enhances stability of repositioned IOL. (From Chan CK, Agarwal A, Agarwal S, Agarwal A. Management of dislocated intraocular implants. In: Nagpal PN, Fine IH, eds. *Ophthalmology Clinics of North America, Posterior Segment Complications of Cataract Surgery*. Philadelphia: W. B. Saunders; 2001:681. Reprinted with permission.)

Some important features of this technique include:[7,8]

1. The horizontal meridians are chosen for the location of the anterior sclerotomies for easier manipulation of the forceps, haptics, and sutures during the repositioning process.
2. The locations of the anterior sclerotomies determine the final position of the IOL. Previous anatomic studies have reported the ciliary sulcus to be between 0.46 mm to 0.8 mm from the limbus.[53] Thus the distance of 1 mm to 1.5 mm from the limbus places the anterior sclerotomies close to the external surface of the ciliary sulcus. Making the anterior sclerotomies at less than 1 mm from the limbus increases the risk of injuring the anterior chamber angle or the iris root.

The following steps are taken to ease the passage of the haptics through the anterior sclerotomies and reduce the chance of haptic breakage:

1. The anterior sclerotomies should have adequate size. If necessary, they may be widened before haptic reinternalization.
2. Fine nonangled positive action intraocular forceps are used for the haptic manipulation to give the surgeon the maximal "feel" and "control". Excessive pinching of the haptics is avoided during the passage of the haptics.

These measures may also be taken to prevent the decentering and tilting of the IOL:

1. The anterior sclerotomies are made at 180° from each other.
2. The sutures are tied at equal distance from the ends of both haptics.

A four-point-fixation option: To enhance more stability, two separate polypropylene sutures can be tied on each haptic, and the associated needles are anchored on the two "corners" of each anterior sclerotomy. This allows a stable configuration of four-point fixation of the IOL (Figure 26-8).

This repositioning technique combines the best features of the external and the internal approaches, while avoiding any intricate and cumbersome intraocular manipulations. With the easy placement of the anchoring sutures in an "opened" environment and the maintenance of the integrity of the globe in a "closed" environment, this technique allows a precise and secure fixation of the dislocated IOL in the ciliary sulcus on a consistent basis.[7-9]

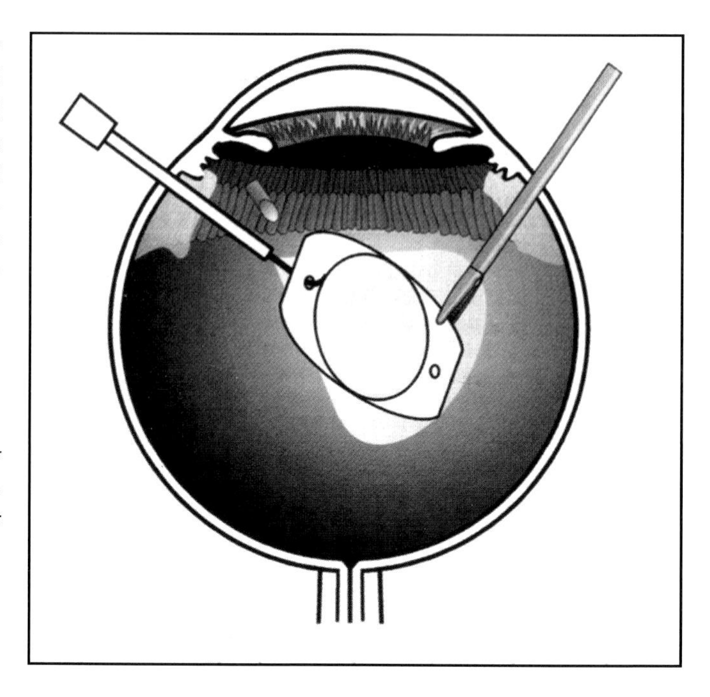

Figure 26-9. The slippery plate implant may be lifted on its edge or hooked through a positioning hole with a lighted pick, and then grasped with intraocular forceps for its repositioning or removal. (From Chan CK, Agarwal A, Agarwal S, Agarwal A. Management of dislocated intraocular implants. In: Nagpal PN, Fine IH, eds. *Ophthalmology Clinics of North America, Posterior Segment Complications of Cataract Surgery*. Philadelphia: W. B. Saunders; 2001: 681. Reprinted with permission.)

One-Piece Silicone Plate Intraocular Lens

An excellent method of removing a one-piece plate haptic IOL is the use of diamond-tipped forceps or manipulation with a lighted pick (Figure 26-9).

Conclusion

There are multiple surgical options for managing a malpositioned IOL. The surgeon must be familiar with the various techniques and be able to adopt the appropriate technique most suitable for the particular circumstance at hand.

Key Points

1. Disturbing visual symptoms such as diplopia, metamorphopsia, and hazy images are associated with a dislocated intraocular lens (IOL). If not properly managed, a malpositioned IOL may also induce sight-threatening ocular complications, including persistent cystoid macular edema, intraocular hemorrhage, retinal breaks, and retinal detachment.
2. Chandelier illumination combined with a panoramic viewing system and bimanual techniques vastly enhances the ease of removal or repositioning of the dislocated IOL.
3. One excellent method is the use of a diamond tipped forceps to hold the IOL and bring it anteriorly after vitrectomy.
4. Diamond-tipped forceps are valuable surgical tools to manipulate the malpositioned IOL for surgical corrections.
5. None of the suturing methods (including the temporary haptic externalization technique) work well for the one-piece silicone IOL with plate haptics.

References

1. Agarwal A, Agarwal S, Agarwal A. Phakonit: lens removal through a 0.9 mm incision. In: Agarwal A, ed. *Phacoemulsification, Laser Cataract Surgery and Foldable IOLs.* 1st ed. Delhi, India: Jaypee Brothers; 1998.
2. Agarwal A, Agarwal A, Agarwal S. No anesthesia cataract surgery. In: Agarwal A, ed. *Phacoemulsification, Laser Cataract Surgery and Foldable IOLs.* 2nd ed. Delhi, India: Jaypee Brothers; 2000.
3. Chang S. Perfluorocarbon liquids in vitreo-retinal surgery. *International Ophthalmology Clinics-New approaches to vitreo-retinal surgery.* 1992;32(2):153.
4. Maguire AM, Blumenkranz MS, Ward TG, Winkelman JZ. Scleral loop fixation for posteriorly dislocated intraocular lenses. Operative technique and long-term results. *Arch Ophthalmol.* 1991;109:1754.
5. Little BC, Rosen PH, Orr G, Aylward GW. Trans-scleral fixation of dislocated posterior chamber intraocular lenses using a 9–0 microsurgical polypropylene snare. *Eye.* 1993;7:740.
6. Chang S, Coll GE. Surgical techniques for repositioning a dislocated intraocular lens, repair of iridodialysis, and secondary intraocular lens implantation using innovative 25-gauge forceps. *Am J Ophthalmol.* 1995;119:165.
7. Chan CK. An improved technique for management of dislocated posterior chamber implants. *Ophthalmol.* 1992;99:51.
8. Chan CK, Agarwal A, Agarwal S, Agarwal A. Management of dislocated intraocular implants. In: Nagpal PN, Fine IH, eds. *Ophthalmology Clinics of North America, Posterior Segment Complications of Cataract Surgery.* Philadelphia: W. B. Saunders; 2001:681.
9. Thach AB, Dugel PU, Sipperley JO, et al. Outcome of sulcus fixation of dislocated PCIOLs using temporary externalization of the haptics. Paper presented at AAO Annual Meeting; 1998; New Orleans, La.
10. Schneiderman TE, Johnson MW, Smiddy WE, et al. Surgical management of posteriorly dislocated silicone plate haptic intraocular lenses. *Am J Ophthalmol.* 1997;123:629.
11. Johnson MW, Schneiderman TE. Surgical management of posteriorly dislocated silicone plate intraocular lenses. *Curr Opin Ophthalmol.* 1998;9:11.

12. Williams DF, Del Piero EJ, Ferrone PJ, et al. Management of complications in eyes containing two intraocular lenses. *Ophthalmol.* 1998;105:2017.
13. Wong KL, Grabow HB. Simplified technique to remove posteriorly dislocated lens implants. *Arch Ophthalmol.* 2001;119:273.
14. Lakshminarayanan K, Venkataraman M. *Physics*. Madras India: KCS Desikan & Co; 1992.
15. Leopold LB, Davis KS. Life Science Library Water. Time Life International BV; 1974, USA.
16. Lapp RE. Life Science Library Matter. Time Life International BV; 1974, USA.
17. Subramanyam N, Lal B. *A Textbook of B.Sc. Physics*. Delhi, India: S. Chand & Company Ltd; 1985.
18. Glaser BM, Carter JB, Kuppermann BD, Michels RG. Perfluoro-octane in the treatment of giant retinal tears with proliferative vitreo-retinopathy. *International Ophthalmology Clinics—New Approaches to Vitreo-retinal Surgery*. 1992;32(2):1–14.
19. Nabih M, Peyman GA, Clark Jr LC, et al. Experimental evaluation of perfluorophenanthrene as a high specific gravity vitreous substitute: A preliminary report. *Ophthalmic Surg.* 1989;20:286.
20. Blinder KJ, Peyman GA, Paris CL, et al. Vitreon, a new perfluorocarbon. *Br J Ophthalmol.* 1991;75:240.
21. Shapiro MJ, Resnick KI, Kim SH, Weinberg A. Management of the dislocated crystalline lens with a perfluorocarbon liquid. *Am J Ophthalmol.* 1991;112:401.
22. Liu K, Peyman GA, Chen M, Chang K. Use of high density vitreous substitute in the removal of posteriorly dislocated lenses or intraocular lenses. *Ophthalmic Surg.* 1991;22:503.
23. Lewis H, Blumenkranz MS, Chang S. Treatment of dislocated crystalline lens and retinal detachment with perfluorocarbon liquids. *Retina*. 1992;12:299.
24. Rowson NJ, Bacon AS, Rosen PH. Perfluorocarbon heavy liquids in the management of posterior dislocation of the lens nucleus during phakoemulsification. *Br J Ophthalmol.* 1992;176(3):169.
25. Greve MD, Peyman GA, Mehta NJ, Millsap CM. Use of perfluoroperhydrophenanthrene in the management of posteriorly dislocated crystalline and intraocular lenses. *Ophthalmic Surg.* 1993;24(9):593.
26. Lewis H, Sanchez G. The use of perfluorocarbon liquids in the repositioning of posteriorly dislocated intraocular lenses. *Ophthalmol.* 1993;100:1055.
27. Elizalde J. Combined use of perfluorocarbon liquids and viscoelastics for safer surgical approach to posterior lens luxation [poster]. The Vitreous Society 17th Annual Meeting; Sept 21–25, 1999; Rome, Italy.
28. Flynn HW Jr. Pars plana vitrectomy in the management of subluxated and posteriorly dislocated intraocular lenses. *Graefes Arch Clin Exp Ophthalmol.* 1987;225:169.
29. Flynn HW Jr., Buus D, Culbertson WW. Management of subluxated and posteriorly dislocated intraocular lenses using pars plana vitrectomy instrumentation. *J Cataract Refract Surg.* 1990;16:51.
30. Jacobi KW, Krey H. Surgical management of intraocular lens dislocation into the vitreous: case report. *J Am Intraocul Implant Soc.* 1983;9:58.
31. Mittra RA, Connor TB, Han DP, et al. Removal of dislocated intraocular lenses using pars plana vitrectomy with placement of an open-loop, flexible anterior chamber lens. *Ophthalmol.* 1998;105:1011.
32. McCannel MA. A retrievable suture idea for anterior uveal problems. *Ophthalmic Surg.* 1976;7(2):98.
33. Stark WJ, Bruner WE. Management of posteriorly dislocated intraocular lenses. *Ophthalmic Surg.* 1980;11:495.
34. Sternberg P Jr, Michels RG. Treatment of dislocated posterior chamber intraocular lenses. *Arch Ophthalmol.* 1986;104:1391.
35. Girard LJ. Pars plana phacoprosthesis (aphakic intraocular implant): a preliminary report. *Ophthalmic Surg.* 1981;12:19.

36. Girard LJ, Nino N, Wesson M, et al. Scleral fixation of a subluxated posterior chamber intraocular lens. *J Cataract Refract Surg*. 1988;14:326.
37. Smiddy WE. Dislocated posterior chamber intraocular lens. A new technique of management. *Arch Ophthalmol*. 1989;107:1678.
38. Campo RV, Chung KD, Oyakawa RT. Pars plana vitrectomy in the management of dislocated posterior chamber lenses. *Am J Ophthalmol*. 1989;108:529.
39. Anand R, Bowman RW. Simplified technique for suturing dislocated posterior chamber intraocular lens to the ciliary sulcus [letter]. *Arch Ophthalmol*. 1990;108:1205.
40. Stark WJ, Goodman G, Goodman D, Gottsch J. Posterior chamber intraocular lens implantation in the absence of posterior capsular support. *Ophthalmic Surg*. 1988;19:240.
41. Hu BV, Shin DH, Gibbs KA, Hong YJ. Implantation of posterior chamber lens in the absence of posterior capsular and zonular support. *Arch Ophthalmol*. 1988;106:416.
42. Shin DH, Hu BV, Hong YJ, Gibbs KA. Posterior chamber lens implantation in the absence of posterior capsular support [letter]. *Ophthalmic Surg*. 1988;19:606.
43. Dahan E. Implantation in the posterior chamber without capsular support. *J Cataract Refract Surg*. 1989;15:339.
44. Pannu JS. A new suturing technique for ciliary sulcus fixation in the absence of posterior capsule. *Ophthalmic Surg*. 1988;19:751.
45. Spigelman AV, Lindstrom RL, Nichols BD, et al. Implantation of a posterior chamber lens without capsular support during penetrating keratoplasty or as a secondary lens implant. *Ophthalmic Surg*. 1988;19:396.
46. Drews RC. Posterior chamber lens implantation during keratoplasty without posterior lens capsule support. *Cornea*. 1987;6:38.
47. Wong SK, Stark WJ, Gottsch SD, et al. Use of posterior chamber lenses in pseudophakic bullous keratopathy. *Arch Ophthalmol*. 1987;105:856.
48. Waring GO III, Stulting RD, Street D. Penetrating keratoplasty for pseudophakic corneal edema with exchange of intraocular lenses. *Arch Ophthalmol*. 1987;105:58.
49. Shin DH. Implantation of a posterior chamber lens without capsular support during penetrating keratoplasty or as a secondary lens [letter]. *Ophthalmic Surg*. 1988;19:755.
50. Lindstrom RL, Harris WS, Lyle WA. Secondary and exchange posterior chamber lens implantation. *J Am Intraocul Implant Soc*. 1982;8:353.
51. Bloom SM, Wyszynski RE, Brucker AJ. Scleral fixation suture for dislocated posterior chamber intraocular lens. *Ophthalmic Surg*. 1990;21:851.
52. Friedberg MA, Pilkerton AR. A new technique for repositioning and fixating a dislocated intraocular lens. *Arch Ophthalmol*. 1992;110:413.
53. Duffey RJ, Holland EJ, Agapitos PJ, Lindstrom RL. Anatomic study of transsclerally sutured intraocular lens implantation. *Am J Ophthalmol*. 1989;108:300.
54. Milauskas AT. Posterior capsule opacification after silicone lens implantation and its management. *J Cataract Refract Surg*. 1987;13:644.
55. Milauskas AT. Capsular bag fixation of one-piece silicone lenses. *J Cataract Refract Surg*. 1990;16:583.
56. Joo CK, Shin JA, Kim JH. Capsular opening contraction after continuous curvilinear capsulorrhexis and intraocular lens implantation. *J Cataract Refract Surg*. 1996;22:585–590.

The authors have no proprietary or financial interests in any commercial products mentioned in this chapter.

Please see Cliffhanger video on enclosed CD-ROM.

Chapter 27

INFECTIOUS ENDOPHTHALMITIS

Clement K. Chan, MD, FACS; Steven G. Lin, MD

INTRODUCTION

Despite numerous recent advances in its treatment, infectious endophthalmitis continues to be one of the most serious complications in ophthalmology. The infectious organism associated with endophthalmitis causes prominent ocular inflammation and toxic reaction, leading to severe intraocular tissue damages and the consequential marked visual loss. Infectious endophthalmitis can be broadly divided into five types: 1) acute or early-onset postoperative (usually after cataract extraction), 2) chronic or late-onset, 3) bleb-related, 4) post-traumatic, and 5) endogenous or metastatic.[1] The majority of endophthalmitis cases encountered by the practicing clinician consist of the first type: acute endophthalmitis after cataract extraction and intraocular lens (IOL) insertion[1] However, any ocular surgery, including the relatively "non-penetrating" ones (eg, strabismus, refractive procedures, transscleral fixation of a posterior chamber implant-PCIOL) may result in endophthalmitis.[1–10]

CLINICAL FEATURES

The preliminary diagnosis of acute postoperative bacterial endophthalmitis must be based on clinical grounds alone, so that the clinician may initiate prompt intervention in time for an optimal outcome.[8,11] The classic presentation of acute postoperative bacterial endophthalmitis includes a red and painful eye associated with frequent headaches and prominent visual loss during the second to the seventh day after surgery.[1,11] The rapidly progressive symptoms are accompanied by diffuse lid and corneal edema, conjunctival discharge, as well as anterior chamber and vitreous infiltrates.[1,11] The increasing intraocular proteinaceous infiltrates frequently result in the layering of a fibrin clot within the bottom of the anterior chamber, known as a hypopyon.[11] Invasion of the retina and optic nerve by the infecting organism invariably leads to progressive disc and retinal edema and hemorrhage, posterior fibrin deposits, as well as tissue necrosis. The eventual severe retinal destruction results in profound visual loss. The necrotic retina is also prone to develop retinal breaks and detachments during and subsequent to the course of the endophthalmitis.[12] Whether other clinical features are present or not, the cardinal sign and the only consistent and reliable indicator of postoperative endophthalmitis is unexplained vitreous inflammation and opacification.[8] In the Endophthalmitis Vitrectomy Study (EVS), pain was absent in 25% of cases and hypopyon was lacking in 14% of cases.[8,13] Typical clinical signs may also be masked and their onset delayed on account of postoperative antibiotic and corticosteroid usage, as well as the low virulence of the causative organism.[1,14,15]

Organisms Associated With Acute Postoperative Endophthalmitis

The most common microbial isolate from acute postoperative endophthalmitis is a gram-positive organism; specifically, a coagulase-negative *Staphylococcus.*[1,15–18] The EVS reported 70% of the isolates to be coagulase-negative micrococci (predominantly staphylococci).[18] Twenty-four point two (24.2%) of the isolates consisted of other gram-positive organisms as follow: 9.9% *Staphylococcus aureus,* 9.0% *Streptococcus* species, 2.2% *Enterococcus* species, and 3.1% miscellaneous gram-positive species (0.6% *Propionibacterium* species, 1.2% *Corynebacterium* species, 0.6% *Bacillus* species, and 0.6% *Diphtheroid.*)[18] Gram-negative organisms were isolated in 5.9% of the cases in the EVS (1.9% *Proteus mirabilis,* 1.2% *Pseudomonas* species, 0.6% *Morganella morganii,* 0.6% *Citrobacter diversus,* 0.3% *Serratia marcescens,* 0.6% *Enterobacter* species, and 0.3% *Flavobacterium* species.)[18-50] It is possible that the EVS may have underestimated the rate of gram-negative infection for postoperative endophthalmitis by excluding eyes with corneal opacities severe enough to preclude a vitrectomy.[8] Table 27-1 outlines a typical spectrum of microbial isolates associated with acute postoperative endophthalmitis (reported in the EVS), as well as distinctive spectra of microbial isolates associated with other types of endophthalmitis.[1,6,16-18,36,41–46,49]

Delayed-Onset Endophthalmitis

Chronic or late-onset endophthalmitis is defined as the presentation of indolent intraocular inflammation one or more months after ocular surgery. Traditionally, fungal endophthalmitis has often been cited as an example of late-onset endophthalmitis.[1,11,19] However, recent reports have also implicated other organisms associated with this category of endophthalmitis.[20–27] In their review of 19 cases of delayed-onset pseudophakic endophthalmitis, Fox and associates reported 63% of those cases to be due to *Propionibacterium acnes,* 16% to *Candida parapsilosis,* 16% to *Staphylococcus epidermidis,* and 5% to *Corynebacterium* species.[26] Ficker et al isolated *Staphylococcus epidermidis* and *Achromobacter* species from eyes with chronic bacterial endophthalmitis.[27]

Propionibacterium Endophthalmitis

In 1986, Meister and associates described the syndrome of *Propionibacterium acnes* endophthalmitis with delayed onset after extracapsular cataract extraction (ECCE) with posterior chamber intraocular lens (PCIOL) implantation.[20] *Propionibacterium* is a gram-positive, nonspore-forming, pleomorphic and anaerobic bacillus. It is ubiquitous in nature and a common component of the bacterial flora of the ocular and periocular tissues, including the conjunctiva and the sebaceous follicles.[20,32] It is an opportunistic pathogen frequently associated with a low-grade, delayed-onset, and persistent endophthalmitis after cataract extraction with an intraocular implant.[20–26] The typical clinical presentation may include

Table 27-1.

Protocol for Intravitreal Antibiotic Preparation

***Vancomycin Hydrochloride:* 1 mg in 0.1 ml**

1. Add 10 ml of diluent to 500-mg powder in vial, resulting in 50 mg/ml concentration.
2. Insert 2 ml (100 mg) or reconstituted drug into 10-ml sterile empty vial, and add 8 ml of diluent, resulting in a final solution of **10 mg/ml.***

Ceftazidime Hydrochloride: 2.25 mg in 0.1 ml

1. Add 10 ml of diluent to 500-mg powder in vial to result in 50 mg/ml concentration.
2. Insert 1 ml (50 mg) of reconstituted drug into a 10-ml sterile empty vial, and mix with 1.2 ml of diluent, for a final solution of **22.5 mg/ml.***

Cefazolin sodium: 2.25 mg in 0.1 ml

1. Add 2 ml of diluent to 500-mg powder in vial to result in concentration of 225 mg/ml.
2. Insert 1 ml (22.5 mg) of reconstituted drug into a 10-ml sterile empty vial, and mix with additional 9 ml of diluent, for a final solution of **22.5 mg/ ml.***

Amikacin sulfate: 0.2 to 0.4 mg in 0.1 ml

1. Original vial contains 500 mg in 2 ml (250 mg/ml) solution.
2. Add 0.8 ml (200 mg) solution into a 10-ml sterile empty vial, and mix with additional 9.2 ml of diluent, to achieve a concentration of 200 mg in 10 ml (20mg/ml).
3. Withdraw 0.2 ml (4 mg) and mix with 0.8 ml of diluent in a second sterile empty vial to achieve final solution of **0.4 mg/ml*;** or withdraw 0.1 ml (2 mg) and mix with 0.9 ml of diluent to achieve a final solution of **0.2 mg/ml.***

Gentamicin sulfate: 0.1 to 0.2 mg in 0.1 ml

1. Original vial contains 80 mg in 2 ml (40 mg/ml) solution.
2. Add 0.1 ml (4 mg) solution into a 10-ml sterile empty vial, and mix with 3.9 ml of diluent to achieve a solution of 4 mg in 4 ml or **1mg/1ml *;** or add 0.2 ml (8 mg) solution into a 10-ml sterile empty vial, and mix with 3.9 ml of diluent to achieve a solution of 8 mg in 4 ml or **2 mg/1 ml***

Clindamycin phosphate: 1 mg in 0.1 ml

1. Original vial contains a 600 mg in 4 ml solution (15 0 mg/1 ml)
2. Add 0.2 ml (30 mg) solution into a 10-ml sterile empty vial and mix with 2.8 ml of diluent to achieve a solution of 30 mg in 3 ml or **10 mg/ml.***

Chloramphenicol sodium succinate: 2 mg in 0.1 ml

1. Original vial contains 1000-mg powder.
2. Add 10 ml of diluent to reconstitute 1000-mg powder for a concentration of 100 mg /ml.
3. Withdraw 1 ml of reconstituted drug (100 mg) and mix with 4 ml of diluent in a 10-ml sterile empty vial to achieve a final solution of **20 mg/1ml.***

continued

Table 27-1, continued.

Protocol for Intravitreal Antibiotic Preparation

***Amphotericin B*: 0.005 mg in 0.1 ml**

1. Original vial contains 50-mg powder.
2. Add 10 ml of diluent to reconstitute the 50-mg powder into a concentration of 5 mg/ml.
3. Add 0.1 ml (0.5 mg) of reconstituted solution into a 10-ml sterile empty vial, and mix with 9.9 ml of diluent to achieve a final solution of **0.05 mg/ 1ml.***

***Miconazole*: 0.025 mg in 0.1 ml**

1. Original ampule contains 20 ml of 10 mg/ml solution.
2. Remove glass particles and impurities by passing solution into a 5-mm filter needle.
3. Add 0.25 ml (2.5 mg) of filtered solution into a 10-ml sterile empty vial, and mix with 9.75 ml of diluent to achieve a final solution of 2.5 mg in 10 ml or **0.25 mg/1 ml.***

Recommendation: For optimal results, the drug dilution and preparation should be performed by trained personnel in the controlled environment of a hospital pharmacy.[1,51] Nonbacteriostatic sterile water is used as diluent for Vancomycin and Amphotericin B. For all others, nonbacteriostatic sterile water or 0.9 % sodium chloride solution is used as diluent.[1,108]

* For all medications, the volume from the final solution for intravitreal injection is 0.1 ml drawn into a tuberculin syringe and delivered with a 27-or 30-gauge needle at the pars plana.[1,52]

an indolent course of chronic low-grade iridocyclitis with one or more of the following signs: large white granulomatous or nongranulomatous keratic precipitates, hypopyon, beaded fibrin strands in the anterior chamber, vitritis, intraretinal hemorrhages and infiltrates, and a prominent whitish plaque on the residual lens capsule.[20–26] The last feature is considered to be a hallmark sign of *P. acnes* endophthalmitis.[25,32] Previous biopsies of lens capsules with the whitish exudates have yielded *P. acnes* on histological studies and cultures, proving that they contain foci of sequestered *P. acnes* organisms.[21–25,32] The delayed activation and proliferation of the sequestered organisms result in a chronic and indolent course of endophthalmitis. Since *P. acnes* is a low virulent and fastidious bacillus, it is difficult to isolate and grow in culture.[20] Specimens of suspected cases of *P. acnes* endophthalmitis should be promptly inoculated into anaerobic media. *P. acnes* may not appear in culture until 5 days or more after inoculation.[20] It has been pointed out that the *P. acnes* organisms isolated from eyes with acute postoperative endophthalmitis may constitute a less resilient form than those from eyes with the delayed-onset or chronic type of endophthalmitis.[33] Unlike the chronic *P. acnes* infection, the acute type is usually easily eradicated with intravitreal antibiotic injections alone and has a low recurrence rate.[1,33] In contrast, the chronic *P. acnes* endophthalmitis frequently requires a vitrectomy and capsulectomy to eliminate the sequestered organisms.[20,25,32]

Diagnostic Workup and Microbiological Studies

When managing an eye with suspected endophthalmitis, the clinician must first perform a careful evaluation. It is important to pay close attention to certain ocular features that may modify the course and influence the management of the infection: eg, wound leak and dehiscence, iris and vitreous prolapse, flat anterior chamber, corneal and suture abscess, bleb defects, eroding scleral suture associated with a sutured posterior chamber implant, etc.[1,8] A successful outcome entails the correction of the above abnormalities besides effective antimicrobial therapy. One must also differentiate endophthalmitis from other conditions with similar clinical features, such as a corneal ulcer and aseptic anterior uveitis with a hypopyon, and vitreous infiltration due to sterile posterior uveitis or retained lens fragments, phacoanaphylactic uveitis, etc. In addition, a search for concomitant conditions that may complicate the course of the endophthalmitis is an important part of the workup, eg, superimposed retinal breaks or detachment, choroidal detachment, located lens fragments, and intraocular foreign body, etc. Ancillary diagnostic tools such as ultrasonography may contribute to the diagnostic workup.[1,8]

Techniques of Specimen Collection

Aqueous and vitreous specimens may be obtained in an office setting or at the time of a vitrectomy. In the former situation, careful administration of local anesthesia (topical, subconjunctival, peribulbar, or retrobulbar) and sterile prepping with 5% povidone-iodine solution are recommended.[1,8,13,53] A small volume of aqueous specimen (0.1 to 0.2 ml) is then carefully withdrawn via a 27- or 30-gauge needle at the limbus into a tuberculin syringe. The vitreous specimen may be obtained with one of the following two methods:[8,13,53]

Needle Tap

A 22- to 27-gauge needle attached to a tuberculin syringe is inserted through the pars plana into the vitreous cavity for gentle aspiration of 0.1 to 0.3 ml of liquid vitreous. Excessive force must be avoided to prevent vitreoretinal traction. A "dry tap" requires the conversion to a mechanized biopsy.

Mechanized Vitreous Biopsy

A one-, two-, or three-port pars plana vitrectomy with a mechanized 20-gauge vitrectomy probe is employed for the biopsy. A small volume of undiluted specimen (up to 0.3 ml) from the anterior vitreous is collected into a sterile syringe connected to the aspiration line of the vitrectomy probe through gentle manual suction by a surgical assistant during the vitrectomy. Diluted specimens collected into a larger syringe or into a vitrectomy cassette may also be concentrated either with the suction filtered technique or the centrifuged method (Figure 27-1).[1,8,54,55] The former involves passing the diluted specimens in an upper sterile chamber through a membrane filter with 0.45-micron pores into a lower chamber connected to suction. With the aid of sterile forceps and scissors or knives, the membrane filter containing the concentrated specimens is then cut into small pieces for direct inoculation on solid and into liquid media for cultures (see Figure 27-1).[1,54] Concentrated specimens scraped off the surface of the membrane filter are also applied on slides for preparation of various stains. The alternative centrifuged method requires the transfer of the diluted specimens into a sterile centrifuge tube for high-speed centrifuge. The sediments from the cen-

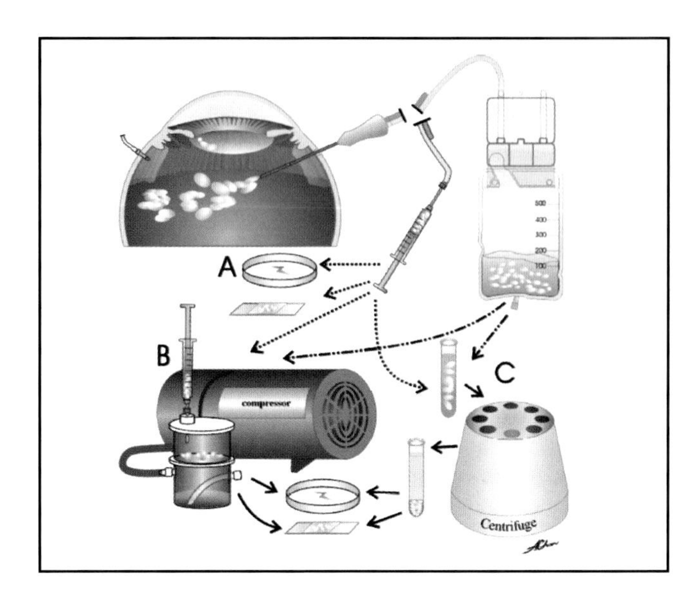

Figure 27-1. Methods of collecting specimens. **A**. Undiluted aqueous and vitreous specimens may be directly inoculated onto culture media and used for smear preparation; **B**. Diluted vitreous specimen collected into a syringe or a cassette is either first concentrated by vacuuming the diluted fluid in a sterile upper chamber through a 0.45-mm membrane filter into a lower sterile chamber (suction filter method); **C**. concentrated in a sterile centrifuge tube after performing high-speed centrifuge (centrifuge method). Small cut segments of the membrane filter with the concentrated specimens or the sediments from the centrifuged tube are innoculated into culture media and applied on slides for smear preparation.

trifuged tube are then processed for microbiological stains and cultures (Figure 27-1). In 1993, Donahue and associates reported a significant increase in positive yield with culturing the contents of a vitrectomy cassette after concentration of the specimen in comparison to culturing the specimen from a needle tap or a limited mechanized vitreous biopsy (76% versus 43%).[55] In the EVS, some degree of culture growth was achieved from 82.8% of the tested vitrectomy cassette specimens, and the vitrectomy cassette fluid was the only source of a positive culture for 8.9% of eyes.[53] The EVS found that the vitrectomy cassette specimen had prognostic significance equivalent to growth from other intraocular sources.[56]

Treatment of Endophthalmitis

The two fundamental therapeutic modalities for treating infectious endophthalmitis in the modern world comprise of antimicrobial therapy and vitrectomy. When appropriate, they may be supplemented with anti-inflammatory therapy for reducing damages induced by the infection. Applying effective strategies for antimicrobial therapy constitutes the most critical aspect of the management of endophthalmitis.

ANTIMICROBIAL THERAPY

Topical and Subconjunctival

PROPHYLACTIC THERAPY

Multiple studies have demonstrated that preoperative application of antiseptics and antibiotics with a broad-spectrum antimicrobial coverage reduces the eyelid and conjunctival bacterial counts, resulting in decreased potential for postoperative endophthalmitis.[57–60] Apt and associates reported that a single preoperative application of half-strength (5%) povidone-iodine solution in the conjunctival cul-de-sac was equivalent to a 3-day course of prophylactic topical combination solution of neomycin sulfate, polymyxin B sulfate, and gramicidin in reducing the bacterial colonies.[57–59]

THERAPY AFTER THE ONSET OF ENDOPHTHALMITIS

With the exception of mild infections, topical and subconjunctival drug delivery usually constitutes only adjunctive antimicrobial therapy after the onset of endophthalmitis. However, they are essential for certain conditions that may accompany the endophthalmitis (ie, bleb infection, corneal ulcer, wound or suture abscess, etc.)[1,8] A typical regimen of supplemental topical therapy for acute postoperative bacterial endophthalmitis includes frequent application of antibiotics with appropriate antibacterial coverage, as well as repeated administration of anti-inflammatory and cycloplegic drugs. Steroid is avoided for fungal cases. The use of customized fortified doses of topical antimicrobial drugs (eg, 45 to 50 mg per ml of vancomycin, 50 mg per ml of cefazolin, cefamandole or ceftazidime, 50 mg per ml of ampicillin, 50 mg per ml of clindamycin, 1% solution of methicillin, 8 to 15 mg per ml of tobramycin, 10 to 20 mg per ml of gentamicin or amikacin, 0.15 to 0.5% of amphotericin B, or 10 mg per ml of miconazole, etc.) has been a common practice in the course of treating the endophthalmitis.[8,13] However, the potential benefit of the fortified doses over the regular doses remains controversial and unproven. Another common practice is supplemental subconjunctival therapy (eg, 25 mg of vancomycin, 100 to 125 mg of cefazolin, or ceftazidime, 75 mg of cefamandole, 100 mg of ampicillin or methicillin, 20 to 40 mg of gentamicin, tobramycin or amikacin, 30 mg of clindamycin, or 5 mg of miconazole.)[1,8,13] The degree of synergy between subconjunctival and intravitreal antimicrobial therapy is unknown.

Intravitreal Antimicrobial Therapy

For all categories of endophthalmitis besides the endogenous type, the mainstay of therapy is prompt and direct intravitreal injections of antimicrobial drugs.[1,8] It is imperative that the intravitreal antimicrobial therapy first provides comprehensive coverage for the gram-positive organisms, since they constitute the majority of the microbial isolates associated with endophthalmitis (94% in the EVS).[1,8,18]

The following antibiotic combinations are the current recommended initial empiric intravitreal antibiotic regimens for acute postoperative bacterial endophthalmitis in a clinical setting:[1,8,13]

1. Vancomycin 1.0 mg/ 0.1 ml and ceftazidime 2.25 mg/ 0.1 ml, or
2. Vancomycin 1.0 mg/ 0.1 ml and amikacin (100 to 400 micrograms/ 0.1 ml) for beta-lactam sensitive patients.

Table 27-1 provides detailed protocol for the preparation and dosages of commonly used intraocular drugs for endophthalmitis.

Systemic Antimicrobial Therapy

Although the EVS found systemic antimicrobial therapy provide no additional benefit to intravitreal therapy for acute postoperative endophthalmitis, its role for other types of endophthalmitis is more important.[13,61] Concomitant intravitreal and systemic antibiotic therapy besides vitrectomy remains to be the standard of care (based on clinical experience but without experimental support) for most bleb-related and trauma-induced endophthalmitis.[34,36,41,61] For endogenous endophthalmitis, appropriate systemic (especially intravenous) therapy with maximal doses for intravitreal penetration is the key for a successful outcome.[49,61] Intravenous antibiotic therapy is generally required for two weeks for most endogenous cases, and as long as four or more weeks for endocarditis cases.[50]

Corticosteroid Therapy

The use of intravitreal corticosteroids for non-fungal endophthalmitis remains controversial due to a lack of randomized controlled studies.[8,62] The potential benefits of corticosteroid therapy for endophthalmitis include inhibition of macrophage and neutrophil migration, stabilization of lysosomal membranes resulting in decreased degranulation of inflammatory cells (neutrophils, mast cells, macrophages, basophils), and reduction in prostaglandin synthesis and capillary permeability due to inhibition of phospholipase A_2.[62] However, its potential harmful effects and limitations include possible reduction in the killing power of inflammatory cells, changes in the bioavailability and doses of the intravitreal antibiotics, potentiation of the infection in the absence of appropriate antibiotic therapy, risk of retinal toxicity due to medication errors, and inability to counteract bacterial toxin-induced damages.[62] The standard clinical dose of intravitreal dexamethasone is 400 micrograms per 0.1 ml, although the optimal dose has not been determined.[1,8,63,64] Besides intravitreal injections, other routes of steroid therapy include subconjunctival injections (4 to 12 mg of dexamethasone or 40 mg of triamcinolone or depomedrol) and systemic therapy (1 mg/kg/day for 5 days followed by rapid tapering).[8,13,62] When fungal endophthalmitis is suspected, most authorities advocate the avoidance of corticosteroid.

Vitrectomy

Indications for Vitrectomy

The theoretical advantages of vitrectomy include the removal of infectious organisms with their toxins and inflammatory mediators, clearing of vitreous opacities and sequestered abscess pockets, collection of abundant specimens for cultures, elimination of vitreous membranes to avoid vitreoretinal traction, allowing increased space for intraocular drug administration, and possible improved diffusion of intravitreal antibiotics.[1,13] For chronic endophthalmitis due to the *Propionibacterium* species, intravitreal antibiotics alone may not be sufficient. Frequently, a vitrectomy combined with a partial or complete removal of the lens capsule with sequestered organisms (sometimes including the implant), is required for a successful outcome.[20,23,25,26,32]

Vitrectomy Techniques

A three-port pars plana vitrectomy using standard 20-gauge instruments and concentrating on the "core" vitreous is usually recommended, although a one- or two-port approach may be sufficient for a limited vitreous biopsy.[8] A portable battery-driven 23-gauge vitrector is also commercially available for a limited vitreous biopsy.[8] The greater

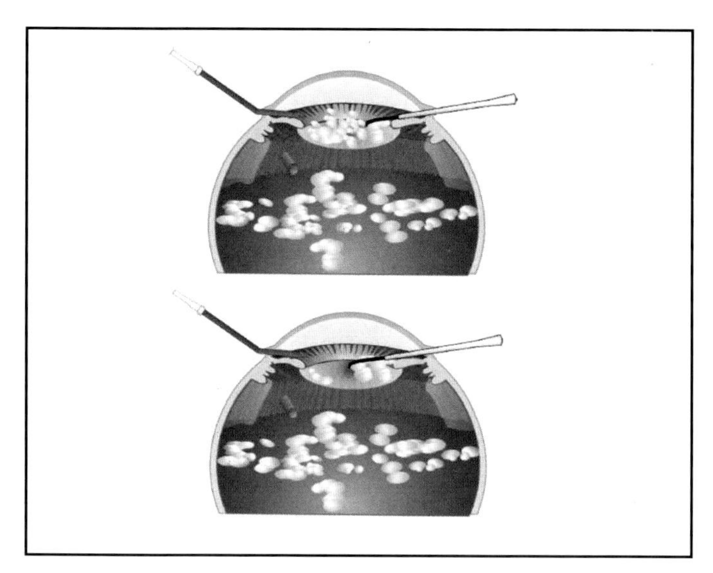

Figure 27-2. Anterior chamber washout before vitrectomy. The technique of eliminating cloudy fibrin deposits, membranes, and hyphema from the anterior chamber is illustrated. A microsurgical hook or pick inserted at the limbus is used to scrape off the cloudy material from the IOL and iris surface before removing them with a vitrectomy probe from the anterior chamber. A separate probe also inserted at the limbus for anterior chamber infusion is often necessary to prevent chamber collapse. The posterior infusion fluid is not turned on until adequate media clarity is achieved to ascertain the proper location of the tip of the posterior infusion cannula.

potential for surgical complications associated with increased tissue vulnerability induced by the endophthalmitis requires the surgeon to be well versed with vitreoretinal techniques and vigilant throughout the vitrectomy. The use of a long infusion cannula (eg, 6 mm) is often advantageous in preventing subretinal and choroidal infusion for pseudophakic eyes and post-traumatic eyes requiring a lensectomy, in light of multiple predisposing factors for such a complication with endophthalmitis (eg, limited intraocular tissue visibility, increased choroidal congestion, frequent hypotony, etc.) To further avoid such a complication, the surgeon must ensure that the tip of the infusion cannula is well within the vitreous cavity before turning on the infusion fluid. For a case with very cloudy media, the surgeon may confirm this by gently rubbing the tip of a microvitreoretinal blade inserted through one of the superior sclerotomies against the tip of the infusion cannula. Frequently, a separate anterior chamber washout via a limbal approach is required to eliminate cloudy fibrin deposits and hyphema from the anterior chamber initially, before sufficient anterior media clarity is attained for a pars plana vitrectomy. Various microsurgical hooks and picks may be inserted through the limbus to scrape off the anterior chamber infiltrates or membranes layered on the surface of the implant and the iris before removing them with a vitrectomy probe from the anterior chamber (Figure 27-2). A separate anterior infusion line may be required during the anterior chamber washout to prevent chamber collapse. When performing a core vitrectomy, care must be taken to apply only gentle intraocular movements and avoid vigorous surgical maneuvers that may induce vitreoretinal traction, such as aggressive epiretinal membrane retrieval and fibrin clean up. Despite the intentional avoidance of their direct removal during the vitrectomy, the posterior epiretinal fibrin deposits and dense retinal hemorrhages tend to gradually dissolve following the injections of intravitreal antimicrobial and anti-inflammatory medications after surgery. Keeping the intraocular instruments well within the anterior and central vitreous cavity and staying away from the fragile infected retina during surgery, will reduce the chance of retinal complications. Vitreous specimen for microbial investigation is either collected into a syringe connected to the aspiration line of the vitrectomy probe or into a cassette of the vitrectomy machine (see Figure 27-1).[8] Finally, the eye is made sufficiently soft to allow space for injections of medications and the sclerotomies are closed tightly to avoid fluid leaks, before the administration of intravitreal drugs at the end of the surgery.

TASS

Toxic Anterior Segment Syndrome (TASS) is being more widely reported after first being recognized as a specific entity in 1992 (Monson et al.). The classic features of TASS are early and intense postoperative inflammation after anterior segment surgery without vitreal involvement. Frequent topical steroids every 30 to 60 minutes are usually effective, with improvement within the first 24 to 48 hours. Vitritis is almost never associated with TASS and indicates infectious endophthalmitis.

Key Points

1. The infectious organism associated with endophthalmitis causes prominent ocular inflammation and toxic reaction, leading to severe intraocular tissue damages and the consequential marked visual loss.
2. The classic presentation of acute postoperative bacterial endophthalmitis includes a red and painful eye associated with frequent headaches and prominent visual loss during the second to the seventh day after surgery.
3. Chronic or late-onset endophthalmitis is defined as the presentation of indolent intraocular inflammation one or more months after ocular surgery.
4. Propionibacterium is a gram-positive, nonspore-forming, pleomorphic and anaerobic bacillus. It is ubiquitous in nature and a common component of the bacterial flora of the ocular and periocular tissues, including the conjunctiva and the sebaceous follicles.
5. Aqueous and vitreous specimens may be obtained in an office setting or at the time of a vitrectomy.
6. The two fundamental therapeutic modalities for treating infectious endophthalmitis in the modern world comprise of antimicrobial therapy and vitrectomy.

References

1. Forster RK. Endophthalmitis. In: Tasman W, Jaeger EA, eds. *Duane's Clinical Ophthalmology*. Vol 4. Philadelphia, PA: Lippincott-Raven; 1996:1-29.
2. Heilskov T, Joondeph BC, Olsen KR, et al. Case report: late endophthalmitis after transscleral fixation of a posterior chamber intraocular lens. *Arch Ophthalmol.* 1989;107:1427.
3. Christy NE, Lall P. Postoperative endophthalmitis following cataract surgery. *Arch Ophthalmol.* 1973;90:361–366.
4. Kattan HM, Flynn HW Jr, Pflugfelder S, et al. Nosocomial endophthalmitis survey. *Ophthalmology.* 1991;98:227–238.

5. Leveille AS, McMullan FD, Cavanagh HD. Endophthalmitis following penetrating keratoplasty. *Ophthalmology.* 1983;90:38–39.
6. Brinton GS, Topping TM, Hyndiuk RA, et al. Posttraumatic endophthalmitis. *Arch Ophthalmol.* 1984;102:547–550.
7. Boldt HC, Pulido JS, Blodi CF, et al. Rural endophthalmitis. *Ophthalmology.* 1989;96:1722–1726.
8. Han DP. Acute-onset postoperative endophthalmitis: current recommendations. In syllabus: Subspecialty Day 1998. Retina: management of posterior segment complications of anterior segment surgery.
9. Starr MB. Prophylactic antibiotics for ophthalmic surgery. *Surv Ophthalmol.* 1983;27:353–373.
10. Javitt JC, Vitale S, Canner JK, et al. National outcomes of cataract extraction. *Arch Ophthalmol.* 1991;109:1085–1089.
11. Wilson FM, Wilson II FM. Postoperataive uveitis. In: Tasman W, Jaeger EA, eds. *Duane's Clinical Ophthalmology*. Vol 4. Philadelphia, PA: Lippincott-Raven; 1996.
12. Nelson PT, Marcus DA, Bovino JA. Retinal detachment following endophthalmitis. *Ophthalmology.* 1985;92:1112–1117.
13. Endophthalmitis Vitrectomy Study Group. Results of the Endophthalmitis Vitrectomy Study. A randomized trial of immediate vitrectomy and intravenous antibiotics for the treatment of postoperative bacterial endophthalmitis. *Arch Ophthalmol.* 1995;113:1479–1496.
14. Bode DD, Gelender H, Forster RK. A retrospective review of endophthalmitis due to coagulase-negative *staphylococci. Br J Ophthalmol.* 1985;69:915–919.
15. Ormerod LD, Ho DD, Becker LE, et al. Endophthalmitis caused by the coagulase-negative *staphylococci*: I. Disease spectrum and outcome. *Ophthalmology.* 1993;100:715–723.
16. Forster RK, Abbott RL, Gelender H. Management of infectious endophthalmitis. *Ophthalmology.* 1980;87:313–319.
17. Puliafito CA, Baker AS, Haaf J, et al. Infectious endophthalmitis. *Ophthalmology.* 1982;89: 921–929.
18. Han DP, Wisniewski SR, Wilson LA, et al. Spectrum and susceptibilities of microbiologic isolates in the Endophthalmitis Vitrectomy Study. *Am J Ophthalmol.* 1996;112:1–17.
19. Theodore FH. Symposium: Postoperative endophthalmitis: etiology and diagnosis of fungal postoperative endophthalmitis. *Ophthalmology.* 1978;85:327–340.
20. Meisler DM, Palestine AG, Vastine DW, et al. Chronic Propionibacterium endophthalmitis after cataract extraction and intraocular lens implantation. *Am J Ophthalmol.* 1986;102:733–739.
21. Jaffe GJ, Whitcher JP, Biswell R, et al. Propionibacterium acnes endophthalmitis seven months after extracapsular cataract extraction and intraocular lens implantation. *Ophthalmic Surg.* 1986;17:791–793.
22. Roussel TJ, Culbertson WW, Jaffe NS. Chronic postoperative endophthalmitis associated with Propionibacterium acnes. *Arch Ophthalmol.* 1987;105:1199–1201.
23. Meisler DM, Zakov ZN, Bruner WE, et al. Endophthalmitis associated with sequestered intraocular Propionibacterium acnes [letter]. *Am J Ophthalmol.* 1987;104:428–429.
24. Brady SE, Cohen EJ, Fischer DH. Diagnosis and treatment of chronic postoperative bacterial endophthalmitis. *Ophthalmic Surg.* 1988;19:580–584.
25. Meisler DM, Mandelbaum S. Propionibacterium-associated endophthalmitis after extracapsular cataract extraction. Review of reported cases. *Ophthalmology.* 1989;96:54–61.
26. Fox GM, Joondeph BC, Flynn HW Jr, et al. Delayed-onset pseudophakic endophthalmitis. *Am J Ophthalmol.* 1991;111:163–173.
27. Ficker L, Meredith TA, Wilson LA, et al. Chronic bacterial endophthalmitis. *Am J Ophthalmol.* 1987;103:745–748.
28. Roussel TJ, Olson ER, Rice T, et al. Chronic postoperative endophthalmitis associated with Actinomyces species. *Arch Ophthalmol.* 1991;109;60–62.

29. Zimmerman PL, Mamalis N, Alder JB, et al. Chronic Nocardia asteroides endophthalmitis after extracapsular cataract extraction. *Arch Ophthalmol.* 1993;111:837–840.
30. Pettit TH, Olson RJ, Foos RY, et al. Fungal endophthalmitis following intraocular lens implantation. *Arch Ophthalmol.* 1980;98:1025–1039.
31. Stern WH, Tamura E, Jacobs RA, et al. Epidemic post-surgical Candida parapsilosis endophthalmitis. *Ophthalmology.* 1985;92:1701–1709.
32. Zambrano W, Flynn HW Jr, Pflugfelder SC, et al. Management options for Propionibacterium acnes endophthalmitis. *Ophthalmology.* 1989;96:1100–1105.
33. Winward KE, Pflugfelder SC, Flynn HW Jr, et al. Postoperative Propionibacterium endophthalmitis. *Ophthalmology.* 1993;100:447–451.
34. Ciulla TA, Beck AD, Topping TM, et al. Blebitis, early endophthalmitis, and late endophthalmitis after glaucoma-filtering surgery. *Ophthalmology.* 1997;104:986–995.
35. Brown RH, Yang LH, Walker SD, et al. Treatment of bleb infection after glaucoma surgery. *Arch Ophthalmol.* 1994;112:57–61.
36. Mandelbaum S, Forster RK, Gelender H, et al. Late onset endophthalmitis associated with filtering blebs. *Ophthalmology.* 1985;92:964–972.
37. Parrish R, Minckler D. Late endophthalmitis-Filtering surgery time bomb? [editorial]. *Ophthalmology*. 1996;103:1167–1168.
38. Wolner B, Liebermann JM, Sassan JW, et al. Late bleb-related endophthalmitis after trabeculectomy with adjunctive 5-fluorouracil. *Ophthalmology.* 1991;98:1053–1060.
39. Higginbotham EJ, Stevens RK, Musch D, et al. Bleb-related endophthalmitis after trabeculectomy with mitomycin C. *Ophthalmology.* 1996;103:650–656.
40. Jett BD, Jensen HG, Atkuri RV, et al. Evaluation of therapeutic measures for treating endophthalmitis caused by isogenic toxin producing and toxin- nonproducing Enterococcus faecalis strains. *Invest Ophthalmol Vis Sci.* 1995;36:9–15.
41. Parrish CM, O'Day D. Traumatic endophthalmitis. *Int Ophthalmol Clin.* 1987;27:112–119.
42. Bohigan GM, Olk RJ. Factors associated with a poor visual result in endophthalmitis. *Am J Ophthalmol.* 1986;101:332–334.
43. Schemmer GB, Driebe WT. Posttraumatic Bacillus cereus endophthalmitis. *Arch Ophthalmol.* 1987;105:342–344.
44. Rowsey JJ, Newsom DL, Sexton DJ, et al. Endophthalmitis: current approaches. *Ophthalmology.* 1982;89:1055–1066.
45. Affeldt JC, Flynn HW, Forster RK, et al. Microbial endophthalmitis resulting from ocular trauma. *Ophthalmology.* 1987;94:407–413.
46. Peyman GA, Raichand M, Bennett TO, et al. Management of endophthalmitis with pars plana vitrectomy. *Br J Ophthalmol.* 1980;64:472–475.
47. O'Day, Smith RS, Gregg CR. The problem of Bacillus species infection with special emphasis on the virulence of Bacillus cereus. *Ophthalmology.* 1981;88:833–838.
48. Bouza E, Grant S, Jordan MC, et al. Bacillus cereus endogenous panophthalmitis. *Arch Ophthalmol.* 1979;97:498–499.
49. Greenwald MJ, Wohl LG, Sell CH. Metastatic bacterial endophthalmitis: a contemporary reappraisal. *Surv Ophthalmol.* 1986;31:81–101.
50. Okada AA, Johnson P, Liles C, et al. Endogenous bacterial endophthalmitis. *Ophthalmology.* 1994;101:832–838.
51. Jeglum EL, Rosenberg SB, Benson WE. Preparation of intravitreal drug doses. *Ophthalmic Surg.* 1981;12:355–359.
52. Bohigan GM. Intravitreal antibiotic preparation. In: *External Diseases of the Eye.* Fort Worth, TX: Alcon Laboratories; 1980:64-67.

53. Barza M, Pavan PR, Doft BH, et al. Evaluation of microbiological diagnostic techniques in postoperative endophthalmitis in the Endophthalmitis Vitrectomy Study. *Arch Ophthalmol.* 1997;115:1142–1150.
54. Forster RK. Symposium: Postoperative endophthalmitis: etiology and diagnosis of bacterial postoperative endophthalmitis. *Ophthalmology.* 1978;85:320–326.
55. Donahue SP, Kowalski RP, Jewar BH, et al. Vitreous cultures in suspected endophthalmitis: Biopsy or vitrectomy? *Ophthalmology.* 1993;100:452–455.
56. Endophthalmitis Vitrectomy Study Group. Microbiologic factors and visual outcome in the Endophthalmitis Vitrectomy Study. *Am J Ophthalmol.* 1996;122–830–846.
57. Isenberg SJ, Apt L, Yoshimori R, et al. Chemical preparation of the eye in ophthalmic surgery. IV. Comparison of povidone-iodine on the conjunctiva with a prophylactic antibiotic. *Arch Ophthalmol.* 1985;103:1340–1342.
58. Apt L, Isenberg S, Yoshimori R, et al. Chemical preparation of the eye in ophthalmic surgery III. Effect of povidone-iodine on the conjunctiva. *Arch Ophthalmol.* 1984;102:728–729.
59. Apt L, Isenberg SJ, Yoshimori R, et al. Outpatient topical use of povidone-iodine in preparing the eye for surgery. *Ophthalmology.* 1989;96:289–292.
60. Speaker MG, Menikoff JA. Prophylaxis of endophthalmitis with topical povidone-iodine. *Ophthalmology.* 1991;98:1769–1775.
61. Sternberg P Jr, Martin DF. Management of endophthalmitis in the post-Endophthalmitis Vitrectomy Study era. [editorial]. *Arch Ophthalmol.* 2001;119: 754–755.
62. Han DO. Corticosteroids in the management of postoperative endophthalmitis. In Syllabus: Subspecialty Day-Retina 2000: Management of posterior segment disease, Drugs and Bugs, pp 229–234, Dallas.
63. Das T, Jalali S, Gothwal VK, et al. Intravitreal dexamethasone in exogenous bacterial endophthalmitis: results of a prospective randomised study. *Br J Ophthalmol.* 1999;83:1050–1055.
64. Kwak HW, D'Amico DJ. Evaluation of the retinal toxicity and pharmacokinetics of dexamethasone after intravitreal injection. *Arch Ophthalmol.* 1992;110:259–266.

Chapter 28

Cystoid Macular Edema

Soosan Jacob, MS, DNB, FRCS, MNAMS, FERC;
Amar Agarwal, MS, FRCS, FRCOphth

Introduction

Since its recognition as a distinct entity by Irvine in 1953[1] and its elaborate clinical description by Gass and Norton in 1966,[2–4] aphakic and pseudophakic cystoid macular edema (CME), commonly referred to as the Irvine Gass syndrome, has continued to perplex ophthalmologists in terms of its pathogenesis, its peculiar clinical manifestations, and its treatment. It is one of the most frequent and troublesome problems following cataract surgery with or without intraocular lens (IOL).

Macular Edema

The extracellular space of the retina normally constitutes a small proportion of its total volume. Active transport of electrolytes and larger molecules from the retina across the retinal pigment epithelium to the blood maintains this situation. Disruption of either the inner or outer blood-retinal barrier leads to leakage of plasma proteins and water, which leads to expansion of the extracellular fluid space of the retina. This is often accompanied by accumulation of fluid in the macular area, especially in the outer plexiform layer and inner nuclear layer. Retinal edema localized to the macula is called macular edema. More generalized leakage leads to diffuse thickening of the posterior pole. Accumulation of fluid in cystic spaces leads to CME.

Cystoid Macular Edema

The macula is the most commonly involved part of the retina because of its peculiar anatomy characterized by an abundance of axons (nerve fiber layer of Henle), paucity of glial tissue, which holds the retinal elements together, relative lack of vasculature, and greater metabolic activity.

Theories Explaining Aphakic and Pseudophakic Cystoid Macular Edema

Vitreous Traction Theory

Constant constriction and dilatation of the pupil creates pulling on the anterior vitreous strands, which is transmitted to the vitreous base and thence to the macula by presumed vitreous connections between the posterior hyaloid and the surface of the macula. This is the vitreous tug syndrome.[3,15–17] Vitreoretinal adhesion is strongest at those regions where the internal limiting lamina is thinnest, ie, the fovea and vitreous base.[18–21] In these regions, the Muller cell attachment plaques to the Internal limiting membrane are most prominent. Thus it appears that the continuity of structure between the collagen fibrils of the vitreous and the Muller cells of the retina[22] could directly transmit any movement, displacement, or traction in the vitreous to the Muller cells of the macula. Since Muller cells are not only transretinal structural elements but also serve a vital metabolic role,[23] any damage to these cells could alter other components of the macula. Chronic Muller cell irritation may also lead to the local release of a variety of mediators, which in turn facilitates leakage.

Inflammation Theory

Eyes with CME nearly always demonstrate signs of intraocular inflammation and also respond to steroid therapy. Clinical observations associating aphakic CME with intraocular inflammation have been made for many years.[1,5,24,25] Aqueous humor contains biochemically active principles called Aqueous Biotoxic Complex (ABC) factors,[26] which manifest biotoxic effects when it leaves its natural reservoir. If large amounts of it are produced or if there is a reduction in its absorption by the ciliary epithelium, these diffuse posteriorly through the collapsed liquefied vitreous gel. The liquefied vitreous anterior to the retina hence assumes chemical and osmotic properties quite unlike those normally present, which results in an outpouring of fluid from the perimacular capillaries.The lower incidence of CME after extracapsular cataract extraction (ECCE) may be due to the presence of an intact posterior capsule, which acts as a diffusion barrier.[26] The ABC factors may be prostaglandins that are synthesized de novo. Since the eye does not contain the enzyme 15-PG dehydrogenase to deactivate prostaglandins, their removal is dependent on an active transport pump called the Bito's pump located in the ciliary epithelium.[26] This pump is inoperable (overburdened or inhibited) for at least 3 weeks after ocular trauma.[27] The inflammatory state persists for longer periods when vitreous is adherent to the cataract wound causing pupillary distortion[28] (Figure 28–1).

Anoxia Theory

This theory is not yet proved. An association between CME and systemic conditions, eg, hypertension, arteriosclerotic heart disease, and diabetes mellitus is seen in which anoxia could be a predisposing factor for CME.[28,29]

Theories Concerning the Origin of Cysts of Cystoid Macular Edema

Intracellular Theory

Yanoff et al[30] and Fine and Brucker[31] proposed that cysts develop from degenerating Muller's cells. Initially, these cells demonstrate edema, which gradually increases until the cytoplasm of the cells begin to develop vacuoles. The edematous cells gradually expand until the cell walls break and adjoining cells from larger cavities leading to the cysts in CME. A breakdown of the blood-retinal barrier or anoxia is the primary cause of the edema.

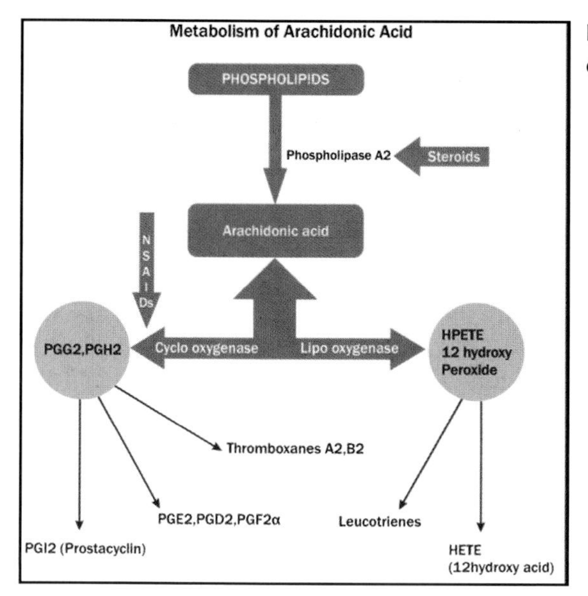

Figure 28-1. Metabolism of arachidonic acid.

Extracellular Theory

Gass, Anderson, and Davis[32] proposed that cysts arise from expansion of the extracellular spaces of the retina by serous exudation within the outer plexiform layer and inner nuclear layer. This involves leakage of serous exudates from perifoveal intraretinal capillaries and sometimes from disc capillaries. The exudates form small puddles in the OPL of Henle, which acts like a sponge because of the peculiar structure of the macula. This theory is supported by the highly reversible function of a CME eye, which argues against cellular death and disruption and also the visible lack of occluded capillaries in the macula, which argues against the presence of anoxia.

Cystoid Macular Edema and Anterior Chamber Intraocular Lens—Possible Pathophysiology

Chronic anterior uveal irritation may either stimulate production of intraocular inflammatory substances or may retard the absorption or removal of these substances by the nonpigmented epithelium of the ciliary body. An ACIOL that can press against the anterior surface of the iris or apply constant pressure on the face of the ciliary body could trigger constant anterior uveal inflammation. Older style IOLs situated with in the pupil (intracameral) that either rest upon the pupillary margin or have haptics sutured to the iris stroma possess the same, if not greater, propensity to elicit chronic uveal irritation.[14] Hence, intracameral and ACIOLs are more likely to stimulate CME than are PCIOLs.[14,34]

Incidence of CME

Irvine[1] originally reported an incidence of 2%, but the incidence of angiographic CME is much higher, occurring approximately after 40% of intracapsular cataract extractions.[14]

Also, if it occurs in one eye, there is almost a 70% probability of it affecting the second eye as well after cataract surgery.[14] Phacoemulsification with "in the bag" IOL placement has been reported to have an incidence as low as 0.5%.[14] Eyes with a primary posterior capsulotomy had a significantly higher incidence of angiographic CME approximately 21.5% as compared to 5.6% in eyes with intact capsules[37] in one series, whereas in another series no statistically significant difference was found in the incidence of angiographic CME 6 weeks or 6 months postoperatively.[38] The incidence of clinically significant pseudophakic CME after Nd: YAG laser posterior capsulotomy was around 1.23% in one study.[39]

Clinical Appearance of Cystoid Macular Edema

Slit Lamp Examination

This is done with Hruby Lens, 90 D lens, 78 D lens, or the Goldmann 3 mirror contact lens. Advantages are the use of slit lamp optics and stereopsis. Biomicroscopic examination with Hruby lens or a fundus contact lens or a 90 D lens shows a characteristic honeycomb lesion with one or more larger cystoid spaces centrally and any number of smaller, oval spaces around them. Cystoid spaces are best seen using red free light, which makes the inner walls visible. The optical section of the convex anterior walls of the cysts can be seen overlying optically empty vesicles, tightly packed together with their interfaces presenting a spidery pattern. With the slit beam, it is possible to see a network of interlacing, fine refractile lines by retroillumination. The retina may be markedly thickened and the lesion may be as large as 1.5 to 2 disc diameters. Some cases may be associated with disc edema.

Direct Ophthalmoscopy

This usually shows a loss of foveal reflex. Monochromatic light is better for detecting subtle macular changes, hence red free light can be used. Using the macular aperture, the beam is passed slowly back and forth across the macula. The septa may be observed by retroillumination, ie, just adjacent to the edge of the light beam. Disadvantages are the lack of stereoscopic view and the difficulty of recoding and transmitting information.

Indirect Ophthalmoscopy

This is useful in ruling out other causes of CME.

Anterior Segment Examination

This usually shows signs of inflammation. The anterior hyaloid face may be intact or broken and the vitreous usually shows cells and vitreous opacities and posterior vitreous detachment.

Fundus Fluorescein Angiography

This is used to confirm and document macular changes and for deciding the management and also for follow-up. In CME, within 1 to 2 minutes of dye injection, leakage into the macula is seen (Figure 28-2). A stellate pattern with feathery margins is seen by 5 to 15 minutes usually, but sometimes takes up to 30 minutes. The pattern seen on FFA is called the flower petal appearance (Figure 28-3). The dark septae in the macular area that compartmentalize the pattern are because of the Muller's fibers. The spaces appear to intercommunicate. Usually there is considerable leakage of dye into the vitreous and aqueous

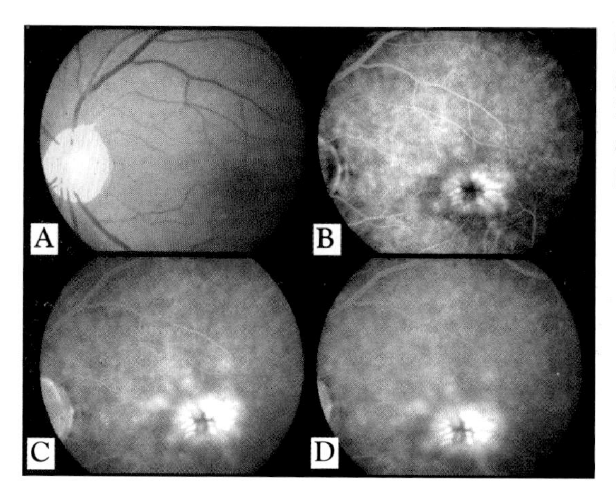

Figure 28-2. A. Color fundus photograph of cystoid macular edema. **B**. Shows capillary leakage in the macular area. **C**. Early flower petal appearance. **D**. Late flower petal appearance.

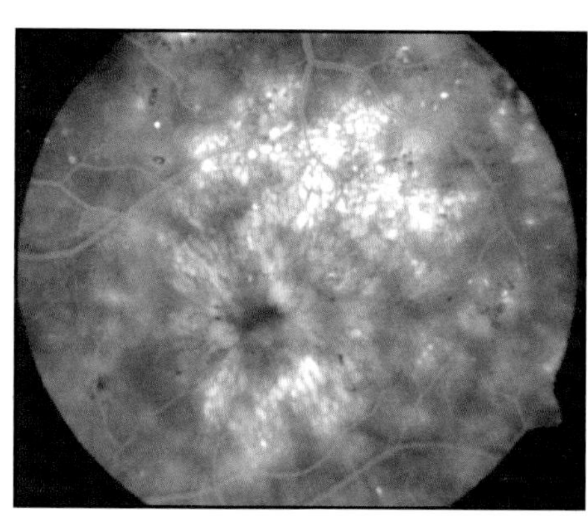

Figure 28-3. Fundus fluorescein photograph of cystoid macular edema (flower petal appearance).

anteriorly. In some patients with disc edema, there may be leakage of dye into the optic nerve and peripupillary retina.

Various FFA grading systems have been used for CME:[40,41]

Grade 0: No edema
Grade 1+: Capillary leakage
Grade 2+: Partial petaloid ring
Grade 3+: Complete petaloid ring

Level 1: Edema less than perifoveal
Level 2: Minimal perifoveal edema
Level 3: Moderate perifoveal edema (1 DD)
Level 4: Severe perifoveal edema

Optical Coherence Tomography

Loss of foveal contour is seen with retina edema, thickening and fluid accumulation in the form of cystic spaces predominantly in the outer plexiform and inner nuclear layers. Tissue bands, probably representing the stretched Muller cells, are seen between the cystic spaces (Figure 28-4).

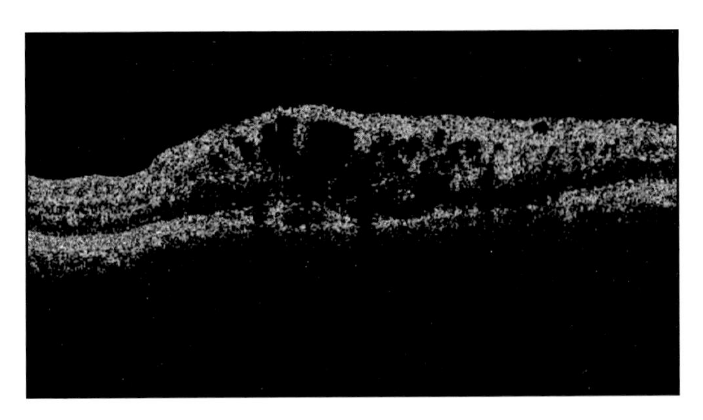

Figure 28-4. OCT of a cystoid macular edema case. Line scan of the macula shows loss of foveal contour. Increased retinal thickness in the macula with multiple large optically clear low reflective cystic spaces with septae seen in the inner retina.

Macular Function Tests in Cystoid Macular Edema

Best corrected visual acuity (BCVA) and visual acuity with pin hole, two point discrimination, and Maddox Rod test, all indicate decreased macular function. Amsler grid chart may show central distortion of the grids or a relative central scotoma. The automated perimeter has special macular programs that may show central scotoma. Any blanks or scotoma in the central area on entoptic imagery implies macular involvement. Potential Acuity Meter (PAM) can be used for differentiating between visual loss from anterior segment disease and macular disease. Longer recovery time, up to 90 to 180 seconds on macular photostress test, implies macular dysfunction even though the area may appear anatomically normal. The normal recovery time is 55 seconds. Difference between the two eyes is also significant.

In cases of opaque media, the visual acuity can be determined with clinical interferometers. Electrophysiology[42] may also show changes in CME. Foveal ERG is a test of the temporal responsiveness of the central 10 degree of the retina and requires integrity of the outer retinal layers, especially Muller's cells. FERG is usually abnormal in 35% of CME eyes. Pattern ERG reflects the inner retinal layer function. It is usually abnormal in 53% of CME eyes. Over half of the PERG abnormal eyes had no associated FERG abnormalities.

Sequela of Cystoid Macular Edema

Permanent macular degeneration may arise secondary to prolonged chronic CME. The cystoid spaces of the macula may coalesce together so that all retinal elements disappear except for the internal limiting membrane.[14] After the internal limiting membrane also disintegrates, a lamellar hole is formed which may be one-fourth to one-third disc diameter in size.[44] Surrounding intact cystoid spaces may be seen. In the presence of a lamellar hole, visual acuity may continue to be good because of the retention of some percipient elements.[26] Rarely does CME progress to a full-thickness macular hole.

On-Off Phenomenon

CME tends to be cyclic in nature, so that sometimes on withdrawing treatment following good response to therapy, CME may relapse again. This is called the on-off phenomenon.[41,47]

PROPHYLACTIC TREATMENT

1. Steady and gentle preoperative ocular compression.
2. Avoiding ICCE and unplanned ECCE.
3. Gentle tissue handling and avoiding excessive instrumentation.
4. Avoiding complications like posterior capsular rent, vitreous loss, iris prolapse, etc.
5. Proper management of vitreous loss with thorough anterior vitrectomy.
6. In-the-bag IOL placement.
7. IOL with chemically inert haptics and high quality optics with good surface finish and correct dimensions.
8. Avoiding photoxicity by using coaxial light only when red reflex is essential and using oblique illumination at all other times. Also by using a pupil occluder, decreasing the intensity of illumination, and by rotating the macula away from light during suturing and also by using an IOL with UV absorbing optics.
9. Pharmacological prophylaxis with postoperative steroids and nonsteroidal anti-inflammatory drugs (NSAIDs) through topical, subconjunctival, sub-Tenon, or systemic routes. The use of steroids and NSAIDs decreases the amount of intraocular inflammatory substances released at the time of surgery.[48]

THERAPY FOR ESTABLISHED CYSTOID MACULAR EDEMA

Medical Therapy

1. Topical steroids: Given 4 to 6 times per day.
2. Repository steroid injections: Methyl prednisolone acetate suspension (Depo-Medrol) or triamcinolone acetonide (Kenalog), usually 40 mg (1 ml) is given subconjunctivally once a month. It is not to be used in eyes with a known propensity for steroid induced rise in intraocular pressure (IOP).
3. Systemic steroids: Efficacy is not known as yet. Dosage: 40 to 100 mg per day or every alternate day.
4. Topical NSAIDs: Topical indomethacin 1%, Ketorolac 0.5%, Diclofenac 0.1%, and Flurbiprofen 0.03% can be tried. Studies have shown an improvement in vision, but an on-off phenomenon[41] may be seen.
5. Oral NSAID therapy: Indomethacin 25 mg tid after meals can be tried. Other drugs are suprofen, fenoprofen, ibuprofen, piroxicam. All these can cause gastric irritation.
6. Hyperbaric oxygen: Some patients receiving 2.2 atm, oxygen for 1.5 hours twice daily for 7 days and then 2 hours daily for 14 days may show improvement. Hyperbaric oxygen may help heal injured capillary complexes by causing constriction of the macular capillaries along with stimulating collagen formation, which seals these spaces.[49]
7. Acetazolamide: It facilitates transport of water across the RPE from the subretinal space to the choroid.[50] Dosage is 250 to 500 mg bid or qid.[51,52]

Medical therapy can also be tried for many elderly patients and for unwilling patients who do not want further surgery.

ND-YAG Laser Vitreolysis

This avoids an invasive procedure. Elevated vitreous strands are transected using Nd-YAG laser.[8,53] Bisecting vitreous membranes that are adherent to the anterior surface of the iris may be difficult without producing small hemorrhages that diffuse into the aqueous and make accurate focussing impossible. Therefore, laser treatment is primarily used in those cases in which vitreous strands bridge the margin of the pupil to the undersurface of the cataract wound without adhering to the anterior surface of the iris.[53]

Surgical Therapy

For Aphakic Cystoid Macular Edema

Vitrectomy: The goal of the surgery is to remove all formed vitreous elements from the anterior segment to restore the anatomy of the iris and pupil to a state as near normal as possible. Technique[28]—the edges of the condensed sheets of solid vitreous adherent to the anterior surface of the iris are carefully identified with the slit lamp preoperatively and with the operating microscope intraoperatively. Then a plane of dissection is created between the sheet of vitreous and the anterior surface of the iris by the to and fro swings of a microcyclodialysis spatula introduced at 90 degrees to the edge. The sheet is then removed by advancing a vitrectomy instrument beneath it. This is done until all formed vitreous is removed and the pupil is restored to normal. Next, a shallow vitrectomy is performed at the level of the pupil to prevent new strands of vitreous from finding their way to the incision site postoperatively. If a pars plana approach is used, a complete posterior vitrectomy can also be done.

For Pseudophakic Cystoid Macular Edema With Anterior Chamber IOL

1. With relatively round pupil: Removal of the ACIOL with anterior vitrectomy is done. The surgical aphakia is corrected either with a sulcus IOL if adequate posterior capsular rim remains (but the disadvantage here is irritation to the uveal tissue) or a scleral fixated IOL. Other solutions are contact lenses, epikeratoplasty, excimer laser, or peripheral intrastromal corneal ring.
2. With moderate pupillary distortion from disrupted vitreous or malpositioned haptics: Anterior vitrectomy and anterior segment restoration is done. The IOL may be left in situ or exchanged.

For Pseudophakic Cystoid Macular Edema With PCIOL

1. With pupillary distortion: Anterior segment restoration with a core pars plana vitrectomy is done.
2. With in-the-bag IOL, intact posterior capsule, normal mobile pupil, no peripheral anterior synechiae: Here a pars plana vitrectomy could be performed to remove the vitreous sump or vitreous traction from the macula, but the sump theory is not yet proved, hence it is better not to operate. If done to release vitreo macular traction, such traction should be confirmed preoperatively by biomicroscopic examination with posterior pole contact lens. This situation is rare and hence surgical intervention should be uncommon.[14] But before resorting to surgery in such cases, other causes for CME should be ruled out and a complete course of medical therapy should have been tried.

Key Points

1. Chronic anterior uveal irritation may either stimulate production of intra ocular inflammatory substances or may retard the absorption or removal of these substances by the non-pigmented epithelium of the ciliary body.
2. Biomicroscopic examination with Hruby lens, a fundus contact lens, or a 90 D lens shows a characteristic honeycomb lesion with one or more larger cystoid spaces centrally and any number of smaller, oval spaces around them. Cystoid spaces are best seen using red free light, which makes the inner walls visible.
3. In CME, within 1 to 2 minutes of dye injection, leakage into the macula is seen. A stellate pattern with feathery margins is seen by 5 to 15 minutes usually, but sometimes takes up to 30 minutes. The pattern seen on FFA is called the flower petal appearance.
4. Rarely does CME progress to a full-thickness macular hole.
5. The goal of vitrectomy is to remove all formed vitreous elements from the anterior segment to restore the anatomy of the iris and pupil to a state as near normal as possible.

References

1. Irvine SR. A newly defined vitreous syndrome following cataract surgery, interpreted according to recent concepts of the structure of the vitreous. *Am J Ophthalmol.* 1953;36:599.
2. Gass JDM, Norton EWD. Cystoid macular edema and papilloedema following cataract extraction: fluorescein fundoscopic and angiographic study. *Arch Ophthalmol.* 1966;76:646.
3. Tolentino FI, Schepens CL. Edema of the posterior pole after cataract extractions: a biomicroscopic study. *Arch Ophthalmol.* 1965;74:781.
4. Iliff CE. Treatment of the vitreous tug syndrome. *Am J Ophthalmol.* 1966;62:856.
5. Gass JDM, Norton EWD. A follow-up study of cystoid macular edema following cataract extraction. *Trans Am Acad Ophthal Otolaryngol.* 1969;73:665.
6. Machemer R, Parel JM, Buettner H. A new concept for vitreous surgery. I. Instrumentation. *Am J Ophthalmol.* 1972;73:1.
7. Miyake K. Prevention of cystoid macular edema after lens extraction by topical indomethacin. (I) A preliminary report. *Albrecht bon graefes Arch Klin Ophthalmol.* 1977;203:81.
8. Katzen LE, Fleischman JA, Trokel S. YAG laser treatment of cystoid macular edema. *Am J Ophthalmol.* 1983;95:589.
9. Shahidi M, Ogura Y. Correlation of retinal thickness with visual acuity in cystoid macular edema. *Arch Ophthalmol.* 1991;109(8):1115.
10. Hee MR, Puliafito CA, Wong C, et al. Quantitative assessment of macular edema with optical coherence tomography. *Arch Ophthalmol.* 1995;113:1019.
11. Arend O, Remky A, Elsner AE, et al. Quantification of cystoid changes in diabetic maculopathy. *Invest Ophthalmol Vis Sci.* 1995;36:608.
12. Brenda and Tripathi. *Wolff's Anatomy of the Eye and Orbit.* 8th ed. Chapman and Hall Ltd; 1997.
13. Duke Elder S. *System of Ophthalmology, Vol. X—Diseases of the Retina.* St. Louis: C.V. Mosby; 1967.
14. Ryan SJ. *Retina.* 2nd ed. St. Louis: C.V. Mosby.

15. Jaffe NS. Vitreous traction at the posterior pole of the fundus due to alterations in the vitreous posterior. *Trans Am Acad Ophthalmol Otolaryngol.* 1967;71:642.
16. Reese AB, Jones IS, Cooper WC. Macular changes secondary to vitreous traction. *Trans Am Ophthalmol Soc.* 1966;64:123.
17. Maumenee AE. Further advances in the study of the macula. *Arch Ophthalmol.* 1967;78:51.
18. Eisner G. Biomicroscopy of the peripheral fundus. *Surv Ophthalmol.* 1972;17:1.
19. Foos RY. Vitreoretinal juncture: topographic variations. *Invest Ophthalmol Vis Sci.* 1972;11:801.
20. Grignolo A. Fibrous components of the vitreous body. *Arch Ophthalmol.* 1952;47:760.
21. Hogan MJ. The vitreous, its structure and relation to the ciliary body and retina. *Invest Ophthalmol Vis Sci.* 1963;2:418.
22. Mann I. *The Development of the Human Eye*. New York: Grune and Stratton; 1964: 162.
23. Lessell S, Kuwabara T. Phosphatase histochemistry of the eye. *Arch Ophthalmol.* 1964;71:851.
24. Hitchings RA, Chisholm IH, Bird AC. Aphakic macular edema: incidence and pathogenesis. *Invest Ophthalmol.* 1975;14:68.
25. Irvine AR, Bresky R, Crowder BM, et al. Macular edema after cataract extraction. *Ann Ophthalmol.* 1971;3:1234.
26. Jaffe N. *Cataract Surgery and its Complications*. 6th ed. St. Louis: CV Mosby; 1977.
27. Bito LZ, Salvador EV. Intraocular fluid dynamics. III. The site and mechanism of prostaglandin transfer across the blood intraocular fluid barriers. *Exp Eye Res.* 1972;14:233.
28. Fung WE. The national, prospective, randomized vitrectomy study for chronic aphakic cystoid macular edema. Progress report and comparison between the control and nonrandomized groups. *Surv Ophthalmol.* 1984;28:569.
29. Tso MO. Animal modeling of cystoid macular edema. *Surv Ophthalmol.* 1984;28:512.
30. Yanoff M, Fine BS, Brucker AJ, et al. Pathology of human cystoid macular edema. *Surv Ophthalmol.* 1984;28:505.
31. Fine BS, Brucker AJ. Macular edema and cystoid macular edema. *Am J Ophthalmol.* 1981;92:466.
32. Gass JDM, Anderson DR, Davis EB. A clinical, fluorescein angiographic, and electron microscopic correlation of cystoid macular edema. *Am J Ophthalmol.* 1985;100:82.
33. Taylor DM, Sachs SW, Stern AL. Aphakic cystoid macular edema. Long-term clinical observations. *Surv Ophthalmol.* 1984;28:437.
34. Stark WJ, Maumenee EA, Fagadau W, et al. Cystoid macular edema in pseudophakia. *Surv Ophthalmol.* 1984;28:442.
35. Moses L. Cystoid macular edema and retinal detachment following cataract surgery. *J Am Intraocul Implant Soc.* 1979;5:326.
36. Keates RH, Steinert RF, Puliafito CA, Maxwell SK. Long-term follow-up of Nd:YAG laser posterior capsulotomy. *J Am Intraocul Implant Soc.* 1984;10:164.
37. Kraff MC, Sanders DR, Jampol LM, et al. Effect of primary capsulotomy with extracapsular surgery on the incidence of pseudophakic cystoid macular edema. *Am J Ophthalmol.* 1984;98:166.
38. Wright PL, Wilkinson CP, Balyeat HD, et al. Angiographic cystoid macular edema after posterior chamber lens implantation. *Arch Ophthalmol.* 1988;106:740.
39. Steinert RF, Puliafito CA, Kumar SR, et al. Cystoid macular edema, retinal detachment, and glaucoma after Nd: YAG laser posterior capsulotomy. *Am J Ophthalmol.* 1991;112:373.
40. Cunha-Vaz JG, Travassos A. Breakdown of the blood retinal barriers and cystoid macular edema, *Surv Ophthalmol.* 1984;28:485.
41. Yannuzzi, LA. A perspective on the treatment of aphakic cystoid macular edema. *Surv Ophthalmol.* 1984;28:540.
42. Salzman J, Seiple W, Carr R, Yannuzzi L. Electrophysiological assessment of aphakic cystoid macular edema. *Br J Ophthalmol.* 1986;70:819.

43. Nussenblatt RB, Kaufman SC, Palestine AG, et al. Macular thickening and visual acuity: measurement in patients with cystoid macular edema. *Ophthalmology.* 1987;94:1134.
44. Gass JDM. Lamellar macular hole: a complication of cystoid macular edema after cataract extraction—a clinicopathologic case report. *Trans Am Ophthalmol Soc.* 1975;73:231.
45. Gass JDM. *Stereoscopic Atlas of Macular Diseases: Diagnosis and Treatment.* 3rd ed. St. Louis: Mosby Year Book; 1987.
46. Jampol LM, Sanders DR, Kraff MC. Prophylaxis and therapy of aphakic cystoid macular edema. *Surv Ophthalmol.* 1984;28:535.
47. Flach AJ, Jampol LM, Weinberg D, et al. Improvement in visual acuity in chronic aphakic and pseudophakic cystoid macular edema after treatment with topical 0.5% ketorolac tromethamine. *Am J Ophthalmol.* 1991;112:514.
48. Jampol LM. Pharmacologic therapy of aphakic and pseudophakic cystoid macular edema: 1985 update. *Ophthalmology.* 1985;92:807.
49. Ploff DS, Thorn SR. Preliminary report on the effect of hyperbaric oxygen on cystoid macular edema. *J Cataract Refract Surg.* 1987;13:136.
50. Marmor MF, Maack T. Enhancement of retinal adhesion and subretinal fluid absorption by acetazolamide. *Invest Ophthalmol Vis Sci.* 1982;23:121.
51. Cox SN, Hay E, Bird AC. Treatment of chronic macular edema with acetazolamide. *Arch Ophthalmol.* 1988;106;1190.
52. Tripathi RC, Fekrat S, Tripathi BJ, et al. A direct correlation of the resolution of pseudophakic cystoid macular edema with acetazolamide therapy. *Ann Ophthalmol.* 1991;23:127.
53. Steinert RF, Wasson PJ. Neodymium: YAG laser anterior vitreolysis for Irvine-Gass cystoid macular edema. *J Cataract Refract Surg.* 1989;15:304.

V

Bimanual Phacoemulsification

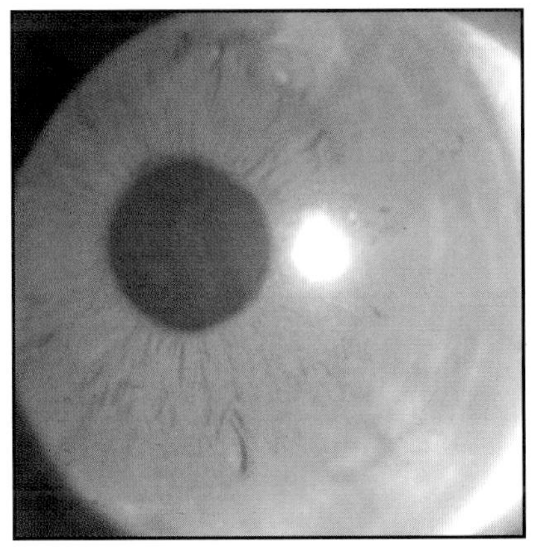

Slit lamp photo of a patient after microphakonit (700 micron cataract surgery).

Chapter 29

Bimanual Phacoemulsification: Surgical Technique

Amar Agarwal, MS, FRCS, FRCOphth

History

Phakonit (bimanual phaco) was first done on August 15, 1998 by the author.[1,2] The cataract was removed through a bimanual phaco technique. It was performed without any anesthesia. The first live phakonit was performed on August 22, 1998 at Pune, India by the author at the Phako & Refractive surgery conference. This was done in front of 350 ophthalmologists.

The problem with this technique was to find an intraocular lens (IOL) that would pass through such a small incision. Then on October 2, 2001, the author did a case of phakonit with the implantation of a rollable IOL. This was done in the Chennai (India) hospital. The lens used was a special lens from Thinoptx (USA). This lens used a fresnel principle and was designed by Wayne Callahan. The first such ultrathin lens was implanted by Jairo Hoyos. The authors then modified this into a special 5 mm optic rollable IOL.

Terminology

The name "phakonit" represents *phako* being done with a needle (*n*) opening via an incision (*i*) and with the phako tip (*t*). This name also indicates that it is phako being done with a needle incision technology.

Synonyms

1. Bimanual phaco
2. Microincision cataract surgery
3. Microphaco
4. Bimanual microphaco
5. Sleeveless phaco

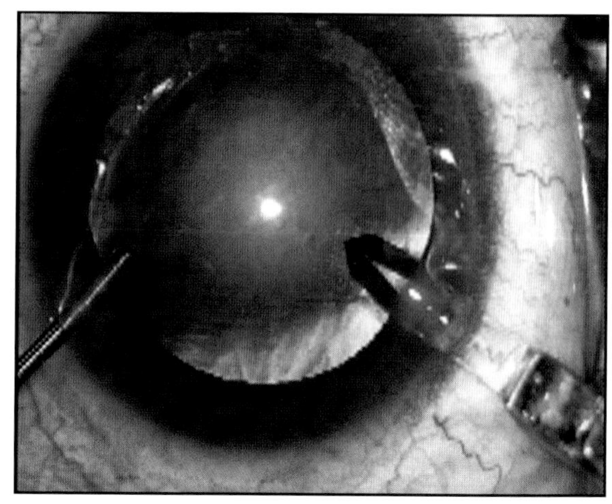

Figure 29-1. Clear corneal incision made with a special knife (MicroSurgical Technology [MST], Redmond, Wash). Note the left hand has a globe stabilization rod to stabilize the eye (Geuder, Germany). This knife can create an incision from sub 1 mm to 1.2 mm.

Phakonit Technique for Cataracts

Anesthesia

Phakonit can be done under any type of anesthesia. The author does the surgery under no anesthesia in which no anesthetic drops are instilled in the eye nor is any intracameral anesthetic injected inside the eye. This is "no anesthesia cataract surgery". The author has discovered that there is no difference between topical anesthesia cataract surgery and no anesthesia cataract surgery. If there is a difficult case, the author uses a peribulbar block.

Incision

In the first step, a needle with viscoelastic is pierced in the eye in the area where the side port has to be made. The viscoelastic is then injected inside the eye. This will distend the eye so that the clear corneal incision can be made. Now a temporal clear corneal incision is made. A special knife can be used for this purpose (Figure 29-1). Note in Figure 29-1, the left hand holds a globe stabilization rod (Geuder, Germany). This helps to stabilize the eye while creating the clear corneal incision. The special knife is held in the dominant hand. This knife has been designed by Mateen Amin. It creates an incision from sub 1 mm or 1.2 mm, depending on which size knife is chosen by the surgeon. If one is using a sub 1 mm knife, then one should use a 22 gauge irrigating chopper and a 0.7 mm phaco needle. This keratome and other instruments for phakonit are made by Huco (Switzerland), Gueder (Germany), and MST (Redmond, Wash).

Rhexis

A rhexis of about 5 to 6 mm is then performed. This is done with a needle (Figure 29-2). In the left hand a straight rod is held to stabilize the eye. This is the globe stabilization rod. The advantage of this is that the movements of the eye are controlled as one is working without any anesthesia. MST has designed an excellent rhexis forceps for phakonit (Figure 29-3). This goes through a 1 mm incision. Those comfortable with a forceps in phako can use this special forceps in phakonit. At present, there is no forceps for microphakonit as the incision is too small (see Chapter 30).

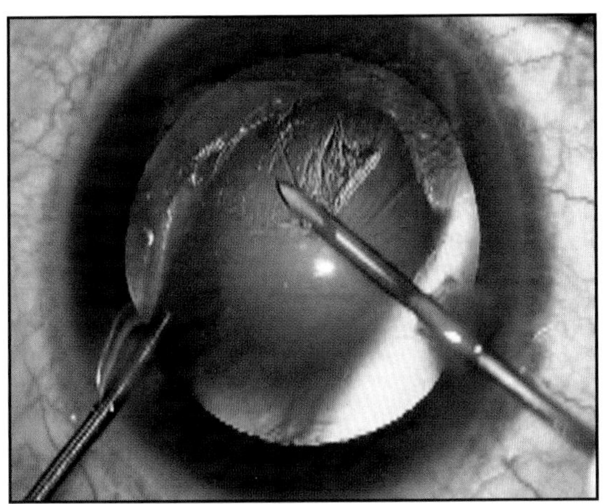

Figure 29-2. Rhexis started with a needle.

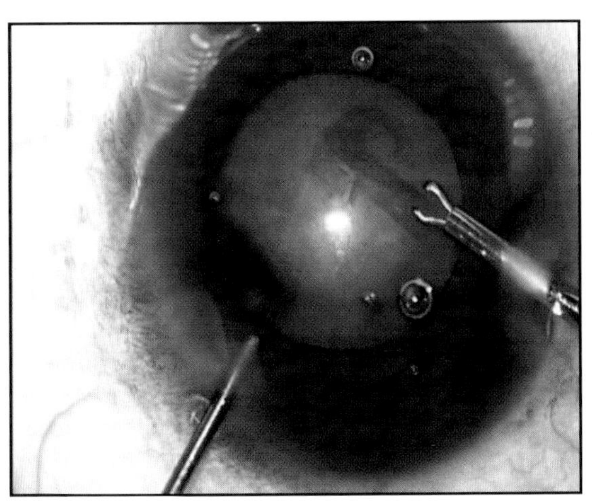

Figure 29-3. MST rhexis forceps used to perform the rhexis in a mature cataract. Note the trypan blue (Blurhex) staining the anterior capsule.

Hydrodissection

Hydrodissection is performed and the fluid wave passing under the nucleus checked. One should always check for rotation of the nucleus.

Phakonit

After enlarging the side port, a 20- or 21-gauge irrigating chopper connected to the infusion line of the phaco machine is introduced with the foot pedal on position 1. There are various irrigating choppers. In Figure 29-4, you will notice two types of irrigating choppers that we have designed. On the left is the Agarwal irrigating chopper made by MST. This is incorporated in the Duet system. The irrigating chopper on the right is made by Geuder. Notice in the right figure the opening for the fluid is end opening, whereas the one on the left has two openings in the side. The surgeon can decide which type of irrigating chopper they would like to use.

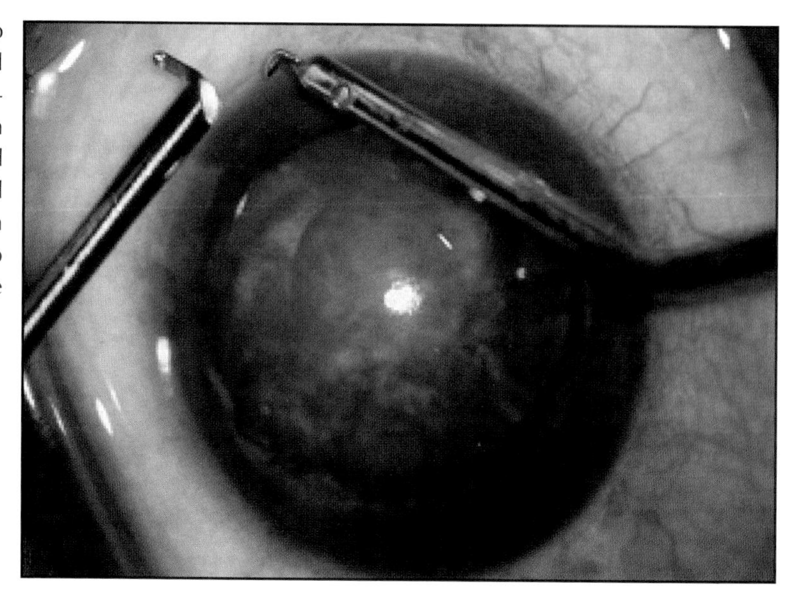

Figure 29-4. Two types of Agarwal irrigating choppers. The one on the left has an end opening for fluid (MST). The one on the right has two openings on the sides (Geuder).

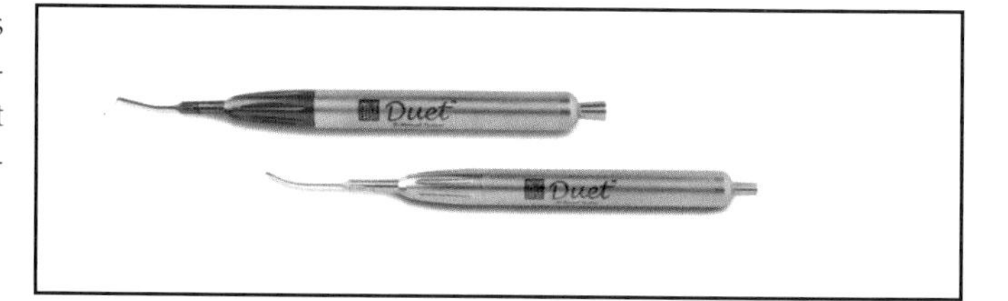

Figure 29-5. Duet handles from MST, USA. The advantage of these handles is that one can change the irrigating chopper tips.

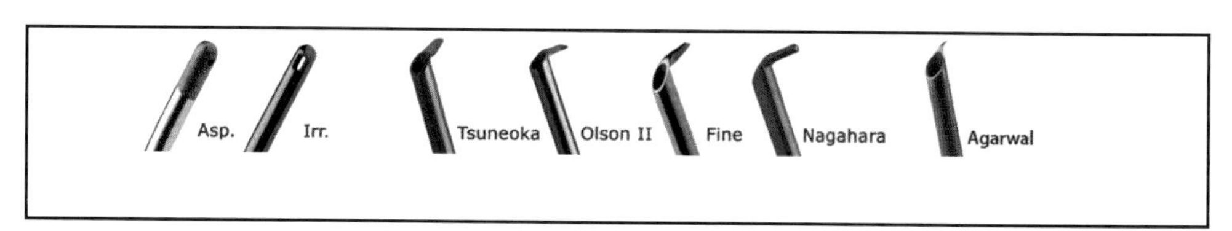

Figure 29-6. Various irrigating chopper tips designed by various surgeons. These can be fixed onto the Duet handles (MST).

The Agarwal irrigating chopper designed by Larry Laks has been made by MST. This is incorporated in the Duet system (Figure 29-5). Other excellent irrigating choppers by various surgeons are made by the same company (Figure 29-6).

The phaco probe is connected to the aspiration line and the phaco tip without an infusion sleeve is introduced through the clear corneal incision (Figures 29-7 and 29-8). Using the phaco tip with moderate ultrasound power, the center of the nucleus is directly embedded starting from the superior edge of rhexis with the phaco probe directed obliquely downwards towards the vitreous. The settings at this stage are 50% phaco power, flow rate 24 ml/min, and 110 mmHg vacuum. When nearly half of the center of nucleus is embedded, the foot pedal is moved to position 2, as it helps to hold the nucleus due to vacuum rise. To avoid undue pressure on the posterior capsule, the nucleus is lifted a bit and with

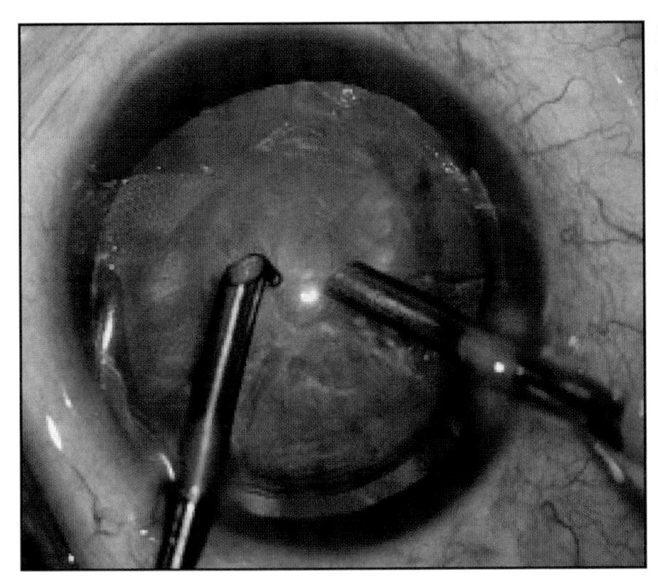

Figure 29-7. Phakonit irrigating chopper and phako probe without the sleeve inside the eye.

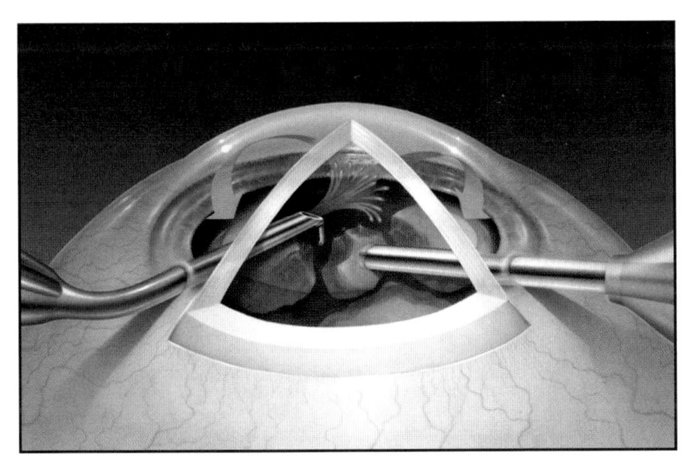

Figure 29-8. Phakonit. Notice the irrigating chopper with an end opening. (Photo courtesy of Larry Laks, MST.)

the irrigating chopper in the left hand the nucleus chopped. This is done with a straight downward motion from the inner edge of the rhexis to the center of the nucleus and then to the left in the form of a laterally reversed L shape. Once the crack is created, the nucleus is split till the center. The nucleus is then rotated 180° and cracked again so that the nucleus is completely split into two halves.

The nucleus is then rotated 90 degrees and embedding done in one half of the nucleus with the probe directed horizontally. With the previously described technique, three pie-shaped quadrants are created in one half of the nucleus. Similarly, three pie-shaped fragments are created in the other half of the nucleus. With a short burst of energy at pulse mode, each pie shaped fragment is lifted and brought at the level of iris where it is further emulsified and aspirated sequentially in pulse mode. Thus the whole nucleus is removed.

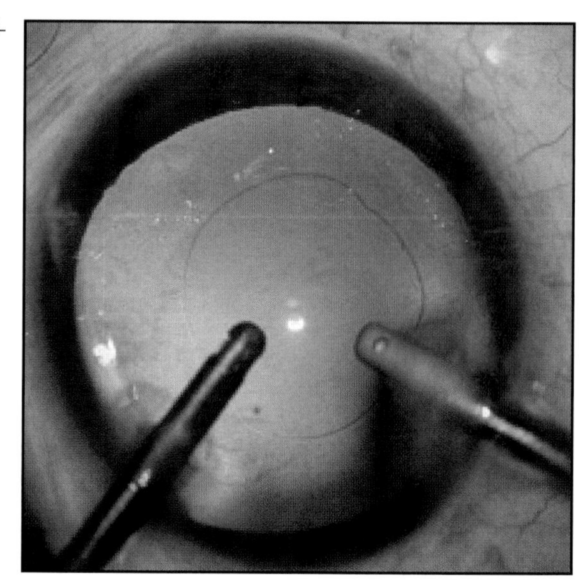

Figure 29-9. Bimanual irrigation aspiration completed.

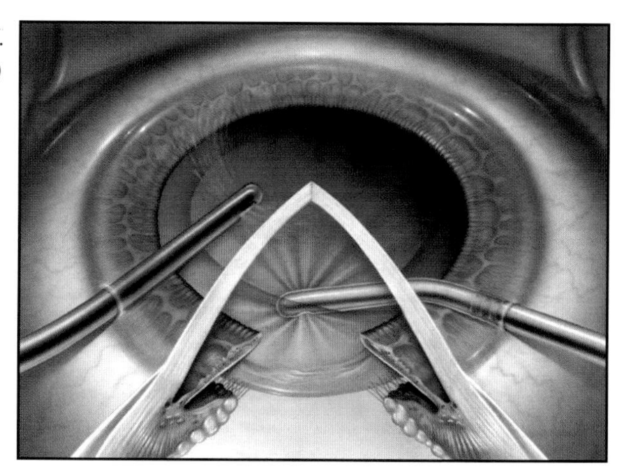

Figure 29-10. Soft tip I/A from MST. (Photo courtesy of Larry Laks, MST.)

Cortical wash-up is the done with the bimanual irrigation aspiration (I/A) technique (Figure 29-9). MST has also designed a soft tip I/A, which is very safe for the posterior capsule (Figure 29-10).

Phakonit With Cut Sleeve

During phakonit, another unique problem faced was that of splashing of the fluid from the base of the phaco needle outside the incision during emulsification. This happened because fluid in contact with the base of the vibrating phaco needle during emulsification was churned, thus releasing droplets of fluid. These fluid droplets could hamper the surgeon's view directly or by getting deposited on the microscope objective.

To eliminate wound burns we should have some way of cooling the corneal wound of entry. This is usually taken care by the fluid that leaks out of the eye from the main wound as the naked phaco needle without the sleeve does not provide a watertight wound. To provide irrigation to the anterior chamber, we use the irrigating chopper through the side port connected to the irrigating bottle, along with an air pump specially devised for this purpose. To prevent the splashing of fluid during emulsification from the base of the phaco needle, we use the cut sleeve around the base of the phaco needle. We cut the sleeve so that it covers only the base of the phaco needle and does not enter the eye. Thus we are able to prevent the splashing of fluid during emulsification.

During phakonit surgery, fluid is constantly leaking out of the eye from the main wound of entry, as the incision around the phaco needle without the sleeve is not watertight. This fluid is coming from the irrigating chopper connected to the air injector. If we connect another fluid irrigating line to the phaco needle with cut sleeve, fluid travels from the base of the phaco needle towards the wound of entry from outside. This stream of fluid meets the stream coming from inside the eye at the corneal entry wound, causing turbulence and fluid collection in the operating field. This reduces visibility during surgery. Moreover, since the wound is cooled internally by the fluid leaking from the eye outwards, there is no need for this second irrigation line. More importantly, when we connect the second irrigation line to the phaco handpiece with the cut sleeve, the irrigation is always on but we need it only during emulsification. Hence, it is better to have an assistant drop cooled BSS at the external wound only during emulsification. We advocate "phakonit with cut sleeve without irrigation" to eliminate water splashing during phakonit to improve visibility during the surgery.

Air Pump

One of the real problems in phakonit when we started it was destabilization of the anterior chamber during surgery. This was solved to a certain extent by using an 18-gauge irrigating chopper. A development made by Sunita Agarwal was to use an anti-chamber collapser,[4,5] which injects air into the infusion bottle. This is an air pump (see Chapter 2). This pushes more fluid into the eye through the irrigating chopper and also prevents surge. Thus we were not only able to use a 20-gauge irrigating chopper but also solve the problem of destabilization of the anterior chamber during surgery. This increases the steady-state pressure of the eye, making the anterior chamber deep and well maintained during the entire procedure. It even makes phacoemulsification a relatively safe procedure by reducing surge even at high vacuum levels. Thus this can be used not only in phakonit but also in phacoemulsification.

Cruise Control

The Cruise Control is a disposable, flow-restricting (0.3-mm internal diameter) device that is placed in between the phaco handpiece and the aspiration tubing of any phaco machine. The goal is very similar to that of the flare tip (Alcon, Fort Worth, Texas): combining a standard phaco tip opening with a narrower shaft to provide more grip with less surge. This has been popularized by David Chang and I. Howard Fine for phakonit surgery. STAAR Surgical (Monrovia, Calif) introduced this disposable Cruise Control device, which can be used with any phaco machine.

Phakonit can be Done With Any Phaco Machine

It is not necessary that only a top end phaco machine is required. The key is to use any machine already present and start Phakonit. The parameters are:

1. Power—50% phaco power. Start in the continuous mode and once chopping has been done then shift to the pulse mode.

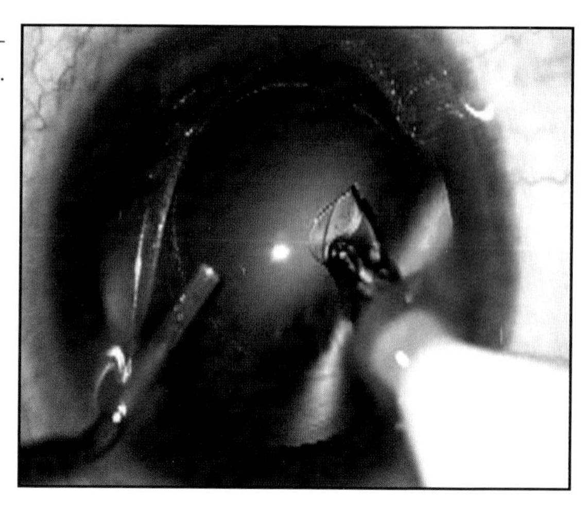

Figure 29-11. Thinoptx roller cum injector inserting the IOL in the capsular bag.

2. Suction—100 mmHg. One has to use the air pump or anti chamber collapser so that no surge occurs. In other words, some sort of forced gas infusion has to be used. One can do without it but the problem will come in difficult cases and one has to go slower.
3. Flow rate—20–24 ml/min. This is what we use for an Alcon or AMO machine.
4. Phaco needle—if one uses a 0.8 mm phaco needle with a 21-gauge irrigating chopper, then one can do a sub 1 mm cataract surgery.
5. Irrigation over corneal incision. It is better than not applying it. You can feel very safe with it as it negates the possibility of a corneal burn.

Thinoptx Rollable Intraocular Lens

Thinoptx has patented technology that allows the manufacture of lenses with plus or minus 30 D of correction on the thickness of 100 microns. The Thinoptx technology, developed by Wayne Callahan, Scott Callahan, and Joe Callahan, is not limited to material choice, but is achieved instead of an evolutionary optic and unprecedented nano-scale manufacturing process. The lens is made from off-the-shelf hydrophilic material, which is similar to several IOL materials already on the market. The key to the Thinoptx lens is the optic design and nano-precision manufacturing. The basic advantage of these lenses is that they are ultra-thin lenses. The author modified this lens to make a special 5 mm optic rollable IOL.

Thinoptx has made a special injector that not only rolls the lens but also inserts the lens. This way we do not need to use our fingers for rolling the lens. In Figure 29-11, you will notice this special injector injecting the IOL in the capsular bag. The tip of the nozzle is kept at the edge of the incision.

Topography

We also performed topography with the Orbscan to compare cases of phakonit and phaco and we found that the astigmatism in phakonit cases is much less compared to phaco (Figure 29-12). Stabilization of refraction is also faster with phakonit compared to phaco surgery. Table 29-1 compares the differences between phaco and phakonit.

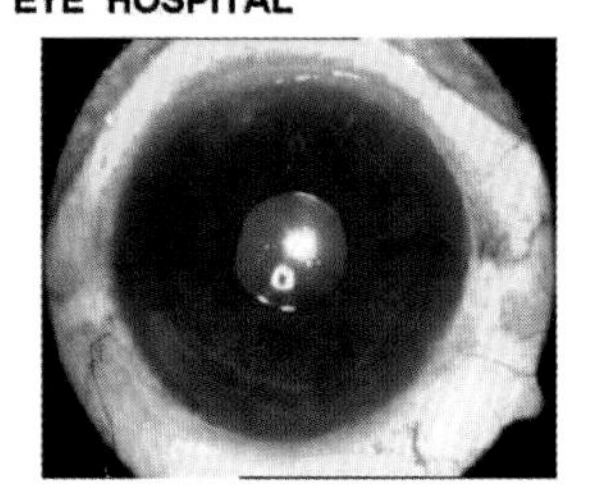

Figure 29-12. Comparison between phako foldable and phakonit thinoptx IOL. The figure on the left shows a case of phako with a foldable IOL and the figure on the right shows phakonit with a thinoptx rollable IOL.

Table 29-1.
Phaco Versus Phakonit

Feature	*Phaco*	*Phakonit*
1. Incision size	3 mm	Sub 1.4 mm
2. Air pump	Not mandatory	Better
3. Hand usage	Single-handed phaco possible	Two hands (bimanual)
4. Nondominant hand entry and exit	Last to enter and first to exit	First to enter and last to exit
5. Capsulorrhexis	Needle or forceps	Better with needle
6. IOL	Foldable IOL	Rollable IOL
7. Astigmatism	Two unequal incisions create astigmatism	Two equal ultrasmall incisions negate the induced astigmatism
8. Stability of refraction	Later than phakonit	Earlier than phaco
9. Iris prolapse-intraoperative	More chances	Fewer chances due to smaller incision

AcriTec Intraocular Lens

The Acrylic IOL is manufactured by the AcriTec company in Berlin, Germany. This lens is a sterile, foldable IOL made of hydrophobic acrylate. The IOL consists of highly purified biocompatible hydrophobic acrylate with chemically bonded UV-absorber. It is a single piece foldable IOL like a plate-haptic IOL. The lens is sterilized by autoclaving. The lens comes in a sterile vial filled with water and wrapped in a sterile pouch.

Intraoperative Protocol for Vancomycin Prophylaxis

One can inject vancomycin inside the eye at the end of the surgery to prevent endophthalmitis from occurring. For this the intraoperative protocol is:

1. 250 mg vial of vancomycin is taken to be dissolved in 25 ml of Ringer lactate (RL) or BSS.
2. This will give a concentration of 1 mg in 0.1 ml.
3. At the end of the surgery, insert 0.1 ml of vancomycin containing 1 mg into the capsular bag behind the IOL. If needed, additional BSS/RL can be injected into the eye to make the eye firm.

Conversion to Phaco or ECCE

While performing phakonit, if the surgeon experiences difficulties like corneal edema on table or continuous destabilization of the anterior chamber, one should convert to phaco or extracapsular cataract extraction (ECCE). One should not be egotistic about this, as the patient's vision is of utmost importance.

There will be slight difficulty in doing phaco as the side-port incision is 1 mm and while doing phaco there will be fluid leakage. In such a case, one can suture the side-port incision to make things easy. The normal chopper will be able to pass through a sutured side port and there will not be leakage. While converting to ECCE, suturing of the clear corneal incisions should be done. The ECCE should then be performed as usual from the superior end through a scleral incision after cutting the conjunctiva.

If phakonit is continued with destabilization of the anterior chamber, there can be permanent endothelial damage. Therefore, it is more prudent to convert in such cases.

Summary

There are various problems that are encountered in any new technique. With time, these will have to be solved. The important point is that today we have broken the 1 mm barrier for cataract removals. This can be done easily by separating the phaco needle from the infusion sleeve. As the saying goes: "We have miles to go before we can sleep."

Key Points

1. Phakonit can be done under any type of anesthesia. This author prefers the no anesthesia cataract surgery technique. In this technique, no anesthetic drops are instilled in the eye nor any intracameral anesthetic injected inside the eye. If there is a difficult case, we use a peribulbar block.
2. The rhexis is preferably performed with a needle. In the left hand a straight rod is held to stabilize the eye. This is the globe stabilization rod. The advantage of this is that the movements of the eye can be controlled as one is working without any anesthesia.
3. Using the phaco tip with moderate ultrasound power, the center of the nucleus is directly embedded starting from the superior edge of rhexis with the phaco probe directed obliquely downwards towards the vitreous. The settings at this stage are 50% phaco power, flow rate 24 ml/min, and 110 mmHg vacuum.
4. When embedding is done until the center of the nucleus, the foot pedal is moved to position 2, as it helps to hold the nucleus due to vacuum rise.
5. To avoid undue pressure on the posterior capsule, the nucleus is lifted a bit and with the irrigating chopper in the left hand the nucleus chopped. This is done with a straight downward motion from the inner edge of the rhexis to the center of the nucleus and then to the left in the form of an inverted L shape.
6. The air pump increases the steady-state pressure of the eye, making the anterior chamber deep and well maintained during the entire procedure. It even makes phacoemulsification a relatively safe procedure by reducing surge even at high vacuum levels.
7. The air pump should be used not only in phakonit but also in phacoemulsification.
8. We advocate "phakonit with cut sleeve" to eliminate water splashing during phakonit to improve visibility during the surgery.
9. It is not necessary that only a top end phaco machine is required. The key is to use any machine already present and start phakonit.
10. One can inject vancomycin inside the eye at the end of the surgery to prevent endophthalmitis from occurring.
11. If one is performing phakonit and cannot complete the case, one can either convert to phaco or to ECCE.

References

1. Agarwal S, Agarwal A, Sachdev MS, Mehta KR, Fine IH, Agarwal A. In: Agarwal A, ed. *Phacoemulsification, Laser Cataract Surgery and Foldable IOLs*. 2nd ed. Delhi, India: Jaypee Brothers; 2000.
2. Boyd B, Agarwal S, Agarwal A, Agarwal A. *LASIK and Beyond LASIK*. Panama: Highlights of Ophthalmology; 2000.
3. Ronge LJ. *Clinical Update: Five Ways to Avoid Phaco Burns*. 1999.
4. Fishkind WJ. The Phaco Machine: How and why it acts and reacts. In: Agarwal A. *Textbook of Ophthalmology*. New Delhi, India: Jaypee Brothers; 2000.
5. Seibel SB. The fluidics and physics of phaco. In: Agarwal A, ed. *Phacoemulsification, Laser Cataract Surgery and Foldable IOLs*. 2nd ed. Delhi, India: Jaypee Brothers; 2000: 45.
6. Agarwal A. No anesthesia cataract surgery with karate chop. In: Agarwal A, ed. *Phacoemulsification, Laser Cataract Surgery and Foldable IOLs*. 2nd ed. Delhi, India: Jaypee Brothers; 2000: 217.

Chapter 30

MICROPHAKONIT

Amar Agarwal, MS, FRCS, FRCOphth

HISTORY

On August 15th, 1998, the author performed 1 mm cataract surgery by a technique called phakonit[1–13] (phako being done with needle incision technology). Dr. Jorge Alio coined the term MICS or microincision cataract surgery[14] for all surgeries including laser cataract surgery and phakonit. Dr. Randall Olson first used a 0.8 mm phaco needle and a 21-gauge irrigating chopper and called it microphaco.[15–18]

On May 21, 2005, for the first time a 0.7 mm phaco needle tip with a 0.7 mm irrigating chopper was used by the author to remove cataracts through the smallest incision possible as of now. This is called microphakonit.

MICROPHAKONIT (0.7 MM) NEEDLE TIP

When we wanted to go for a 0.7 mm phaco needle, we wondered whether the needle would be able to hold the energy of the ultrasound. We gave this problem to Larry Laks from MST (Redmond, Wash) to work on. He then made this special 0.7 mm phaco needle (Figure 30-1). As you will understand, if we go smaller from a 0.9 mm phaco needle to a 0.7 mm phaco needle, the speed of the surgery would go down. This is because the amount of aspiration flow rate would be less.

It was decided to solve this problem by working on the wall of the 0.7 mm phaco needle. There is a standard wall thickness for all phaco tips. If we say the outer diameter is a constant, the resultant inner diameter is an area of the outer diameter minus the area of the wall.

The inner diameter will regulate the flow rate/perceived efficiency, which can be good or bad, depending on how you look at it. In order to increase the allowed aspiration flow rate from what a standard 0.7mm tip would be, Larry Laks had the walls made thinner, thus increasing the inner diameter. This would allow a case to go, speed wise, closer to what a 0.9mm tip would go (not exactly the same, but closer). With the gas-forced infusion it would work very well. Finally we decided to go for a 30° tip to make it even better.

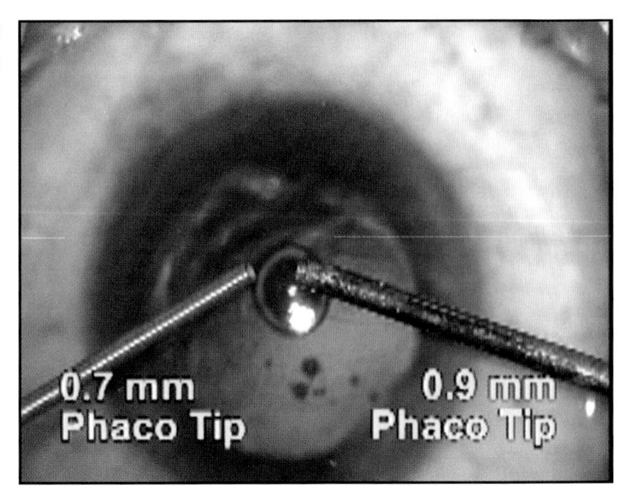

Figure 30-1. A 0.7 mm phaco tip (microphakonit) as compared to a 0.9 mm phaco tip (phakonit).

Microphakonit (0.7 mm) Irrigating Chopper

There are two types of 20-gauge (0.9 mm) irrigating choppers that we have designed. One is the Agarwal irrigating chopper made by MST. The opening for the fluid is an end opening This is incorporated in the Duet system. The other irrigating chopper is made by Geuder, Germany. This has two openings in the side. The surgeon can decide which design of irrigating chopper he would like to use. There are advantages and disadvantages to both types of irrigating choppers. The end opening chopper has an advantage of more fluid coming out of the chopper. The disadvantage is that there is a gush of fluid that might push the nuclear pieces away. The advantage of the side opening irrigating chopper is that there is good control as the nuclear pieces are not pushed away. The disadvantage is that the amount of fluid coming out of it is much less. That is why if one is using the side opening irrigating chopper, one should use an air pump or gas-forced infusion.

MST increased flow in their irrigating chopper by removing the flow restrictions incorporated in other irrigating choppers as a by-product of their attachment method. They also had control of incisional outflow by making all the instruments one size and created a matching knife of the proper size and geometry.

When we decided to go smaller (Figure 30-2) we decided to go for an end-opening irrigating chopper. The reason is as the bore of the irrigating chopper was smaller the amount of fluid coming out of it would be less, and so an end-opening chopper would maintain the fluidics better. With gas-forced infusion we thought we would be able to balance the entry and exit of fluid into the anterior chamber and that is what happened.

We measured the amount of fluid coming out of the various irrigating choppers with and without an air pump using a lower end Alcon Universal II phaco machine (Table 30-1). We also measured the values using the simple aquarium air pump (external gas-forced infusion) and the Accurus machine giving internal gas-forced infusion. When using the Infinity Alcon machine with the air pump, we get 65 cc/min through the 700 micron irrigating chopper.

The microphakonit irrigating chopper that we have designed is basically a sharp chopper with a sharp cutting edge and helps in karate chopping or quick chopping. It can chop any type of cataract.

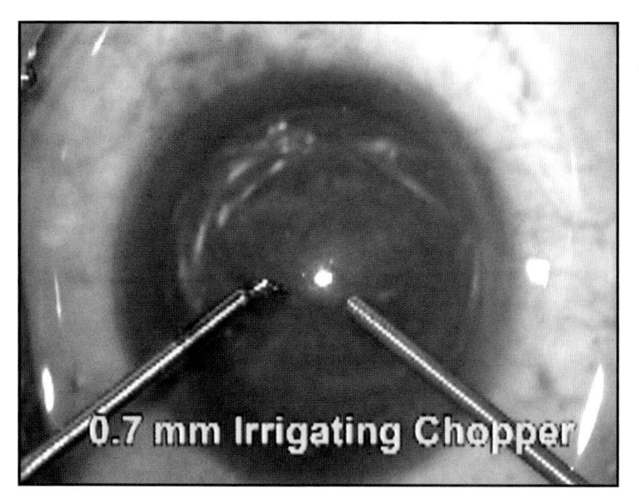

Figure 30-2. A 0.7 mm irrigating chopper.

Table 30-1.

Fluid Exiting From Various Irrigating Choppers (Values in ml/minute)

Irrigating Chopper	*Without Gas Forced Infusion*	*With Gas Forced Infusion Using the Accurus Machine at 50 mm Hg*	*With Gas Forced Infusion Using the Accurus Machine at 75 mm Hg*	*With Gas Forced Infusion Using the Accurus Machine at 100 mm Hg*	*Air Pump With Regulator At Low*	*Air Pump With Regulator At High*
0.9 mm Side Opening	25	36	42	48	37	51
0.9 mm End Opening	34	51	57	65	52	68
0.7 mm End Opening	27	39	44	51	41	54

Air Pump and Gas-Forced Infusion

The main problem in phakonit was the destabilization of the anterior chamber during surgery. We solved it to a certain extent by using an 18-gauge irrigating chopper. Then Sunita Agarwal suggested the use of an antichamber collapser,19 which injects air into the infusion bottle (see Chapter 2). This pushes more fluid into the eye through the irrigating chopper and also prevents surge (Figures 30-3 and 30-4). Thus, we were able to use a 20- or 21-gauge irrigating chopper as well as solve the problem of destabilization of the anterior chamber during surgery. Now with a 22-gauge (0.7 mm) irrigating chopper it is extremely essential that gas-forced infusion be used in the surgery. This is also called external gas-forced infusion.

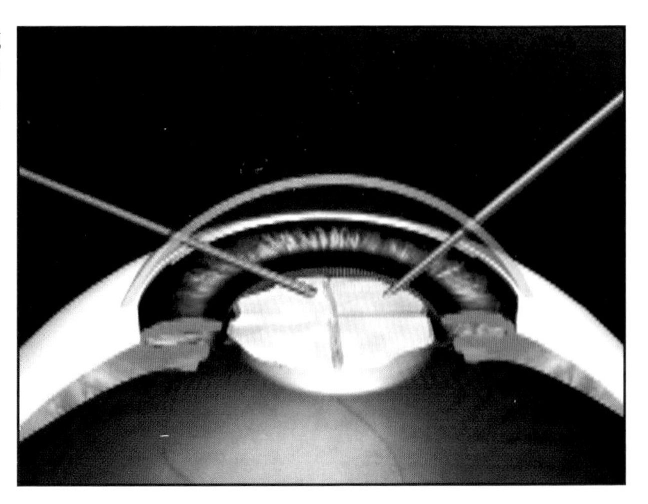

Figure 30-3. Illustration showing normal anterior chamber when case is started. Air pump is not used.

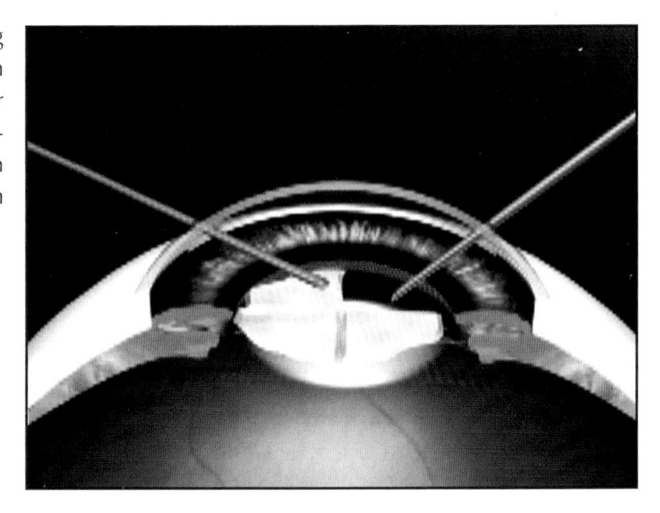

Figure 30-4. Illustration showing surge and chamber collapse when nucleus is being removed. Air pump is not used. Note the chamber depth has come down. When we use the air pump this problem does not occur.

When the surgeon uses the air pump contained in the same phaco machine, it is called internal gas forced infusion (IFI). To solve the problem of infection we use a millipore filter connected to the machine. The advantages of the internal forced Infusion over the external are:

1. The surgeon doesn't have to incorporate an external air pump to the surgical system to obtain the advantages of the forced infusion.
2. The surgeon can control all the parameters (forced infusion rate, ultrasonic power modulations and vacuum settings) in the same panel of the surgical system he or she is working with.
3. The forced infusion rate can be actively and digitally controlled during the surgery, adjusting the parameters to the conditions and/or the surgical steps of each individual case.

When we decided to use the 0.7 mm MST Duet set, we decided to use the internal gas-forced infusion of the Accurus machine to measure the pressure of air exactly. This is from Alcon (Fort Worth, Tex). The advantage of this was that we could regulate the amount of air entering into the infusion bottle and thus titrate the system in such a way that there is no surge or collapse of the anterior chamber. When we are using a 0.7 mm irrigating chopper, the problem is that the amount of fluid entering the eye is not enough. To solve this problem, gas-forced infusion is a must.

The anterior vented gas-forced infusion system (AVGFI) of the Accurus surgical system helps in the performance of phakonit. This was started by Arturo Pérez-Arteaga. The AVGFI is a system incorporated in the Accurus machine that creates a positive infusion pressure inside the eye. It consists of an air pump and a regulator that are inside the machine. The air is pushed inside the bottle of intraocular solution, and so the fluid is actively pushed inside the eye without raising or lowering the bottle. The control of the air pump is digitally integrated in the Accurus panel. We preset the infusion pump at 100 mmHg when we are performing microphakonit.

As you will notice in Table 30-1, if we use the air pump at high it is equal to using the Accurus machine at about 100 mmHg pressure, and if we use the air pump at low it is equal to using the Accurus machine at 50 mmHg pressure. Some air pumps come with such a regulator so that one can have more air coming out of them. The regulator has a switch for low and high pressure. In microphakonit, we always use the regulator at high mode. The cost of the air pump is about $2 to $10, depending on the country. This can be bought from an aquarium shop. If one uses an air pump, one can connect a millipore filter to it to prevent any infection. Alternatively, one can use a gas-forced internal infusion system using the Accurus machine. In such a case, preset the pump at 100 mmHg.

Bimanual 0.7 mm Irrigation/Aspiration System

Bimanual irrigation/aspiration (I/A) is done with the bimanual I/A instruments. These instruments are also designed by MST. The previous set we used was the 0.9 mm set. Now with microphakonit we use the new 0.7 mm bimanual I/A set (Figures 30-5 and 30-6) so that after the nucleus removal we need not enlarge the incision.

Duet Handles

All these instruments of the 0.7 mm set fit onto the handles of the Duet system. So if a surgeon already has the handles and is using it for phakonit, they need to get only the tips and can use the same handles for microphakonit.

Differences Between 0.9 mm and 0.7 mm Sets in Cataract Surgery

Table 30-2 indicates the differences between the two techniques.

Technique

Incision

The incision is made with a keratome. This can be done using a sapphire knife or a stainless steel knife. One should be careful when one is making the incision so that the incision is a bit long as one would be using gas-forced infusion in microphakonit. Before making

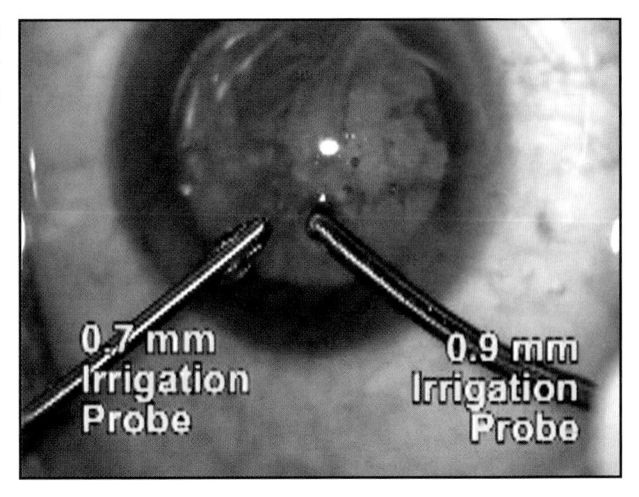

Figure 30-5. 0.7 mm irrigation probe used for bimanual I/A compared to the 0.9 mm irrigation probe.

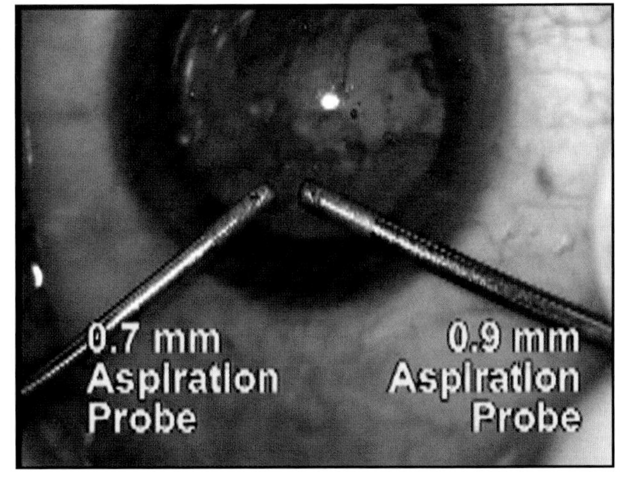

Figure 30-6. 0.7 mm aspiration probe used for bimanual I/A compared to the 0.9 mm aspiration probe.

the incision, a needle with viscoelastic is taken and pierced in the eye in the area where the side port has to be made. The viscoelastic is then injected inside the eye. This will distend the eye so that the clear corneal incision can be made easily. Make one clear corneal incision between the lateral rectus and inferior rectus and the other between the lateral rectus and superior rectus. This way one is able to control the movements of the eye during surgery.

Rhexis

The rhexis is then performed of about 5 to 6 mm. This is done with a needle. In the left hand a straight rod is held to stabilize the eye. This is the globe stabilization rod. The advantage of this is that the movements of the eye can be controlled if one is working without any anesthesia or under topical anesthesia.

Table 30-2.
Differences Between Phakonit and Microphakonit

Features	*Phakonit*	*Microphakonit*
Irrigating chopper	0.9 mm	0.7 mm
Phaco needle	0.9 mm	0.7 mm
Control in surgery	Good	Better control
Valve construction	Extremely important	Not very important as incision is much smaller
Iris prolapse	Can occur if valve is bad	Very rare
Intraoperative Floppy iris syndrome	Can be managed	Much better to manage as incision is much smaller and there is better control
Hydrodissection	Can be done from both incisions	To be careful as very little space is there for escape of fluid
Air pump (gas forced infusion) (GFI)	Can be done without it though better with it	Mandatory. 0.7 mm irrigating choppers even with higher end machines need GFI
Flow rate	Can keep any value	Do not keep it very high. 20-24 ml/min
Bimanual I/A	0.9 mm	0.7 mm

Hydrodissection

Hydrodissection is performed and the fluid wave passing under the nucleus checked. Check for rotation of the nucleus. The advantage of microphakonit is that one can do hydrodissection from both incisions so that even the subincisional areas can get easily hydrodissected. The problem is as there is not much escape of fluid one should be careful in hydrodissection as if too much fluid is passed into the eye one can get a complication.

Microphakonit

The 22 (0.7 mm) gauge irrigating chopper connected to the infusion line of the phaco machine is introduced with foot pedal on position 1. The phaco probe is connected to the aspiration line and the 0.7 mm phaco tip without an infusion sleeve is introduced through the clear corneal incision (Figure 30-7). Using the phaco tip with moderate ultrasound power, the center of the nucleus is directly embedded starting from the superior edge of rhexis with the phaco probe directed obliquely downwards towards the vitreous. The settings at this stage are 50% phaco power, flow rate 20 ml/min, and 100 to 200 mmHg vacuum. Using the karate chop technique, the nucleus is chopped (Figure 30-8). Thus the whole nucleus is removed (Figure 30-9). Cortical wash-up is then done with the bimanual

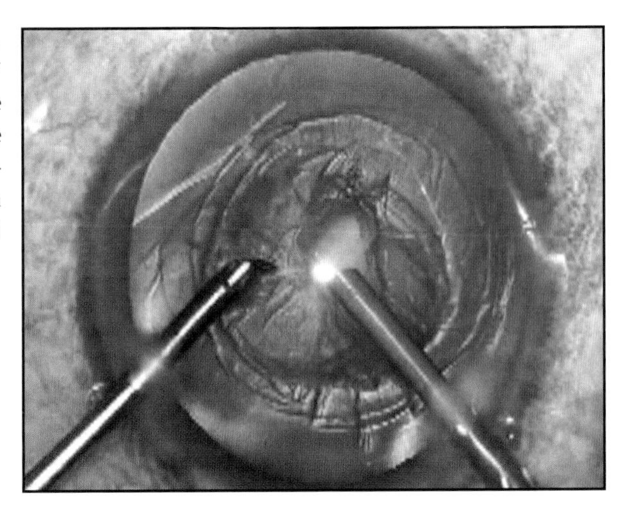

Figure 30-7. Microphakonit started. 0.7 mm irrigating chopper and 0.7 mm phako tip without the sleeve inside the eye. All instruments are made by MST. The assistant continuously irrigates the phaco probe area from outside to prevent corneal burns.

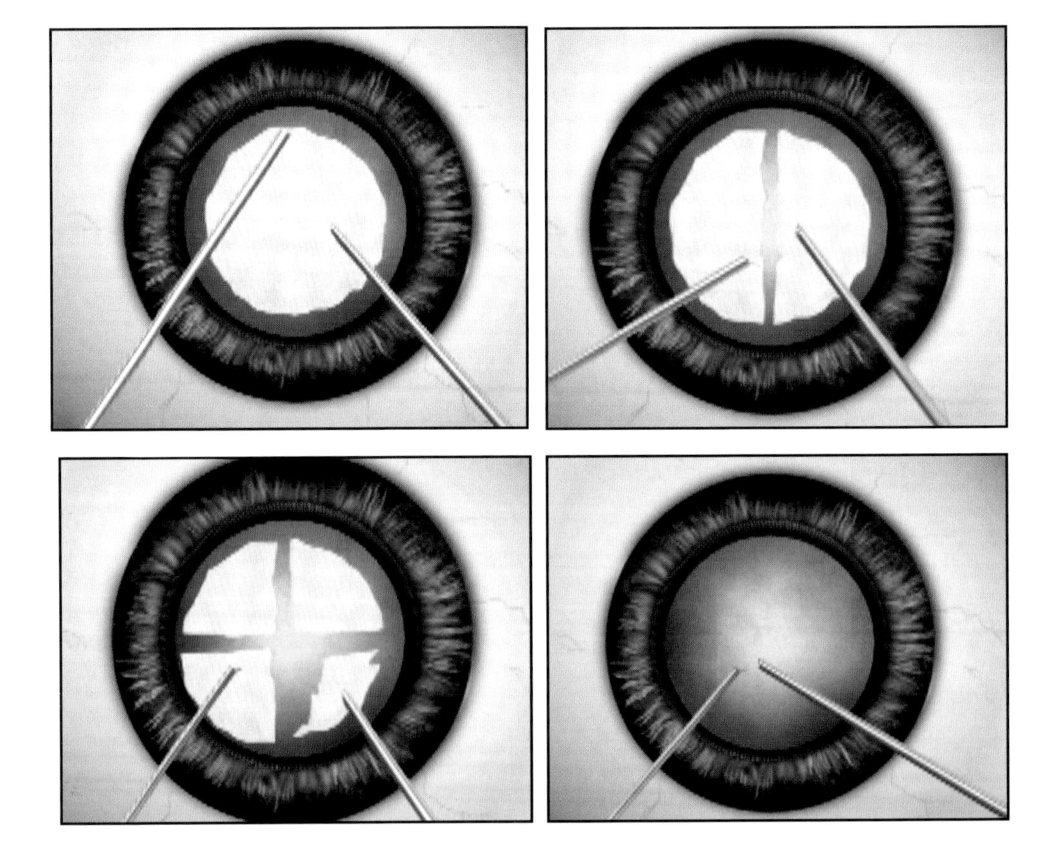

Figure 30-8. Illustration showing the nucleus removal.

I/A (0.7 mm set) technique (Figures 30-10 and 30-11). During this whole procedure of microphakonit gas-forced infusion is used.

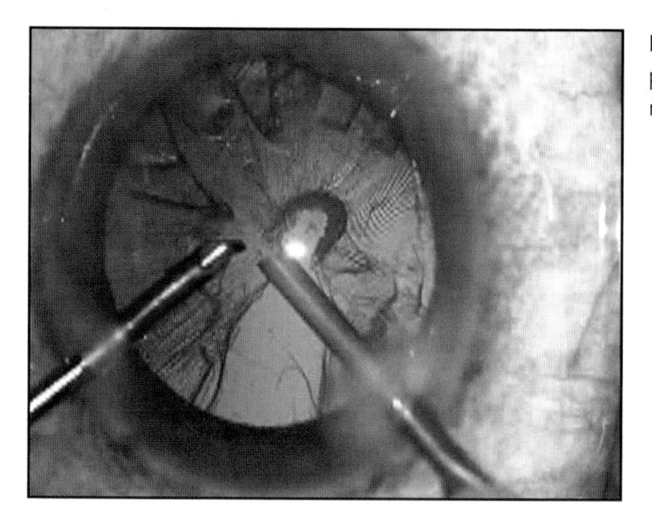

Figure 30-9. Microphakonit completed. The nucleus has been removed.

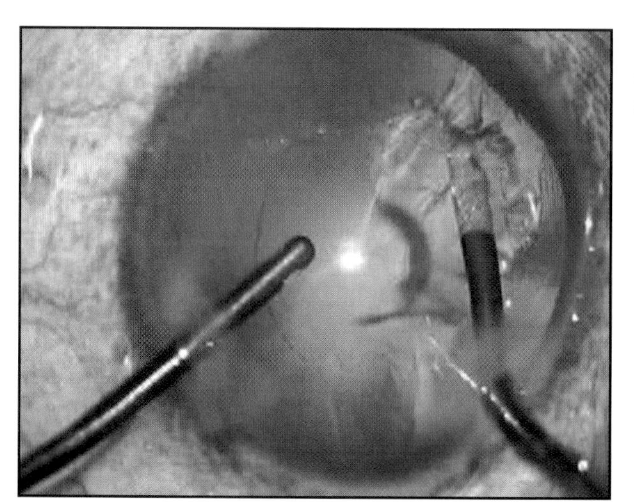

Figure 30-10. Bimanual irrigation aspiration started with the 0.7 mm set.

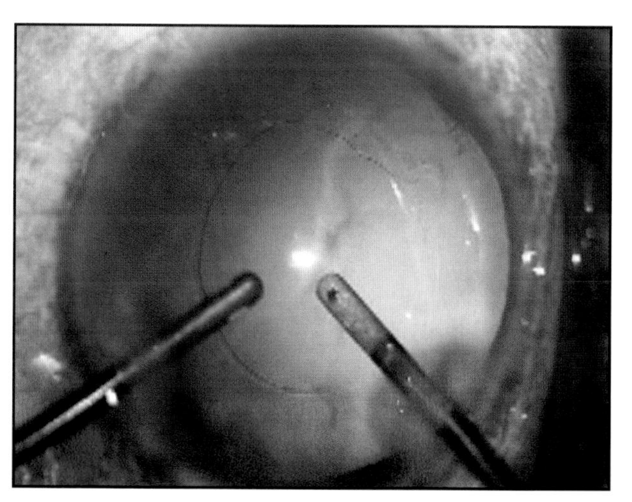

Figure 30-11. Bimanual irrigation aspiration completed.

SUMMARY

With microphakonit a 0.7 mm set is used to remove the cataract. At present this is the smallest one can use for cataract surgery. With time one would be able to go smaller with better and better instruments and devices. The problem at present is the IOL. We have to get good quality IOLs going through sub 1mm cataract surgical incisions so that the real benefit of microphakonit can be given to the patient.

KEY POINTS

1. In order to increase the allowed aspiration flow rate from what a standard 0.7 mm tip would be, Larry Laks (MST) had the walls made thinner, thus increasing the inner diameter. This would allow a case to go, speed wise, closer to what a 0.9 mm tip would go (not exactly the same, but closer).
2. The microphakonit irrigating chopper is basically a sharp chopper that has a sharp cutting edge and helps in karate chopping or quick chopping. It can chop any type of cataract.
3. The advantage of microphakonit is that one can do hydrodissection from both incisions so that even the subincisional areas can get easily hydrodissected.
4. With microphakonit, a 0.7 mm set is used to remove the cataract. At present, this is the smallest one can use for cataract surgery. With time, one would be able to go smaller with better and better instruments and devices.

REFERENCES

1. Agarwal A, Agarwal S, Agarwal At. No anesthesia cataract surgery. In: Agarwal A, ed. *Phacoemulsification, Laser Cataract Surgery and Foldable IOLs*. 1st ed. Delhi, India: Jaypee Brothers; 1998:144.
2. Pandey S, Werner L, Agarwal A, Agarwal S, Agarwal At, Apple D. No anesthesia cataract surgery. *J Cataract Refract Surg*. 2001;28:1710.
3. Agarwal A, Agarwal S, Agarwal At. Phakonit: a new technique of removing cataracts through a 0.9 mm incision. In: Agarwal A, ed. *Phacoemulsification, Laser Cataract Surgery and Foldable IOLs*. 1st ed. Delhi, India: Jaypee Brothers; 1998:139.
4. Agarwal A, Agarwal S, Agarwal At. Phakonit and laser phakonit: lens surgery through a 0.9 mm incision. In: Agarwal A, ed. *Phacoemulsification, Laser Cataract Surgery and Foldable IOLs*. 2nd ed. Delhi, India: Jaypee Brothers; 2000:204.
5. Agarwal A, Agarwal S, Agarwal At. Phakonit. In: Agarwal A, ed. *Phacoemulsification, Laser Cataract Surgery and Foldable IOLs*. 3rd ed. Delhi, India: Jaypee Brothers; 2003:317.
6. Agarwal A, Agarwal S, Agarwal At. Phakonit and laser phakonit. In: Boyd B, Agarwal A, et al, eds *LASIK and Beyond LASIK*. Panama: Highlights of Ophthalmology; 2000:463.
7. Agarwal A, Agarwal S, Agarwal At. Phakonit and laser phakonit: cataract surgery through a 0.9 mm incision. In: Boyd B, Agarwal A, et al, eds. *Phako, Phakonit and Laser Phako*. Panama: Highlights of Ophthalmology; 2000:327.
8. Agarwal A, Agarwal S, Agarwal At. The Phakonit Thinoptx IOL. In: Agarwal A, ed. *Presbyopia*. Thorofare, NJ: SLACK Incorporated; 2002:187.

9. Agarwal A, Agarwal S, Agarwal At. Antichamber collapser. *J Cataract Refract Surg*. 2002;28:1085.
10. Pandey S, Werner L, Agarwal A, Agarwal S, Agarwal At, Hoyos J. Phakonit: cataract removal through a sub 1.0 mm incision with implantation of the Thinoptx rollable IOL. *J Cataract Refract Surg*. 2002;28:1710.
11. Agarwal A, Agarwal S, Agarwal At. Phakonit: phacoemulsification through a 0.9 mm incision. *J Cataract Refract Surg*. 2001;27:1548.
12. Agarwal A, Agarwal S, Agarwal At. Phakonit with an Acritec IOL. *J Cataract Refract Surg*. 2003;29:854.
13. Agarwal S, Agarwal A, Agarwal At. *Phakonit with Acritec IOL*. Panama: Highlights of Ophthalmology; 2000.
14. Alio J. What does MICS require? In: Alio J. *MICS*. Panama: Highlights of Ophthalmology. 2004:1.
15. Soscia W, Howard JG, Olson RJ. Microphacoemulsification with Whitestar. A wound-temperature study. *J Cataract Refract Surg*. 2002;28:1044.
16. Soscia W, Howard JG, Olson RJ. Bimanual phacoemulsification through two stab incisions. A wound-temperature study. *J Cataract Refract Surg*. 2002;28:1039.
17. Olson R. Microphaco chop. In: Chang D. *Phaco Chop*. Thorofare, NJ: SLACK Incorporated; 2004:227.
18. Chang D. Bimanual phaco chop. In: Chang D. *Phaco Chop*. Thorofare, NJ: SLACK Incorporated; 2004:239.
19. Agarwal A. Air pump. In: Agarwal A, ed. *Bimanual Phaco: Mastering the Phakonit/MICS Technique*. Thorofare, NJ: SLACK Incorporated; 2005.

Please see Sub 1 mm Cataract Surgery video on enclosed CD-ROM.

Chapter 31

Complications of Bimanual Phacoemulsification

Amar Agarwal, MS, FRCS, FRCOphth; Mahipal Singh Sachdev, MBBS(AIIMS), MD Ophthal(AIIMS); Clement K. Chan, MD, FACS

Introduction

More complications[1-5] may be encountered by a new phakonit surgeon who has just begun to do phakonit, as a longer learning curve is often associated with this technique in comparison to other methods.

Wound Construction

The importance of a perfectly constructed wound in phakonit surgery cannot be overstated. A well-constructed wound is the key to achieving a flawless self-sealing wound that requires no sutures. A well-constructed wound can be closed by any method with good results. A poorly constructed wound can be a continued source of astigmatism, filtration, irritation, hemorrhage, and corneal trauma despite a satisfactory wound closure.

Complications Related to Nucleus (Emulsification Technique)

While manipulating with the micromanipulator, great care should be taken not to sink it through the soft nuclei and especially into the posterior capsule. Phacoemulsification energy must be substantially reduced when fragments are small, or they will bounce off the tip when the power is activated.

When removing the nuclear chips, it is advisable to shift to pulsed mode to reduce the "chattering" of the chip. Moreover, the posterior capsule is covered during the entire emulsification process by the outer nucleus, which acts as a thick layer of foam rubber separating the firm inner nucleus from the capsular bag.

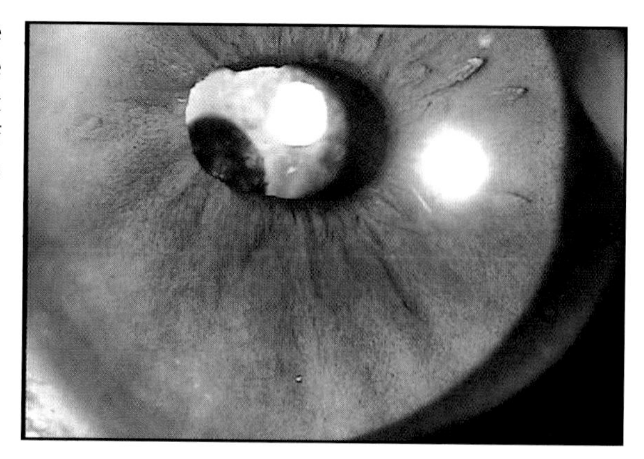

Figure 31-1. Capsular phimosis. Note the anterior capsular rim in the central pupillary zone. The treatment of this complication is enlargement of the opening with the YAG laser. (Photo courtesy of Dr. D.P. Prakash.)

If the phacoemulsification tip does not emulsify the nucleus properly, correction of one or more of the following responsible conditions is required:

1. The titanium needle is not tightly screwed to the handpiece.
2. The aspiration system is partially blocked by a piece of nucleus.
3. The ultrasound setting is too low for a particular piece of nucleus.

Moreover, the handpiece temperature should be monitored at all times, and it should not be allowed to become too warm. After cortical aspiration, meticulous anterior capsular vacuuming should be performed to eliminate residual lenticular peri-equatorial epithelial cells that could lead to capsular phimosis (Figure 31–1).

CORNEAL COMPLICATIONS

Many corneal complications may occur especially with beginners. They are summarized in Table 31–1.

Transient postoperative superior corneal edema is usually present in cases of phakonit for the beginners (Figure 31-2). Moreover, adequate incision construction, proper instrumentation, and avoidance of false passages reduce the occurrence and hasten the resolution of corneal edema. Incisional burns can be averted by avoiding too tight an incision, using cold balanced salt solution (4°C) as irrigating fluid, and minimizing the phaco time.

Moreover, diffuse corneal haze (Figure 31-3) or loss of corneal clarity is a common problem encountered during phakonit surgery. Topical medications should be used judiciously, as their prolonged and frequent instillation may induce superficial punctate keratopathy.

Descemet's detachment and Descemet's tears may also occur occasionally. The anterior tip of the incision should be lifted up when the instruments are inserted. Descemet's tears can also be prevented by using sharp instruments. The probe tip should be inserted with the bevel down. The side-port entry should also be made with a beveled instrument in a similar fashion, and any mechanical damage to the Descemet's membrane should be avoided.

Corneal endothelium damages can be further prevented by decreasing the effective emulsification time and confining the procedure to the nucleus with the minimal required ultrasonic energy in the posterior chamber. Only high-quality ophthalmic fluids, ie, sodium hyaluronate and other similar viscoelastics, and balanced salt solution. etc. should be used.

In the event of a postoperative corneal decompensation, anti-inflammatory and cycloplegic agents should be applied to counteract the associated inflammation and achieve cycloplegia, respectively. Hyperosmotics may also be useful for decongesting microcystic corneal edema. In the event of irreversible corneal endothelial damages, however, penetrating keratoplasty may be undertaken.

Table 31-1.
Corneal Complications of Phakonit

Epithelial	• Abrasions • Filamentary keratitis • Toxic keratopathy
Corneal burns	• Thermal • Cautery
Infection	• Bacterial wound infection • Fungal wound infection • Herpetic keratitis
Sterile ulcerations and Stromal melting	• Rheumatoid arthritis • Collagen vascular disease • Keratoconjunctivitis sicca
Sterile Descemet's membrane	• Blunt blade injury • Oblique instrument insertion • Incomplete insertion of instruments • Injection of viscoelastic, air, or irrigation fluids
Endothelial damage	1. Poor endothelial preoperative cell count 2. Intraocular mechanical damage • Anterior chamber collapse • Instruments • Irrigating fluid disturbances • Anterior chamber emulsification • Lens nucleus/nucleus fragment touch • IOL touch • Foreign matter 3. Toxicity • Irrigating solutions • Povidone Iodine 4. Chronic endothelial touch • IOL • Vitreous 5. Faulty IOL • Closed loop anterior chamber IOL • Iris supported IOL • Poorly coated surfaces 6. Ingrowth of cells • Epithelial • Fibrous
Corneal complications (postoperative)	• Endothelial decompensation • Striate keratopathy • Bullous keratopathy

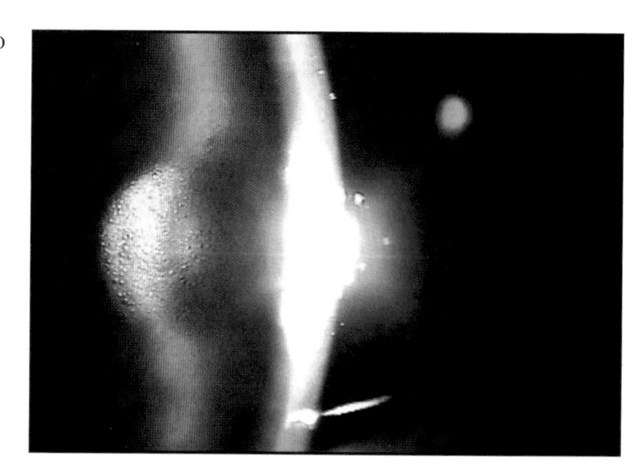

Figure 31-2. Corneal edema. (Photo courtesy of Dr. D.P. Prakash.)

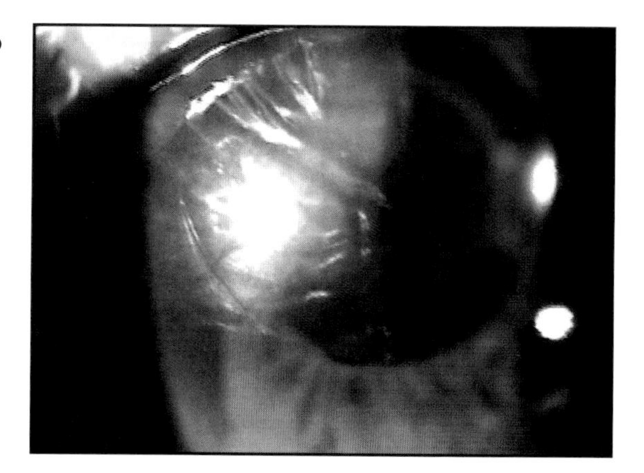

Figure 31-3. Striate keratopathy. (Photo courtesy of Dr. D.P. Prakash.)

Iris Injury

Injury to both the superior and inferior portions of the iris may occur during phakonit. Iris fluttering should always be prevented during phacoemulsification. While performing phacoemulsification, the bevel of the phaco needle should be pointed upwards and maintained parallel to the iris plane throughout the process.

Vitreous Loss

The closed system inherent with the ultra-small incisional wound of phakonit limits vitreous loss and enhances the surgeon's ability to perform an adequate vitrectomy. The constant pressure in the anterior chamber due to the closed system associated with phakonit reduces the tendency of anterior vitreous prolapse. The small incision also limits the amount of vitreous extrusion from the eye. Zonular dehiscence may occur if an attempt is made to rotate the nucleus after an inadequate hydrodissection, partially due to the lack of capsular flexibility upon stress.

Unplanned posterior capsulotomy that violates the anterior vitreous hyaloid face tends to induce vitreous loss. Factors which inhibit early recognition of a posterior capsular rent by the surgeon, ie, obstruction of view by a large and opaque nuclear fragment, may increase the tendency for greater vitreous loss.

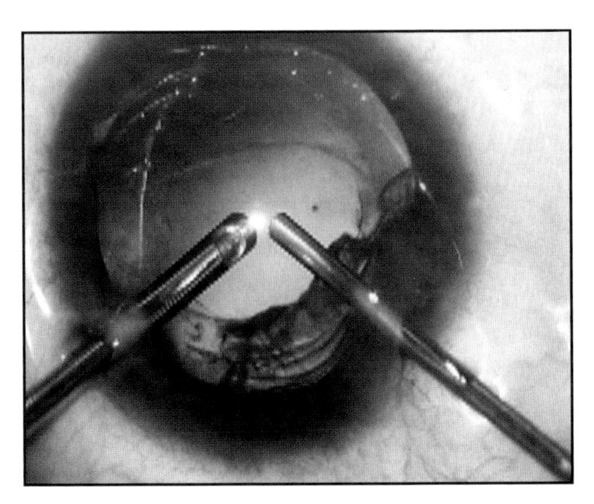

Figure 31-4. Bimanual vitrectomy. Please note separate vitrectomy probe and infusion cannula.

In the event of a posterior capsular rent with no vitreous loss, vitrectomy may not be required. Nevertheless, the flow rate and infusion should be decreased to avoid subsequent anterior vitreous herniation. However, a vitrectomy is mandatory when vitreous loss is confirmed. A single vitrectomy probe with a coaxial cannula should generally be avoided in favor of a bimanual vitrectomy technique using separate infusion cannula and vitrectomy probe (Figure 31-4). A coaxial infusion probe may require enlargement of the original incisional wound. Coaxial infusion also tends to open up the posterior capsular flap and hydrate the vitreous more than a separate infusion cannula, thus permitting more anterior vitreous prolapse. With the bimanual technique, a limited anterior vitrectomy is performed and the main body of the vitreous is not disturbed. During the procedure, vitreous should be aspirated downwards below the plane of the posterior capsule. Irrigation should be gentle and limited to the anterior chamber. Following vitrectomy, a posterior IOL may be inserted in front of the anterior capsule in the ciliary sulcus, if an adequate capsular rim is present. Vitreous loss can be prevented or minimized by avoiding phacoemulsification on the posterior surface of the nucleus. Improper vitrectomy can result in postoperative malpositioning of the IOL (Figure 31-5), and severe intraocular inflammation (Figure 31-6).

Nuclear Dislocation

If the posterior capsular rent is large, the nucleus may migrate into the posterior vitreous cavity. Since an exposed nucleus is strongly antigenic and may cause a severe ocular phacoanaphylactic or phacotoxic reaction, its removal is mandatory. A soft nucleus can be removed with a vitrectomy probe alone, but a hard one requires posterior phacofragmentation, usually via a pars plana approach. An alternative method for removing a large and hard nuclear fragment is floating it anteriorly with perfluorocarbon liquids (PFCL) after a posterior vitrectomy. The anteriorly displaced lens fragment can then be delivered out of an enlarged corneal-scleral limbal wound. One can also use the FAVIT technique for removing dropped nuclear pieces.[6]

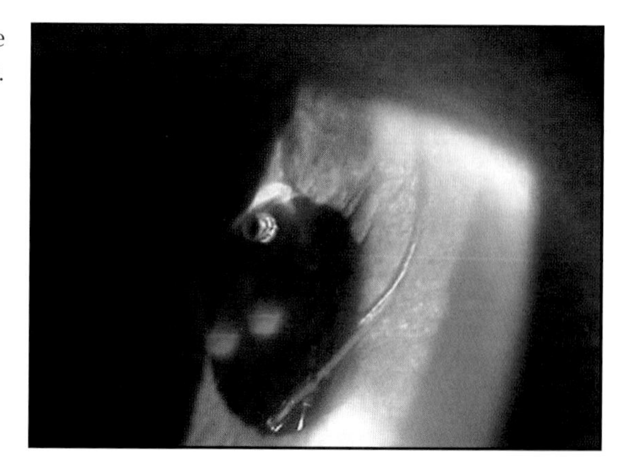

Figure 31-5. Haptic of an IOL in the anterior chamber. (Photo courtesy of Dr. D.P. Prakash.)

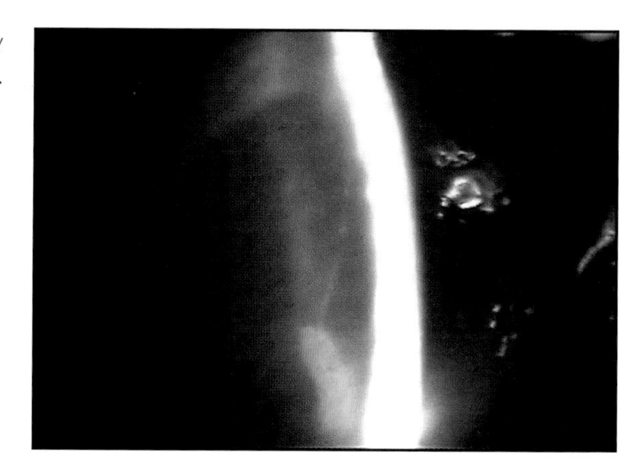

Figure 31-6. Severe inflammatory reaction in the anterior chamber. (Photo courtesy of Dr. D.P. Prakash.)

Expulsive Hemorrhage

Expulsive suprachoroidal hemorrhage rarely occurs in conjunction with a 1-mm incision associated with phakonit. This small beveled incision is self-sealing, and therefore usually prevents extrusion of intraocular contents associated with the suprachoroidal hemorrhage. In the event of a hemorrhagic choroidal detachment, the performance of a posterior sclerotomy to allow posterior release of the suprachoroidal hemorrhage and a rapid closure of the wounds minimize the chance of an expulsive hemorrhage.

Conversion to Extracapsular Cataract Extraction

Upon the first sign of excessive corneal clouding or anterior vitreous prolapse, the surgeon should consider converting phakonit to extracapsular cataract extraction (ECCE), in order to enhance the likelihood of achieving good functional visual outcome. Conversion should be undertaken preferably before excessive corneal endothelial damages and capsular rupture occur.

Planned conversion to ECCE is better than forced conversion. The surgeon should enlarge the limbal wound for extracapsular delivery of the nucleus from the posterior chamber, upon the first sign of anterior vitreous herniation. A lens loop or equivalent instrument

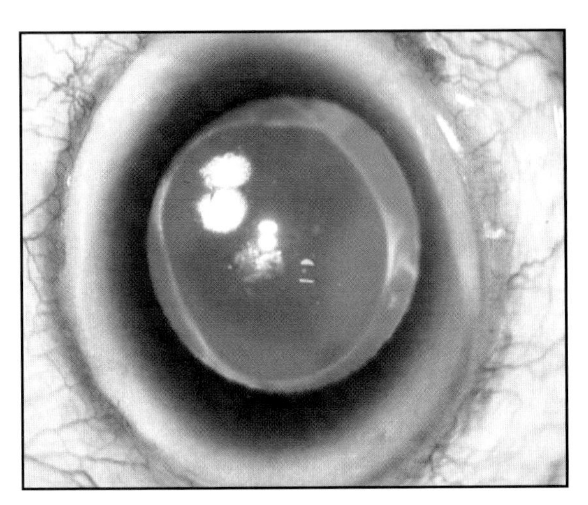

Figure 31-7. IOL opacification.

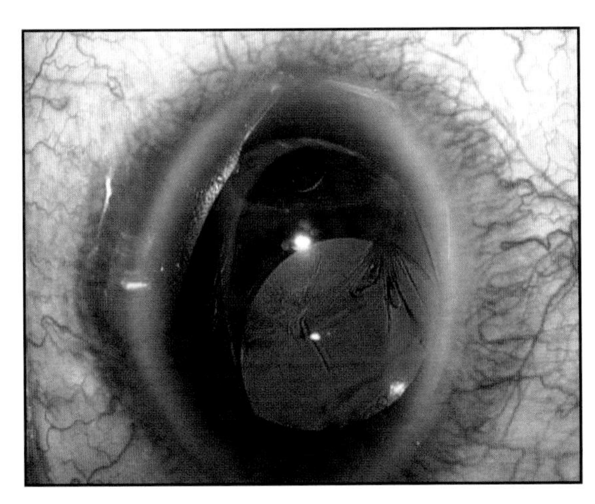

Figure 31-8. IOL decentration.

may be inserted under the nucleus for its expression out of the eye. After the nucleus is out, an irrigation-aspiration handpiece with a 0.5 mm tip is employed with low vacuum for lenticular cortical clean-up. However, lens fragments dislocated into the vitreous cavity are left alone for subsequent management with vitreoretinal techniques. The cataract surgeon unfamiliar with vitreoretinal techniques should refer the patient to a vitreoretinal surgeon. Attempts in removing posteriorly dislocated lens fragments without proper vitreoretinal techniques tend to cause retinal complications. In the event of vitreous loss, cortical aspiration may be difficult, and a vitrectomy probe is usually a better tool for completing the cortical clean-up.

Miscellaneous IOL Problems

A number of problems may be associated with the IOL itself. For instance, defective IOL due to improper manufacturing may cause increased tendency for Opacification of the IOL (Figure 31-7). The IOL may also decenter or tilt (Figure 31-8), and extrude (Figure 31-9).

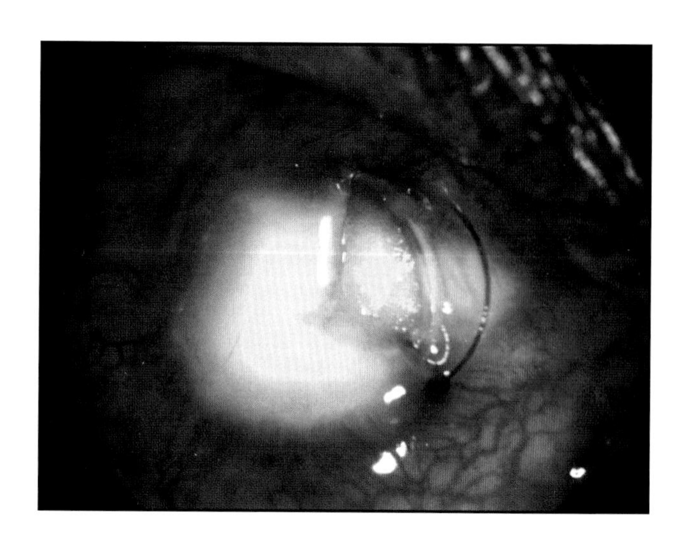

Figure 31-9. IOL extrusion.

Key Points

1. A poorly constructed wound can be a source of astigmatism, filtration, irritation, hemorrhage, and corneal trauma despite a satisfactory wound closure.
2. The handpiece temperature should be monitored at all times, and it should not be allowed to become too warm.
3. In the event of postoperative corneal decompensation, anti-inflammatory and cycloplegic agents should be applied to counteract the associated inflammation and achieve cycloplegia, respectively. Hyperosmotics may also be useful for decongesting microcystic corneal edema. In the event of irreversible corneal endothelial damages, however, penetrating keratoplasty may be undertaken.
4. A single vitrectomy probe with a coaxial cannula should generally be avoided in favor of a bimanual vitrectomy technique using separate infusion cannula and vitrectomy probe.
5. A true expulsive suprachoroidal hemorrhage through the 1-mm incision associated with phakonit is rare.

References

1. Agarwal A, Agarwal S, Agarwal A. Phakonit: lens removal through a 0.9 mm incision. In: Agarwal A, ed. *Phacoemulsification, Laser Cataract Surgery and Foldable IOLs*. 1st ed. Delhi, India: Jaypee Brothers; 1998.
2. Agarwal A, Agarwal A, Agarwal S. No anesthesia cataract surgery. In: Agarwal A, ed. *Phacoemulsification, Laser Cataract Surgery and Foldable IOLs*. 2nd ed. Delhi, India: Jaypee Brothers; 2000.
3. Chang S. Perfluorocarbon liquids in vitreoretinal surgery. *International Ophthalmology Clinics-New approaches to vitreoretinal surgery*. 1992;32(2):153.
4. Chan CK. An improved technique for management of dislocated posterior chamber implants. *Ophthalmol*. 1992;99:51.
5. Chan CK, Agarwal A, Agarwal S, Agarwal A. Management of dislocated intraocular implants. In: Nagpal PN, Fine IH, eds. *Ophthalmology Clinics of North America, Posterior Segment Complications of Cataract Surgery*. Philadelphia: W.B. Saunders; 2001:681.
6. Agarwal A, Siraj AA. FAVIT—a new method to remove dropped nuclei. In: Agarwal S, Agarwal A, Sachdev MS, et al, eds. *Phacoemulsification, Laser Cataract Surgery and Foldable IOLs*. 2nd ed. Delhi, India: Jaypee Brothers; 2000.

Index

WAIT

...There's More!

SLACK Incorporated's Health Care Books and Journals offers a wide selection of products in the field of Ophthalmology. We are dedicated to providing important works that educate, inform and improve the knowledge of our customers. Don't miss out on our other informative titles that will enhance your collection.

Handbook of Ophthalmology
Amar Agarwal, MS, FRCS, FRCOphth
752 pp., Soft Cover, 2006, ISBN 1-55642-685-2,
Order #66852, **$64.95**

The Handbook of Ophthalmology is a pocket-sized, ready reference book that provides a compact review of diagnostic eye disorders. Presented in an outline format, including color images and photographs, the detailed information inside this resource for ophthalmic conditions is perfect for everyone involved with ophthalmology, from residents to advanced surgeons.

Bimanual Phaco: Mastering the Phakonit/MICS Technique
Amar Agarwal, MS, FRCS, FRCOphth
296 pp., Hard Cover, 2005, ISBN 1-55642-717-4,
Order #67174, **$119.95**

This break-through text covers all aspects of bimanual phaco and how one can master the technique. *Bimanual Phaco* will explain how to manage complications and the implantation of various ultra-small incision IOLs. With world-renowned contributions from 25 of the world's experts in cataract surgery, key points at the end of each chapter, and over 200 color photographs and illustrations, *Bimanual Phaco* will launch today's surgeon into the future and the new era of 1 mm cataract surgery.

Presbyopia: A Surgical Textbook
Amar Agarwal, MS, FRCS, FRCOphth
256 pp., Hard Cover, 2002, ISBN 1-55642-577-5,
Order# 65775, **$111.95**

The Little Eye Book: A Pupil's Guide to Understanding Ophthalmology
Janice K. Ledford, COMT and Roberto Pineda, II, MD
160 pp., Soft Cover, 2002, ISBN 1-55642-560-0,
Order #65600, **$19.95**

Quick Reference Dictionary of Eyecare Terminology, Fourth Edition
Janice K. Ledford, COMT and Joseph Hoffman
424 pp., Soft Cover, 2004, ISBN 1-55642-711-5,
Order #67115, **$28.95**

Fundus Fluorescein and Indocyanine Green Angiography: A Textbook and Atlas
Amar Agarwal, MS, FRCS, FRCOphth
320 pp., Hard Cover, 2007, ISBN 1-55642-787-5,
Order #67875, **$119.95**

Refractive Surgery Nightmares
Amar Agarwal, MS, FRCS, FRCOphth
250 pp., Hard Cover, 2007, ISBN 1-55642-788-3,
Order #67883, **$169.95**

Please visit

www.slackbooks.com

to order any of these titles!

24 Hours a Day...7 Days a Week!

Attention Industry Partners!

Whether you are interested in buying multiple copies of a book, chapter reprints, or looking for something new and different — we are able to accommodate your needs.

Multiple Copies

At attractive discounts starting for purchases as low as 25 copies for a single title, SLACK Incorporated will be able to meet all your of your needs.

Chapter Reprints

SLACK Incorporated is able to offer the chapters you want in a format that will lead to success. Bound with an attractive cover, use the chapters that are a fit specifically for your company. Available for quantities of 100 or more.

Customize

SLACK Incorporated is able to create a specialized custom version of any of our products specifically for your company.

Please contact the Marketing Manager of the Health Care Books and Journals for further details on multiple copy purchases, chapter reprints or custom printing at 1-800-257-8290 or 1-856-848-1000.

**Please note all conditions are subject to change.*

CODE: 328

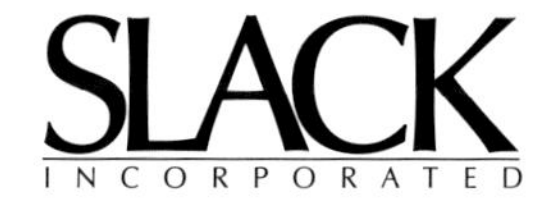

SLACK Incorporated • Health Care Books and Journals

6900 Grove Road • Thorofare, NJ 08086

1-800-257-8290 or 1-856-848-1000

Fax: 1-856-853-5991 • E-mail: orders@slackinc.com • Visit www.slackbooks.com

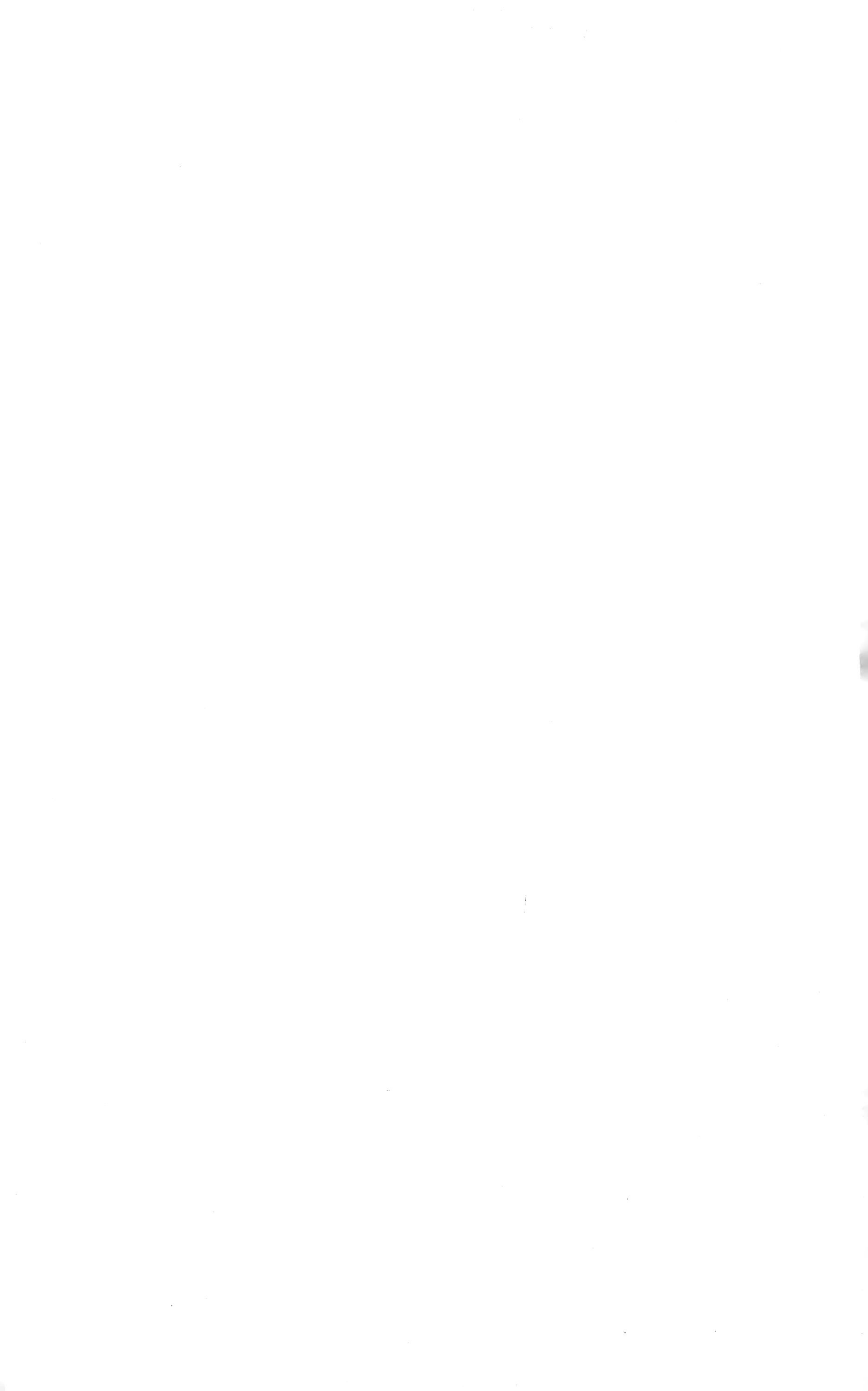